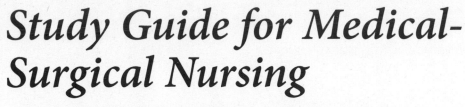

Study Guide for Medical-Surgical Nursing
Concepts for Interprofessional Collaborative Care

Ninth Edition

Donna D. Ignatavicius, MS, RN, CNE, ANEF
Speaker and Curriculum Consultant for
Academic Nursing Programs;
Founder, Boot Camp for Nurse Educators;
President, DI Associates, Inc.
Littleton, Colorado

M. Linda Workman, PhD, RN, FAAN
Author and Consultant
Cincinnati, Ohio

Cherie R. Rebar, PhD, MBA, RN, COI
Professor of Nursing
Wittenberg University
Springfield, Ohio

Clinical Nursing Judgment Study Guide prepared by

Linda A. LaCharity, PhD, RN
Retired Accelerated Program Director
and Assistant Professor
College of Nursing
University of Cincinnati
Cincinnati, Ohio

Candice K. Kumagai, RN, MSN
Former Instructor in Clinical Nursing
School of Nursing
University of Texas at Austin
Austin, Texas

Reviewer

Susan J. Eisel, BSN, MSEd
Associate Professor
Nursing
Mercy College of Ohio
Toledo, Ohio

ELSEVIER

3251 Riverport Lane
St. Louis, Missouri 63043

STUDY GUIDE FOR MEDICAL-SURGICAL NURSING: ISBN: 978-0-323-46162-7
CONCEPTS FOR INTERPROFESSIONAL COLLABORATIVE CARE,
NINTH EDITION

Notices

Knowledge and best practice in this field are constantly changing. As new research and experience broaden our understanding, changes in research methods, professional practices, or medical treatment may become necessary.

Practitioners and researchers must always rely on their own experience and knowledge in evaluating and using any information, methods, compounds, or experiments described herein. In using such information or methods, they should be mindful of their own safety and the safety of others, including parties for whom they have a professional responsibility.

With respect to any drug or pharmaceutical products identified, readers are advised to check the most current information provided (i) on procedures featured or (ii) by the manufacturer of each product to be administered and to verify the recommended dose or formula, the method and duration of administration, and contraindications. It is the responsibility of practitioners, relying on their own experience and knowledge of their patients, to make diagnoses, to determine dosages and the best treatment for each individual patient, and to take all appropriate safety precautions.

To the fullest extent of the law, neither the Publisher nor the authors, contributors, or editors assume any liability for any injury and/or damage to persons or property as a matter of products liability, negligence or otherwise, or from any use or operation of any methods, products, instructions, or ideas contained in the material herein.

Executive Content Strategist: Lee Henderson
Senior Content Development Manager: Laurie Gower
Senior Content Development Specialist: Laura Goodrich
Publishing Services Manager: Deepthi Unni
Project Manager: Apoorva V
Design Direction: Muthukumaran Thangaraj

Printed in United States of America

Last digit is the print number: 9 8 7 6 5 4 3 2

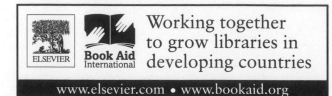

Preface

The *Study Guide for Medical-Surgical Nursing: Concepts for Interprofessional Collaborative Care,* 9th Edition, is a companion publication for Ignatavicius and Workman's *Medical-Surgical Nursing: Patient-Centered Collaborative Care,* 9th Edition. This Study Guide, written by experts in the fields of adult medical-surgical nursing and nursing education, will help to ensure mastery of the textbook content and help you learn about collaborative practice in the care of the adult medical-surgical patient.

The 9th Edition has been carefully revised and updated for an increased emphasis on clinical decision-making.

The overall organization of the *Study Guide for Medical-Surgical Nursing: Concepts for Interprofessional Collaborative Care* directly corresponds to the unit/chapter name and number in the textbook so that you or your instructor can readily select the corresponding learning exercises in the Study Guide. Chapters are focused on

- **Study/Review Questions** that are designed to encourage prioritizing, clinical decision making, and application of the steps of the nursing process. Questions have been updated to focus on the question formats of the NCLEX examination and emphasize the NCLEX priorities of delegation, management of care, and pharmacology.

Answers to the Study/Review Questions are provided in the back of the Study Guide. Case Studies and answer guidelines for the Case Studies are available on the Evolve website at http://evolve.elsevier.com/Iggy/.

The *Study Guide for Medical-Surgical Nursing: Concepts for Interprofessional Collaborative Care* is a practical tool to help you prepare for classroom examinations and standardized tests as well as a review for clinical practice. This improved format will help you review and apply medical-surgical content and help you prepare for the NCLEX Examination.

Contents

Chapter 1 Overview of Professional Nursing Concepts for Medical-Surgical Nursing 1

Chapter 2 Overview of Health Concepts for Medical-Surgical Nursing 4

Chapter 3 Common Health Problems of Older Adults 9

Chapter 4 Assessment and Care of Patients with Pain.. 12

Chapter 5 Principles of Genetics and Genomics... 21

Chapter 6 Principles of Rehabilitation for Chronic and Disabling Health Problems 25

Chapter 7 Care of Patients at End-of-Life 31

Chapter 8 Principles of Emergency and Trauma Nursing.. 34

Chapter 9 Care of Patients with Common Environmental Emergencies 44

Chapter 10 Principles of Emergency and Disaster Preparedness...................................... 56

Chapter 11 Assessment and Care of Patients with Impaired Fluid and Electrolyte Balances 62

Chapter 12 Assessment and Care of Patients with Impaired Acid-Base Balances 74

Chapter 13 Principles of Infusion Therapy... 80

Chapter 14 Care of Preoperative Patients... 90

Chapter 15 Care of Intraoperative Patients 95

Chapter 16 Care of Postoperative Patients... 100

Chapter 17 Principles of Inflammation and Immunity 107

Chapter 18 Care of Patients with Arthritis and Other Connective Tissue Diseases 114

Chapter 19 Care of Patients with HIV Disease 124

Chapter 20 Care of Patients with Hypersensitivity (Allergy) and Autoimmunity 131

Chapter 21 Principles of Cancer Development 136

Chapter 22 Care of Patients with Cancer... 141

Chapter 23 Care of Patients with Infection 149

Chapter 24 Assessment of the Skin, Hair, and Nails.. 154

Chapter 25 Care of Patients with Skin Problems 163

Chapter 26 Care of Patients with Burns 173

Chapter 27 Assessment of the Respiratory System 185

Chapter 28 Care of Patients Requiring Oxygen Therapy or Tracheostomy 194

Chapter 29 Care of Patients with Noninfectious Upper Respiratory Problems 202

Chapter 30 Care of Patients with Noninfectious Lower Respiratory Problems 211

Chapter 31 Care of Patients with Infectious Respiratory Problems 222

Chapter 32 Care of Critically Ill Patients with Respiratory Problems 233

Chapter 33 Assessment of the Cardiovascular System... 245

Chapter 34 Care of Patients with Dysrhythmias... 256

Chapter 35 Care of Patients with Cardiac Problems... 271

Chapter 36 Care of Patients with Vascular Problems 282

Chapter 37 Care of Patients with Shock 298

Chapter 38 Care of Patients with Acute Coronary Syndromes 306

Chapter 39 Assessment of the Hematologic System 320

Chapter 40 Care of Patients with Hematologic Problems 324

Chapter 41 Assessment of the Nervous System 331

Chapter 42 Care of Patients with Problems of the Central Nervous System: The Brain 337

Chapter 43 Care of Patients with Problems of the Central Nervous System: The Spinal Cord 343

Chapter 44 Care of Patients with Problems of the Peripheral Nervous System 350

Chapter 45 Care of Critically Ill Patients with Neurologic Problems 358

Chapter 46 Assessment of the Eye and Vision 368

Chapter 47 Care of Patients with Eye and Vision Problems 372

Chapter 48 Assessment and Care of Patients with Ear and Hearing Problems 376

Chapter 49 Assessment of the Musculoskeletal System 384

Chapter 50 Care of Patients with Musculoskeletal Problems 390

Chapter 51 Care of Patients with Musculoskeletal Trauma 397

Chapter 52 Assessment of the Gastrointestinal System 407

Chapter 53 Care of Patients with Oral Cavity Problems 413

Chapter 54 Care of Patients with Esophageal Problems 418

Chapter 55 Care of Patients with Stomach Disorders 424

Chapter 56 Care of Patients with Noninflammatory Intestinal Disorders 430

Chapter 57 Care of Patients with Inflammatory Intestinal Disorders 436

Chapter 58 Care of Patients with Liver Problems 442

Chapter 59 Care of Patients with Problems of the Biliary System and Pancreas 448

Chapter 60 Care of Patients with Malnutrition: Undernutrition and Obesity 453

Chapter 61 Assessment of the Endocrine System 460

Chapter 62 Care of Patients with Pituitary and Adrenal Gland Problems 465

Chapter 63 Care of Patients with Problems of the Thyroid and Parathyroid Glands 473

Chapter 64 Care of Patients with Diabetes Mellitus 480

Chapter 65 Assessment of the Renal/Urinary System 492

Chapter 66 Care of Patients with Urinary Problems 501

Chapter 67 Care of Patients with Kidney Disorders 511

Chapter 68 Care of Patients with Acute Kidney Injury and Chronic Kidney Disease 521

Chapter 69 Assessment of the Reproductive System 533

Chapter 70 Care of Patients with Breast Disorders 539

Chapter 71 Care of Patients with Gynecologic Problems 547

Chapter 72 Care of Patients with Male Reproductive Problems 554

Chapter 73 Care of Transgender Patients 562

Chapter 74 Care of Patients with Sexually Transmitted Infections 567

Answer Key 575

1 CHAPTER

Overview of Professional Nursing Concepts for Medical-Surgical Nursing

1. Which nursing action **best** exemplifies the concept of patient-centered care?
   a. Uses sterile technique to establish a peripheral intravenous catheter
   b. Assesses the patient's values and attitudes about advanced directives
   c. Checks the patient's vital signs and compares them to baseline values
   d. Administers breathing treatments according to the scheduled time

2. For which circumstance would the nurse alert the Rapid Response Team?
   a. Patient is newly diagnosed with multiple organ failure.
   b. Patient has difficulty breathing and intense chest pain.
   c. Patient has severe pain and ordered medication is not available.
   d. Patient is threatening to leave the hospital against medical advice.

3. An older patient, who was treated for a hip fracture, is being discharged from the hospital and transferred to a long-term care facility. What would be included in managing the transition of this patient?
   a. A list of the patient's valuables and property that were at the hospital
   b. Available balance of Medicare benefits after hospital costs are covered
   c. Family's preferences regarding advanced directives and living will
   d. Discharge care instructions related to the hip fracture and surgical site

4. Which health care workers are likely to be members of a Rapid Response Team? **Select all that apply.**
   a. Critical care nurse
   b. Respiratory therapist
   c. Phlebotomist
   d. Social worker
   e. Intensivist
   f. Pastoral caregiver

5. What is the **best** way for the nurse to assess the patient's understanding after teaching?
   a. Have the patient teach important points to the family.
   b. Ask the patient to repeat back the information.
   c. Quiz the patient on relevant points of the information.
   d. Repeat the important points to the patient.

6. Which type of evidence would be rated **highest** on a level of evidence scale?
   a. A nurse researcher studies a select number of nutritional factors among childhood cohorts who are matched for age.
   b. A nurse researcher randomly selects children from a walk-in clinic and describes their daily dietary intake.
   c. A nurse researcher studies selected children with specific dietary needs and instructs them about nutritious meals.
   d. A nurse researcher conducts a meta-analysis of all randomized controlled dietary studies among children.

7. Which occurrence would be considered a sentinel event?
   a. A 23-year-old post partum woman is admitted for abdominal pain and dies of sepsis.
   b. A 69-year-old man has a cardiac arrest in the cafeteria and is admitted to intensive care.
   c. A 5-year-old is admitted for injuries and the father admits to repeatedly beating the child.
   d. A 28-year-old man commits vehicular homicide and is accompanied by police to the hospital.

8. Which nursing action exemplifies the goal of case management in an acute care setting?
   a. Making sure the patient's dietary choices meet prescribed nutritional needs
   b. Coordinating inpatient and community-based care before discharge
   c. Monitoring the patient's vital signs and noting trends of change over time
   d. Reviewing the patient's hospital bill for accuracy and any excessive charges

9. Which nursing actions possess a high risk for contributing to error and patient harm? **Select all that apply.**
   a. Caring for several unstable patients who require complex nursing and medical interventions
   b. Requesting the assistance of another staff member to turn a patient
   c. Administering cardiac medications before evaluating vital signs
   d. Preparing medications while trying to answer a student's questions about laboratory results
   e. Recognizing a patient's change in mental status but assuming that it is transitory
   f. Taking a verbal order over the phone from a health care provider regarding a patient's code status

10. Which situation is an example of a nursing intervention that addresses the Institute of Medicine/Quality and Safety Education for Nurses (IOM/QSEN) health care disparities competency?
    a. Nurse recognizes that the patient's mannerisms are sexually offensive.
    b. Nurse administers pain medication as scheduled, before the patient requests it.
    c. Nurse listens with sensitivity while the lesbian patient talks about discrimination.
    d. Nurse advises an abused woman about legal protection, such as a restraining order.

11. According to ethical principles, which patient has been provided social justice?
    a. Patient with no health insurance receives the same care as all other patients.
    b. Patient gets a bath and a back rub at the exact time that the nurse promised.
    c. Patient decides what will be included in the advanced directives.
    d. Patient agrees with the nurse's advice to eat a healthy and balanced diet.

12. When using the Situation, Background, Assessment, Recommendation (SBAR) method of communication, the nurse would include which information in the B section?
    a. Recommend fingerstick glucose monitoring.
    b. Patient states he feels dizzy and lightheaded.
    c. Admission diagnosis is new-onset type 2 diabetes.
    d. Blood pressure is 130/90 mm Hg; heart rate is 89 beats per minute.

13. Which tasks should the nurse delegate to an unlicensed assistive personnel (UAP)? **Select all that apply.**
    a. Turn patient every 2 hours.
    b. Evaluate patient's skin during bathing.
    c. Feed patient breakfast and lunch.
    d. Assist patient with morning care.
    e. Take and record patient's vital signs.
    f. Discontinue IV infusion.

14. Which occurrence does The Joint Commission's National Patient Safety Goals designate as a high-risk issue?
    a. Being exposed to infectious diseases in the workplace
    b. Violating privacy of patients' confidential information
    c. Administering medication that is not familiar to the nurse
    d. Failing to review patients' food allergies before serving meals

15. Which patient is **most likely** to experience inequality in health care?
    a. A 73-year-old transgender female who is asking for directions to the public restroom
    b. A 56-year-old woman who has liver failure and wants to be on the transplant list
    c. A 34-year-old man seeking treatment for a broken wrist sustained by falling from a motorcycle
    d. A 17-year-old female who wants a pregnancy test but is unaccompanied by a parent

2 CHAPTER

Overview of Health Concepts for Medical-Surgical Nursing

1. The patient's recent history includes several episodes of nausea and vomiting. Which medical-surgical concept is the nurse's **highest** priority?
   a. Acid-base imbalance
   b. Cellular regulation
   c. Gas exchange
   d. Perfusion

2. The patient has a pH of 7.49. Which is an example of compensation for the imbalance of this concept?
   a. Kidneys reabsorb bicarbonate.
   b. Respiratory rate increases.
   c. Kidneys excrete H+ ions.
   d. Lungs decrease CO_2 excretion.

3. Which is an example of an intervention to prevent acid-base imbalance?
   a. Patient with type 2 diabetes avoids carbohydrates.
   b. Patient with COPD quits smoking.
   c. Patient with alkalosis uses daily antacids.
   d. Patient with heart disease consumes hamburgers daily for lunch.

4. Which are risk factors for impaired cellular regulation? **Select all that apply.**
   a. Adult 45-50 years old
   b. Poor nutrition
   c. Radiation therapy
   d. Excessive exercise
   e. Smoking cigarettes
   f. Exposure to pollution

5. The nurse is providing care for a patient with adenocarcinoma of the lungs. Which medical-surgical concept is the nurse's **highest** priority?
   a. Acid-base imbalance
   b. Gas exchange
   c. Cellular regulation
   d. Immunity

6. The nurse plans to teach primary prevention to a patient to promote cellular regulation and prevent impaired cellular regulation. Which topics would the nurse include? **Select all that apply.**
   a. Prevent skin cancer by minimizing exposure to sunlight.
   b. Prevent colon cancer by eating a diet low in fiber and saturated fats.
   c. Stop smoking to prevent oral or lung cancer.
   d. Get regular exercise to help prevent all types of cancers.
   e. Be aware of family illness history and screen for risk factors.
   f. Avoid exposure to environmental hazards to prevent all types of cancers.

7. The nurse is caring for a patient who is a smoker with a history of polycythemia and immobility issues. Which medical-surgical concept is the nurse's **highest** priority for this patient?
   a. Gas exchange
   b. Clotting
   c. Fluid and electrolyte imbalance
   d. Comfort

8. Which condition is an example of an imbalance concept that results in decreased clotting?
   a. Atrial fibrillation
   b. Polycythemia
   c. Cirrhosis of the liver
   d. Venous thromboembolism

9. The patient is admitted with a venous thrombosis in a deep vein of the leg. The chances of which event does the nurse recognize are increased as a physiologic consequence of the impaired clotting?
   a. Pulmonary embolus
   b. Superficial phlebitis
   c. Hemorrhagic stroke
   d. Epistaxis

10. Which are signs and symptoms of impaired clotting? **Select all that apply.**
    a. Purpural lesions
    b. Localized redness
    c. Ecchymosis
    d. Prolonged bleeding
    e. Swelling and warmth
    f. Hematuria

11. Which statement by a patient indicates the need for **additional** teaching about the risk for increased clotting?
    a. "I will cross my legs only when sitting down."
    b. "I will drink plenty of fluids so that I will stay hydrated."
    c. "I will avoid sitting for long periods of time."
    d. "I will notify my health care provider if I see redness or swelling in my leg."

12. The nurse assesses a patient for impaired cognition and finds that the confusion is recent, with a rapid onset. Which type of impaired cognition does the nurse recognize for this patient?
    a. Delirium
    b. Amnesia
    c. Dementia
    d. Fluctuating confusion

13. Which nursing interventions are appropriate when caring for a patient with late-stage dementia? **Select all that apply.**
    a. Frequently reorient the patient.
    b. Provide a safe environment.
    c. Teach the patient what is real and what is unreal.
    d. Observe for delusions or hallucinations.
    e. Teach family that the patient should not operate machinery.
    f. Allow the patient to make his or her own decisions.

14. The nurse is caring for a postoperative patient whose surgery occurred that morning. Which cause is **most likely** responsible for the alteration in the medical-surgical concept of comfort?
    a. Stress
    b. Nausea
    c. Pain
    d. Anxiety

15. The nurse is assessing a patient for altered bowel elimination related to constipation. Which finding would the nurse expect?
    a. Overactive bowel sounds
    b. Hypoactive bowel sounds
    c. Distention of the bladder
    d. Skin breakdown

16. A patient has altered bowel elimination related to diarrhea. Which are appropriate nursing care interventions for this patient? **Select all that apply.**
    a. Protect the perineal and buttock area with a barrier cream.
    b. Encourage the patient to consume foods high in calcium such as cheese and yogurt.
    c. Check the patient's weight each day for weight loss.
    d. Restrict fluid intake to help decrease episodes of diarrhea.
    e. Keep the patient's skin clean and dry.
    f. Carefully document all intake and output.

17. Which intervention should the nurse delegate to the unlicensed assistive personnel (UAP) when caring for a patient with altered bowel elimination related to urinary incontinence?
    a. Instruct the patient about use of protective briefs.
    b. Assess the patient's skin for redness or breakdown.
    c. Monitor the patient for symptoms of electrolyte imbalance.
    d. Assist the patient to the bathroom every 2 hours.

18. The nurse is assessing a patient with altered fluid volume related to excess fluids. Which sign or symptom would the nurse expect to find?
    a. Weak, thready pulses
    b. Increased blood pressure
    c. Decreased heart rate
    d. Decreased urine output

19. Which patient is most at risk for an alteration in fluid and electrolyte balance?
    a. 85-year-old with chronic kidney disease
    b. 72-year-old with constipation
    c. 63-year-old with small burn to right forearm
    d. 51-year-old with diet high in fruits and vegetables

20. Which processes are essential for the medical-surgical concept of normal gas exchange to occur?
    a. Osmosis and respiration
    b. Diffusion and absorption
    c. Ventilation and diffusion
    d. Absorption and osmosis

21. Which statement about risk factors for impaired gas exchange is accurate?
    a. Only acute problems result in decreased ventilation to cause impaired gas exchange.
    b. Short-term immobility can lead to severely impaired gas exchange.
    c. Retention of excess carbon dioxide can lead to a respiratory alkalosis.
    d. With age, pulmonary alveoli lose some elasticity, causing a decrease in gas exchange.

22. The nurse is caring for a patient with impaired gas exchange. Which interventions are appropriate in the care of this patient? **Select all that apply.**
    a. Instruct the patient to get vaccinations to prevent influenza and pneumonia.
    b. Elevate the patient's bed into the high Fowler's position.
    c. Remind the patient to wash hands thoroughly after using the commode.
    d. Administer bronchodilators as ordered by the health care provider.
    e. Remind the patient to use incentive spirometry every hour while awake.
    f. Keep oxygen in place by nasal cannula at all times.

23. Which statement about the medical-surgical concept of immunity is accurate?
    a. Natural active immunity occurs when an antibody enters the body and the body creates antigens to fight off the antibody.
    b. Artificial active immunity occurs via a vaccination or immunization.
    c. Natural passive immunity occurs via a specific transfusion, such as immunoglobulins.
    d. Artificial passive immunity occurs when antibodies are passed from a mother to the fetus through the placenta, colostrum, or breast milk.

24. Which are common risk factors for impaired immunity? **Select all that apply.**
    a. Lack of some immunizations in adults
    b. Prescription and use of corticosteroid drugs
    c. Substance abuse disorders in adults
    d. Younger age in adults
    e. From lower socioeconomic groups in adults
    f. Undergoing radiation therapy in adults

25. The nurse is caring for a patient with impaired immunity related to a suppressed immune system. Which intervention can the nurse delegate to the unlicensed assistive personnel (UAP)?
    a. Teach the patient to avoid contact with large crowds.
    b. Monitor white blood cell levels each time the patient has a CBC drawn.
    c. Assess the patient for allergies to prescribed medications.
    d. Remind the patient to wash hands carefully before each meal.

26. Which patient is at **highest** risk for impaired mobility?
    a. Patient with unrepaired hip fracture
    b. Patient with mild heart failure
    c. Post-cardiac-catheterization patient on bedrest
    d. Patient with fractured right radius

27. Which are common physiologic complications for a patient with impaired mobility? **Select all that apply.**
    a. Pressure ulcers
    b. Changes in sleep-wake cycle
    c. Constipation
    d. Sensory deprivation
    e. Muscle atrophy
    f. Urinary calculi

28. The patient has impaired mobility. Which intervention should the nurse delegate to the unlicensed assistive personnel (UAP)?
    a. Assess skin for redness or breakdown.
    b. Turn and reposition the patient every 2 hours.
    c. Teach the patient and family about the need for adequate nutrition.
    d. Instruct the patient on how and when to use incentive spirometry.

29. The nurse is caring for a patient with impaired nutrition related to bulimia nervosa. Which are appropriate interventions for the care of this patient? **Select all that apply.**
    a. Administer high-protein nutrient supplements.
    b. Assess for dry skin and dry or brittle hair.
    c. Encourage regular, strenuous exercise at least twice a day.
    d. Stress the need for intake of high-fat foods for weight gain.
    e. Monitor serum albumin and prealbumin levels.
    f. Provide teaching about bariatric surgery.

30. The patient has impaired nutrition related to lactose intolerance. Which complication will the nurse teach this patient about?
    a. Generalized edema
    b. Iron deficiency anemia
    c. Osteoporosis
    d. Constipation

31. Which is a modifiable risk factor for the medical-surgical concept of perfusion?
    a. Age
    b. Obesity
    c. Gender
    d. Genetics

32. Which are signs of impaired central perfusion? **Select all that apply.**
    a. Dizziness
    b. Decreased hair distribution
    c. Pallor of extremities
    d. Difficulty breathing
    e. Chest pain
    f. Cyanosis of extremities

33. The patient has impaired sensory perception related to smell and taste. Which question would the nurse ask this patient?
    a. "Have you ever had a stroke or brain injury of any kind?"
    b. "Did you listen to loud music when you were young?"
    c. "Do you have any dry mouth side effects with your antidepressant drug?"
    d. "How recently was the prescription on your eyeglasses changed?"

34. Which drugs are ototoxic and can cause impaired sensory perception related to hearing? **Select all that apply.**
    a. Salicylates
    b. Diuretics
    c. Antihistamines
    d. Antiepileptic drugs
    e. Aminoglycosides
    f. Chemotherapy drugs

35. Which is an example of a secondary intervention to promote sensory perception?
    a. Using protective earplugs
    b. Wearing safety goggles
    c. Avoiding hypertension by taking antihypertensive drugs
    d. Having regular eye examinations

36. Which statement about the concept of sexuality is most accurate?
    a. Sexuality and reproduction are the same.
    b. The major goal of sexuality is the conception of a child.
    c. Intimacy, self-concept, and role relationships are related to sexuality.
    d. The concept of sexuality is perceived in the same manner by most people.

37. Which patient is **most** at risk for impaired sexuality?
    a. A 20-year-old female with a history of an abortion
    b. A 45-year-old male with erectile dysfunction
    c. A 65-year-old male with history of prostate disease
    d. A 85-year-old female who has been a widow for 10 years

38. Which is the **most** common form of impaired tissue integrity?
    a. Pressure ulcers
    b. Burns
    c. Growths or lesions
    d. Injury or trauma

39. The nurse assesses a patient with impaired tissue integrity. The patient has a wound that extends through the epidermis and dermis. Which term **best** describes this wound?
    a. Full thickness
    b. Partial thickness
    c. Pressure ulcer
    d. Cellulitis

40. The nurse is caring for a patient who is at risk for impaired tissue integrity. Which interventions will promote tissue integrity and prevent impaired tissue integrity? **Select all that apply.**
    a. Keep the patient's skin clean and dry.
    b. Provide a healthy diet including protein.
    c. Give the patient protein shakes after each meal.
    d. Assist the patient to reposition in bed every 4 hours.
    e. Place a gel pad on the chair before getting the patient out of bed.
    f. Moisturize skin when needed to prevent excessively dry skin.

3 CHAPTER

Common Health Problems of Older Adults

1. The home health nurse is reviewing the charts of newly assigned patients. Which patient is **most likely** to need an assessment for geriatric failure to thrive?
   a. A 66-year-old with heart failure, chronic renal failure, and signs of liver failure
   b. An 89-year-old who has a pacemaker and must use a walker and a hearing aid
   c. A 73-year-old who has osteoporosis, history of fractures, and significant fallophobia
   d. A 69-year-old with depression, weight loss, and impaired physical functioning

2. The nurse is caring for an older adult patient. What are the **best** interventions to help reduce relocation stress in this patient? **Select all that apply.**
   a. Explain all procedures to the patient before they occur.
   b. Reorient the patient frequently to location.
   c. Initially, encourage family and friends to keep their visits to a minimum.
   d. Provide opportunity and time for the patient to participate in decision making.
   e. Arrange for familiar keepsakes to be at the patient's bedside.
   f. Change room assignment several times and assess for preferred choice.

3. Which older adult is demonstrating a health-enhancing behavior that the nurse should reinforce?
   a. A 70-year-old farmer wears sunscreen whenever sun exposure exceeds 6 hours per day.
   b. A 66-year-old man with a family history of heart problems takes an aspirin twice a day.
   c. A 65-year-old nurse exercises regularly three to five times a week.
   d. An 88-year-old woman eats one serving of vegetables four times a week.

4. The older patient tells the nurse that his teeth are in poor condition, so he tends to eat soft foods such as mashed potatoes, macaroni with cheese, and ice cream. Which question is the nurse **most likely** to ask to identify a probable physiologic consequence of the patient's dietary patterns?
   a. "Do you have any problems with your bowel movements?"
   b. "Are you experiencing weight loss?"
   c. "Have you had any changes in your ability to accomplish ADLs?"
   d. "Would you like me to help you make an appointment with the dentist?"

5. The older patient is homebound, so the nurse will focus on helping the patient to maintain functional fitness. Which exercise is the nurse **most likely** to suggest?
   a. During the winter months, go to the mall and walk around.
   b. Attend an exercise class at a senior citizens' center.
   c. Walk on a treadmill 3-5 times per week for 60 minutes.
   d. Maintain independent performance of ADLs.

6. Which older adult has the **greatest** risk for falls?
   a. A 73-year-old who takes frequent walking excursions
   b. An 81-year-old who frequently calls for help to change position
   c. A 68-year-old who uses a cane when ambulating
   d. A 90-year-old who has decreased sensation in the lower extremities

7. The nurse is caring for a confused older patient who is at risk for falls. Which interventions should the nurse implement to ensure the patient's safety? **Select all that apply.**
   a. Remind the patient to use ambulatory devices as needed.
   b. Instruct the patient to limit activity as much as possible.
   c. Provide appropriate lighting in the patient's environment.
   d. Make sure the patient's eyeglasses are clean and functional.
   e. Implement facility-specific fall protocols.
   f. Position the bed against the wall so the patient can get out of bed on only one side.

8. The patient requires physical restraints. Which intervention should the nurse perform for this patient?
   a. Check the patient every 30-60 minutes.
   b. Release the restraints at least every 4 hours.
   c. Turn up the television volume to provide distraction.
   d. Minimize communication with the patient.

9. The charge nurse is reviewing all the medication administration records for the long-term care facility. For older patients, which medication is the nurse **most likely** to question?
   a. Tricyclic antidepressant
   b. Antipsychotic
   c. Antianxiety agent
   d. Sedative-hypnotic

10. According to the Beers Criteria, the nurse would question an order for which medication in an older adult?
    a. Promethazine
    b. Thiothixen
    c. Risperidone
    d. Haloperidol

11. The creatinine clearance test result for an older female patient is 70 mL/min. How would the nurse handle the findings of this diagnostic test?
    a. Consult the pharmacy to determine if the patient's drugs are harmful to the liver.
    b. Notify the health care provider because serum drug levels could become toxic.
    c. Notify the health care provider because drug doses will need to be increased.
    d. Document the level in the patient's record as within the normal range.

12. Which intervention would the nurse use if the older adult is suffering from delirium?
    a. Talk to the patient using a calm voice.
    b. Prohibit visitors until the delirium abates.
    c. Remove and safely store personal items.
    d. Apply restraints to keep the patient safe.

13. The older patient reports early morning insomnia, excessive daytime sleeping, poor appetite, a lack of energy, and an unwillingness to participate in social and recreational activities. Which screening tool is the nurse **most likely** to use **first**?
    a. Confusion Assessment Method (CAM)
    b. Geriatric Depression Scale—Short Form (GDS-SF)
    c. CAGE questionnaire
    d. Brief Abuse Screen for the Elderly

14. In planning care for the older adult with dementia, the nurse identifies which intervention as the **first priority** goal of care?
    a. Prevent cognitive decline.
    b. Reorient on a regular basis.
    c. Prevent injury.
    d. Assist with ambulation.

15. The unlicensed assistive personnel (UAP) tells the nurse that an older gentleman was wearing a bra and women's panties when he was first admitted to the unit. What instructions would the nurse give to the UAP?
    a. "Show me the bra and panties, and then I will confront the patient."
    b. "Store the bra and panties away, and I'll talk to the family later on."
    c. "Pretend like you never saw the lingerie, and treat the patient like a male."
    d. "Assist the patient to dress, and allow him to select his own clothing."

16. On assessment of a newly admitted older patient, the nurse notes cigarette burns on the lower abdomen. Which term **best** describes this finding?
    a. Neglect
    b. Physical abuse
    c. Psychological abuse
    d. Mistreatment

17. The patient is both confused and agitated. Which action is **most important** at this time?
    a. Place the patient in a quiet, supervised area.
    b. Check the patient every 2 hours.
    c. Sedate the patient using IV medication.
    d. Apply soft wrist restraints for a limited time.

18. Which task should the nurse delegate to unlicensed assistive personnel when caring for an older adult?
    a. Instruct the patient to drink at least 2 liters of fluids each day.
    b. Assess the patient's skin every 2 hours during repositioning.
    c. Assist the patient with tray preparation and feeding at mealtimes.
    d. Teach the patient how to balance the diet with healthy food selections.

19. The nurse is using the Fulmer SPICES framework to assess an older adult. Which question would the nurse ask when using SPICES?
    a. Do you use a hearing aid?
    b. How do you like to be addressed?
    c. Have ever been treated for mental illness?
    d. Have you had any recent falls?

20. An older resident living in a long-term care facility is usually mildly confused, talkative, outgoing, and cheerful but today is suddenly quiet, apathetic, lethargic, unaware, and withdrawn. What action would the nurse take **first**?
    a. Call the health care provider and report the sudden change in behavior.
    b. Take a full set of vital signs and check pulse oximeter and glucometer readings.
    c. Draw blood specimen and have it checked for electrolyte and fluid imbalances.
    d. Verbally and physically stimulate the resident until behavior returns to normal.

CHAPTER 4

Assessment and Care of Patients with Pain

1. The nurse is working at a walk-in clinic and has interviewed several patients. Which patient has the **most common** reason for seeking medical care?
   a. Has a family history of angina
   b. Has a personal history of chronic pain
   c. Has drug addiction and is seeking pain medication
   d. Has a desire to avoid pain or injury during exercise

2. The nurse is performing a pain assessment on a patient who had abdominal surgery. He was just transferred from the intensive care unit to the medical surgical unit. Which question would the nurse ask?
   a. "You are probably having pain at the incision site. Right?"
   b. "How bad is your pain? Is it better compared to before?"
   c. "Can you tell me about any pain or discomfort you are having?"
   d. "Do you think you can walk, or would you like pain medication first?"

3. The patient reports that he has chronic lower back pain that is not relieved by the prescribed medication and that the primary care provider is unwilling to prescribe anything stronger. Who should the nurse consult **first**?
   a. Pharmacist
   b. Physical therapist
   c. Pain resource nurse
   d. Alternate health care provider

4. Which patient has the **highest** risk for inadequate pain management?
   a. 56-year-old man who had major abdominal surgery for a stab wound
   b. 78-year-old woman who was transferred to a nursing home after hip surgery
   c. 10-year-old child who had a tonsillectomy and whose parents can't speak English
   d. 24-year-old postpartum woman with a history of drug abuse

5. Which patient has chronic noncancer pain?
   a. A 17-year-old male after an appendectomy
   b. A 64-year-old male with back pain related to tumor growth
   c. A 48-year-old female who has persistent pain related to interstitial cystitis
   d. A 5-year-old female with stomach cramps related to food poisoning

6. A patient with chronic leg pain reports pain level at 7/10, so the nurse administers a prn medication. Which observation **best** suggests that the functional goal of therapy is being met?
   a. Patient appears relaxed while talking with family members.
   b. Pulse, blood pressure, and respirations are not elevated.
   c. Patient ambulates independently down the hall without distress.
   d. Patient asks for additional food between lunch and dinner.

7. Despite the nurse's best efforts, the patient's wife continuously asks the nurse to reassess her husband's pain and to give him additional medication. What is the **best** rationale for using the concept of "self-report"?
   a. The wife's behavior indicates that she is overly anxious.
   b. The concerns of the wife make accurate pain assessment very difficult.
   c. The patient's relationship with his wife is interfering with the plan of care.
   d. The patient is the only one who can describe his experience of pain.

8. Which patient is **most likely** to report pain that would be considered acute?
   a. Has a history of peripheral vascular disease; foot is suddenly cold and blue
   b. Has a history of diabetic neuropathy; reports burning sensation in lower leg
   c. Has a history of old ankle fracture; reports recent diagnosis of osteoarthritis
   d. Has a history of osteosarcoma in the femur with amputation above tumor site

9. In assessing pain in an older adult patient, what is a major barrier to accurate assessment?
   a. Many older adults are reluctant to report pain.
   b. Pain sensation decreases with age.
   c. Pain scales are inaccurate for older adults.
   d. Most older adults have some cognitive impairment.

10. The nurse is caring for a patient on the first postoperative day. The patient denies pain, but his blood pressure and pulse are elevated and he is diaphoretic and anxious. What should the nurse do **first**?
    a. Believe and document the patient's self-report of "denies pain."
    b. Call the health care provider and report the vital signs, diaphoresis, and anxiety.
    c. Assess the patient for postoperative complications or barriers to reporting pain.
    d. Ask a family member if the patient would typically be stoic during pain or discomfort.

11. The older patient tells the home health nurse that he took two tablets of arthritis-strength extended release acetaminophen at 6:00 am and two tablets of hydrocodone at 2:00 pm and that he plans to take one dose of an over-the-counter product that contains acetaminophen, doxylamine succinate, and dextromethorphan to sleep at night. What would the nurse do **first**?
    a. Call poison control, because the patient has exceeded the recommended dose of acetaminophen.
    b. Tell the patient to call the health care provider and report all medications that he takes.
    c. Educate the patient about the acetaminophen in each product and the maximum dosage/day.
    d. Record the medications, frequency, and dosage in the medication reconciliation record.

12. The nurse knows that acute pain serves a biologic purpose. How does the nurse apply this knowledge in caring for a patient with a history of cardiac problems who now reports severe chest pain?
    a. Immediately administers supplemental oxygen
    b. Calmly reassures that acute pain is usually temporary
    c. Efficiently assesses for anxiety or panic attack
    d. Quickly obtains an order for prn pain medication

13. A patient with rheumatoid arthritis reports having chronic pain for years with an exacerbation that started in the morning. Which observation indicates the patient has a physiologic adaptation to pain?
    a. Pupils are dilated.
    b. Breathing is shallow.
    c. Pulse rate is 70/min.
    d. Temperature is 98.6°F (37°C).

14. The nurse is caring for several patients who will receive pain medication. Which patient is **most likely** to receive around-the-clock oral opioids?
    a. Patient with fibromyalgia
    b. Patient with chronic cancer pain
    c. Patient with Crohn's disease
    d. Patient who had a stroke

15. Which patient is **most likely** to receive a prescription for gabapentin?
    a. A patient who has persistent burning and tingling sensation in the lower extremities
    b. A patient who reports a gnawing and burning discomfort in the epigastric area between meals
    c. A patient who expresses fear, anxiety, and uncertainty related to episodes of angina
    d. A patient who has intractable pain related to malignant spread of cancer

16. Nociception involves the normal function of physiologic systems and four processes. When the nurse suggests listening to music as a distraction, which process is the target of the intervention?
    a. Transduction
    b. Transmission
    c. Perception
    d. Modulation

17. Which patient is having pain that is unlikely to respond to **first-line** opioid and nonopioid medication?
    a. 62-year-old woman who fractured her wrist
    b. 70-year-old woman with postherpetic neuralgia
    c. 50-year-old man with a recently inserted chest tube
    d. 45-year-old man who sustained burns to the hands

18. Which behavior exemplifies the nurse's primary role in assessing and managing the patient's pain?
    a. Administers pain medication as ordered if pain is sufficient to warrant therapy
    b. Listens to the patient's self-report and forms an opinion about the veracity of the description
    c. Observes for concurrent verbal reports and nonverbal signs to substantiate presence of pain
    d. Listens to and accepts the self-report of pain and assesses patient's preferences and values

19. What are physiologic responses that indicate a patient is experiencing acute pain? **Select all that apply.**
    a. Diaphoresis
    b. Somnolence
    c. Bradypnea
    d. Hypotension
    e. Tachycardia
    f. Dilated pupils

20. What is the **best** type of pain scale to use for children or for adult patients who have language barriers or reading problems?
    a. 0 to 10 numeric rating scale
    b. FACES (smile to frown)
    c. Vertical presentation scale
    d. Pasero Opioid-Induced Sedation Scale

21. The nurse asks the patient with cancer, "Sir, where is your pain?" The patient repeatedly responds, "It hurts all over." What is the **best** rationale for taking the extra time to help the patient to identify specific areas that hurt?
    a. Documentation is incomplete as a legal document if the nurse charts "hurts all over."
    b. Formulating an achievable therapeutic goal is very difficult for a vague complaint.
    c. Health care provider cannot prescribe appropriate medication for relief of generalized pain.
    d. Patient understands the origin, and new or increasing pain raises the suspicion of metastasis.

22. Using the concept of comfort, which application creates the **greatest** concern related to the use of the patient-controlled analgesia (PCA) infusion device?
    a. Pendant
    b. Demand
    c. Lockout
    d. Proxy

23. The nurse is assessing an elderly patient who has "pain all over." Which strategy would the nurse use to help the patient identify which areas of the body are painful?
    a. Start with gentle palpation on the abdomen and chest.
    b. Focus on the hand and fingers of one extremity.
    c. Direct the patient to find one area that does not hurt.
    d. Provide examples and comparisons of severe pain.

24. The home health nurse is reviewing the older adult's medication and sees that naproxen is prescribed. Which question is the nurse **most likely** to ask in order to assess for adverse effects?
    a. "Have you noticed unusual fatigue, restlessness, or feelings of depression?"
    b. "Do you notice dry mouth, dizziness, mental clouding, or weight gain?"
    c. "Are you experiencing constipation, itching, or excessive sleepiness?"
    d. "Have you had any gastric discomfort, vomiting, bleeding, or bruising?"

25. The nursing student is using the Wong-Baker FACES pain rating scale to assess the pain of a 4-year-old child. The nurse would intervene if the student performed which action?
    a. Points to the smiling face and tells the child that this face has "no pain"
    b. Tells the child that FACES helps nurses understand how he is feeling
    c. Points to the tearful face and tells the child that the picture means "worst pain"
    d. Observes the child's facial expression and matches it to a face on the scale

26. The nurse is assessing the patient for chronic pain or discomfort. Which is the **best** question to use to elicit the quality of the pain?
    a. "Am I correct in assuming that you are having pain?"
    b. "Would you describe the pain as sharp?"
    c. "Is the pain really bad right now?"
    d. "How would you describe your pain?"

27. Based on evidence-based practice, what is the **best** choice for managing chronic pain for a 73-year-old female with osteoarthritis?
    a. Acetaminophen is the primary drug of choice.
    b. Tramadol is the first-line choice for this patient.
    c. Long-term use of an oral NSAID, such as ibuprofen, is the best.
    d. Topical NSAIDs and nonpharmacologic measures should be tried first.

28. The nurse is assisting a surgical patient with pain management. Which outcome statement **best** demonstrates that the short-term goal is being met 45 minutes after receiving pain medication?
    a. Patient reports that the pain level is 6/10.
    b. Patient tolerates the dressing change without grimacing.
    c. Patient declines a prn anxiolytic medication.
    d. Patient asks for assistance to go to the bathroom.

29. The patient reports a vivid childhood memory of having severe pain during and after a dental procedure and expresses reluctance to visit the dentist even for routine cleanings. What should the nurse do?
    a. Refer the patient for psychological counseling before seeking dental care.
    b. Obtain an order for antianxiety medication and suggest relaxation techniques.
    c. Suggest talking to a dentist about current pain management techniques.
    d. Advise patient that past fears should not interfere with good health practices.

30. The nurse is interviewing a patient who frequently comes to the clinic to obtain medication for chronic back pain. The patient states, "I know you guys think I am faking, but I hurt and I am really sick of your attitude." What is the **best** response?
    a. "Sir, tell me about your pain and how it is affecting your life."
    b. "Sir, you can speak to a pain specialist if you would prefer."
    c. "Sir, I see you are frustrated, but you are unfairly judging me."
    d. "Sir, we are trying our best; let's just continue the interview."

31. Which nursing action indicates that the nurse is performing the **first** step of the Hierarchy of Pain Measures?
    a. Premedicates before a dressing change
    b. Uses a standard pain assessment tool
    c. Compares vital signs before and after pain medication
    d. Starts with a low dose and observes for behavioral changes

32. A patient needs morphine 2 mg IV push. The drug is available as 5 mg/mL. How many mL would the nurse administer? _____ mL of morphine.

33. The nurse is assessing a patient with severe dementia who resides in a long-term care facility. A score of 9 is obtained using the Pain Assessment in Advanced Dementia Scale. Based on assessment findings, which action will the nurse take?
    a. Speak calmly to the patient and explain that repositioning will make him more comfortable.
    b. Gently reassure the patient and continue routine observation for discomfort or pain.
    c. Assess the patient for the source of the pain and immediately inform the health care provider.
    d. Contact the family and ask how the patient would typically respond to discomfort.

34. The home health nurse is visiting a 73-year-old diabetic patient who was recently discharged after surgery. While reviewing a list of the patient's medications, the nurse sees that there are several different classes of analgesics listed. Which action is the nurse **most likely** to take?
    a. Assesses patient's understanding of the multimodal treatment plan and ability to comply
    b. Contacts the health care provider to discontinue medications that contribute to polypharmacy
    c. Emphasizes that medications with more side effects are the last choice for pain
    d. Advises the patient not to take any NSAIDs because of irritation of gastric mucosa

35. Which drug can cause adverse effects, particularly in an older adult, because of an accumulation of toxic metabolites?
    a. Ibuprofen
    b. Morphine
    c. Meperidine
    d. Acetaminophen

36. The nurse is giving discharge instructions about multimodal analgesia to a daughter who will care for her elderly father at home while he recovers from surgery. The daughter suggests that the single best medication should be recommended for convenience and to save money. What is the **best** response?
    a. "The doctor always prescribes this combination of medications as the best therapy."
    b. "Elderly people frequently do better with fewer medications; let me call the doctor."
    c. "Just see how it goes for your dad. It is likely that you can gradually decrease the medication."
    d. "Combining different analgesics gives greater relief with lower doses and fewer side effects."

37. The patient has a severe burn on the hand and forearm and reports pain that is severe and escalating. The nurse anticipates that pain medication will be administered via which route?
    a. Oral
    b. Intravenous
    c. Intranasal
    d. Subcutaneous

38. The postanesthesia care unit reports to the nurse in the medical-surgical unit that the patient received 2 mg of intravenous morphine with relief. When is the patient likely to be transitioned to oral analgesics?
    a. Upon arrival to the medical-surgical unit
    b. When the health care provider writes postoperative orders
    c. When the patient is able to tolerate oral intake
    d. When the intravenous access is discontinued

39. A patient is prescribed morphine sulfate. Which nursing interventions decrease the risk of constipation? **Select all that apply.**
    a. Give foods that are soft, such as white bread or white rice.
    b. Encourage an increase in water and fluid intake.
    c. Administer a stool softener every morning.
    d. Obtain an order for a bulk laxative.
    e. Encourage movement, activity, and walking.
    f. Teach to keep a record of bowel movements

40. A new, inexperienced nurse sees that the patient is receiving around-the-clock medication but also has orders for prn analgesic every 4-6 hours as needed. How will the new nurse determine when a prn dose is given?
    a. Administer a dose every 6 hours to ensure adequate relief.
    b. Call the health care provider and ask for specific parameters for prn dosing.
    c. Look at the medication administration record to see what the previous nurse gave.
    d. Assess the patient for breakthrough pain and anticipate painful procedures.

41. The health care provider informs the nurse that a young patient should receive morphine for severe pain but that caution is needed because the patient is opioid naïve. Which consideration is the **most important** in caring for and observing this patient?
    a. Decreased analgesia may occur because the patient is opioid naïve.
    b. Respiratory depression is a problem only for elderly adults with respiratory disorders.
    c. Excessive sedation can progress to clinically significant respiratory depression.
    d. A standing order for a prn one-time dose of naloxone is needed for adverse effects.

42. Which patient is **least likely** to be a good candidate for patient-controlled analgesia?
    a. 32-year-old male with severe burns and a history of drug abuse
    b. 16-year-old male with multiple injuries sustained during an accident
    c. 34-year-old female with functional blindness who had abdominal surgery
    d. 25-year-old female with intermittent lucidity after a severe head injury

43. The nurse is assessing a patient who is receiving opioid medication via a patient-controlled analgesia device. The patient is very drowsy and difficult to arouse. What should the nurse do **first**?
    a. Wake the patient and tell the patient to stop pushing the button so frequently.
    b. Stay with the patient and discontinue the basal rate.
    c. Let the patient sleep but increase the frequency of assessment.
    d. Obtain an order for exclusive use of nonopioid medication.

44. Based on the concept of comfort, what is the expected physiologic consequence of taking a mu opioid agonist?
    a. An increase in dosage yields an increase in pain relief.
    b. There is a dose ceiling effect, so comfort is readily achieved.
    c. Analgesia is reversed at the peak effect.
    d. Peak comfort is typically 15-20 minutes after administration.

45. The nurse is caring for a patient who has an epidural catheter for pain management. Which information is appropriate in the care of this patient?
    a. Pain assessments are performed less frequently if epidural catheters are used for pain management.
    b. Morphine and hydromorphone may be used with a local anesthetic such as bupivacaine.
    c. Epidural catheters are used exclusively to deliver single bolus doses during surgical procedures.
    d. The patient will be confined to bed during the therapy because of lower extremity weakness.

46. The patient has a history of rheumatoid arthritis and is also being treated for acute pain from a wrist fracture. Which medication is **most likely** to be prescribed to reduce the pain and discomfort caused by inflammation?
    a. Morphine
    b. Acetaminophen
    c. Ibuprofen
    d. Bupivacaine

47. The nurse is reviewing the patient's medication list and sees that acetaminophen and celecoxib are scheduled to be administered at the same time. What should the nurse do?
    a. Call the health care provider for an order to stagger the administration of these two pain medications.
    b. Ask the patient which one he prefers to take; administer the preferred drug and assess for relief.
    c. Give the acetaminophen because it is less likely to cause gastric irritation and bleeding.
    d. Administer the medications as ordered because they can be given together without ill effects.

48. The nurse sees that during the night the patient received lorazepam for anxiety, promethazine for nausea, and hydromorphone for pain. Which assessment is the **most important** to conduct?
    a. Closely monitor liver enzymes to identify early indicators of adverse effects.
    b. Watch for symptoms of cardiotoxicity, such as tingling and cardiac dysrhythmias.
    c. Use the Pasero Opioid-Induced Sedation Scale and check respiratory status.
    d. Watch for gastrointestinal distress, decreased platelet count, and bleeding.

49. An older patient requires an NSAID for inflammatory pain. The nurse would seek an order for what type of additional medication to accompany the NSAID therapy?
    a. Anxiolytic, such as alprazolam
    b. Nonopioid analgesic, such as acetaminophen
    c. Proton pump inhibitor, such as lansoprazole
    d. Anticonvulsant, such as pregabalin

50. Which concept is **most** closely aligned with how a transcutaneous electrical nerve stimulation (TENS) unit works to decrease pain?
    a. Comfort
    b. Sensory perception
    c. Cognition
    d. Cellular regulation

51. The nurse is assessing the patient's use of transdermal fentanyl and discovers that the patient is making several errors. Which behavior is **most likely** to result in fentanyl-induced respiratory depression?
    a. Patient is folding the patch in half.
    b. Patient is saving the old used patches.
    c. Patient is placing a heating pad over the patch.
    d. Patient is using adhesive tape over the patch.

52. The patient reports pruritus related to taking an opioid medication. What medication prescription would the nurse obtain to help the patient to manage this side effect?
    a. Reduced opioid dose
    b. Over-the-counter antihistamine
    c. Topical steroid
    d. Antianxiety medication

53. The nurse is reviewing the medication list for a patient who had open heart surgery. The nurse is likely to query the prescription for which medication because prostaglandin inhibition is associated with adverse cardiovascular effects?
    a. Duloxetine
    b. Acetaminophen
    c. Naproxen
    d. Morphine

54. The patient reports that he has been taking hydrocodone as prescribed by his provider and uses over-the-counter acetaminophen whenever he needs additional pain relief. Which laboratory test indicates the adverse and additive effects of these two medications?
    a. Decreased clotting times
    b. Decreased hematocrit
    c. Elevated white blood cell count
    d. Elevated liver enzymes

55. The patient with chronic cancer pain has been taking oral morphine for several months. The health care provider suggests a very low dose of nalbuphine for relief of opioid-induced pruritus. What would the nurse frequently assess for?
    a. Higher risk for respiratory depression
    b. Severe pain or withdrawal symptoms
    c. Hemodynamic adverse effects
    d. Bleeding and increased clotting time

56. A patient develops a physical dependence after taking an opioid as prescribed for postsurgical pain. What is the recommended approach for dealing with the dependence?
    a. Immediate discontinuation of the opioid
    b. Administering an antagonist, such as naloxone
    c. Gradual reduction of the opioid as pain decreases
    d. Referral to a substance specialist for treatment

57. The patient is receiving the first dose of transdermal fentanyl, and the health care provider informs the nurse that the dosage will be titrated until the patient experiences adequate pain control. How much time does the nurse expect will pass between dosage changes?
    a. Between 5 and 15 minutes if the patient has severe pain
    b. At least 24 hours before the next dose
    c. Approximately 2-3 days for transdermal applications
    d. Depends on the ordered frequency of the patch change

58. A patient with chronic cancer pain has been taking opioids for several months and now reports needing increasing doses to achieve pain relief. What is the **most likely** explanation of the need for increasing amounts of medication for this patient?
    a. Patient is addicted to opioids.
    b. Disease is progressing.
    c. A different opioid is needed.
    d. Patient has a tolerance for opioids.

59. A modified-release opioid is ordered for a patient who is currently NPO (nothing by mouth) and receiving nutrition and fluids through a small-bore nasogastric (NG) tube. What should the nurse do?
    a. Crush the medication and mix it with water to instill through the NG tube.
    b. Contact the health care provider for an order to administer the medication rectally.
    c. Have the patient swallow the medication with a very small amount of water.
    d. Hold the medication and document that the patient is NPO for foods and fluids.

60. Which assessment would the nurse perform to determine if a patient would be an appropriate candidate for using imagery as a distraction therapy?
    a. Determine if touch and physical proximity are culturally acceptable.
    b. Ensure that the patient can speak, read, and write English.
    c. Assess environmental factors that contribute to discomfort or annoyance.
    d. Confirm that the patient can follow a logical and sustained conversation.

61. Acetaminophen is the **first-line** medication for which patient?
    a. Needs relief from pain related to a minor surgical procedure
    b. Has chronic pain and discomfort due to rheumatoid arthritis
    c. Experiences burning and tingling in legs due to diabetes
    d. Has intermittent abdominal cramping due to Crohn's disease

CHAPTER 5

Principles of Genetics and Genomics

1. What is the **major** reason nurses need to understand the genetic basis for diseases?
   a. Nurses must be prepared to offer genetic counseling at the bedside.
   b. Most serious adult-onset diseases have a genetic component.
   c. Patients read about genetics and ask questions about this topic.
   d. Many adult-onset diseases can lead to genetic anomalies.

2. What are autosomes?
   a. Structures composed of two Xs as the sex chromosomes
   b. The organized arrangements of chromosomes in one cell
   c. The proteins needed to generate chromosome pairs
   d. Chromosomes not involved in gender determination

3. Which statement **best** reflects the correct explanations by the health care professional who is providing genetic counseling?
   a. "This test will tell us everything about you!"
   b. "We are going to perform this testing because you asked for it, and it won't affect your family in any way."
   c. "I'm here to provide information so that you can make an informed decision about genetic testing."
   d. "The results of this genetic testing will be sent to your health insurance carrier immediately."

4. A patient asks you to explain the term "microbiome." Which explanation is **most** accurate?
   a. Microbiome is a new genetics concern because it refers to microorganisms that are pathogenic.
   b. Microbiome is the genomes of all the microorganisms that coexist in and on a person.
   c. Microbiome is the microorganisms that are responsible for the occurrence of mutations.
   d. Microbiome is the microorganisms that move from place to place within the human body.

5. When assessing for genetic risks, which factors indicate that a client may have an **increased** genetic risk for a disease or disorder? **Select all that apply.**
   a. A close family member has an identified genetic problem.
   b. A patient tells you that he was exposed to a carcinogenic substance during a war.
   c. A patient has been diagnosed with two different types of cancer.
   d. A patient's sister had breast cancer at age 24.
   e. A patient's father was diagnosed with rheumatic fever at 10 years of age.
   f. A patient tells you that she never exercises.

6. Which disorders have a genetic pattern of inheritance? **Select all that apply.**
   a. Malignant hyperthermia
   b. Gallstones
   c. Cystic fibrosis
   d. Acute lymphocytic leukemia
   e. Polycystic kidney disease
   f. Sickle cell disease

7. What is the smallest functional unit of DNA?
   a. Chromosome
   b. Allele
   c. Nucleotide
   d. Gene

8. A newborn infant inherits a type A allele from his mother and a type B allele from his father. What type of blood will the infant have?
   a. Type A
   b. Type B
   c. Type AB
   d. Type O

9. A child has 2 identical alleles for pointed ears. Which term **best** describes the child's likelihood of developing pointed ears?
   a. The child is homozygous and will develop pointed ears.
   b. The child is heterozygous and may develop pointed ears.
   c. The child has dominant alleles and will develop pointed ears.
   d. The child has codominant alleles and may develop pointed ears.

10. A person's hair is curly. Which statement is true about this person's alleles for hair type?
    a. The person must have two identical alleles for curly hair.
    b. The person may have one allele for curly hair and one allele for straight hair.
    c. The person's parents must both have the phenotype of curly hair.
    d. The person must have two recessive alleles for curly hair.

11. A person's genetic sequence for a specific protein has a variation or mutation. Which statements express what may happen to that person? **Select all that apply.**
    a. Function of the protein may be reduced.
    b. Function of the protein may be the same.
    c. Function of the protein may be eliminated.
    d. Function of the protein may be completely different.
    e. Function of the protein may be normal or expected.
    f. Function of the protein may be enhanced.

12. The patient is of Caucasian heritage. Which **heritage-based** precaution is essential when the health care provider prescribes warfarin for this patient?
    a. Teach the patient to use a soft-bristled toothbrush.
    b. Assess the patient for signs of abnormal bleeding every shift.
    c. Instruct the UAP to avoid the use of a regular razor during morning care.
    d. Monitor the patient's international normalized ratio (INR) more frequently.

13. Which criteria are used to determine if inheritance is autosomal dominant (AD)? **Select all that apply.**
    a. The trait appears in every other generation.
    b. The risk for the affected person to pass the trait to a child is 50% with each pregnancy.
    c. Unaffected people do not have affected children.
    d. The trait is found equally in males and females.
    e. For the trait to be expressed, both alleles must be dominant.
    f. The trait will appear in every other child.

14. The patient has the gene for Huntington disease (HD). What is her risk for developing this disease?
    a. The HD gene has low penetrance and the patient is unlikely to develop the disease.
    b. The patient must have two genes for HD for the disease to develop.
    c. The HD gene is autosomal dominant; the patient has a moderate risk for developing the disease.
    d. The HD gene has high penetrance and the patient's risk is almost 100%.

15. Which statement about autosomal recessive patterns of inheritance is accurate?
    a. The trait appears in every generation.
    b. The children of two affected parents will always be affected.
    c. About 50% of a family will be affected by the trait.
    d. The trait is found more commonly in female than male family members.

16. Which statement about a sex-linked recessive pattern of inheritance is accurate?
    a. The trait cannot be passed down from mother to son.
    b. The incidence is much higher in females than males in a family.
    c. Female carriers have a 50% risk with each pregnancy of passing the gene to their children.
    d. Transmission of the trait is from mother to all daughters, who will become carriers.

17. The adult patient from Ethiopia with high blood pressure is prescribed metoprolol 50 mg twice a day. What **major** concern must the nurse monitor for with this patient?
    a. The patient is at risk for sudden severe hypotension.
    b. The patient may develop a severe allergic reaction to this drug.
    c. The patient's blood pressure may not respond to this drug.
    d. The patient may develop orthostatic hypotension.

18. Which feature is **"key"** when a genetics counselor is providing a patient with genetics counseling?
    a. The counseling should be nondirective.
    b. The counselor provides information and advice to the patient.
    c. The counseling should be provided by an advanced practice nurse.
    d. The counselor provides risks, benefits, and suggestions for early diagnosis.

19. The patient desires genetic testing for the Huntington disease (HD) gene but does not want other members of his family to know the results. Which ethical issue would be violated if the patient's family were informed of these results?
    a. The right to know versus the right not to know
    b. Confidentiality
    c. Coercion
    d. Privacy

20. What is the role of the medical-surgical nurse in genetic testing? **Select all that apply.**
    a. Ensure that the patient's rights are respected.
    b. Provide complete information on the results of the testing.
    c. Refer the patient to a genetics counseling expert.
    d. Always be present when the patient receives genetic counseling.
    e. Teach patients about the nature of genetic testing.
    f. Warn the patient about the likelihood of genetic anomalies.

21. For a patient with a genetic predisposition to develop type 2 diabetes mellitus, which factor increases the risk that the patient will be diagnosed with this disease?
    a. Patient lives sedentary lifestyle.
    b. Grandfather has type 1 diabetes.
    c. Mother has coronary artery disease.
    d. Patient consumes high-fat diet.

22. Which statements about gene mutation are accurate? **Select all that apply.**
    a. All gene mutations are serious and potentially deadly.
    b. Gene mutations that increase risk of a disorder are susceptibility genes.
    c. Mutations that occur in the body cells (somatic) can be passed from parents to children.
    d. Germline mutations (sex cells) cannot be passed from parents to children.
    e. Gene mutations that decrease risk for a disorder are protective genes.
    f. Somatic cell gene mutations may cause increased risk for cancer in cells.

23. An adult patient prescribed antibiotics for an acute infection develops severe bloody diarrhea. Which phenomenon is this an example of?
    a. Gene mutation
    b. Inheritance alteration
    c. Altered microbiome
    d. Allergic reaction

24. For which adult disorders is carrier genetic testing performed? **Select all that apply.**
    a. Sickle cell disease
    b. Huntington disease
    c. Tay-Sachs disease
    d. Breast cancer
    e. Alzheimer's disease
    f. Hemophilia

6 CHAPTER

Principles of Rehabilitation for Chronic and Disabling Health Problems

1. Which statement **best** describes a chronic health problem?
   a. A physical or mental problem that causes disability
   b. A health condition that has existed for at least 3 months
   c. A specialty focused on the care of patients with long-term care problems
   d. A condition that occurs in patients over the age of 65 years

2. Which problem is the **leading** cause of trauma and death in young and middle-aged adults?
   a. Stroke
   b. Cancer
   c. Arthritis
   d. Accidents

3. As a result of a car accident, an adult patient is unable to perform certain activities of daily living (ADLs) such as bathing without assistance. This is an example of which concept?
   a. Disability
   b. Handicap
   c. Impairment
   d. Rehabilitation

4. The rehab patient wears street clothes and makes decisions about how her day will be planned. Which type of rehab setting is this patient in? **Select all that apply.**
   a. Custodial nursing home
   b. Short-term rehabilitation facility
   c. Skilled nursing facility
   d. Acute care facility
   e. Assisted living facility
   f. Specialized rehabilitation clinic

5. Which responsibilities are part of the nurse's role as a member of the rehabilitation team? **Select all that apply.**
   a. Advocates for the patient and family
   b. Creates a therapeutic rehabilitation milieu
   c. Delegates patient care only to the unlicensed assistive personnel (UAP)
   d. Plans for continuity of care when the patient is discharged
   e. Coordinates rehabilitation team activities
   f. Directs all members of the rehabilitation team

6. The patient needs help with self-feeding, bathing, and dressing. Which rehabilitation team member would **best** help the patient to develop these skills?
   a. Physical therapist
   b. Rehabilitation nurse
   c. Rehabilitation case manager
   d. Occupational therapist

7. What statement best describes the primary goal of the rehabilitation team?
   a. To rely on a specific plan of care standardized to the medical diagnosis
   b. To identify and use one conceptual framework to serve as the sole model for the practice of rehabilitation nursing
   c. To restore and maintain the patient's function to the best extent possible
   d. To enable patients and their families to identify strategies to successfully meet short-term goals

8. What are the nurse's responsibilities regarding the skin care assessment of the rehabilitation patient? **Select all that apply.**
   a. Identification of actual or potential interruptions of skin integrity
   b. Keeping track of patient urination patterns and bowel movements
   c. Assessment of the skin for all patients under his or her care
   d. Education of the patient in how to inspect his or her own skin
   e. Thorough documentation of the integrity of the skin
   f. Measuring depth and diameter of any open skin areas

9. Which factors will the nurse assess when implementing a position change schedule for an older adult? **Select all that apply.**
   a. Ability of the patient to change positions
   b. Condition of the patient's skin with each position change
   c. Presence of abnormal breath sounds
   d. Type of injury the patient sustained
   e. Age of the patient
   f. Frailty in older adults

10. The patient is at risk for impaired skin integrity. For which action performed by the unlicensed assistive personnel (UAP) must the nurse intervene?
    a. UAP assists the patient to turn in bed every 2 hours.
    b. UAP carefully cleans and dries skin after incontinence episode.
    c. UAP rubs and massages a reddened area on the patient's hip.
    d. UAP uses pillows to support the patient when turned on his side.

11. Which statement by a nursing student providing care for a patient with impaired skin integrity on a pressure-relieving mattress requires intervention by the clinical instructor?
    a. "The purpose of this mattress is to reduce pressure on the patient's skin."
    b. "Because my patient is on a pressure-relieving mattress, I will only turn her every 6 hours."
    c. "I will do a careful skin assessment while giving my patient her morning bath."
    d. "With assistance, I will get my patient up in the chair as ordered by the health care provider."

12. For which **priority** common gastrointestinal problem should the nurse create a plan to prevent for a rehab patient?
    a. Constipation
    b. Diarrhea
    c. Emaciation
    d. Electrolyte imbalance

13. A patient with decreased cardiac output is entering a rehabilitation program. What will the nurse expect to find during the assessment of this patient?
    a. Fatigue and need for rest periods
    b. Ability to ambulate without angina
    c. Feeling rested upon awakening from sleep
    d. Ability to move from sitting to standing position easily

14. A patient with paraplegia is entering a rehabilitation program. What does the nurse focus on **first** in assessing this patient?
    a. Family and cultural background
    b. Baseline hemoglobin and hematocrit measurements
    c. Habits of bowel elimination before illness
    d. Manual dexterity, muscle control, and mobility

15. A patient with a neurogenic bladder is to be taught how to perform intermittent self-catheterization. Before beginning the teaching-learning sessions, what will the nurse assess in this patient **first**?
    a. Motor function of both upper extremities
    b. Type of neurogenic bladder the patient has
    c. Client's gender
    d. Age of the client

16. To maintain the skin integrity of a patient in a rehabilitation unit, what does the nurse assess? **Select all that apply.**
    a. Sensation of the skin
    b. Placement of clear dressings over reddened areas
    c. Ability to move extremities
    d. Presence or absence of exudate and odor
    e. Ability to change position as needed
    f. Photographs taken of patient skin on admission

17. Which statements correctly describe the Functional Independence Measure (FIM)? **Select all that apply.**
    a. It is a basic indicator of the severity of a disability.
    b. It tries to measure what a person should do, whatever the diagnosis or impairment.
    c. It tries to measure what a person actually does, whatever the diagnosis or impairment.
    d. The assessment may be performed by various health care disciplines.
    e. Categories for assessment are self-care, sphincter control, mobility and locomotion, communication, and cognition.
    f. Evaluations may be done at specified times during therapy to determine patient progress.

18. Which of the following are activities of daily living? **Select all that apply.**
    a. Bathing
    b. Using a telephone
    c. Dressing
    d. Ambulating
    e. Preparing food
    f. Using a toilet

19. What **best** describes the purpose of a vocational assessment for a patient in rehabilitation?
    a. Assist the patient to find meaningful training, education, or employment after discharge from a rehabilitation setting.
    b. Evaluate and retrain patients with deficits that distort consonant and vowel sound production.
    c. Identify resources to assist with patient injuries that cause deficits in cognition.
    d. Demonstrate improvements in physical, social, cognitive, and emotional functions.

20. The nurse reviews with a patient the results of manual muscle testing performed by physical therapy. What ability of the patient does this procedure determine?
    a. Body flexibility and muscle strength
    b. Range of motion and resistance against gravity
    c. Muscle strength and amount of pain on movement
    d. Voluntary versus involuntary muscle movement

21. While performing a psychosocial assessment on a patient newly admitted to the rehabilitation unit, the nurse discovers that the patient's only support system is a married son who lives 2,500 miles away. Which **priority** complication must the nurse monitor for?
    a. Anxiety
    b. Fear
    c. Depression
    d. Panic

22. When assisting a patient with hemiplegia to dress, what does the nurse instruct the patient to do when putting on his shirt?
    a. Put on a shirt by first placing the affected arm in the sleeve, followed by the unaffected arm.
    b. Put on a shirt by first placing the unaffected arm in the sleeve, followed by the affected arm.
    c. Button the buttons; then slide the shirt over the head and put on both sleeves.
    d. Use the strong arm to lift the shirt over both arms and then pull the shirt over the head.

23. Which assistive device would the nurse recommend for a rehabilitation patient who can no longer tie shoes?
    a. Hook-and-loop fastener
    b. Long-handled reacher
    c. Velcro shoe closer
    d. Extended shoehorn

24. A patient with impaired physical mobility must be monitored for which early potential complication?
    a. Pressure ulcers
    b. Renal calculi
    c. Osteoporosis
    d. Fractures

25. Which practices are followed by and taught to staff for safe patient handling and mobility (SPHM)?
    a. Maintain a narrow, stable base with your feet.
    b. Put the bed at the correct height, hip level while providing direct care and waist level when moving patients.
    c. Keep the patient or work directly in front of you to prevent your spine from rotating.
    d. Keep the patient about 2 to 3 feet from your body to prevent reaching.

26. The nurse's facility follows a no-lift or limited-lift policy to prevent musculoskeletal injury to staff. Which methods for patient transfer can the nurse use? **Select all that apply.**
    a. Independent movement of the patient when he or she is able
    b. Mechanical full-body lift that is either ceiling- or wall-mounted or portable
    c. Following facility guidelines for safe patient transfer
    d. No transfers for patients who are unable to move independently
    e. Multiple staff assistance when physically lifting a patient
    f. Use of electric-powered, portable sit-to-stand devices

27. Which methods to prevent pressure ulcers resulting from immobility are best to teach patients and their significant others? **Select all that apply.**
    a. Change position often to relieve pressure on all bony prominences.
    b. Maintain good skin care by keeping the skin clean and dry.
    c. Inspect the skin at least once a day for problems such as reddened areas that do not fade readily.
    d. Use pressure-relieving devices as a substitute for changing position.
    e. Eat foods high in protein, carbohydrates, and vitamins for sufficient nutrition.
    f. Massage reddened areas to facilitate bloodflow with oxygen and nutrient delivery.

28. Which assistive-adaptive device would be recommended for a patient with a weak hand grasp?
    a. Gel pad
    b. Foam buildups
    c. Hook-and-loop fastener straps
    d. Buttonhook

29. When teaching a patient with hemiplegia about energy conservation techniques, which method does the nurse include?
    a. Using a walker instead of a cane
    b. Scheduling physical therapy immediately before eating
    c. Using a bedside commode to facilitate defecation
    d. Scheduling recreational activities in afternoon or evening

30. Which statement is true about the use of mechanical pressure-relieving devices?
    a. They effectively eliminate the need to turn patients.
    b. Patients still require regular repositioning.
    c. They prevent pressure ulcers in debilitated patients.
    d. They have been shown to be ineffective against pressure ulcers.

31. A patient has a lower motor neuron injury below T12. This injury results in which type of neurogenic bladder?
    a. Reflex or spastic
    b. Flaccid
    c. Uninhibited
    d. Inhibited

32. A patient with a flaccid bladder will have which urinary elimination problem?
    a. Incontinence and inability to empty the bladder completely
    b. Incontinence caused by inability to wait until on a commode or bedpan
    c. Urinary retention and dribbling because of overflow of urine
    d. Incontinence due to loss of sensation

33. Which statements are correct principles for performing an intermittent catheterization? **Select all that apply.**
    a. A catheter is inserted every few hours.
    b. It is usually performed after the Valsalva or Credé maneuver.
    c. A residual of less than 100-150 mL increases the interval between catheterizations.
    d. The maximum time interval between catheterizations is 4 hours.
    e. The patient uses sterile technique at home.
    f. A specialized appliance to help perform the procedure can be used at home when problems with manual dexterity occur.

34. Which medication would a patient with a mild overactive bladder **most likely** be given?
    a. Dantrolene sodium
    b. Bethanechol chloride
    c. Oxybutynin
    d. Trimethoprim

35. Which patient is **most likely** to have a flaccid bladder dysfunction?
    a. 28-year-old man with a crushed pelvis
    b. 54-year-old man with Guillain-Barré syndrome
    c. 18-year-old woman with a displaced cervical fracture
    d. 48-year-old woman who has multiple sclerosis

36. For which patient with constipation does the nurse avoid performing digital stimulation?
    a. Patient with myocardial infarction who is starting cardiac rehabilitation
    b. Patient with bowel incontinence resulting from cognition deficit
    c. Patient with a spinal cord injury resulting from a diving accident
    d. Patient with a spinal cord injury resulting from a motor vehicle accident

37. Which intervention would the nurse delegate to an unlicensed assistive personnel (UAP) when caring for a patient with an overactive bladder?
    a. Perform an intermittent catheterization every 4 hours.
    b. Toilet the patient every 2 hours during the day and every 3 to 4 hours at night.
    c. Assess the patient's bladder for fullness after each voiding.
    d. Perform a bladder scan at the bedside after each intermittent catheterization.

38. The older patient has a diagnosis of hypertension for which he is prescribed antihypertensive drugs. Before assisting this patient to rise from bed, which **priority** assessment should be completed by the nurse?
    a. Blood pressure in both arms
    b. Gait assessment
    c. Orthostatic vital signs
    d. Chest pain with activity

39. The unlicensed assistive personnel (UAP) is assisting a rehab patient with activities of daily living (ADLs) in the morning. What is the **priority** instruction the nurse should give the UAP?
    a. Encourage the patient to do as much self-care as possible.
    b. Bathe the patient but let the patient dress and feed himself.
    c. Let the patient inform you about the help he needs.
    d. Stress to the patient that his ADLs need to be completed as soon as possible.

40. In the long-term care setting, which are foci for the coordinated efforts of restorative nursing programs? **Select all that apply.**
    a. Dressing
    b. Passive range of motion
    c. Communication
    d. Nutrition
    e. Walking
    f. Bed mobility

41. Which assistive device is useful for a patient in rehabilitation who becomes easily fatigued while walking?
    a. Broad-based cane
    b. Walker with a seat
    c. Wheelchair
    d. Scooter

42. What is the **first** step to patient safety when providing gait training with assistive devices such as walkers and canes?
    a. Apply a transfer belt around the patient's waist.
    b. Guide the patient to a standing position.
    c. Ensure that the patient's body is well balanced.
    d. Instruct the patient to take small steps.

43. Which description characterizes the uninhibited bowel pattern dysfunction?
    a. Defecation occurring suddenly and without warning
    b. Defecation occurring infrequently and in small amounts
    c. Frequent defecation, urgency, and complaints of hard stool
    d. Intermittent constipation and diarrhea

Care of Patients at End-of-Life

1. Which patient has a disorder that would be considered among the **leading causes** of death in the United States?
   a. Has a history of alcohol abuse
   b. Has Alzheimer's disease
   c. Is positive for human immunodeficiency virus (HIV)
   d. Has pancreatitis

2. The terminally ill patient has an advance directive living will, which indicates that no heroic measures such as cardiopulmonary resuscitation (CPR) and intubation should be performed. She also has a do not resuscitate (DNR) order in her chart written by the health care provider. As the patient nears death, her daughter tells the nurse that she wants everything possible done to save her mother's life. What is the nurse's **best** action?
   a. Call a code and bring the crash cart to the patient's bedside.
   b. Inform the health care provider of this change in the plan of care.
   c. Respect the patient's wishes and ask the chaplain to stay with the daughter.
   d. Inform the daughter that further interventions are not warranted.

3. Which patient and family have the **best** understanding of home hospice?
   a. Family believes that the dying patient receives care at home if there are no funds for hospitalization.
   b. Family expects that the patient will resist hospice; therefore, an involuntary order is requested.
   c. The dying patient and family want to focus on facilitating quality of life.
   d. The patient and family expect an RN to provide around-the-clock nursing care.

4. The unlicensed assistive personnel (UAP) tells the nurse that the dying patient is manifesting a death rattle. Which action would the nurse perform?
   a. Instruct the UAP to initiate postmortem care.
   b. Notify the family that the patient has died.
   c. Turn the patient on the side to reduce gurgling.
   d. Tell the UAP that this is expected and nothing can be done.

5. To qualify for Medicare hospice benefits, a criterion for admission is that the patient's prognosis must be limited to what amount of time?
   a. 2 weeks or less
   b. 3 months or less
   c. 6 months or less
   d. 1 year or less

6. Under what circumstances should the nurse contact the patient's health care proxy?
   a. Patient has a sudden and unexpected episode of dizziness.
   b. Patient is discovered at 4:00 am in a comatose state.
   c. Patient refuses to eat unless he gets a beer with dinner.
   d. Patient needs catheterization for a urine specimen.

7. Which action is an example of active euthanasia for a dying patient?
   a. Discontinuing the mechanical ventilator
   b. Terminating the intravenous fluids
   c. Suspending telemetry heart monitoring
   d. Giving a large dose of intravenous morphine

8. The nurse is caring for a 92-year-old postsurgical patient who has a do-not-attempt-to-resusitate (DNAR) order. When the nurse assesses the patient, he is diaphoretic and hyperalert and reports mild left anterior chest pain with shortness of breath. What should the nurse do **first**?
   a. Sit with the patient, talk calmly, and be gently present.
   b. Administer oxygen and alert the Rapid Response Team.
   c. Notify the person who has durable power of attorney for health.
   d. Monitor for cardiac or respiratory arrest and call the family.

9. When the nurse assesses the dying patient, inadequate perfusion is suspected because the patient's lower extremities are cold, mottled, and cyanotic. Which intervention should the nurse perform?
   a. Place the lower extremities in a dependent position.
   b. Give warm oral or intravenous fluids.
   c. Cover the patient with a warm blanket.
   d. Gently rub the extremities to stimulate circulation.

10. Which patient statement **best** represents the symptom that is the **most** distressing and feared by terminally ill patients?
    a. "I get really nervous when I can't catch my breath."
    b. "My family will be so upset if I can't recognize them."
    c. "I'm hoping my doctor prescribes a lot of pain medication."
    d. "When I get nauseated, I won't be able to eat or drink."

11. The terminally ill patient is nearing death. His wife expresses concern that he has no appetite and eats very little. What is the nurse's **best** response to this concern?
    a. Teach the wife about risk of aspiration and explain that loss of appetite is normal when a patient nears death.
    b. Encourage the wife to feed the patient as much as he will take to maintain adequate nutrition.
    c. Request that the health care provider order a dietary nutrition consult to include foods that the patient prefers.
    d. Keep fluids and finger foods at the bedside for easy access whenever the patient is hungry or thirsty.

12. The terminally ill patient who is near death has loud, wet respirations that are disturbing to the family. Which interventions by the nurse are appropriate at this time? **Select all that apply.**
    a. Auscultate lung sounds and obtain an order for a chest x-ray.
    b. Place a small towel under the patient's mouth.
    c. Use oropharyngeal suctioning to remove the secretions.
    d. Administer an ordered anticholinergic drug to dry the secretions.
    e. Assist the patient to cough and deep-breathe to mobilize secretions.
    f. Reposition the patient onto one side to reduce gurgling.

13. Which intervention should be done when performing postmortem care?
    a. Place the head of the bed at 30 degrees.
    b. Remove pillows from under the head.
    c. Remove dentures and carefully clean and store them.
    d. Place pads under the hips and around the perineum.

14. A family member calls the nurse into the patient's room and says, "I think Mom just died." What should the nurse do **first**?
    a. Notify the nursing supervisor to have the body moved to the morgue.
    b. Ascertain that the patient does not rouse to verbal or tactile stimuli.
    c. Make sure that the health care provider has completed and signed the death certificate.
    d. Provide privacy for the family and significant others with the deceased.

15. A hospice patient is deteriorating and the family is concerned about his restlessness and agitation. Which intervention should the nurse perform?
    a. Notify the primary health care provider and request orders for transfer to the hospital.
    b. Assess for pain, provide analgesics, and make the patient as comfortable as possible.
    c. Initiate IV hydration to provide the patient with necessary fluids.
    d. Encourage the family to assist the patient to eat in order to gain energy.

16. The nurse is caring for a terminally ill cancer patient who is near death. The patient reports an uncomfortable feeling of breathlessness. Which therapy is the nurse **most likely** to administer?
    a. 5 mg of morphine sulfate
    b. 10 mg of furosemide
    c. 2 liters of oxygen per nasal cannula
    d. Albuterol via a metered-dose inhaler

17. The nurse is reviewing the dying patient's medication record and sees that one tablet of hyoscyamine 0.125 mg was administered 2 hours ago. Which assessment will the nurse perform in order to determine if the medication is effective?
    a. Assess for agitation and restlessness.
    b. Ask the patient if the nausea has decreased.
    c. Palpate the bladder to assess for urinary retention.
    d. Observe for oral secretions or wet-sounding respirations.

18. While caring for a patient of the Orthodox Jewish faith who is dying, what cultural concept should the nurse keep in mind?
    a. Traditionally, Jewish cultures are male-dominated.
    b. Expression of grief is open, especially among women.
    c. A person who is extremely ill and dying should not be left alone.
    d. Family members are likely to avoid visiting the terminally ill family member.

19. A dying patient is receiving morphine for severe pain. The health care provider informs the nurse that the patient is at risk for acute renal failure. What assessment will the nurse perform in order to determine if the kidney is failing to excrete the morphine metabolites?
    a. Assess the patient for adequate pain relief.
    b. Observe for signs of confusion or delirium.
    c. Auscultate the lungs for crackles or wheezes.
    d. Observe the color, clarity, and amount of urine.

20. The dying patient reports shortness of breath and has an oxygen saturation of 90%. He refuses oxygen therapy but requests that the nurse obtain a fan to increase the circulation of air. Based on the concept of comfort, what should the nurse do **first**?
    a. Explain that the use of a fan will not increase the oxygen saturation level.
    b. Try a nonpharmacologic intervention, such as position change or distraction.
    c. Call the health care provider and report the refusal of oxygen therapy.
    d. Offer morphine and advise the patient that a fan will be provided.

21. Which patient is a candidate for proportionate palliative sedation?
    a. Patient is having refractory symptoms of distress that are not responding to treatments.
    b. Patient is seeking options and alternatives to passive euthanasia.
    c. Patient is extremely anxious that pain and suffering will not be adequately addressed.
    d. Patient is convinced that established palliative protocols will hasten death.

8 CHAPTER

Principles of Emergency and Trauma Nursing

1. Which emergency department (ED) scenario represents a concern that has been addressed by the Core Measure Sets for the ED that are established by The Joint Commission?
   a. Patient lacks health insurance and has no steady source of income.
   b. Patient has waited 7 hours to be transferred to the medical-surgical unit.
   c. Patient with a history of falls sustains a fall in the ED waiting room.
   d. Patient has respiratory arrest and requires emergency intubation.

2. The emergency department (ED) nurse is preparing a **S**ituation, **B**ackground, **A**ssessment, **R**ecommendation (SBAR) report on a patient being admitted for bacterial meningitis. Which points are included in the ED nurse's report to the medical-surgical nurse? **Select all that apply.**
   a. "Patient reports severe headache with high fever that started 4 days ago."
   b. "Patient is currently alert and oriented × 2; speech clear but rambling."
   c. "Patient is very demanding and has used the call bell repeatedly since arriving in the ED."
   d. "IV normal saline into left anterior forearm; received first dose of IV ceftriaxone at 0700."
   e. "Lumbar puncture results are pending, but meningococcal meningitis is suspected."
   f. "Patient has male characteristics but prefers to be called Mrs. Jenny Jones."

3. The emergency department (ED) nurse is attempting to transfer a patient to the medical-surgical unit. When the receiving nurse answers the phone, he says, "You people always dump these admissions on us during shift change." Which response by the ED nurse represents the **best** attempt at respectful negotiation and collaboration?
   a. "I am sorry. I realize you are busy, but we are busy too."
   b. "I am also trying to finish handoff report. Should I call the supervisor?"
   c. "I apologize for the timing. How much time do you need for shift change?"
   d. "I apologize. We just received the bed assignment."

4. The nurse is interviewing a patient who has been verbally aggressive for the past several hours, according to the family. The family states, "He won't hurt anybody." However, the patient is pacing and appears suspicious and angry. Which strategy does the nurse use to conduct the interview?
   a. Sit at eye level with the patient in a quiet, secluded room.
   b. Conduct the interview standing near the door in a quiet room.
   c. Bring the entire family in and have everyone sit in comfortable chairs.
   d. Have the security guard stand by the patient during the interview.

5. The nurse is working alone in triage. It is a busy night and the waiting room is full of people who are restless and unhappy about having to wait. Which situation warrants the nurse to activate the panic button?
   a. The line for patients waiting to be triaged becomes overwhelmingly long.
   b. Emergency medical services calls en route with a patient in full arrest.
   c. Several patients in the waiting room start to complain very loudly.
   d. A person walks in and starts threatening the registration staff with a weapon.

6. The emergency department nurse is caring for a patient who was found in an alley with no identification and no known family. The nurse must give medication to the patient. What is the correct procedure for patient identification?
   a. Emergent conditions prevent identification, so the nurse gives the medication as ordered.
   b. The patient is designated as John Doe and the nurse uses two unique identifiers.
   c. The nurse validates the order with another nurse and both verify that the patient is unidentified.
   d. The nurse gives the medication and identification is made as soon as possible.

7. The nurse is using the SBAR method to give a handoff report to the nurse who will assume care of the patient. What would the nurse say **first**?
   a. "Mr. S. is very uncomfortable, and we should get him admitted as soon as possible."
   b. "Mr. S. has a history of high blood pressure but stopped taking medication 3 months ago."
   c. "Mr. S.'s vital signs are T 98.6°F, P 80/min, R 16/min, and BP 160/80."
   d. "Mr. S. is a 65-year-old male who came to the emergency department for a severe headache."

8. An older adult is in the emergency department (ED) for over 12 hours awaiting transfer to an inpatient bed. The charge nurse delegates turning the patient every 2 hours to the unlicensed assistive personnel (UAP) because the patient is at risk for skin breakdown. The patient is not turned and begins to develop a pressure ulcer. What does the charge nurse do to prevent a recurrence of this type of problem for future patients? **Select all that apply.**
   a. Nothing; in the overall priorities of the ED, the situation is unfortunate but unavoidable.
   b. Make anecdotal notes and counsel all the involved UAPs.
   c. Delegate the duty of turning and repositioning to the family members.
   d. File an incident report and seek assistance at the system level.
   e. Reeducate staff on the need to turn patients at risk for skin breakdown.
   f. Evaluate UAP-patient ratios when patients require frequent turning.

9. An older couple on vacation comes to the emergency department. The man is unable to speak clearly or coherently. His wife is very distraught and states, "He has many allergies and takes many medications, but I can't remember anything right now!" What should the nurse do **first** to quickly obtain drug and allergy information?
   a. Call the patient's family health care provider for a phone report about his drugs and allergies.
   b. Remind the wife to keep a list of the patient's drugs and allergies in her purse.
   c. Call the pharmacy where the patient obtains most of his medications.
   d. Check for a medical alert bracelet and help the wife to look in the patient's suitcase.

10. A patient is brought to the emergency department by friends, who report, "He probably overdosed on downers." The patient has a decreased level of consciousness and a decreased gag reflex; his face and chest are covered with emesis; he demonstrates spontaneous sonorous respirations; and pulse oximetry is 87% on room air. What type of airway management does the nurse expect this patient to receive?
    a. Supplemental oxygen per nasal cannula at 4-6 L/min
    b. Bag-valve-mask and 100% oxygen to assist with ventilatory effort
    c. Nonrebreather mask with high-flow oxygen
    d. Endotracheal intubation with initial high-concentration oxygen

11. The emergency department nurse is caring for several patients, all of whom are currently lying on stretchers awaiting discharge or transfer to a hospital bed. Which patients have the **greatest** risk for falls? **Select all that apply.**
    a. Patient with chronic pain who received 10 mg PO oxycodone for myalgia
    b. Opioid-naïve teenager with a fracture who received 3 mg IV morphine for pain
    c. Middle-aged woman with severe vomiting and frequent watery stools for 3 days
    d. Young child with a fever of 102°F, crying, with an ear infection
    e. Older adult patient with acute dementia secondary to infection
    f. Young woman with heavy vaginal bleeding secondary to a miscarriage

12. For which circumstance would the use of standard precautions be adequate to ensure the safety of the nurse, staff, and other patients?
    a. Performing hygienic care for a patient with copious watery diarrhea
    b. Assisting with intubation of a patient with symptoms of tuberculosis
    c. Initiating a peripheral intravenous access on a patient who is HIV positive
    d. Assessing a child with a fever and rash and known exposure to chickenpox

13. A patient is brought to the emergency department by the family because he has verbally threatened others and attempted to stab the neighbor's dog. What does the nurse do to ensure the safety of the patient and others? **Select all that apply.**
    a. Search the patient's belongings and secure personal effects.
    b. Instruct the patient's family to stay with him and call for help as necessary.
    c. Remove dangerous equipment from the room, such as sharps containers or portable instruments.
    d. Escort the patient to the waiting area, where he can readily be observed by the triage nurse.
    e. Use a metal detector to search for objects that could be used as weapons.
    f. Put the patient into 4-point restraint until a psychiatric consult can be obtained.

14. For which patients would the nurse try to obtain a social service consult? **Select all that apply.**
    a. Toddler who bumped her head on a table; observation for 24 hours is required
    b. Homeless woman who will be discharged with a splint to the lower leg and crutches
    c. Woman who was punched and beaten by her husband and sustained a broken jaw
    d. Man who drove himself to the hospital for a dressing change of an infected wound on his back
    e. Preteen admitted for vaginal bleeding and sexually transmitted infection
    f. Elderly man who lives alone and has no means to obtain medications from the pharmacy

15. Which function represents an appropriate referral to the emergency department (ED) case manager?
    a. Check with the admissions office to get a count of available intensive care beds.
    b. Contact the peripherally inserted central catheter (PICC) nurse, because the patient has bad veins.
    c. Investigate whether the patient is misusing and overusing ED services.
    d. Follow the patient into the community setting and evaluate the home environment.

16. Three people who accompanied a patient to the emergency department (ED) become verbally argumentative and physically threaten each other. Which actions does the ED nurse take to ensure the safety of staff and others? **Select all that apply.**
    a. Tell individuals that they are being filmed.
    b. Follow the hospital's security plan.
    c. Attempt to deescalate the situation.
    d. Quietly ask the individuals to leave.
    e. Identify potential escape routes.
    f. Obtain assistance from the security department as needed.

17. The nurse is evaluating the lower extremities of several patients. Which description represents the **least serious** physical presentation?
    a. Pain in calf; lower leg is swollen and red.
    b. Progressively increasing pain; distal portion is cool and bluish.
    c. Decreased sensation; lower leg has widespread brownish discoloration.
    d. Tight sensation in ankle; skin appears tight, shiny, and edematous.

18. A parent brings her 2-year-old child to the emergency department, stating, "She fell and bumped her head and forearm." Which behavior by the child causes the nurse the **least concern** during the initial triage interview?
    a. Crying and reaching for the parent as the nurse approaches.
    b. Alert and still, quietly watching as the nurse approaches.
    c. Asleep, limp, with even and unlabored respirations.
    d. Crying loudly and inconsolably since she was brought in.

19. The emergency department trauma team is preparing to receive a motor vehicle crash victim with severe chest trauma who is coughing up blood and has a crush injury to the right leg. What type of personal protective equipment (PPE) does the nurse who is assigned to do the recording put on?
    a. No PPE is necessary because the nurse is only recording and not giving direct care.
    b. Gloves only, but handwashing is required before and after all emergency care.
    c. Gown, gloves, eye protection, face mask, cap, and shoe covers.
    d. Patient situation must first be assessed before determining what PPE to wear.

20. The emergency health care provider is currently involved in the care of several critical patients. The emergency nurse must initiate care for patients under interdisciplinary and medical protocols. Which intervention is the **least likely** to be covered by a standing protocol?
    a. Give 50% dextrose IV push for low blood sugar.
    b. Initiate pulse oximetry monitoring and start oxygen therapy.
    c. Ventilate with bag-valve-mask at 100% oxygen and intubate.
    d. Start a peripheral IV with normal saline at 125 mL/hr.

21. Several patients have been waiting for more than 36 hours to be transferred to an inpatient room because the census is high during flu season. The emergency department staff is attempting to meet basic health needs in these circumstances. Which need is the **priority**?
    a. Helping the patients with hygiene
    b. Making sure that patients are fed
    c. Informing patients about admission status
    d. Ensuring safety of environment and care

22. Which patient should be triaged as emergent?
    a. 56-year-old man with severe unilateral back pain and previous history of kidney stones
    b. 23-year-old woman with severe abdominal pain, positive home pregnancy test, and BP 80/40 mm Hg
    c. 6-year-old with a temperature of 101°F and flulike symptoms
    d. 10-year-old girl with vomiting, diarrhea, and abdominal cramps onset 4 hours after eating fish

23. Which patient should be triaged as urgent?
    a. 44-year-old man with a dislocated elbow
    b. 35-year-old man with chest pain and diaphoresis
    c. 85-year-old man with new onset of confusion and BP grossly elevated compared to his usual
    d. 65-year-old woman with redness and swelling on the forearm associated with a bee sting

24. The nurse is trying to prepare an intravenous antibiotic medication for a patient, but the emergency department is very busy, chaotic, and noisy, and the nurse is continuously interrupted. What should the nurse do **first**?
    a. Ask the charge nurse to administer the antibiotic medication or send additional help.
    b. Prioritize the urgency of the medication in relation to the urgency of the interruptions.
    c. Shut the door and proceed through the six rights of medication administration.
    d. Prepare the medication while fielding the interruptions and delegating appropriately.

25. Because of the high risk for health care–acquired urinary tract infections, the nurse would question an order for a catheterized urine specimen for which patient?
    a. 78-year-old female transferred from a long-term care facility for dysuria
    b. 25-year-old female with back pain and hematuria, currently menstruating
    c. 3-year-old with severe dehydration after prolonged diarrhea and vomiting
    d. 43-year-old multiple trauma patient with signs of hypovolemic shock

26. The nurse has administered pain medication to a patient who has a migraine headache. What instructions should be given to unlicensed assistive personnel?
    a. Wait 45 minutes and then ask the patient if the pain is relieved.
    b. Help the patient out of bed, sit him up, then dangle his feet, then assist to stand.
    c. Check the patient frequently to make sure he arouses and is not getting worse.
    d. Ask the patient if he has a ride home; if not, call a family member to make arrangements.

27. Which intervention would be addressed during the primary survey?
    a. Insert a urinary catheter.
    b. Establish patent airway.
    c. Stabilize a fracture.
    d. Insert a nasogastric tube.

28. What is the **fastest** way for the nurse to estimate the systolic blood pressure in a patient with multiple injuries who has just been moved from the transport stretcher to the emergency department resuscitation stretcher?
    a. Palpate for presence of a radial pulse.
    b. Use the automated blood pressure cuff.
    c. Place the patient on a cardiac monitor.
    d. Check for the presence of capillary refill.

29. A patient comes to the emergency department after falling off a roof. He displays absent breath sounds over the left chest, severe respiratory distress, hypotension, jugular vein distention, and tracheal deviation to the right. Based on these assessment findings, for which condition does the nurse anticipate the patient must receive immediate treatment?
    a. Tension pneumothorax
    b. Cardiac arrest
    c. Airway obstruction
    d. Multiple fractured ribs

30. The nurse is helping the health care provider treat a patient with a tension pneumothorax. What type of equipment does the nurse obtain to immediately alleviate this life-threatening condition?
    a. Large adult endotracheal tube
    b. Transvenous pacemaker insertion
    c. Chest tube insertion tray
    d. Tracheostomy tray

31. The nurse's next-door neighbor has sustained a deep laceration to the right upper arm, and there is active bright-red bleeding. What does the nurse do to immediately control the bleeding? **Select all that apply.**
    a. Apply a tourniquet just above the laceration.
    b. Have the neighbor lie flat and elevate the arm.
    c. Apply direct pressure with a thick, dry towel.
    d. Apply sterile gauze and wrap with a gauze roller bandage.
    e. Flush the wound with tap water and apply a thick dressing.
    f. Have the neighbor sit down and splint arm in anatomical position.

32. For which patient is the forensic nurse examiner **most likely** to be consulted?
    a. Elderly patient who died under mysterious circumstances in the emergency department
    b. Prisoner who was injured by a police officer while resisting arrest
    c. Patient who was gang-raped by a group of football players
    d. Patient who accidently received a large dose of opioid medication

33. The nurse is caring for a patient with a head injury whose Glasgow Coma Scale score is 3. This score indicates the patient is **most likely** to do what?
    a. Withdraw from painful stimuli
    b. Open eyes spontaneously
    c. Moan with incoherent speech
    d. Present as totally unresponsive

34. The emergency department clinical nurse specialist (CNS) is designing ways to teach newly hired nurses about priority setting in the triage area. Which strategy is the CNS **most likely** to recommend?
    a. Assign new nurses to triage during low-volume periods.
    b. Pair a new nurse with an experienced nurse in the triage area.
    c. Prepare handouts and tip sheets for the principles of triage.
    d. Have the new nurses observe the triage process for several days.

35. A patient comes to the emergency department with severe respiratory distress. He has a long history of chronic respiratory disease and now requires endotracheal intubation. How does the nurse assess this patient's lung compliance?
    a. Auscultate the lung fields, especially for coarse crackles.
    b. Sense the degree of difficulty in ventilating with a bag-valve-mask.
    c. Monitor the pulse oximeter for decreasing saturation levels.
    d. Count the respiratory rate and observe the respiratory effort.

36. Each patient listed below has entered the emergency department's waiting area. **Place them in order of priority, with 1 being the highest priority and 4 being the lowest priority.**

    _____ a. 3-year-old child with inconsolable high-pitched cry, high fever, headache, and nuchal rigidity

    _____ b. 65-year-old man having diaphoresis with crushing left anterior chest pain

    _____ c. 32-year-old woman reporting upper abdominal pain and vomiting green bile emesis

    _____ d. 16-year-old boy with a broken arm from skateboarding and pulse and sensation intact

37. Based on the nurse's knowledge of normal versus abnormal findings related to age and acuity, which assessment finding is of **greatest** concern to the nurse?
    a. Mottling of extremities in a newborn
    b. Dry skin with tenting in a 72-year-old female
    c. Slow pulse rate in a 35-year-old athletic male
    d. Rapid, shallow respirations in a healthy 18-year-old

38. An elderly patient is brought to the emergency department by the paramedics. The patient is alert but disoriented, and the left lower leg has swelling and deformity; an air splint is in place. Which question is **most essential** to ask the paramedics?
    a. "How did the patient describe the level of his pain?"
    b. "Does the patient normally walk independently?"
    c. "What was the mechanism of injury?"
    d. "What time was the air splint applied?"

39. An older gentleman is brought to the emergency department by a neighbor who tells the nurse, "Mr. S. has been drinking heavily and seems depressed and is saying strange things." What is the **priority** question for the nurse to include in the assessment?
    a. "What makes you think that Mr. S. is depressed?"
    b. "Has Mr. S. expressed any thoughts about suicide or self-harm?"
    c. "How much alcohol has Mr. S. drunk in the past few days?"
    d. "Who would normally provide emotional support for Mr. S?"

40. A patient was involved in a high-speed motor vehicle accident. The health care provider instructs the nurse to prepare for several urgent procedures because of severe injury and physical compromise. Which procedure does the nurse prepare for **first**?
    a. Central line insertion
    b. Peritoneal lavage
    c. Chest tube insertion
    d. Endotracheal intubation

41. A patient sustained a closed tibia-fibula fracture after falling 50 feet while rock climbing. What is the **priority** order for the assessments and interventions that the emergency department nurse would perform for this patient? **Select in order of priority, with 1 being the highest priority.**

    _____ a. Evaluate the neuromuscular status of the left lower extremity.

    _____ b. Assess the head, chest, and abdomen for injuries.

    _____ c. Assess airway, breathing, and circulation.

    _____ d. Immobilize the injured extremity.

    _____ e. Monitor the degree of pain or discomfort.

42. Which factor is **most likely** to hinder the nurse's ability to objectively and accurately perform triage duties?
    a. Nurse has ambiguity about which triage model is the best for selected patients.
    b. Several patients arrive simultaneously at the triage area.
    c. Nurse is personally experiencing compassion fatigue and burnout.
    d. Patient has a complex health history and is a poor historian.

43. A patient comes to the emergency department for gastric distress, vomiting large amounts of dark-brown emesis, and passing small amounts of bright-red blood rectally. Which preexisting health condition is **most likely** to be a factor in determining triage classification?
    a. History of diabetes mellitus
    b. History of anticoagulant use
    c. History of high blood pressure
    d. History of recent alcohol intoxication

44. An elderly man is brought to the emergency department by his son. The patient is alert but is disoriented to person, place, and time and is unable to follow simple instructions. Which question is the **most important** to ask the son?
    a. "Do you think your father would consent to emergency care?"
    b. "Did you bring a list of your father's medications and allergies?"
    c. "When did you first notice your father's disorientation and confusion?"
    d. "Do you have the power of attorney for health for your father?"

45. A patient with a sprained ankle says, "I have been here for 4 hours, and other people who came after me have been taken back to see the doctor. My ankle hurts! Why am I being ignored?" What is the **best** response?
    a. "Sir, other patients have problems that are more serious than yours."
    b. "This is a system fault; if you would like to complain, I'll call a supervisor."
    c. "We have to attend to life-threatening or unstable conditions first."
    d. "Sir, I see that you are frustrated, but please sit down and wait your turn."

46. An experienced nurse is working in triage. For which circumstance is the nurse **most likely** to seek input from the emergency health care provider or advanced practice nurse about acuity level of the patient?
    a. A 65-year-old man is having severe left anterior chest pain and shortness of breath.
    b. A 35-year-old man with history of kidney stones has severe back pain and hematuria.
    c. A 1-year-old child with history of frequent ear infections is screaming and pulling at his ear.
    d. A 23-year-old female with previous good health has sudden, severe flulike symptoms.

47. Based on mechanism of injury, which patient is **most likely** to automatically require trauma team intervention?
    a. Stab wound to the leg
    b. Gunshot wound to the chest
    c. Possible drowning
    d. Unwitnessed cardiac arrest

48. The patient died in the emergency department despite resuscitation efforts. Homicide is suspected. Which nursing action would be incorrect because of the likelihood of forensic investigation?
    a. Invites the family to spend time with the deceased patient
    b. Gives the patient's clothes and other belongings to the family
    c. Declines to give information to friends of the deceased
    d. Leaves intravenous lines and indwelling tubes in place

49. The nurse sees that the emergency provider has written an order to discharge an elderly patient to go home. The patient cannot walk independently and has no relatives. What should the nurse do **first**?
    a. Talk to the provider about the patient's self-care abilities.
    b. Ask the patient if a friend could come to the hospital.
    c. Obtain a taxicab voucher for the patient.
    d. Consult social services for nursing home placement.

50. A patient died in the emergency department after sustaining multiple injuries that occurred during an aggravated assault. The family arrives after the patient is pronounced dead, and they ask to see the body. What does the nurse do?
    a. Explain that viewing the body would be too traumatic because all the tubes must remain in place for the forensic exam.
    b. Remove any tubes or debris that is near the patient's face and then cover the rest of the body with a blanket.
    c. Explain what they will see; dim the lights; leave the patient's face exposed; and cover the rest of the body with a blanket.
    d. Suggest that the family could spend time with their loved one at the mortuary after the medical examiner is finished.

51. The emergency health care provider and the nurse go together to tell the family that a patient died despite resuscitation efforts. What is the **best** way to inform the family?
    a. "We did everything that we could, but Mr. S. expired."
    b. "Mr. S. never woke up, but we are sure that he passed on without discomfort."
    c. "We are sorry to inform you that Mr. S. died due to extensive injuries."
    d. "We want to extend our sympathies because Mr. S. is not with us anymore."

52. Which action would typically be performed by the emergency department bereavement committee?
    a. Assigns a staff nurse to sit with the family during resuscitation efforts of patient
    b. Advocates that one or two family members be allowed at bedside during resuscitation
    c. Provides grief counseling and group support for nurses who care for patients who die
    d. Attends funerals, sends sympathy cards, and makes follow-up calls to family

53. The nurse observes that a homeless woman frequently comes to the emergency department during the winter for symptoms of dizziness and generalized pain. The patient typically stays for several hours, undergoes diagnostic testing, and is discharged with a referral to a primary care provider. What is the nurse's **best** action?
    a. Assess and treat the patient as if she were any other patient.
    b. Offer food and a blanket and encourage her to leave after she warms up.
    c. Develop an individual care plan using an interdisciplinary team approach.
    d. Talk to the patient and attempt to establish validity of symptoms.

54. The nurse is interviewing a homeless patient in the triage area. The patient says, "I'm a nurse too. Flying pictures say God is me. I'm a god, taking noise away." The patient then stands up and kicks over the garbage can. What should the nurse do **first**?
    a. Remain calm and slowly step away from the patient.
    b. Run toward the panic button and immediately push it.
    c. Gently take the patient's arm and lead her to a quiet space.
    d. Call for help and instruct bystanders to get out of the way.

55. The nurse is working at a level III trauma center. A patient involved in a chemical plant explosion arrives with burns, probable closed head injury, extremity fractures, and blunt trauma to the abdomen. What action is the nurse **most likely** to perform in the care of this patient?
    a. Preparing the patient for emergency surgery
    b. Débriding and cleansing the burned areas
    c. Initiating large-bore intravenous access for fluids
    d. Assisting with procedures to diagnose internal hemorrhage

56. The patient was repeatedly kicked and punched in the abdomen. The initial assessment and diagnostic testing reveal no life-threatening damage. The emergency provider tells the nurse that the patient should remain in the emergency department for observation. What is the **most important** action for the nurse to perform?
    a. Administer pain medication in a timely fashion.
    b. Initiate serial abdominal assessments.
    c. Delegate vital signs every 4 hours.
    d. Find a quiet space where the patient can rest.

57. The nurse is working in a large urban hospital. In what circumstance is the nurse **most likely** to refer to the emergency department's (ED's) automated electronic tracking system?
    a. Desires to know if a patient's computerized tomography scan is completed
    b. Is seeking a complete previous medical record for a patient
    c. Needs a medication for a patient that should be coming from the pharmacy
    d. Believes that a patient frequently visits the ED and requests prescriptions for opioids

58. An elderly woman is brought to the emergency department by her son, who tells the nurse," Mom just seems weak, tired, and more confused than usual." Which combination of question and assessment is the nurse **most likely** to perform for this patient?
    a. Ask if she has difficulty sleeping and observe for pedal edema.
    b. Inquire if she has any changes in urination and auscultate the lungs fields.
    c. Question her about appetite changes and check for pupillary response.
    d. Ask if she has noticed a vaginal discharge and observe gait and balance.

59. Which patient is **most likely** to require the skills that the nurse learned during Advanced Cardiac Life Support (ACLS) training?
    a. Patient who was just informed that he will be put on the heart transplant list
    b. Patient who has low oxygen saturation with a history of heart failure and fluid retention
    c. Patient who arrives unresponsive, secondary to unwitnessed cardiac arrest
    d. Patient who is pending transfer to the telemetry unit for atrial fibrillation

60. Which patients are **most likely** to undergo care via triage nurse–initiated protocols? **Select all that apply.**
    a. 36-year-old female with flulike symptoms that started two days ago
    b. 55-year-old male with left anterior chest pain that started after exercising
    c. 88-year-old male with sudden onset of confusion and shallow respirations
    d. 3-year-old female with an earache and a low-grade fever
    e. 45-year-old female with left-sided weakness, slurred speech, and drooling
    f. 18-year-old male with tenderness of testicles that started after sexual intercourse

9

CHAPTER

Care of Patients with Common Environmental Emergencies

1. Which patient has the **most** predisposing factors that are associated with heat-related illness?
   a. Obese older male who drinks beer in the afternoon at a baseball game
   b. Middle-aged female with hypothyroidism who lives in the southern United States
   c. Malnourished young female with an eating disorder who exercises in the morning
   d. Young female with iron-deficiency anemia who is in the first trimester of pregnancy

2. Which person is **best** demonstrating behaviors that would prevent heat-related illness?
   a. Sits in a shaded patio and drinks ice-cold beer and mixed alcohol drinks
   b. Plays touch football in the mid-afternoon wearing a hat and sunscreen
   c. Works in the garden in the morning and frequently rests and takes breaks
   d. Wears short pants and a sleeveless shirt while hiking on a hot day

3. An older patient reports being outside when temperatures reached 110°F (43.4°C) and forgetting to drink water. Now he reports weakness and nausea with dizziness. His body temperature is 98.9°F (37.2°C). What is the **priority** assessment?
   a. Assess for medications that increase risk for heat stroke.
   b. Check for orthostatic hypotension and tachycardia.
   c. Observe skin turgor and other signs of dehydration.
   d. Assess the size and responsiveness of the pupils.

4. The nurse is caring for a patient who was admitted for heat stroke. In reviewing the medication administration record, the nurse sees that the patient received a dose of intravenous benzodiazepine. Based on this information, which action is the nurse **most likely** to perform?
   a. Asks the patient about level of pain or discomfort
   b. Ensures that seizure precautions have been initiated
   c. Assesses the patient for cardiac dysrhythmia
   d. Auscultates the lung fields and assesses respiratory effort

5. During a summer marathon, the temperature is over 100°F (37.8°C) and the humidity is high. Suddenly a runner collapses after running in the race for 1 hour. The runner's body temperature is 105.2°F (40.7°C), and she is confused and sweating. What evidence-based intervention should be used for this patient?
   a. Give oxygen and start several IV lines with normal saline.
   b. Initiate rapid cooling using on-site cold-water immersion.
   c. Have patient rest in a cool environment and drink cold water.
   d. Place in a supine position and call 911.

6. The nurse is participating in a local community sports day. The day is hot and humid, and older adults are walking around. Prevention of heat-related injuries would include which intervention?
   a. Encouraging participants to eat high-energy snacks, such as sports bars
   b. Advising that people with disabilities should not participate
   c. Setting up a shade tent with areas for rest and relaxed activity
   d. Limiting direct sun exposure to 2 hours during the hottest time of the day

7. The nurse is volunteering at the first-aid station at a local community fair. The weather is predicted to be hot and humid. In planning care for people who may experience heat-related illness in this setting, what equipment should the nurse obtain?
   a. Supply of salt tablets and bottles of water
   b. Bags of IV normal saline and IV insertion equipment
   c. Several water spray bottles and a portable fan
   d. Supply of educational pamphlets and sunscreen samples

8. It is the middle of summer, and the weather has been hot and humid for several weeks. Which patient has the **highest** risk for severe heat-related illness?
   a. Young child who is participating in an organized team sport
   b. Well-conditioned athlete who is participating in a marathon
   c. Experienced construction worker who is working on an outdoor structure
   d. Older adult who lives alone and uses a fan during hot weather

9. The nurse has received report on several patients who were seen and treated for heat-related illnesses. The patient who has the **most severe** case of heat-related illness exhibits which signs/symptoms?
   a. Headache, heavy perspiration, temperature of 101°F (38.3°C)
   b. Subjective feeling of illness with nausea and vomiting
   c. Significant sunburn to extremities, face, and neck; temperature of 102°F (38.8°C)
   d. Hot and dry skin, alert, oriented to person, with pulse of 120/min

10. A homeless man is found lying in a vacant lot in the middle of July. He is lethargic and confused, and he has sustained severe sunburns on the exposed areas of his skin. His core temperature is 106°F (41.1°C). Which laboratory test can be used to predict severity and organ damage?
    a. Cardiac troponin I
    b. Creatine kinase
    c. Clotting studies
    d. Complete blood count

11. A young migrant worker has been living in a garden shed for several months. He is brought to the emergency department (ED) and is alert and conversant but appears fearful and confused. His skin is hot and dry, and his lips are cracked and bleeding. His skin turgor is poor, and he is malnourished. His blood pressure is 96/60 mm Hg, pulse is 130, respirations are 30, and temperature is 105°F (40.5°C). In addition to high-flow oxygen, what does the nurse anticipate the ED health care provider will initially order?
    a. IV normal saline and an indwelling urinary catheter
    b. IV Ringer's lactate and a nasogastric tube
    c. IV 5% dextrose and acetaminophen
    d. IV 45% saline and chlorpromazine

12. An older adult man comes to the emergency department for a snakebite. Which assessment finding suggests the **highest** risk for envenomation?
    a. Fang marks with local pain and swelling
    b. Progressive swelling with nausea and vomiting
    c. Localized swelling, with no systemic reactions
    d. Marked swelling and manifestations of coagulopathy

13. A patient sustained a bite from a pit viper and is admitted for observation. Which potential complications does the nurse observe for? **Select all that apply.**
    a. Hemorrhagic bullae
    b. Tingling of scalp, lips, or face
    c. Hypertension
    d. Excessive salivation with drooling
    e. Clotting abnormalities
    f. Seizures

14. The nurse is participating in a summer hike with a group of children. Suddenly the children start screaming, "Snake! Snake!" One little girl is sitting in a tall grassy area, clutching her ankle and crying. What is the **priority** in the field care of this child?
    a. Remove any constricting clothing from the child's leg.
    b. Maintain the child's extremity below the level of the heart.
    c. Move children to a safe area and encourage the child to rest.
    d. Keep the child warm and provide calm reassurance.

15. The nurse is on a backpacking trip. One of the hikers sustains a pit viper bite to the lower leg. Which first-aid measure will the nurse perform while waiting for transportation to the hospital?
    a. Elevate the leg and apply cool packs.
    b. Incise the fang marks with a pocket knife.
    c. Immobilize the leg with a splint in a functional position.
    d. Apply a constricting band proximal to the fang marks.

16. A patient arrives in the emergency department after sustaining a cottonmouth snakebite. What is included in the immediate interventions for this patient?
    a. Assessing for cranial nerve deficits
    b. Applying a pressure bandage
    c. Monitoring blood pressure and cardiac function
    d. Administering packed red blood cells

17. A patient is admitted for a brown recluse spider bite. The nurse observes that the patient has hemorrhagic complications of hematuria, hemoptysis, petechiae, and extensive bruising. These clinical observations indicate to the nurse that the patient may be experiencing which complication associated with the bite?
    a. Disseminated intravascular coagulation
    b. Agranulocytosis
    c. Thrombocytopenia
    d. Aplastic anemia

18. A patient sustained a coral snakebite and developed severe complications. Which diagnostic test results will reveal the physiologic damage that occurs with envenomation?
    a. Complete blood count
    b. Coagulation profile
    c. Creatine kinase
    d. Electrolytes

19. The nurse is assisting a neighbor with a gardening project. The neighbor sustains a snakebite when reaching to move a rock. What is the **best** action to perform to identify the snake?
    a. Crush the body of the snake with a rock but preserve the head.
    b. Note the markings of the snake and seek pictures on the Internet.
    c. Stand at a distance and take a digital picture of the snake.
    d. Trap the snake using a long garden tool and bucket.

20. A patient sustained a coral snakebite and calls the emergency department for instructions. Besides calling for an ambulance, what does the nurse instruct the patient to do?
    a. Apply an ice pack to the wound and refresh every 20 minutes.
    b. Incise the wound to allow the blood to flow freely and then apply sterile dressing.
    c. Snugly wrap with an elastic bandage, check arterial pulse, and apply a splint.
    d. Place a tourniquet that is tight enough to reduce arterial flow of the venom.

21. A patient calls the emergency department for advice on immediate first aid for a brown recluse spider bite on his hand. He denies allergic response or shortness of breath and states that he plans to see his health care provider but is currently about 2 to 3 hours away. What does the nurse advise the patient to do?
    a. Apply a warm pack and elevate the extremity.
    b. Scrub the bite area several times with soap and water.
    c. Apply cold compresses and rest as much as possible.
    d. Apply a snug constricting band at the wrist level.

22. A patient sustained a brown recluse bite and has been admitted for IV antibiotics and wound management. Which laboratory value indicates that the patient may be developing severe systemic complications from the bite?
    a. Increased red blood count
    b. Increased glucose level
    c. Decreased platelet count
    d. Decreased blood urea nitrogen

23. A patient was bitten by a brown recluse spider 4 days ago. The nurse observes prolonged bleeding after venipunctures and notes that the patient has a low platelet count. What do these findings indicate?
    a. Thrombocytopenia
    b. Hemolytic anemia
    c. Aplastic anemia
    d. Agranulocytosis

24. Which complications are related to a black widow spider bite? **Select all that apply.**
    a. Muscle rigidity and spasms of large muscles
    b. Severe tinnitus
    c. Severe abdominal pain
    d. Latrodectism
    e. Hypertension
    f. Seizures

25. The nurse is assessing a patient who reports being bitten by a black widow spider. The patient may have clinical signs and symptoms that mimic which disorder?
    a. Myocardial infarction
    b. Acute abdomen
    c. Acute renal failure
    d. Deep vein thrombosis

26. The nurse is caring for a patient who has been bitten by a black widow spider. Which vital sign change is cause for **greatest** concern?
    a. Patient appears anxious and is intermittently hyperventilating.
    b. Blood pressure (BP) is significantly higher than patient's typical BP.
    c. Temperature is elevated and patient shows signs of dehydration.
    d. Pulse is elevated and patient seems hypervigilant and nervous.

27. A patient reports a scorpion sting to the back of the hand. There is no obvious redness or inflammation at the suspected sting site. Which assessment technique does the nurse use to confirm a bark scorpion sting?
    a. Raise the arm and observe for blanching.
    b. Observe for the stinger embedded in the skin.
    c. Look for puncture marks surrounded by fine hairs.
    d. Gently tap at the suspected sting site to elicit pain.

28. A patient is being treated for a bark scorpion sting. He is currently alert but somewhat confused. He reports localized pain (7/10) at the site and requires frequent oral suction. Vital signs are temperature 102°F (38.8°C), pulse 95/min, respirations 12/min, and blood pressure 140/85 mm Hg. Which medication prescription does the nurse question?
    a. Acetaminophen 650 mg prn (as needed) for fever
    b. Tetanus toxoid 0.5 mL intramuscularly × 1 dose
    c. Morphine 20 mg intravenous push for severe pain
    d. Atropine 0.4 mg subcutaneously for hypersalivation

29. A person is stung by a wasp at a picnic. The person has no difficulty breathing and no history of allergic reaction to bee or wasp stings. What is the **priority** first-aid action for this person?
    a. Place a tourniquet proximal to the sting.
    b. Gently scrape the stinger off with the edge of a credit card.
    c. Apply a warm pack to the area and elevate.
    d. Observe the area for signs of inflammation prior to taking any action.

30. A teenager is brought to the emergency department with a reported bee sting. The nurse observes facial swelling, an audible wheeze, and labored rapid breathing. The teen's friend reports he has been vomiting and having trouble speaking and breathing. What does the nurse anticipate the **priority** medication order will be?
    a. IV normal saline bolus of 400 mL
    b. 50 mg diphenhydramine PO (by mouth)
    c. 0.5 mL of 1:1000 epinephrine IV
    d. 100 mg methylprednisolone sodium succinate IV infusion

31. The health care provider orders IV infusion of epinephrine for an older adult patient for an allergic reaction to a bee sting. In conjunction with the epinephrine administration, which action does the nurse take?
    a. Places the patient on a cardiac monitor
    b. Inserts an indwelling urinary catheter
    c. Obtains an order for an electrocardiogram
    d. Obtains an order for an arterial blood gas

32. The school nurse is preparing for a field trip to a farm with middle school–aged children. What instructions does the nurse provide to the children for bee and wasp sting prevention? **Select all that apply.**
    a. Place all jackets or sweaters in a pile on the ground.
    b. Try to outrun bees if attacked by a swarm.
    c. Keep garbage or leftover food in covered containers.
    d. Inspect clothes and shoes for insects before putting on.
    e. Do not swat at bees or wasps close to you.
    f. Do not place unprotected hands where the eyes cannot see.

33. A patient calls the health care provider's office asking for advice about whether to seek immediate medical attention for a bee sting. She has no shortness of breath or swelling to the face, throat, or lips. Which question will elicit information to assist the patient in making the decision?
    a. "Were you stung by an African 'killer bee'?"
    b. "Is the affected area red, painful, or swollen?"
    c. "Did you receive multiple stings?"
    d. "Were you able to remove the stinger?"

34. At a park, the nurse observes a mother of a toddler attempting to remove the stinger of a bee with tweezers. What should the nurse do?
    a. Instruct the mother to stop, because tweezing the stinger injects additional venom.
    b. Reinforce that removing the stinger with tweezers or by scraping is correct.
    c. Suggest applying an ice pack for local anesthesia before removing the stinger.
    d. Place a bandage over the stinger and suggest immediately going to the hospital.

35. A patient treated for a severe allergic reaction to a bee sting tells the nurse, "The doctor told me that I had to be careful about getting bee stings in the future because I could have another allergic reaction." Based on the patient's statement, what is the nurse's **first** action?
    a. Repeat the information that the health care provider gave her.
    b. Assess the patient's understanding of allergic reactions and first aid.
    c. Advise the patient to obtain a medical alert bracelet.
    d. Ensure that the patient has a prescription for an epinephrine autoinjector.

36. An anaphylactic reaction to a wasp or bee sting manifests as which conditions? **Select all that apply.**
    a. Hypertension
    b. Respiratory distress
    c. Hypoglycemia
    d. Laryngeal edema
    e. Deterioration in mental status
    f. Bronchospasm

37. Which patient would **best** benefit from always carrying an epinephrine autoinjector?
    a. Frequently works outside in the yard or tends to the garden
    b. Lives a long way from the nearest hospital or medical facility
    c. Had a previous severe allergic reaction to a wasp sting
    d. Has a history of severe pain with bee or wasp stings

38. A man who was stung by a wasp is treated and observed for several hours for symptoms of urticaria, pruritus, and swelling of the lips and then discharged home with medication instructions. Which medication is **most likely** to be prescribed to prevent delayed allergic effects?
    a. Epinephrine autoinjector
    b. Acetaminophen as needed
    c. Corticosteroids in tapered doses
    d. Albuterol

39. The nurse is instructing a patient who has a history of severe allergic reaction to bee stings on what to do if he experiences a bee sting in the future. What information does the nurse relay to the patient? **Select all that apply.**
    a. Wear a medical alert bracelet.
    b. Take an antihistamine before trying the EpiPen injection.
    c. Administer epinephrine immediately.
    d. Call 911 to be transported to a medical facility.
    e. Immediately apply a moist warm towel.
    f. Obtain a prescription for prophylactic corticosteroids.

40. A 37-year-old woman was stung by bees while gardening. Which factor is **most likely** to cause her to develop a systemic effect?
    a. Multiple bee stings
    b. Immediate local reaction
    c. Desensitization to the venom
    d. First time incident of bee sting

41. Which person has the **greatest** risk for injury from lightning strike?
    a. Jogger in the park at mid-morning in December
    b. Deer hunter walking through the woods in the evening in October
    c. Golfer out on the green in the late afternoon in June
    d. Camper walking on the beach during the early morning in April

42. Which lightning-strike victim should receive attention **first**?
    a. Teenager who is motionless except for shallow respirations; he has a weak pulse
    b. Middle-aged man, unconscious, with no palpable pulse
    c. Confused older adult woman with apparent paralysis in lower extremities
    d. Child crying, with bleeding from ears, mottled skin, and decreased pulses in left leg

43. A construction worker who was struck by lightning is brought to the emergency department (ED). He was found unconscious, but cardiopulmonary resuscitation was started immediately, and he awoke just before the arrival of emergency medical services personnel. In the ED, he is alert but confused and reports pain to his right hand and foot with fern-like marks. Which assessment tool is the **priority** for this patient?
    a. Glasgow Coma Scale
    b. Pulse oximeter
    c. Cardiac monitor
    d. Rule of nines chart

44. The nurse receives a phone call from a child who says, "Mommy was hit by lightning! She's outside. I'm afraid to touch her! I'll get shocked too!" How does the nurse advise the child?
    a. "There is no danger in touching your mom. You won't get hurt."
    b. "It will be okay, just quickly run outside and see if she is breathing."
    c. "Is there anybody at home with you? I need to speak to an adult."
    d. "You stay in the house, and someone will come to help very soon."

45. A patient was struck by lightning and sustained temporary paralysis of the lower limbs, which resolved with no physical effects, but the patient developed emotional problems. Which mental health disorder is the **most likely** complication?
    a. Generalized anxiety disorder
    b. Schizophrenia
    c. Posttraumatic stress disorder
    d. Acute-onset dementia

46. The nurse is caring for a patient who had cardiac and respiratory arrest after being struck by lightning. The patient was resuscitated, and he is now alert and appears to be progressing toward recovery. The nurse observes tea-colored urine in the urinary drainage bag. What does the nurse suspect?
    a. Chronic renal failure
    b. Dehydration
    c. Urinary tract infection
    d. Rhabdomyolysis

47. The nurse is advising a group of parents who are organizing a winter cross-country skiing trip. In assisting the parents to develop an appropriate winter clothing list, which articles should be taken on the trip? **Select all that apply.**
    a. Synthetic socks
    b. Cotton underwear
    c. Polyester fleece shirt
    d. Windproof outer jacket
    e. Hat made from waterproof, breathable fabric
    f. Sunglasses

48. The day camp nurse is with a group of children who have been participating in hiking, swimming, and crafts. The nurse sees a child who is soaking wet, stumbling, and taking off all her clothes. What does the nurse suspect is wrong with this child?
    a. Water snakebite
    b. High-altitude sickness
    c. Hypothermia
    d. Nearly drowned

49. The nurse is conducting a community presentation on cold weather safety. Which point is the nurse sure to include in the presentation?
    a. Hydration and water intake are not an issue, so pack extra clothes, not extra water.
    b. Wear multiple layers of socks when participating in winter sports.
    c. When driving in cold winter weather, carry extra clothes, food, and fluids.
    d. Hypothermia occurs only in the winter months in the United States.

50. Which signs/symptoms indicate the **most severe** case of hypothermia? **Select all that apply.**
    a. Tachycardia
    b. Depressed respiratory rate
    c. Decreased pain response
    d. Acid-base imbalance
    e. Shivering
    f. Hyperemia and edema after rewarming

51. The nurse is caring for a patient who sustained severe frostbite to the lower leg. The patient reports increasing pain despite receiving analgesic medication 1 hour ago. What should the nurse do **first**?
    a. Ensure that the leg is elevated.
    b. Assess for pulses and muscle weakness.
    c. Obtain an order for additional pain medication.
    d. Ask the patient to wait and see if the medication will work.

52. Several people on a cross-country ski trip return to the ski lodge with mild hypothermia. Which items does the nurse offer or obtain for the hypothermia victims? **Select all that apply.**
    a. Synthetic-fiber hats
    b. Warm blankets
    c. Cups of hot coffee or tea
    d. Polyester fleece shirts
    e. Dry socks and gloves
    f. Electric space heaters

53. A patient arrives at the emergency department after a prolonged cold exposure. The staff avoids rough and vigorous movements during the transfer from stretcher to bed to prevent which complication?
    a. Ventricular fibrillation related to rough handling
    b. Third-degree heart block related to cold autotransfusion
    c. After-drop due to cold blood moving to the central circulation
    d. Pulmonary emboli related to dislodgment of a clot

54. The health care provider orders core warming methods for a conscious patient with moderate hypothermia. What equipment would the nurse obtain to provide this therapy?
    a. Three-way urinary catheter with warmed lavage fluid
    b. Axillary thermometer to monitor core temperature
    c. Bag-valve-mask with warmed humidified oxygen
    d. Several warm blankets and warming pads

55. A man is found lying in an alley in cold weather for an unknown length of time. His hands, toes, and face show evidence of frostbite; otherwise there are no obvious injuries. He is severely obtunded with a pulse of 43 beats/min, respirations of 9/min, and a core temperature of 90°F (32.2°C). What is this patient's **most immediate** physiologic risk?
    a. Acute respiratory distress syndrome
    b. Pulmonary edema
    c. Cardiac arrest
    d. Acute renal failure

56. The nurse has volunteered at a storm shelter to identify potential problems associated with cold-related injuries. Which conditions predispose people to a **greater** risk for cold injury? **Select all that apply.**
    a. Hypothyroidism
    b. Advanced age
    c. Crohn's disease
    d. Alcohol intoxication or substance abuse
    e. Malnutrition
    f. Cold water immersion

57. The nurse is working in a mountain clinic where there is a high incidence of cold-related injuries. Which signs/symptoms indicate the **most severe** case of frostbite?
    a. Large fluid-filled blisters with partial-thickness skin necrosis
    b. Numbness, coldness, and bloodlessness of affected area
    c. Small blisters that contain dark fluid; skin is cool
    d. Pain, numbness, and pallor of the affected area

58. Which measures are correct when rewarming a victim of deep frostbite? **Select all that apply.**
    a. Briskly rub the area to speed the warming process.
    b. Use rapid rewarming in a 104°F-108°F (40°C-42°C) water bath.
    c. Apply a heating pad and adjust temperature to the lowest setting.
    d. Elevate the extremity above the heart level after rewarming.
    e. Administer an opioid analgesic for pain associated with rewarming.
    f. Administer tetanus immunization for prophylaxis.

59. The nurse is conducting a class about cold-weather hiking. What are the **early** signs of frostbite, which hiking partners should frequently observe for?
    a. White, waxy, or pale gray appearance to ears, nose, and cheeks
    b. Edema and redness over the exposed skin
    c. Mottled discoloration of the lower extremities
    d. Small blisters that contain clear fluid and areas that do not blanch

60. The emergency department nurse receives a phone call from someone stating that he and his friend have been out in the cold weather and his friend's fingers of the right hand appear white and waxy. What does the nurse direct the caller to do?
    a. Seek shelter immediately and massage and briskly rub the fingers.
    b. Seek shelter immediately and place the hands under the armpits.
    c. Seek medical attention and place hands on car heating vents while en route.
    d. Seek medical attention and place fingers in cool water while en route.

61. A patient has sustained severe frostbite to the toes and lower legs. He received rewarming therapy in the emergency department and arrives to the medical-surgical unit with a splint on both legs. IV normal saline is infusing at 125 mL/hr. He reports severe pain in the lower extremities. Which health care provider order does the nurse question?
    a. Give morphine 1-2 mg IV push prn for pain in extremities.
    b. Elevate bilateral lower extremities above the level of the heart.
    c. Perform neurologic and circulation checks on bilateral lower extremities every hour.
    d. Apply compression bandage to bilateral lower extremities.

62. The nurse is reviewing the complete blood count (CBC) results for a patient who lives in a high mountain town. The patient's red blood cell count (RBC) is 6.8 million/mm^3. What does this lab value combined with the patient's environment indicate?
    a. Anemia related to a decreased production of erythropoietin
    b. Polycythemia related to chronic hypoxia
    c. Pernicious anemia related to a regional dietary deficiency
    d. Hemolytic anemia related to cold temperature

63. A patient reports having a throbbing headache with nausea and vomiting "like the worst hangover of my life" after recently returning from a hiking trip to the mountains. The nurse suspects high-altitude sickness. Which question helps the nurse gather relevant information about this condition?
    a. "Did you experience any episodes of hypothermia during your trip?"
    b. "How quickly did you ascend to the top of the mountain range?"
    c. "Did you go skiing or hiking in a nearby area?"
    d. "Did you have trouble sleeping while you were in the mountains?"

64. A patient is admitted to the emergency department for high-altitude sickness. In the morning, he appears apathetic and declines to perform basic activities of daily living (ADLs). Later in the shift, the patient is unable to move himself in bed or to independently sit upright. What condition does the nurse suspect?
    a. High-altitude cerebral edema
    b. Severe hypoxemia
    c. Acute mountain sickness
    d. Severe hypothermia

65. What are the **most common** signs/symptoms of high-altitude pulmonary edema? **Select all that apply.**
    a. Tachypnea at rest
    b. Persistent dry cough
    c. Abdominal pain and cramping
    d. Waxy appearance of ears, cheeks, and nose
    e. Cyanotic lips and nail beds
    f. Bradycardia at rest

66. A Foreign Service employee normally lives in a coastal area, but he must take an emergency trip to a high-mountain area. He asks the nurse what he can do if acute mountain sickness occurs when he is at a high altitude. What is the **best** advice?
    a. Rest as much as possible.
    b. If available, administer oxygen.
    c. Take the oral form of furosemide.
    d. Descend to a lower altitude.

67. Which occurrence in the patient treated for acute mountain sickness indicates that treatment with acetazolamide was effective?
    a. Decreased pulse rate and decreased urine output
    b. Increased urine output and increased respiratory rate
    c. Periodic respirations during sleep and decreased pulse
    d. Decreased sleep disturbance and decreased respiratory rate

68. A rescue team is attempting to take the patient to the hospital for symptoms of high-altitude pulmonary edema. The descent to the hospital is delayed due to severe weather conditions. What is the **most important** treatment for this patient during the delay?
    a. Dexamethasone
    b. Furosemide
    c. Oxygen administration
    d. Keep patient as warm as possible

69. Two teenagers bring their friend to the emergency department because "he was drowning." The patient is unconscious but breathing spontaneously, and he is immediately taken to the resuscitation area. Which question is **most important** for the nurse to ask the patient's friends in determining the outcomes for the patient?
    a. "Was this a freshwater or saltwater drowning?"
    b. "Does he have any medical conditions, such as seizures?"
    c. "Was the water contaminated with chemicals or algae?"
    d. "How long was he under the water and not breathing?"

70. What responses does the "diving reflex" cause in the body? **Select all that apply.**
    a. Tachypnea
    b. Metabolic alkalosis
    c. Bradycardia
    d. Decreased cardiac output
    e. Vasoconstriction of vessels in the intestines and kidneys
    f. Increased blood flow into peripheral circulation

71. Several people are looking out across a lake and pointing to a swimmer in the distance who appears to be struggling to stay afloat. What is the correct sequence of emergency steps to take? **Select in order of priority.**

    _____ a. Handle gently to prevent ventricular fibrillation.

    _____ b. Safely rescue the victim.

    _____ c. Begin delivering rescue breaths as soon as possible.

    _____ d. Assess neurologic status.

    _____ e. Assess airway patency.

72. The pathophysiology of drowning involves a washing out of surfactant, which leads to decreased surface tension, increased lung compliance, and increased airway resistance. What disorder is a result of the pathophysiology?
    a. Pulmonary emboli
    b. Pulmonary edema
    c. Chemical pneumonitis
    d. Aspiration pneumonia

73. A college student was drinking beer and dove from a 20-foot ledge into a lake. He was pulled from the lake by a friend and given mouth-to-mouth. The patient is currently in the emergency department, awake, and receiving supplemental oxygen. What type of serial assessment is the nurse **most likely** to initiate for this patient?
    a. Cardiac monitoring for possible myocardial infarction
    b. Level of consciousness and orientation to monitor for alcohol intoxication
    c. Peripheral sensation and movement related to spinal cord injury
    d. Frequent blood glucose checks to monitor for hypoglycemia

74. The emergency department health care team is administering emergency treatment to a drowning victim. Which task can be delegated to unlicensed assistive personnel?
    a. Insert the nasogastric tube.
    b. Advise the family about the patient's status.
    c. Take and report vital signs every 15 minutes.
    d. Assist with the bag-valve-mask during intubation.

75. Which combination of factors is likely to contribute to the **highest** survival rate for drowning victims who are immediately transported to the emergency department for care?
    a. In very cold fresh water for 7 minutes; arrives in ED with pulse of 40
    b. In warm salt water for 12 minutes; arrives in ED with pulse of 150
    c. In very cold salt water for 10 minutes; arrives in ED with no pulse
    d. In warm contaminated water for 6 minutes; arrives in ED with no pulse

76. The nurse is teaching a class on water safety to a group of 5-year-old children. Which point is the nurse **most likely** to emphasize with this group?
    a. Take swimming lessons and learn how to use floatation devices.
    b. Never swim alone; a parent or other adult should always be with you.
    c. Always test the water depth before jumping in head-first.
    d. If your friends don't know how to swim, always watch out for them.

77. What might the nurse notice if the patient has impaired thermoregulation as a result of a cold-related injury? **Select all that apply.**
    a. Hyperemia and edema of fingers or toes
    b. Shivering
    c. Possible atrial fibrillation
    d. Numbness and pain of nose or ears
    e. Profuse diaphoresis
    f. Headache, weakness, nausea, and/or vomiting

78. What should the nurse interpret for the patient with impaired thermoregulation as a result of a cold-related injury? **Select all that apply.**
    a. Temperature
    b. Cardiac assessment
    c. Neurologic assessment
    d. Gastrointestinal assessment
    e. Fluid status
    f. Skin integrity

79. How should the nurse respond to the patient with impaired thermoregulation as a result of a cold-related injury? **Select all that apply.**
    a. Thaw frozen body parts in a warm-water bath and handle gently.
    b. Provide pain control measures.
    c. Advocate for increased drug doses as a result of lowered metabolism.
    d. Administer tetanus prophylaxis and possible antibiotics for open wounds.
    e. Initiate passive external rewarming by covering with blankets.
    f. Prepare patient for possible amputation of frostbitten body part.

80. What should the nurse do in caring for the patient with impaired thermoregulation as a result of a cold-related injury? **Select all that apply.**
    a. Monitor the patient's response to pain medication and rewarming techniques.
    b. Monitor for further injury from rewarming techniques.
    c. Monitor for signs and symptoms of pulmonary edema.
    d. Evaluate the patient and family's knowledge about the injury and treatment plans.
    e. Educate the patient and family on ways to prevent future cold-related injury.
    f. Monitor for signs of high altitude cerebral edema.

10
CHAPTER

Principles of Emergency and Disaster Preparedness

1. For which event would a large urban hospital's emergency management plan typically be activated?
   a. Three-car collision on the freeway
   b. Fight between two local street gangs
   c. School bus involved in an accident
   d. Explosion at a chemical factory

2. Which event would be considered an internal disaster?
   a. A fire in a long-term care facility
   b. Gunfire in the hospital parking lot
   c. A tornado devastates the community
   d. Several people dying from flulike symptoms

3. Which priority intervention would be **more likely** to occur during an internal disaster compared to an external disaster?
   a. Extra staff would be called in to assist.
   b. Emergency management plan would be activated.
   c. Patients and staff would be evacuated.
   d. Staff would don personal protective equipment.

4. A nurse working at a small rural hospital gets a frantic phone call about a rumor of a student attacking other students at a local high school. Which information is the **most important** to determine potential for a multicasualty event versus a mass casualty event?
   a. "How long ago did the event occur?"
   b. "What are the number and severity of the injuries?"
   c. "What are school officials saying about the incident?"
   d. "Have emergency medical services been notified?"

5. The hospital in a small mountain town is updating its emergency management plan to incorporate the "all hazards approach" and to address all credible threats to the area. Which disaster events are the likely priorities in this community's emergency management plan? **Select all that apply.**
   a. Avalanches
   b. Floods
   c. "Active shooter"
   d. Car accidents
   e. Tornados
   f. Pandemic influenza

6. The hospital committee is reviewing the emergency management plan of their small community hospital in a suburban area of a large city. What is a priority to include in **this hospital's** emergency management plan?
   a. Plan for evacuation routes out of the city
   b. Plan for transporting patients to other hospitals
   c. Method to contact the National Disaster Medical System
   d. Stockpiling postexposure prophylactic antibiotics

7. The hospital staff is participating in a disaster drill, and the nurse is assigned to organize personnel who are called in from home. Which task would be appropriate to delegate to unlicensed assistive personnel who usually work in the labor and delivery area?
   a. Stay with "black tag" patients in the holding area.
   b. Talk to the families of the "red tag" patients.
   c. Care for and support the "green tag" patients.
   d. Obtain vital signs of the "yellow tag" patients.

8. A nurse based in Iowa is a volunteer member of the Medical Reserve Corps and has been called to serve in Ohio, where he does not hold an active nursing license. What should the nurse do?
   a. Determine if Ohio has reciprocity with Iowa before accepting deployment.
   b. Decline deployment because his nursing license will not allow him to practice in Ohio.
   c. Prepare for deployment because he will be considered a federal employee with valid licensure.
   d. Delay deployment until he has reviewed the nurse practice act that is specific to Ohio.

9. The nursing director of a long-term care facility is designated as the "incident commander" for the facility's emergency management plan. What is the **priority** action for the incident commander?
   a. Call all the off-duty staff and ask them to come into work.
   b. Take inventory of supplies according to the emergency management plan.
   c. Activate the disaster management process according to the plan.
   d. Call the National Guard to move all patients to other facilities.

10. The nurse is assigned to assist the hospital incident commander during a disaster drill. Which responsibility is appropriate for the nurse in this capacity?
    a. Call all nursing units to determine the number of patients who could potentially be discharged.
    b. Call the physical therapy department and direct therapists to assist in the operating room or the intensive care unit.
    c. Go to the emergency department and assist with the triage of disaster victims to appropriate clinical areas.
    d. Contact the security department and instruct them to control the number of people who attempt to enter the hospital.

11. The nurse serves on a committee that is tasked with developing tools and aids that the medical command physician could use during a disaster event. What is an appropriate project for this purpose?
    a. Make a current list, including contact information, of trauma and orthopedic surgeons.
    b. Make a telephone tree for contacting the nursing and ancillary staff.
    c. Design a triage algorithm that addresses different types of disaster events.
    d. Design an algorithm for contacting the Federal Emergency Management Agency.

12. At 3:00 am, the emergency department charge nurse of a large suburban hospital receives notification that a commercial plane has just crashed outside the city limits. What does the nurse do? **Select all that apply.**
    a. Collaborate with the medical command physician.
    b. Activate the hospital's emergency management plan.
    c. Initiate the staff telephone tree.
    d. Collaborate with the triage officer.
    e. Organize nursing and ancillary services.
    f. Alert the critical incident stress debriefing team.

13. A local news station calls the hospital seeking permission to verify the number of victims and details of a local disaster. What is the nurse's **best** response?
    a. "Please don't bother us now. We are trying to care for the victims."
    b. "We have a lot of stable victims and so far no one has died."
    c. "Please hold and I will connect you to the community relations officer."
    d. "I will connect you with the emergency command center."

14. The emergency management plan is activated because a major earthquake has caused many serious and minor injuries. Which nurse reassignment is **most likely** to meet the needs of the patients while best utilizing available personnel?
    a. Operating room nurse is reassigned to the emergency department to assist in triage.
    b. Emergency department nurse is reassigned to care for patients on the medical-surgical unit.
    c. Critical care nurse is reassigned to the emergency department to care for "black tag" patients.
    d. Performance improvement nurse is reassigned to care for "green tag" patients.

15. A city committee reviews possible scenarios related to a disaster event. Which is an example of the "greatest good for the greatest number of people"?
    a. The city's supply of antibiotics is sent to one hospital that has 25 victims with exposure to a bioterrorism agent.
    b. Twenty victims infected by a bioterrorism agent are placed on life support and mechanical ventilation.
    c. Thirty people with possible exposure to a bioterrorism agent are quarantined, including five children who are asymptomatic.
    d. Elderly community members are treated with prophylactic antibiotics for a bioterrorism agent.

16. The nurse is making a personal emergency preparedness plan. What is the nurse sure to include in the plan?
    a. Make a disaster supply kit with clothing and basic survival supplies.
    b. Resolve the ethical conflicts of family and professional obligations.
    c. Stockpile antibiotics, first-aid supplies, and resuscitation equipment.
    d. Teach family members about radiation and bioterrorism safety issues.

17. A patient comes to the emergency department (ED) worried that he has been exposed to an infectious bioterrorism agent that was sent to him through the mail. What is the **priority** action for the ED nurse to take?
    a. Escort the patient to a quarantined area.
    b. Take a history and assess for symptoms.
    c. Call local police and the Department of Public Health.
    d. Activate the emergency preparedness plan.

18. The nurse is assigned to assist the incident commander who is evaluating the feasibility of deactivating the emergency management plan. The commander directs the nurse to accomplish certain tasks. Which task is the **priority**?
    a. Contact all hospital departments and determine if needs have been met.
    b. Go to the emergency department and supervise inventory and restocking of supplies.
    c. Arrange for temporary sleeping quarters for exhausted staff members.
    d. Assist in the preparations of the critical incident stress debriefing.

19. A multiple-car accident with mass casualties has occurred near an urban hospital. The hospital's emergency preparedness plan is activated. For what purposes is the postplan administrative review conducted?
    a. To focus on the errors that were made and things that went wrong during the plan
    b. To identify employees who need financial assistance or reimbursement
    c. To establish a system of networking and support for the employees
    d. To provide all employees the opportunity to express positive and negative comments

20. To prevent the development of posttraumatic stress disorder (PTSD) in hospital staff, what action is likely to be taken by the facility?
    a. Conducting administrative debriefings
    b. Providing employees with information on PTSD
    c. Offering employees psychological counseling
    d. Conducting critical incident stress debriefings

21. To protect hospital staff from experiencing posttraumatic stress disorder, what are appropriate recommendations by the facility to its employees?
    a. Drink plenty of water and eat healthy snacks.
    b. Avoid putting emotional burden on your family.
    c. Seek counseling when stress becomes debilitating.
    d. Avoid coworkers who dwell on unpleasant details.

22. To promote effective coping for survivors of a mass-casualty event, the nurse uses which principles while interacting with patients in crisis? **Select all that apply.**
    a. Actively listening to feelings and expression of experiences
    b. Reassuring that everything will be okay and things will return to normal
    c. Encouraging exploration about why the event occurred and who caused it
    d. Helping to problem-solve
    e. Conveying caring behaviors
    f. Advocating resumption of daily routines as soon as possible

23. A gang-related incident has occurred involving major casualties from gunshot wounds to 11 victims. Which intervention would be included in the critical stress incident debriefing?
    a. Reviewing mistakes and recommending corrective actions to be taken.
    b. Identifying those who are experiencing posttraumatic stress disorder.
    c. Encouraging unconditional acceptance of all thoughts and feelings.
    d. Encouraging self-acceptance of blame and guilt for errors in judgment.

24. A community hospital is reviewing the activation and implementation of its emergency preparedness plan after a recent mass-casualty event. Which outcome statement reflects the goal of an administrative review?
    a. Emergency preparedness plan was activated in a timely fashion, but telephone tree was outdated and did not include new employees.
    b. Three hundred employees were offered a debriefing session, and two employees have symptoms of posttraumatic stress disorder.
    c. The mass-casualty event was handled well, and we expect to see positive reports in the media and to receive additional funding.
    d. The mass-casualty event resulted in an influx of 35 walking wounded, and 6 patients came via emergency medical transport.

25. After a major city-wide environmental crisis, which type of intervention is **most appropriate** for hospital staff?
    a. Administrative debriefing
    b. Critical incident stress debriefing
    c. Small discussion groups that include family
    d. Mandatory referrals for mental health counseling

26. Which nurse activity would **best** help the hospital to meet The Joint Commission's mandate for emergency preparedness?
    a. Assist in planning drills that include patient simulations.
    b. Help other nurses make a personal emergency preparedness plan.
    c. Attend training classes to learn how to handle hazardous materials.
    d. Identify the credible threats to the safety of the community.

27. The emergency department nurse is instructing a group of unlicensed assistive personnel on how to use personal protective equipment (PPE) when caring for patients who may have been exposed to bioterrorism agents. One of the group is clowning around and making jokes. What should the nurse do **first**?
    a. Suggest that he report to the supervisor if he doesn't settle down and pay attention.
    b. Ask him to demonstrate the use of PPE in the care of a patient with Ebola.
    c. Advise him that PPE is for his safety, but ignoring safety protocols is a personal choice.
    d. Ignore him and continue instructing because clowning around is a coping method for him.

28. A long-term care facility formed a committee to review the facility's emergency preparedness plan. Which element needs to be resolved in order to meet the guidelines of the Life Safety Code, which is published by the National Fire Protection Association?
    a. Fire extinguishers are heavy and difficult to use.
    b. Fire safety training is difficult because of high staff turnover.
    c. Building has one main front door, and side doors are sealed shut.
    d. Many residents are unwilling or incapable of participating in fire drills.

29. Using disaster triage principles, which patient has been correctly triaged and marked with the appropriate color tag?
    a. A toddler who has died of his injuries: green tag
    b. An older woman with a fractured ankle: yellow tag
    c. An older man with shortness of breath and a hemothorax: red tag
    d. A teenager with profuse bleeding from a severe arm laceration: black tag

30. A committee is reviewing the hospital's emergency management plan. In the event of a large-scale multi-casualty event, which group is likely to require the largest amount of physical space to accommodate the number of victims?
    a. Black-tagged patients
    b. Red-tagged patients
    c. Yellow-tagged patients
    d. Green-tagged patients

31. Which disaster situation is **most likely** to increase the complexity of managing the green-tagged patients who are more likely to self-transport from the scene of the incident to the health care facility?
    a. Collapse of a church roof during Sunday services
    b. Human stampede at a poorly controlled music festival
    c. Breach of containment at a nuclear plant
    d. Demonstration with rioting on a college campus

32. Which scenario is **most likely** to require activation of the emergency preparedness plan?
    a. A private six-passenger plane crashes at a large urban airport on Wednesday morning.
    b. There is an outbreak of foodborne illness at a long-term care center on Tuesday afternoon.
    c. An ice storm strikes a city on Monday morning and causes falls and vehicular accidents.
    d. A multi-car accident occurs in front of a small rural hospital after midnight on Sunday.

33. The triage method for multi-casualty or mass response utilizes what sorting methods? **Select all that apply.**
    a. Patients are alphabetized by name.
    b. Health care providers triage most critical patients.
    c. Patients are labeled by number.
    d. Patients are ranked by assessment scores.
    e. Patients are ranked using colored labels.
    f. Patients are categorized as John Does with unique identifiers.

34. The nurse is working in the emergency department (ED) where several local gang members are being treated for gunshot and knife wounds. The nurse hears gunshots in the waiting room, followed by screaming and cries for help. What does the nurse do **first**?
    a. Grab the resuscitation box and run to the waiting room.
    b. Assist all the ambulatory patients to leave through a back entrance.
    c. Alert the ED health care provider that additional trauma victims need care.
    d. Assess the level of threat to self and others and call for help.

35. Following a tornado disaster, a charge nurse is assigned to be the group co-leader of a critical incident stress debriefing session. During the session, a nurse says, "We weren't prepared for this! The administration at this hospital is a joke." What is the **best** response?
    a. "This session is not about pointing fingers or fixing blame."
    b. "Tell us about what you experienced while you were caring for victims."
    c. "Improving the emergency plan will be discussed at the administrative review."
    d. "We are all pretty stressed out. Let's take a deep breath and calm down."

36. Which action meets The Joint Commission's 2015 mandate for the hospital's emergency preparedness plan?
    a. All nursing staff are certified annually in basic and advanced cardiac life support.
    b. Plan is tested twice a year using simulated patients to assess collaboration and command.
    c. Stockpiles of equipment and supplies needed for a pandemic influenza outbreak are inventoried.
    d. Emergency department staff meets annually with administration to review plan and update as needed.

37. A nurse working on a medical-surgical unit is informed by the charge nurse that the emergency preparedness plan has been activated and a large number of injured patients are expected to arrive over the next few hours. Which question is the charge nurse **most likely** to ask?
    a. "Have you read the disaster plan, and do you know your role?"
    b. "Could you check the emergency equipment and see if everything works?"
    c. "Potentially, could any of your patients be immediately discharged?"
    d. "Would you be willing to care for patients in the hallway if there is no other option?"

38. The nurse is using the Impact of Event Scale-Revised (IES-R) to assess an unlicensed assistive personnel (UAP) who was working in a long-term care facility that was devastated by a fire. The IES-R score is high on all subscales. What should the nurse do?
    a. Reinforce the coping strategies that the UAP is successfully using.
    b. Suggest additional coping strategies that the UAP can use to decrease stress.
    c. Refer the UAP to a social worker or a support group for survivors.
    d. Refer the UAP to a psychiatrist or clinical psychologist for additional evaluation.

11 CHAPTER

Assessment and Care of Patients with Impaired Fluid and Electrolyte Balances

1. After a 5-km run on a hot summer day, a diaphoretic patient tells the volunteer nurse that she is very thirsty. What is the nurse's **best** action?
   a. Instruct the patient to sit down.
   b. Apply ice to the patient's axilla areas.
   c. Tell the patient to breathe slowly and deeply.
   d. Offer the patient bottled water to drink.

2. Which findings indicate that a patient may have hypervolemia? **Select all that apply.**
   a. Increased, bounding pulse
   b. Jugular venous distention
   c. Presence of crackles
   d. Excessive thirst
   e. Elevated blood pressure
   f. Orthostatic hypotension

3. What is the term for a difference in concentration of particles that is greater on one side of a permeable membrane than on the other side?
   a. Hydrostatic pressure
   b. Concentration gradient
   c. Passive transport
   d. Active transport

4. A patient's blood osmolarity is 302 mOsm/L. What manifestation does the nurse expect to see in the patient?
   a. Increased urine output
   b. Thirst
   c. Peripheral edema
   d. Nausea

5. An older adult patient at risk for fluid and electrolyte problems is carefully monitored by the nurse for the first indication of a fluid balance problem. What is this indication?
   a. Fever
   b. Elevated blood pressure
   c. Poor skin turgor
   d. Mental status changes

6. What are the consequences for a patient who does not meet the obligatory urine output? **Select all that apply.**
   a. Lethal electrolyte imbalances
   b. Alkalosis
   c. Urine becomes diluted
   d. Toxic buildup of nitrogen
   e. Urine output increases
   f. Acidosis

7. What is the minimum amount of urine output per day needed to excrete toxic waste products?
   a. 200 to 300 mL
   b. 400 to 600 mL
   c. 500 to 1000 mL
   d. 1000 to 1500 mL

8. Which patient is at risk for excess insensible water loss?
   a. Patient with continuous GI suctioning
   b. Patient with slow, deep respirations
   c. Patient receiving oxygen therapy
   d. Patient with hypothermia

9. Patients with which conditions are at greatest risk for deficient fluid volume? **Select all that apply.**
   a. Fever of 103°F (39.4°C)
   b. Extensive burns
   c. Thyroid crisis
   d. Water intoxication
   e. Continuous fistula drainage
   f. Diabetes insipidus

10. The nurse is working in a long-term care facility where there are numerous patients who are immobile and at risk for dehydration. Which task is **best** to delegate to the unlicensed assistive personnel (UAP)?
    a. Offer patients a choice of fluids every 1 hour.
    b. Check patients at the beginning of the shift to see who is thirsty.
    c. Give patients extra fluids around medication times.
    d. Evaluate oral intake and urinary output.

11. The nurse is caring for a postoperative surgical patient in the recovery room. What is the **main** reason for carefully monitoring the patient's urine output?
    a. Decreasing urine output indicates poor kidney function.
    b. Increasing urine output can indicate too much IV fluid during surgery.
    c. Decreasing urine output may mean hemorrhage and risk for shock.
    d. Increasing urine output may mean that kidney function is returning to normal.

12. Which factors affect the amount and distribution of body fluids? **Select all that apply.**
    a. Race
    b. Age
    c. Gender
    d. Height
    e. Body fat
    f. Weight

13. The nurse is caring for a patient with hypovolemia secondary to severe diarrhea and vomiting. In evaluating the respiratory system for this patient, what does the nurse expect to find on assessment?
    a. No changes, because the respiratory system is not involved
    b. Increased respiratory rate, because the body perceives hypovolemia as hypoxia
    c. Hypoventilation, because the respiratory system is trying to compensate for low pH
    d. Normal respiratory rate, but a decreased oxygen saturation

14. The nurse is assessing skin turgor in a 65-year-old patient. What is the correct technique to use with this patient?
    a. Observe the skin for a dry, scaly appearance and compare it to a previous assessment.
    b. Pinch the skin over the back of the hand and observe for tenting; count the number of seconds for the skin to recover position.
    c. Observe the mucous membranes and tongue for cracks, fissures, or a pasty coating.
    d. Pinch the skin over the sternum and observe for tenting and resumption of skin to its normal position after release.

15. The emergency department (ED) nurse is caring for a patient who was brought in for significant alcohol intoxication and minor trauma to the wrist. What will serial hematocrits for this patient likely show?
    a. Hemoconcentration
    b. Normal and stable hematocrits
    c. Progressively lower hematocrits
    d. Decreasing osmolality

16. Which changes on a patient's electrocardiogram (ECG) reflect hyperkalemia?
    a. Tall peaked T waves
    b. Narrow QRS complex
    c. Tall P waves
    d. Normal P-R interval

17. The nurse is caring for several older adult patients who are at risk for dehydration. Which task can be delegated to the unlicensed assistive personnel (UAP)?
    a. Withhold fluids if patients have bowel or bladder incontinence.
    b. Assess for and report any difficulties that patients are having in swallowing.
    c. Stay with patients while they drink fluids and note the exact amount ingested.
    d. Divide the total amount of fluids needed over a 24-hour period and note in medical record.

18. The nurse assessing a patient notes a bounding pulse quality, neck vein distention when supine, presence of crackles in the lungs, and increasing peripheral edema. What fluid disorder do these findings reflect?
    a. Fluid volume deficit
    b. Fluid volume excess
    c. Fluid homeostasis
    d. Fluid dehydration

19. A patient is at risk for fluid volume excess and dependent edema. Which task does the nurse delegate to the UAP?
    a. Massage the legs and heels to stimulate circulation.
    b. Evaluate the effectiveness of a pressure-reducing mattress.
    c. Assess the coccyx, elbows, and hips daily for signs of redness.
    d. Assist the patient to change position every 2 hours.

20. The nurse is reviewing orders for several patients who are at risk for fluid volume overload. For which patient condition does the nurse question an order for diuretics?
    a. Pulmonary edema
    b. Congestive heart failure
    c. End-stage renal disease
    d. Ascites

21. The unlicensed assistive personnel (UAP) reports to the nurse that a patient being evaluated for kidney problems has produced a large amount of pale-yellow urine. What does the nurse do **next**?
    a. Instruct the UAP to measure the amount carefully and then discard the urine.
    b. Instruct the UAP to save the urine in a large bottle for a 24-hour urine specimen.
    c. Assess the patient for signs of fluid imbalance and check the specific gravity of the urine.
    d. Compare the amount of urine output to the fluid intake for the previous 8 hours.

22. On admission, a patient with pulmonary edema weighed 151 lbs; now the patient's weight is 149 lbs. Assuming the patient was weighed both times with the same clothing, on the same scale, and at the same time of day, how many milliliters of fluid does the nurse estimate the patient has lost?
    a. 500
    b. 1000
    c. 2000
    d. 2500

23. The nurse is giving discharge instructions to the patient with advanced heart failure who is at continued risk for fluid volume overload. For which physical change does the nurse instruct the patient to call the health care provider?
    a. Greater than 3 lbs gained in a week or greater than 1 to 2 lbs gained in a 24-hour period
    b. Greater than 5 lbs gained in a week or greater than 1 to 2 lbs gained in a 24-hour period
    c. Greater than 15 lbs gained in a month or greater than 5 lbs gained in a week
    d. Greater than 20 lbs gained in a month or greater than 5 lbs gained in a week

24. The nurse is caring for several patients at risk for falls because of fluid and electrolyte imbalances. Which task related to patient safety and fall prevention does the nurse delegate to the UAP?
    a. Assess for orthostatic hypotension.
    b. Orient the patient to the environment.
    c. Help the incontinent patient to toilet every 1-2 hours.
    d. Encourage family members or significant other to stay with the patient.

25. The nurse is assessing a patient's urine specific gravity. The value is 1.035. How does the nurse interpret this result?
    a. Overhydration
    b. Dehydration
    c. Normal value for an adult
    d. Renal disease

26. What are the functions of potassium in the body? **Select all that apply.**
    a. Regulates hydration status
    b. Controls intracellular osmolarity and volume
    c. Stimulates the secretion of antidiuretic hormone (ADH)
    d. Functions as the major cation of intracellular fluid (ICF)
    e. Regulates glucose use and storage
    f. Helps maintain normal cardiac rhythm

27. What impacts does sodium have on body function? **Select all that apply.**
    a. Maintains electroneutrality
    b. Maintains electrical membrane excitability
    c. Aids in carbohydrate and lipid metabolism
    d. Regulates water balance
    e. Low sodium stimulates secretion of aldosterone
    f. Regulates plasma osmolality

28. The electrolyte magnesium is responsible for which functions? **Select all that apply.**
    a. Formation of hydrochloric acid
    b. Carbohydrate metabolism
    c. Contraction of skeletal muscle
    d. Regulation of intracellular osmolarity
    e. Vitamin activation
    f. Blood coagulation

29. A patient is talking to the nurse about sodium intake. Which statement by the patient indicates an understanding of high-sodium food sources?
    a. "I have bacon and eggs every morning for breakfast."
    b. "We never eat seafood because of the salt water."
    c. "I love Chinese food, but I gave it up because of the soy sauce."
    d. "Pickled herring is a fish, and my doctor told me to eat a lot of fish."

30. Which statement **best** explains how antidiuretic hormone (ADH) affects urine output?
    a. It increases permeability to water in the tubules, causing a decrease in urine output.
    b. It increases urine output as a result of water being absorbed by the tubules.
    c. Urine output is reduced as the posterior pituitary decreases ADH production.
    d. Increased urine output results from increased osmolarity and fluid in the extracellular space.

31. A patient with hyponatremia would have which gastrointestinal findings upon assessment? **Select all that apply.**
    a. Hyperactive bowel sounds on auscultation
    b. Hard, dark-brown stools
    c. Hypoactive bowel sounds on auscultation
    d. Frequent watery bowel movements
    e. Abdominal cramping
    f. Nausea

32. The nurse is caring for a patient with severe hypocalcemia. What safety measures does the nurse put in place for this patient? **Select all that apply.**
    a. Encourage the patient to use a cane when ambulating.
    b. Turn on a bed alarm when the patient is in bed.
    c. Obtain an order for zolpidem (Ambien) to ensure the patient sleeps at night.
    d. Place the patient on a low bed.
    e. Ensure the top side rails are up when the patient is in bed.
    f. Raise all four side rails.

33. Which patients are at risk for developing hyponatremia? **Select all that apply.**
    a. Postoperative patient who has been NPO (nothing by mouth) for 24 hours with no IV fluid infusing
    b. Patient with decreased fluid intake for three days
    c. Patient receiving excessive intravenous fluids with 5% dextrose
    d. Diabetic patient with blood glucose of 250 mg/dL
    e. Patient with overactive adrenal glands
    f. Tennis player in 100°F (37.7°C) weather who has been drinking water

34. The nurse is evaluating the lab results of a patient with hyperaldosteronism. What abnormal electrolyte finding does the nurse expect to see?
    a. Hyponatremia
    b. Hyperkalemia
    c. Hypocalcemia
    d. Hypernatremia

35. The unlicensed assistive personnel (UAP) informs the nurse that a patient with hypernatremia who was initially confused and disoriented on admission to the hospital is now trying to pull out the IV access and indwelling urinary catheter. What is the nurse's **first** action?
    a. Place bilateral soft wrist restraints.
    b. Inform the provider of the patient's change in behavior and obtain an order for restraints.
    c. Assess the patient.
    d. Offer the patient oral fluids.

36. Patients with which conditions are at risk for developing hypernatremia? **Select all that apply.**
    a. Chronic constipation
    b. Heart failure
    c. Severe diarrhea
    d. Decreased kidney function
    e. Profound diaphoresis
    f. Cushing's syndrome

37. The provider has ordered therapy for a patient with low sodium and signs of hypervolemia. Which diuretic is **best** for this patient?
    a. Conivaptan
    b. Furosemide
    c. Hydrochlorothiazide
    d. Bumetanide

38. The nurse is assessing a patient with a mild increase in sodium level. What early manifestation does the nurse observe in this patient?
    a. Muscle twitching and irregular muscle contractions
    b. Inability of muscles and nerves to respond to a stimulus
    c. Muscle weakness occurring bilaterally with no specific pattern
    d. Reduced or absent bilateral deep tendon reflexes

39. The nurse is caring for a patient with hypernatremia caused by fluid loss. What type of IV solution is **best** for treating this patient?
    a. Hypotonic 0.225% sodium chloride
    b. Small-volume infusions of hypertonic (2%-3%) saline
    c. Isotonic sodium chloride (NaCl)
    d. 0.9% sodium chloride

40. Which serum value does the nurse expect to see for a patient with hyponatremia?
    a. Sodium less than 136 mEq/L
    b. Chloride less than 95 mEq/L
    c. Sodium less than 145 mEq/L
    d. Chloride less than 103 mEq/L

41. The nurse is caring for a psychiatric patient who is continuously drinking water. The nurse monitors for which complication related to potential hyponatremia?
    a. Proteinuria/prerenal failure
    b. Change in mental status/increased intracranial pressure
    c. Pitting edema/circulatory failure
    d. Possible occult blood/gastrointestinal bleeding in stool

42. What interventions are appropriate for a patient with hypernatremia caused by reduced kidney sodium excretion? **Select all that apply.**
    a. Hypotonic solutions
    b. 0.45% sodium chloride intravenous infusion
    c. D_5W intravenous infusion
    d. Administration of bumetanide
    e. Ensure adequate water intake
    f. Diuretics such as furosemide

43. The nurse is caring for several patients at risk for fluid and electrolyte imbalances. Which patient problem or condition can result in a relative hypernatremia?
    a. Use of a salt substitute
    b. Presence of a feeding tube
    c. Drinking too much water
    d. Long-term NPO status

44. The nurse is caring for an older adult patient whose serum sodium level is 150 mEq/L. The nurse assesses the patient for which common signs and symptoms associated with this sodium level? **Select all that apply.**
    a. Intact recall of recent events
    b. Increased pulse rate
    c. Rigidity of extremities
    d. Hyperactivity
    e. Muscle weakness
    f. Difficulty palpating peripheral pulses

45. Which precaution or intervention does the nurse teach a patient at continued risk for hypernatremia?
    a. Avoid salt substitutes.
    b. Avoid aspirin and aspirin-containing products.
    c. Read labels on canned or packaged foods to determine sodium content.
    d. Increase daily intake of caffeine-containing foods and beverages.

46. On assessment, the patient has respiratory muscle weakness resulting in shallow respirations. Which electrolyte abnormality would the nurse suspect?
    a. Hypokalemia
    b. Hyperkalemia
    c. Hypocalcemia
    d. Hypercalcemia

47. A patient with renal failure that results in hypernatremia will require which interventions? **Select all that apply.**
    a. Administration of furosemide
    b. Hemodialysis
    c. IV infusion of 0.9% sodium chloride
    d. Dietary sodium restriction
    e. Administration of potassium supplement
    f. Administration of demeclocycline

48. The patient with mild fluid volume overload has been instructed by the provider to follow dietary sodium restriction. What would the nurse teach this patient about sodium restriction?
    a. Do not add salt to ordinary table foods.
    b. Restrict sodium intake to 2 gm per day.
    c. Restrict sodium intake to 4 gm per day.
    d. Do not add salt when cooking or eating.

49. A hospitalized patient who is known to be homeless has been diagnosed with severe malnutrition, end-stage renal disease, and anemia. He is transfused with three units of packed red blood cells. Which potential electrolyte imbalance does the nurse anticipate could occur in this patient?
    a. Hypernatremia
    b. Hyperkalemia
    c. Hypercalcemia
    d. Hypermagnesemia

50. The patient has severe hypokalemia (2.4 mEq/L). For which intestinal complication does the nurse monitor?
    a. Hypoactive bowel sounds
    b. Paralytic ileus
    c. Nausea
    d. Constipation

51. A newly admitted patient with congestive heart failure has a potassium level of 5.7 mEq/L. How does the nurse identify contributing factors for the electrolyte imbalance? **Select all that apply.**
    a. Assess the patient for hypokalemia.
    b. Obtain a list of the patient's home medications.
    c. Assess the patient for hyperkalemia.
    d. Ask about the patient's method of taking medications at home.
    e. Evaluate the patient's appetite.
    f. Auscultate for hypoactive bowel sounds.

52. A young adult patient is in the early stages of being treated for severe burns. Which electrolyte imbalance does the nurse expect to assess in this patient?
    a. Hypernatremia
    b. Hypokalemia
    c. Hypercalcemia
    d. Hyperkalemia

53. A patient with hypokalemia is likely to have which conditions? **Select all that apply.**
    a. Liver failure
    b. Metabolic alkalosis
    c. Cushing's syndrome
    d. Hypothyroidism
    e. Paralytic ileus
    f. Kidney failure

54. The nurse is taking care of a trauma patient who was in a motor vehicle accident. The patient has a history of hypertension, which is managed with spironolactone. This patient is at risk for developing which electrolyte imbalance?
    a. Hyperkalemia
    b. Hypernatremia
    c. Hypokalemia
    d. Hypocalcemia

55. Which serum laboratory value does the nurse expect to see in the patient with hypokalemia?
    a. Calcium less than 8.0 mg/dL
    b. Potassium less than 5.0 mEq/L
    c. Calcium less than 11.0 mg/dL
    d. Potassium less than 3.5 mEq/L

56. The patient's potassium level is 2.5 mEq/L. Which clinical findings does the nurse expect to see when assessing this patient? **Select all that apply.**
    a. General skeletal muscle weakness
    b. Moist crackles and tachypnea
    c. Lethargy
    d. Decreased urine output
    e. Weak hand grasps
    f. Weak, thready pulse

57. The nurse administering potassium to a patient carefully monitors the infusion because of the risk for which condition?
    a. Pulmonary edema
    b. Cardiac dysrhythmia
    c. Postural hypotension
    d. Renal failure

58. The patient with hypokalemia has an IV potassium supplement ordered. Which IV potassium supplement can be administered safely?
    a. KCl 5 mEq in 20 mL NS
    b. KCl 10 mEq in 100 mL NS
    c. KCl 15 mEq in 50 mL NS
    d. KCl 20 mEq in 100 mL NS

59. The nurse is teaching the patient about hypokalemia. Which statement by the patient indicates a correct understanding of the treatment of hypokalemia?
    a. "My wife does all the cooking. She shops for food high in calcium."
    b. "When I take the liquid potassium in the evening, I'll eat a snack beforehand."
    c. "I will avoid bananas, orange juice, and salt substitutes."
    d. "I hate being stuck with needles all the time to monitor how much sugar I can eat."

60. The nurse is caring for a patient who takes potassium and digoxin. For what reason does the nurse monitor both laboratory results?
    a. Digoxin increases potassium loss through the kidneys.
    b. Digoxin toxicity can result if hypokalemia is present.
    c. Digoxin may cause potassium levels to rise to toxic levels.
    d. Hypokalemia causes the cardiac muscle to be less sensitive to digoxin.

61. Which serum laboratory value does the nurse expect to see in a patient with hyperkalemia?
    a. Calcium greater than 8.0 mg/dL
    b. Potassium greater than 3.5 mEq/L
    c. Calcium greater than 11.0 mg/dL
    d. Potassium greater than 5.0 mEq/L

62. A patient has an elevated potassium level. Which assessment findings are associated with hyperkalemia? **Select all that apply.**
    a. Wheezing on exhalation
    b. Numbness in hands and feet and around the mouth
    c. Frequent, watery stools
    d. Irregular heart rate
    e. Circumoral cyanosis
    f. Muscle weakness

63. The nurse is teaching a patient with hypokalemia about foods high in potassium. Which food items does the nurse recommend to this patient? **Select all that apply.**
    a. Soybeans
    b. Lettuce
    c. Cantaloupe
    d. Potatoes
    e. Peaches
    f. Bananas

64. A patient's serum potassium value is below 2.8 mEq/L. The patient is also on digoxin. The nurse quickly assesses the patient for which cardiac problem **before** notifying the provider?
    a. Cardiac murmur
    b. Cardiac dysrhythmia
    c. Congestive heart failure
    d. Cardiac tamponade

65. Which potassium levels are within normal limits? **Select all that apply.**
    a. 2.0 mmol/L
    b. 3.5 mmol/L
    c. 4.5 mmol/L
    d. 5.0 mmol/L
    e. 6.0 mmol/L

66. A patient has hyperkalemia resulting from dehydration. Which additional laboratory findings does the nurse anticipate for this patient?
    a. Increased hematocrit and hemoglobin levels
    b. Decreased serum electrolyte levels
    c. Increased urine potassium levels
    d. Decreased serum creatinine

67. A 65-year-old patient has a potassium laboratory value of 5.0 mEq/L. How does the nurse interpret this value?
    a. High for the patient's age
    b. Low for the patient's age
    c. Normal for the patient's age
    d. Dependent upon the medical diagnosis

68. A patient's potassium level is high secondary to kidney failure. What laboratory changes does the nurse expect to see? **Select all that apply.**
    a. Elevated serum creatinine
    b. Decreased blood pH
    c. Elevated sodium
    d. Low to normal hematocrit
    e. Elevated hemoglobin
    f. Decreased blood urea nitrogen

69. Plasma is part of which body fluid space compartments? **Select all that apply.**
    a. The intracellular compartment
    b. The extracellular compartment
    c. All fluid within the cells
    d. Interstitial fluid
    e. Intravascular fluid
    f. Fluid within joint capsules

70. Which fluid has the highest corresponding electrolyte content?
    a. Intracellular fluid is highest in potassium.
    b. Extracellular fluid is highest in sodium.
    c. Extracellular fluid is highest in sodium and chloride.
    d. Intracellular fluid is highest in magnesium and sodium.

71. Which component has a high content of potassium and phosphorus?
    a. Extracellular fluid
    b. Intracellular fluid
    c. Extracellular fluid and the intravascular space
    d. Intracellular fluid and lymph fluid

72. A patient with low potassium requires an IV potassium infusion. The pharmacy sends a 250-mL IV bag of dextrose in water with 40 mEq of potassium. The label is marked "to infuse over 1 hour." What is the nurse's **best** action?
    a. Obtain a pump and administer the solution.
    b. Double-check the provider's order and call the pharmacy.
    c. Hold the infusion because there is an error in labeling.
    d. Recalculate the rate so that it is safe for the patient.

73. An older adult patient needs an oral potassium solution but is refusing it because it has a strong and unpleasant taste. What is the **best** strategy the nurse can use to administer the drug?
    a. Tell the patient that failure to take the drug could result in serious heart problems.
    b. Ask the patient's preference of juice and mix the drug with a small amount.
    c. Mix the solution into food on the patient's meal tray and encourage the patient to eat everything.
    d. Offer the drug to the patient several times and then document the patient's refusal.

74. A patient has a low potassium level, and the provider has ordered an IV infusion. **Before** starting an IV potassium infusion, what does the nurse assess?
    a. Intravenous line patency
    b. Oxygen saturation level
    c. Baseline mental status
    d. Apical pulse

75. Which foods will the nurse instruct a patient with kidney disease and hyperkalemia to avoid? **Select all that apply.**
    a. Canned apricots
    b. Dried beans
    c. Potatoes
    d. Cabbage
    e. Cantaloupe
    f. Canned sausage

76. The patient with hyperkalemia is prescribed patiromer. Which statement **most accurately** describes the function of this drug?
    a. It works in the kidneys to increase excretion of potassium.
    b. The drug prevents the kidneys from absorbing potassium.
    c. It binds with potassium in the GI tract and decreases its absorption.
    d. The drug increases motility in the GI tract, eliminating potassium in diarrhea stools.

77. By which mechanisms does parathyroid hormone (PTH) increase serum calcium levels? **Select all that apply.**
    a. Releasing free calcium from the bones
    b. Increasing calcium excretion in the urine
    c. Stimulating kidney reabsorption of calcium
    d. Causing vitamin D activation
    e. Increasing calcium absorption in the GI tract
    f. Pulling calcium out of the cells

78. Which assessment findings are related to mild hypercalcemia? **Select all that apply.**
    a. Increased heart rate
    b. Paresthesia
    c. Decreased deep tendon reflexes
    d. Hypoactive bowel sounds
    e. Shortened QT interval
    f. Profound muscle weakness

79. Which nursing interventions apply to patients with hypercalcemia? **Select all that apply.**
    a. Administer IV normal saline (0.9% sodium chloride).
    b. Measure the abdominal girth.
    c. Massage calves to encourage blood return to the heart.
    d. Monitor for ECG changes.
    e. Provide adequate intake of vitamin D.
    f. During treatment, monitor for tetany.

80. The nurse is reviewing the laboratory calcium level results for a patient. Which value indicates mild hypocalcemia?
    a. 5.0 mg/dL
    b. 8.0 mg/dL
    c. 10.0 mg/dL
    d. 12.0 mg/dL

81. A patient with a recent history of anterior neck injury reports muscle twitching and spasms with tingling in the lips, nose, and ears. The nurse suspects these symptoms may be caused by which condition?
    a. Hypocalcemia
    b. Hypokalemia
    c. Hyponatremia
    d. Hypomagnesemia

82. Which conditions cause a patient to be at risk for hypocalcemia? **Select all that apply.**
    a. Crohn's disease
    b. Acute pancreatitis
    c. Removal or destruction of parathyroid glands
    d. Immobility
    e. Use of digitalis
    f. GI wound drainage

83. The nurse is assessing the patient with a risk for hypocalcemia. What is the correct technique to test for Chvostek's sign?
    a. Patient flexes arms against the chest and examiner attempts to pull the arms away from the chest.
    b. Place a blood pressure cuff around the upper arm and inflate the cuff to greater than the patient's systolic pressure.
    c. Tap the patient's face just below and in front of the ear to trigger facial twitching of one side of the mouth, nose, and cheek.
    d. Lightly tap the patient's patellar and Achilles tendons with a reflex hammer and measure the movement.

84. The nurse is caring for several patients with electrolyte imbalances. Which intervention is included in the plan of care for a patient with hypomagnesemia?
    a. Implementing an oral fluid restriction of 1500 mL/day
    b. Implementing a renal diet
    c. Providing moderate environmental stimulation with music
    d. Placing the patient on seizure precautions

85. Which clinical condition can result from hypocalcemia?
    a. Stimulated cardiac muscle contraction
    b. Increased intestinal and gastric motility
    c. Decreased peripheral nerve excitability
    d. Increased bone density

86. Which patient is at greatest risk of developing hypocalcemia?
    a. 30-year-old Asian woman with breast cancer
    b. 45-year-old Caucasian man with hypertension and diuretic therapy
    c. 60-year-old African-American woman with a recent ileostomy
    d. 70-year-old Caucasian man on long-term lithium therapy

87. Which is a preventive measure for patients at risk for developing hypocalcemia?
    a. Increase daily dietary calcium and vitamin D intake.
    b. Increase intake of phosphorus.
    c. Apply sunblock and wear protective clothing whenever outdoors.
    d. Administer calcium-containing IV fluids to patients receiving multiple blood transfusions.

88. The patient who has undergone which surgical procedure is **most** at risk for hypocalcemia?
    a. Thyroidectomy
    b. Adrenalectomy
    c. Pancreatectomy
    d. Gastrectomy

89. Which patient is at greatest risk for chronic hypocalcemia?
    a. 38-year-old man with chronic kidney disease
    b. 50-year-old postmenopausal woman
    c. 62-year-old man with type 2 diabetes
    d. 78-year-old woman with dehydration

90. Which are typical nursing assessment findings for a patient with hypocalcemia? **Select all that apply.**
    a. Positive Chvostek's sign
    b. Hypertension
    c. Diarrhea
    d. Prolonged ST interval
    e. Elevated T wave
    f. Positive Trousseau's sign

91. Which intervention does the nurse implement for a patient with hypocalcemia?
    a. Encourage activity by the patient as tolerated, including weight-lifting.
    b. Encourage socialization and active participation in stimulating activities.
    c. Keep a tracheostomy tray at the bedside for emergency use.
    d. Provide adequate intake of vitamin D and calcium-rich foods.

92. A patient with hypocalcemia needs supplemental diet therapy. Which foods does the nurse recommend, providing both calcium and vitamin D? **Select all that apply.**
    a. Tofu
    b. Cheese
    c. Eggs
    d. Broccoli
    e. Milk
    f. Salmon

93. A patient shows a positive Trousseau's or Chvostek's sign. The nurse prepares to give the patient which urgent treatment?
    a. IV calcium
    b. Calcitonin
    c. IV potassium chloride
    d. Large doses of oral calcium

94. Which are appropriate interventions for a patient who has hypercalcemia? **Select all that apply.**
    a. Administer IV normal saline (0.9% sodium chloride).
    b. Administer hydrochlorothiazide (HCTZ).
    c. Ensure adequate hydration.
    d. Administer calcium-based antacid for GI upset.
    e. Discourage weight-bearing activity such as walking.
    f. Provide continuous cardiac monitoring.

95. The nurse caring for a patient with hypercalcemia anticipates orders for which medications? **Select all that apply.**
    a. Magnesium sulfate
    b. Calcitonin
    c. Furosemide
    d. Plicamycin
    e. Calcium gluconate
    f. Aluminum hydroxide

96. The nurse instructs the unlicensed assistive personnel (UAP) to use precautions with moving and using a lift sheet for which patient with an electrolyte imbalance?
    a. Young woman with diabetes and hyperkalemia
    b. Patient with psychiatric illness and hyponatremia
    c. Older woman with hypocalcemia
    d. Child with severe diarrhea and hypomagnesemia

97. Which are major causes of hypomagnesemia? **Select all that apply.**
    a. Inadequate intake of magnesium
    b. Inadequate intake of sodium
    c. Use of potassium-sparing diuretics
    d. Decreased kidney excretion of magnesium
    e. Prescription of loop diuretics
    f. Cessation of alcohol intake

98. The health care provider orders magnesium sulfate (MgSO$_4$) for a patient with severe hypomagnesemia. What is the **preferred** route of administration for this drug?
    a. Oral
    b. Subcutaneous
    c. Intramuscular
    d. Intravenous

99. In addition to magnesium levels, which other lab values should the nurse be sure to monitor when a patient has hypomagnesemia?
    a. Sodium and potassium
    b. Potassium and calcium
    c. Calcium and sodium
    d. Chloride and sodium

100. The nurse is assessing a patient with severe hypermagnesemia. Which assessment findings are associated with this electrolyte imbalance?
    a. Bradycardia and hypotension
    b. Tachycardia and weak palpable pulse
    c. Hypertension and irritability
    d. Irregular pulse and deep respirations

101. A patient in the hospital has a severely elevated magnesium level. Which intervention should the nurse complete **first**?
    a. Discontinue oral magnesium.
    b. Administer furosemide (Lasix).
    c. Discontinue parenteral magnesium.
    d. Administer calcium to treat bradycardia.

102. A patient has a magnesium level of 0.8 mg/dL. Which treatment does the nurse expect to be ordered for this patient?
    a. Intramuscular magnesium sulfate
    b. Increased intake of fruits and vegetables
    c. Oral preparations of magnesium sulfate
    d. IV magnesium sulfate and discontinuation of diuretic therapy

103. The nurse monitors the effectiveness of magnesium sulfate by assessing which factor every hour?
    a. Deep tendon reflexes
    b. Vital signs
    c. Serum laboratory values
    d. Urine output

104. Which condition places a patient at risk for hypocalcemia, hyperkalemia, and hypernatremia?
    a. Hypothyroidism
    b. Diabetes mellitus
    c. Chronic kidney disease
    d. Adrenal insufficiency

105. A patient with congestive heart failure is receiving a loop diuretic. The nurse monitors for which electrolyte imbalances? **Select all that apply.**
    a. Hypocalcemia
    b. Hypercalcemia
    c. Hyponatremia
    d. Hypernatremia
    e. Hypokalemia
    f. Hyperkalemia

106. The patient with a serum magnesium level of 2.9 mEq/L develops bradycardia with a prolonged P-R interval and a widened QRS. What is the nurse's **best first** action?
    a. Start an IV with 5% dextrose at 100 mL/hr.
    b. Notify the health care provider immediately.
    c. Auscultate the patient's apical heart rate.
    d. Prepare to administer supplemental magnesium by IV.

12 CHAPTER

Assessment and Care of Patients with Impaired Acid-Base Balances

1. Changes from normal pH can have what effects on which body functions? **Select all that apply.**
   a. Alter fluid and electrolyte balance
   b. Increase effectiveness of drugs
   c. Reduce function of hormones
   d. Increase function of enzymes
   e. Increase excitability of the heart muscle
   f. Cause increased activity of the GI tract

2. A patient with chronic obstructive pulmonary disease (COPD) has just developed respiratory distress. Vital signs are pulse oximetry 88% on 2 L nasal cannula oxygen, dyspnea at rest, and respirations 32 per minute. The patient reports shortness of breath. Which statements apply to this clinical situation? **Select all that apply.**
   a. Interference in alveolar-capillary diffusion results in carbon dioxide retention.
   b. The nurse should instruct the patient to use pursed-lip breathing.
   c. Position the patient with the head of the bed at less than 20 degrees.
   d. Interference in alveolar-capillary diffusion results in acidemia.
   e. The nurse should explain to the patient that rapid breathing will relieve the shortness of breath.
   f. Use of an as-needed bronchodilator may relieve the shortness of breath.

3. Which body pH level can be **fatal**?
   a. 7.22
   b. 7.11
   c. 7.05
   d. 6.85

4. Which statement about compensation for acid-base imbalance is accurate?
   a. The respiratory system is less sensitive to acid-base changes.
   b. The respiratory system can begin compensation within seconds to minutes.
   c. The renal system is less powerful than the respiratory system.
   d. The renal system is more sensitive to acid-base changes.

5. The unlicensed assistive personnel (UAP) notifies the nurse that the patient with emphysema receiving oxygen at 2 L via nasal cannula is short of breath after morning care. What is the nurse's **first** action?
   a. Notify the health care provider immediately.
   b. Ask the UAP to check the patient's SaO_2 level.
   c. Instruct the UAP to check vital signs.
   d. Document the incident in the patient's chart.

6. A patient with bilateral lower lobe pneumonia is diagnosed with respiratory acidosis based on arterial blood gas (ABG) results. What is the **likely** cause of the patient's respiratory acidosis?
   a. Underelimination of carbon dioxide from the lungs
   b. Buffering of extracellular fluid by ammonium
   c. Overelimination of carbon dioxide from the lungs
   d. An increased bicarbonate level due to respiratory elimination of acid

7. A patient is admitted to the hospital for diabetic ketoacidosis. Which arterial blood gas (ABG) results should the nurse expect? **Select all that apply.**
   a. pH 7.32
   b. $PaCO_2$ 55 mm Hg
   c. Bicarbonate (Bicarb) 18 mEq/L
   d. pH 7.46
   e. Bicarbonate (Bicarb) 29 mEq/L
   f. $PaCO_2$ 44 mm Hg

8. A patient has been admitted to the emergency department (ED) with diabetic ketoacidosis. On intake assessment, the patient cannot recall the medications she takes. What **first** action does the nurse take?
   a. Instruct the patient to compare a hospital list of medications to her home medications.
   b. Ask the patient's significant other to bring the patient's medications from home.
   c. Request that the patient complete a meal recall for the past 24 hours.
   d. Teach the patient about the importance of keeping a list of current medications in her purse.

9. A patient who has pancreatitis with nausea and vomiting will likely have which related alterations in acid-base balance? **Select all that apply.**
   a. Overproduction of hydrogen ions
   b. Metabolic acidosis
   c. Serum pH value that is directly related to the concentration of hydrogen ions
   d. Underproduction of bicarbonate
   e. Metabolic alkalosis
   f. Respiratory acidosis

10. Which statements correctly apply to acid-base balance in the body? **Select all that apply.**
    a. Renal mechanisms are stronger in regulating acid-base balance but slower to respond than respiratory mechanisms.
    b. The immediate binding of excess hydrogen ions occurs primarily in the red blood cells.
    c. Combined acidosis is less severe than either metabolic acidosis or respiratory acidosis alone.
    d. Respiratory acidosis is caused by a patent airway.
    e. Acid-base balance occurs through control of hydrogen ion production and elimination.
    f. Buffers are the third-line defense against acid-base imbalances in the body.

11. The nurse is interpreting the arterial blood gas (ABG) results of a patient with acute respiratory insufficiency. As the $PaCO_2$ level increases, which result would the nurse expect?
    a. Decreased pH
    b. Decreased Bicarb
    c. Increased PaO_2
    d. Increased pH

12. The nurse is admitting a patient with acute kidney injury to the medical unit. Which ABG results would she expect for this patient?
    a. Respiratory acidosis
    b. Metabolic acidosis
    c. Respiratory alkalosis
    d. Metabolic alkalosis

13. Which blood pH value does the nurse interpret as within normal limits?
    a. 7.27
    b. 7.37
    c. 7.47
    d. 7.5

14. Which conditions could cause a patient to develop acidosis? **Select all that apply.**
    a. Sepsis
    b. Hypovolemic shock
    c. Use of a mechanical ventilator
    d. Prolonged nasogastric suctioning
    e. Hypoventilation
    f. Severe diarrhea

15. Which patient with the highest risk for acidosis must the nurse care for **first**?
    a. Patient in mild pain with a kidney stone
    b. Patient with chronic obstructive pulmonary disease and pulse oximetry 88% on 2 L oxygen
    c. Patient who had a seizure prior to admission with pulse oximetry of 91%
    d. Patient with a rectal tube in place for frequent diarrhea

16. A patient's arterial blood gas (ABG) results show an increase in pH. Which condition is **most likely** to contribute to this laboratory value?
    a. Mechanical ventilation
    b. Diabetic ketoacidosis
    c. Nasogastric suction
    d. Diarrhea

17. Which patient is most likely to have a decrease in bicarbonate?
    a. Patient with pancreatitis
    b. Patient with hypoventilation
    c. Patient who is vomiting
    d. Patient with emphysema

18. A patient has a new onset of shallow and slow respirations. While the patient's body attempts to compensate, what happens to the patient's pH level?
    a. Increases
    b. Decreases
    c. Stabilizes
    d. Fluctuates

19. A patient is at risk for acid-base imbalance. Which laboratory value indicates that the patient has metabolic acidosis?
    a. $Paco_2 = 55$ mm Hg
    b. $HCO_3^- = 17$ mEq/L
    c. Lactate = 2.5 mmol/L
    d. pH = 7.35

20. Which type of medication increases an older adult patient's risk for acid-base imbalance?
    a. Antilipidemics
    b. Hormonal therapy
    c. Diuretics
    d. Antidysrhythmics

21. Which medication usage could cause metabolic acidosis?
    a. Aspirin overdose
    b. Overuse of antacids
    c. Prolonged use of antihistamines
    d. Vitamin overdose

22. Which nursing assessment finding indicates a worsening of respiratory acidosis?
    a. Decreased respiratory rate
    b. Decreased blood pressure
    c. Use of accessory respiratory muscles
    d. Pale nail beds

23. Which patient is **most likely** to develop respiratory acidosis?
    a. Patient who is anxious and breathing rapidly
    b. Patient with multiple rib fractures
    c. Patient with IV normal saline bolus
    d. Patient with increased urinary output

24. Which patients require assessment related to inadequate chest expansion that would place them at risk for respiratory acidosis? **Select all that apply.**
    a. Patient with lordosis
    b. Patient with emphysema
    c. Severely obese patient on prolonged bedrest
    d. Patient in the first trimester of pregnancy
    e. Patient 2 days postoperative for laparoscopic cholecystectomy
    f. Patient with ascites

25. The nurse reviews the electrocardiogram (ECG) and cardiovascular status of a patient. Which findings are **early** changes associated with acidosis?
    a. Decreased heart rate with hypertension
    b. Hypotension and faint peripheral pulses
    c. Increased heart rate and increased cardiac output
    d. Peaked T waves and wide QRS complexes

26. Which system should be assessed **first** for a patient at risk for acidosis?
    a. Cardiovascular system
    b. Neuromuscular system
    c. Central nervous system
    d. Respiratory system

27. Which arterial blood gas (ABG) results indicate that a patient's acid-base imbalance is a respiratory acidosis? **Select all that apply.**
    a. pH 7.31
    b. $PaCO_2$ 58 mm Hg
    c. Bicarbonate (Bicarb) 17 mEq/L
    d. PaO_2 75 mm Hg
    e. Serum potassium 4.5 mEq/L
    f. $PaCO_2$ 31 mm Hg

28. The nurse is testing the muscle strength of a patient at risk for acid-base imbalance. Which technique does the nurse use to test arm strength?
    a. Asks the patient to hold the arms straight out in front, and the nurse observes for drift
    b. Asks the patient to squeeze the nurse's hand
    c. Asks the patient to pick up an object that weighs at least 10 lbs
    d. Tries to separate the patient's clasped hands

29. The nurse assesses an acidotic patient's lower extremities for strength as part of the nursing shift assessment. What finding does the nurse expect to see?
    a. Bilateral weakness
    b. Weakness on the dominant side
    c. No change from baseline
    d. Cramping, but no weakness

30. The nurse observes tall peaked T waves on the ECG of a patient with metabolic acidosis. **Before** notifying the health care provider, the nurse would assess the results of which laboratory test?
    a. Serum calcium
    b. Serum glucose
    c. Serum potassium
    d. Serum magnesium

31. Which signs and symptoms would the nurse expect to assess in a patient with metabolic acidosis? **Select all that apply.**
    a. Kussmaul respirations
    b. Shallow, rapid respirations
    c. Warm, flushed skin
    d. Skin pale to cyanotic
    e. Elevated $PaCO_2$
    f. Decreased bicarbonate

32. What interventions are included in the plan of care for a patient with metabolic ketoacidosis? **Select all that apply.**
    a. Monitor ABG levels for decreasing pH level.
    b. Maintain patent IV access.
    c. Administer fluids as prescribed.
    d. Monitor for irritability and muscle tetany.
    e. Monitor loss of bicarbonate through the gastrointestinal tract such as with diarrhea.
    f. Administer IV 50% dextrose as needed.

33. What is the **priority** intervention for a patient with diabetic ketoacidosis?
    a. Administer bicarbonate.
    b. Administer oxygen.
    c. Administer insulin.
    d. Administer potassium.

34. What are the hallmark laboratory findings of respiratory alkalosis?
    a. High pH and low PaO_2
    b. High pH and low $PaCO_2$
    c. High pH and high bicarbonate
    d. High pH and high $PaCO_2$

35. Which statement made by the patient indicates that he or she may have an alkaline condition?
    a. "I am more and more tired and can't concentrate."
    b. "I have tingling in my fingers and toes."
    c. "My feet and ankles are swollen."
    d. "I am short of breath all of the time."

36. Which patient is most likely to develop respiratory alkalosis?
    a. Hypoxic patient
    b. Patient with a body cast
    c. Fearful patient having a panic attack
    d. Morbidly obese patient

37. Which type of electrolyte imbalance does the nurse expect to see in a patient with metabolic alkalosis?
    a. Hyperkalemia
    b. Hypophosphatemia
    c. Hyperchloremia
    d. Hypocalcemia

38. Which patient is most likely to develop metabolic alkalosis as a result of base excess?
    a. Patient taking thiazide diuretics
    b. Patient who is having nasogastric suction
    c. Patient with severe vomiting
    d. Patient who had a massive blood transfusion

39. The nurse is assessing a patient with metabolic alkalosis. Which neuromuscular finding is the **most** ominous and warrants immediate notification of the health care provider?
    a. Muscle cramps
    b. Muscle twitching
    c. Hyperactive deep tendon reflexes
    d. Tetany

40. The nurse is caring for a patient with metabolic alkalosis secondary to diuretic medication. Which equipment does the nurse obtain to administer the correct therapy to this patient?
    a. Oxygen tubing and cannula or mask
    b. IV catheter and IV start kit
    c. Foley catheter and drainage bag
    d. Antiemetic drug and emesis basin

41. Which occurrence can be a result of hyperventilation?
    a. Hypocalcemia
    b. Anxiety
    c. Respiratory alkalosis
    d. Respiratory acidosis

42. Which patient showing symptoms of an acid-base imbalance must the nurse see **first**?
    a. Patient who exhibits increased heart rate of 110/min and increased cardiac output
    b. Patient showing activity weakness and lethargy
    c. Patient who has a reduced attention span
    d. Patient who has asymptomatic bradycardia with a heart rate of 57/min

43. A patient has taken antacids for the past 3 days to relieve "heartburn." What alteration in acid-base balance would the nurse expect for this patient?
    a. Respiratory alkalosis
    b. Metabolic acidosis
    c. Metabolic alkalosis
    d. Respiratory acidosis

44. A patient with anemia has completed a blood transfusion of 2 units of packed red blood cells. Which imbalance should the nurse monitor for **after** the blood transfusion?
    a. Metabolic alkalosis
    b. Respiratory acidosis
    c. Metabolic acidosis
    d. Respiratory alkalosis

45. A patient has had diarrhea for the past 2 days. Which acid-base abnormalities would the nurse monitor for? **Select all that apply.**
    a. Overelimination of bicarbonate
    b. Respiratory alkalosis
    c. Metabolic acidosis
    d. Underelimination of hydrogen ions
    e. Overproduction of hydrogen ions
    f. Elevated potassium

46. A patient who has advanced muscular dystrophy may develop which complications related to the disease? **Select all that apply.**
    a. Hyperventilation
    b. Hypoventilation
    c. Underproduction of bicarbonate
    d. Respiratory acidosis
    e. Underelimination of hydrogen ions
    f. Decreased chest wall movement

47. A patient who has a decreased amount of hydrogen ions and a decreased amount of carbon dioxide in the body will have what response?
    a. Decreased rate and depth of respirations
    b. Decreased renal absorption of hydrogen ions
    c. Increased rate and depth of respirations
    d. Decreased renal excretions of bicarbonate

48. A patient's ABG results reveal respiratory acidosis. How does the body compensate for this imbalance?
    a. Loss of bicarbonate
    b. Regular, unlabored respirations
    c. Hypoventilation
    d. Renal reabsorption of bicarbonate

49. The nurse is caring for a patient with excessive alcohol ingestion and salicylate intoxication. What is the **most likely** acid-base imbalance this patient will have?
    a. Bicarbonate underelimination
    b. Bicarbonate loss
    c. Metabolic acidosis
    d. Metabolic alkalosis

50. Which ABG results would the nurse interpret as metabolic alkalosis?
    a. pH 7.30, $Paco_2$ 66, bicarbonate 38, Pao_2 70
    b. pH 7.52, $Paco_2$ 45, bicarbonate 36, Pao_2 95
    c. pH 7.55, $Paco_2$ 24, bicarbonate 20, Pao_2 95
    d. pH 7.28, $Paco_2$ 24, bicarbonate 15, Pao_2 95

51. Which arterial blood gas results would the nurse interpret as within normal limits?
    a. pH 7.28, $Paco_2$ 24, bicarbonate 15, Pao_2 95
    b. pH 7.45, $Paco_2$ 41, bicarbonate 25, Pao_2 97
    c. pH 7.35, $Paco_2$ 24, bicarbonate 15, Pao_2 95
    d. pH 7.30, $Paco_2$ 66, bicarbonate 38, Pao_2 70

52. A patient has a low pH level. Which other concurrent change does the nurse expect to see in this patient?
    a. Elevated serum sodium level
    b. Elevated serum potassium
    c. Decreased serum chloride level
    d. Decreased serum calcium level

53. Which assessment finding indicates that a patient with chronic respiratory acidosis is responding favorably to treatment?
    a. Nail beds pale, extremities cool
    b. Respiratory stridor with inspiration
    c. Expectorating clear, thin mucus
    d. Diffuse crackles auscultated bilaterally

54. To ensure the safety of a patient with metabolic alkalosis, which task is best delegated to the unlicensed assistive personnel (UAP)?
    a. Watch the patient when he or she eats or drinks anything.
    b. Sit with the patient to prevent wandering.
    c. Assist the patient to the bathroom as needed.
    d. Remove all sharp objects from the bedside table.

55. Which arterial blood gas (ABG) value indicates an alkaline condition?
    a. $Paco_2$ = 66
    b. Bicarbonate = 16
    c. pH = 7.55
    d. pH = 7.32

56. Which conditions cause the underproduction of bicarbonate? **Select all that apply.**
    a. Heavy exercise
    b. Kidney failure
    c. Liver failure
    d. Seizure activity
    e. Dehydration
    f. Diarrhea

13 CHAPTER

Principles of Infusion Therapy

1. Which activities are performed by infusion nurses? **Select all that apply.**
   a. Develop evidence-based policies and procedures.
   b. Insert and maintain peripheral and central venous catheters.
   c. Develop new products for more effective infusion therapy.
   d. Consult on product selection and purchasing decisions.
   e. Monitor patient outcomes of infusion therapy.
   f. Provide education to staff, patients, and families.

2. The nurse is preparing to start an infusion of dextrose 10% in water (D10W). Why would the nurse infuse the solution through a central line?
   a. Osmolarity of the solution could cause phlebitis or thrombosis.
   b. The patient could be at risk for fluid overload.
   c. Viscosity of the solution would slow the infusion.
   d. This solution should not be mixed with other drugs or solutions.

3. Intravenous therapy with a hypotonic fluid is ordered for the patient. The nurse would plan to start which solution?
   a. 0.9% NaCl
   b. 0.45% NaCl
   c. 5% dextrose and 0.9% saline
   d. Lactated Ringer's solution

4. A patient with lung cancer is to receive his first chemotherapy treatment. Which IV access methods are appropriate for this patient? **Select all that apply.**
   a. Peripheral IV access
   b. Peripherally inserted central catheter (PICC)
   c. Dialysis catheter
   d. Tunneled central venous catheter
   e. Implanted port
   f. Intraarterial catheter

5. A patient has a peripherally inserted central catheter (PICC) placed and receives IV cisplatin. The drug has infiltrated into the tissue, and redness is observed in the right lower side of the neck. What is the nurse's **first** action?
   a. Apply cold compresses to the site of swelling.
   b. Stop the infusion and disconnect the IV line from the administration set.
   c. Aspirate the drug from the IV access device.
   d. Monitor the patient and document.

6. The nurse is preparing to give a patient IV drug therapy. What information does the nurse need before administering the drug? **Select all that apply.**
   a. Indications, contraindications, and precautions for IV therapy
   b. Appropriate dilution, pH, and osmolarity of solution
   c. Rate of infusion and dosage of drugs
   d. Percentage of adverse events for the drug
   e. Compatibility with other IV medications
   f. Parameters to monitor related to immediate drug effects

7. The charge nurse is reviewing IV therapy orders. What information **must** be included in each order? **Select all that apply.**
   a. Specific type of solution
   b. Rate of administration
   c. Specific drug dose to be added to the solution
   d. Method for diluting drugs for the solution
   e. Specific type of administration equipment
   f. Frequency of drug administration

8. The nurse must insert a short peripheral IV catheter. To decrease the risk of deep vein thrombosis or phlebitis, which area of the arm should be chosen for insertion of the IV catheter?
   a. Wrist
   b. Hand
   c. Forearm
   d. Antecubital area

9. A patient requires IV therapy via a peripheral line. What factors does the nurse consider when inserting the peripheral IV? **Select all that apply.**
   a. Use either an upper or lower extremity for the insertion site.
   b. For older adults, start with more distal sites, such as the hand veins.
   c. For active adults, start with more proximal sites, such as the forearm.
   d. Choose the patient's nondominant arm.
   e. Do not use the arm if the patient had a mastectomy on that side.
   f. If the vein is hard and cordlike, use an indirect approach.
   g. Avoid placing an IV on the anterior surface of the wrist.

10. While assessing a patient's IV site, the nurse identifies signs and symptoms of infiltration. What is the **first** action that the nurse implements for this patient?
    a. Elevate the extremity.
    b. Apply a sterile dressing if weeping from the tissue has occurred.
    c. Remove the IV access.
    d. Stop the IV infusion.

11. After completing the insertion of a peripherally inserted central catheter (PICC), which entries does the nurse make in the documentation? **Select all that apply.**
    a. Type of dressing applied
    b. Response of the family to IV access
    c. Type of IV access device used
    d. How long it took to place the IV access
    e. Vein that was used for insertion
    f. Length of catheter, the insertion site, and tip location

12. The nurse is selecting a site for peripheral IV insertion. Which patient condition influences the choice of left versus right upper extremity?
    a. Pneumothorax with a chest tube on the right side
    b. Myocardial infarction with pain radiating down the left arm
    c. Right hip fracture with immobilization and traction in place
    d. Regular renal dialysis with a shunt in the left upper forearm

13. The nurse is attempting to insert a peripheral IV when the patient reports tingling and a feeling like "pins and needles." What does the nurse do **next**?
    a. Change to a short-winged butterfly needle.
    b. Stop immediately, remove the catheter, and choose a new site.
    c. Ask the patient to wiggle the fingers to stimulate circulation.
    d. Pause the procedure and gently massage the fingers.

14. A patient has been on prolonged steroid therapy. In assessing the patient for an IV insertion site, what finding does the nurse expect to see?
    a. Ecchymosis and possibly a hematoma
    b. Skin that is thick, tough, dry, and difficult to puncture
    c. Edema or puffiness, making visualization of veins difficult
    d. Rash with excoriation from scratching, which limits site selection

15. Under what circumstance does the nurse elect to use one secondary set to administer multiple medications instead of a secondary set to administer each medication?
    a. When multiple intermittent medications are required
    b. To eliminate the cost of using multiple secondary sets
    c. When the nurse is using the back-priming method
    d. When the medications are compatible

16. When using an intermittent administration set to deliver medications, how often does the Infusion Nurses Society (INS) recommend that the set be changed?
    a. Every 24 hours
    b. Every shift
    c. Every morning
    d. After every dose

17. The nurse is supervising a student nurse who is preparing an IV bag with IV administration tubing. For which action by the student nurse **must** the nurse intervene?
    a. The student touches the drip chamber.
    b. The sterile cap from the distal end of the set is removed.
    c. The distal end is attached to a needleless connector.
    d. The student touches the tubing spike.

18. The nurse is caring for a patient with a peripherally inserted central catheter (PICC) line. According to recommendations by the Infusion Nurses Society (INS), which technique does the nurse use in maintaining this type of catheter?
    a. Flush the catheter with 10 mL heparinized saline after each dose of IV medication.
    b. Use 10 mL of sterile saline to flush before and after medication.
    c. Avoid flushing the catheter more than twice a week.
    d. Flush the catheter every 12 hours using a 20-mL syringe.

19. A patient has a peripherally inserted central catheter (PICC) placed by an IV therapy nurse at the bedside. Before using the catheter, how is its placement verified?
    a. The provider who ordered the procedure verifies placement.
    b. The line is aspirated gently, and the nurse watches for blood return.
    c. A chest x-ray is taken, which shows the catheter tip in the lower superior vena cava.
    d. The line is slowly flushed with 10 mL of saline while the nurse notes the ease of flow.

20. A patient requires a nontunneled percutaneous central catheter. What is the nurse's role in this procedure?
    a. Insert the catheter using sterile technique.
    b. Place the patient in Trendelenburg position.
    c. Read the chest x-ray to validate placement.
    d. Select and prepare the insertion site.

21. A patient requires an infusion of packed red blood cells (PRBCs). Which factor allows the nurse to infuse the PRBCs through the patient's peripherally inserted central catheter PICC?
    a. Length of the PICC allows infusion within 6 hours.
    b. The nurse is unable to obtain an infusion pump.
    c. Lumen size of the PICC is 4 Fr or larger.
    d. PRBCs can be warmed before infusion.

22. Which patient is the most likely candidate for a tunneled central venous catheter?
    a. Patient with trauma from a motor vehicle accident
    b. Patient in need of IV antibiotics for several weeks
    c. Patient in need of permanent parenteral nutrition
    d. Patient in need of intermittent chemotherapy

23. Which nursing interventions are implemented when caring for a patient with an implanted port? **Select all that apply.**
    a. Before puncture, palpate the port to locate the septum.
    b. Use a large-bore needle to access the port.
    c. Flush the port before each use.
    d. Use a noncoring needle to access the port.
    e. Flush the port at least once a month.
    f. Check for blood return before giving any drug through a port.

24. A 65-year-old patient has been receiving IV $D_5 1/2$ NS (normal saline) at 100 mL/ hr for the past 3 days, along with IV antibiotic therapy. The patient reports chills and a headache. On assessment, the patient's temperature is elevated. What complication do these assessment findings suggest?
    a. Catheter-related infection in the blood
    b. Allergic reaction to the antibiotics
    c. Phlebitis
    d. Fluid volume overload

25. Which disadvantage accompanies the placement of a large-bore peripheral IV catheter?
    a. Increased bloodstream infections
    b. Increased occurrence of phlebitis
    c. Decreased time to need for catheter replacement
    d. Decreased size of vein to accommodate catheter

26. What is the minimum size peripheral IV catheter through which a blood transfusion can be infused?
    a. 24 gauge
    b. 22 gauge
    c. 20 gauge
    d. 18 gauge

27. A patient has a central line inserted in the vena cava. The nurse assesses the patient for which potential complications related to the procedure? **Select all that apply.**
    a. Phlebitis
    b. Hemothorax
    c. Air embolism
    d. Cardiac tamponade
    e. Arterial puncture
    f. Bloodstream infection

28. The nurse is assessing a patient's vascular access for phlebitis. The IV site shows erythema with swelling and pain. Based on Infusion Nurse Society (INS) standards, which grade of phlebitis would the nurse document?
    a. Grade 0
    b. Grade 1
    c. Grade 2
    d. Grade 3

29. A triple-lumen catheter central line is inserted in a patient. What does the nurse do **immediately after** the procedure?
    a. Start IV fluids, but at a slower rate to prevent any fluid overload.
    b. Watch and wait for any complications before using the site.
    c. Obtain a portable chest x-ray and hold IV fluids until results are obtained.
    d. Assess the patient including vital signs; if the patient is stable, start IV fluids.

30. When providing care for an older patient receiving IV fluids through a central line at 150 mL/hr, the nurse finds the patient has shortness of breath, cough, puffiness around the eyes, and crackles. What does the nurse do **next**?
    a. Place the patient in an upright position, administer oxygen, slow the IV rate, and notify the care provider.
    b. Assess for patency of the catheter, change the tubing, and resume IV fluids.
    c. Notify the provider, remove the central line, apply pressure, and place the patient in a semi-Fowler's position.
    d. Notify the provider, place the patient in Trendelenburg position, and administer urokinase to unclot the catheter.

31. Which interventions by the staff nurse are **essential** to prevent an infection in a patient with a central line? **Select all that apply.**
    a. Assess the dressing and insertion site of the central line.
    b. Employ aseptic technique when administering medications and changing tubing.
    c. Change the catheter every 72 hours and tubing every 24 hours.
    d. Monitor the patient's temperature for any elevation and give acetaminophen as needed.
    e. Use sterile technique when assisting the HCP with insertion of a central line.
    f. Use proper handwashing and nonsterile gloves before coming into contact with a central line.

32. A patient with an implanted port is discharged home to receive long-term therapy on an outpatient basis. How frequently must the implanted port be flushed between courses of therapy?
    a. Daily
    b. Weekly
    c. Monthly
    d. When therapy resumes

33. The nurse is preparing to deliver IV infusion therapy through an implanted port. What technique does the nurse use to access the port?
    a. Palpate the port, scrub skin, and access with a noncoring (Huber) needle.
    b. Scrub the port with alcohol and access with a needleless device.
    c. Scrub the port with Betadine and flush using a 10-mL syringe.
    d. Palpate the port, scrub skin, and access with a winged butterfly needle.

34. A patient is to be discharged home with an implanted port and needs discharge instructions on prescribed medication administration. Which instructions must the nurse give to the patient and family member who will be assisting the patient? **Select all that apply.**
    a. The device must be flushed every 24 hours.
    b. When the port is not accessed, an occlusive dressing should be applied.
    c. The skin will be punctured over the port when the port is accessed.
    d. When the port is not accessed, no dressing needs to be applied.
    e. The port must be flushed after each use.
    f. Check for blood return after medication administration.

35. The nurse is preparing to administer IV infusion therapy to a patient. When is the choice of using a glass container appropriate?
    a. When the patient needs a rapid infusion of fluids
    b. When the patient needs emergency transportation
    c. When the nurse must accurately read the container
    d. When the drug is incompatible with a plastic container

36. A patient requires a 2-month course of IV antibiotics to treat a resistant infection. Which device is chosen for this therapy?
    a. Short peripheral catheter
    b. Midline catheter
    c. Nontunneled percutaneous central catheter
    d. Peripherally inserted central catheter (PICC)

37. The nurse is attaching an administration set to a central venous catheter. Which type of equipment **decreases** the risk of accidental disconnection or leakage?
    a. Slip lock connector
    b. Luer-Lok connector
    c. Extension set
    d. Needleless connector

38. The nurse is adding a filter to an IV administration setup. Where is the **best** place to add the filter to the IV line?
    a. As close to the solution container as possible
    b. Immediately below the infusion pump
    c. At any convenient connection point
    d. As close as possible to the catheter hub

39. Which safety measures does the nurse apply to decrease the risk of catheter-related bloodstream infection (CR-BSI) related to needleless systems? **Select all that apply.**
    a. Clean needleless system connections vigorously every 24 hours.
    b. Tape connections between tubing sets.
    c. Clean all needleless connections vigorously for at least 60 seconds before connecting.
    d. Use evidence-based hand hygiene guidelines from the CDC and OSHA.
    e. Use needleless systems only when necessary.
    f. Discard needleless equipment in a biohazard container.

40. A patient is receiving IV therapy via an infusion pump. What is the **priority** nursing responsibility related to the equipment?
    a. Ensure the IV pump is programmed correctly.
    b. Monitor the patient's infusion site and rate.
    c. Check the equipment at the end of the infusion.
    d. Position the container for gravity flow.

41. Which characteristics apply to IV infusion pumps? **Select all that apply.**
    a. Deliver fluids under pressure
    b. Rely on gravity to create fluid flow
    c. Can be pole-mounted or ambulatory and portable
    d. Are best for accurate infusion
    e. Count drops to regulate flow
    f. Decrease drug errors through smart technology

42. Which content must the nurse be sure to teach a patient before central line insertion, specific to prevention of catheter-related bloodstream infection (CR-BSI)? **Select all that apply.**
    a. The type of catheter used
    b. Hand hygiene and aseptic technique for care of the catheter
    c. How to remove the catheter when it is no longer needed
    d. Activity limitations
    e. Signs and symptoms of complications
    f. That there is no alternative to the catheter placement or therapy

43. The nurse is assessing a patient's IV insertion site. What must the nurse look for during the assessment? **Select all that apply.**
    a. Observe for redness and swelling.
    b. Check that the dressing is clean and dry.
    c. Ensure that the dressing is adherent to the skin.
    d. Observe for yellow discoloration.
    e. Observe for hardness or drainage.
    f. Check for blood patency and blood return.

44. A patient's central venous IV site is covered with a transparent membrane dressing. How often does the nurse change this dressing?
    a. Every 24 hours
    b. Every 48 hours
    c. Every 5 to 7 days
    d. The dressing does not need changing

45. A patient is ordered to receive peripheral parenteral nutrition (PPN). What type of access device is appropriate for this patient?
    a. Peripheral 20-gauge IV needle
    b. Nontunneled percutaneous central catheter
    c. Peripheral 22-gauge IV needle
    d. Peripherally inserted central catheter (PICC)

46. An external long-term IV catheter is required for hemodialysis of a hospitalized patient. Which statements are true about this external long-term IV access device? **Select all that apply.**
    a. Should not be used for administration of other fluids or medications except in an emergency
    b. Is required for hemodialysis because it has a large lumen
    c. Can often cause a common problem of venous thrombosis
    d. Features a port to access the catheter through
    e. Is a tunneled catheter with large lumen needed for long-term hemodialysis
    f. Requires aspiration of the previously instilled heparin before being used

47. The nurse has removed the dressing from a patient's central venous catheter site. To monitor the catheter position, what does the nurse do?
    a. Gently push the catheter into the insertion site.
    b. Slightly retract the catheter and observe the position.
    c. Mark the catheter with a pen to monitor the length.
    d. Note the length of the catheter external to the insertion site.

48. The nurse is caring for a patient with a central venous catheter. When changing the administration set or connectors, what measures will the nurse use to prevent air emboli? **Select all that apply.**
    a. Positions the patient flat so the catheter site is below the heart
    b. Uses the pinch clamp that can be closed during the procedure
    c. Uses sterile technique when handling the equipment
    d. Has an assistant apply pressure at the insertion site
    e. Asks the patient to perform the Valsalva maneuver by holding the breath and bearing down
    f. Times the IV set change to the expiratory cycle when the patient is spontaneously breathing

49. After assessing the patency of a patient's IV catheter, the nurse attempts to flush the catheter and meets resistance. What does the nurse do **next**?
    a. Get a larger-sized syringe and repeat the flush attempt.
    b. Use a heparinized solution and repeat the flush attempt.
    c. Gently force-flush the catheter using the push-pause method.
    d. Stop the flush attempt and discontinue the IV.

50. The nurse is flushing a patient's short peripheral IV catheter. What solution and volume does the nurse typically use for this procedure?
    a. 3 mL of normal saline
    b. 5 mL of heparin
    c. 10 mL of normal saline
    d. 30 mL of bacteriostatic saline

51. The patient is ready for discharge. Which actions must the nurse follow to remove the patient's peripheral catheter? **Select all that apply.**
    a. Hold pressure on the site until hemostasis is achieved.
    b. Flush the peripheral catheter with normal saline before removing.
    c. Assess the catheter tip to make sure it is intact and completely removed.
    d. Rapidly withdraw the catheter from the skin.
    e. Remove the peripheral catheter dressing.
    f. Document catheter removal and the appearance of the IV site.

52. While attempting to remove a PICC line, the nurse feels resistance. What technique does the nurse use **first** to attempt to resolve this problem?
    a. Gently pull on the catheter while the patient holds his or her breath.
    b. Place a cold pack on the extremity and give the patient a cold drink.
    c. Use simple distraction techniques and deep breathing.
    d. Place the patient in Trendelenburg position.

53. The nurse is assessing a short peripheral catheter after removal, and it appears that the catheter tip is missing. What does the nurse do **next**?
    a. Notify the health care provider.
    b. Assess the patient for symptoms of emboli.
    c. Apply firm pressure to the insertion site.
    d. Assess the extremity for coldness, cyanosis, or numbness.

54. Which instruction does the nurse give to an unlicensed assistive personnel (UAP) who has been delegated to check blood pressure on six patients being infused with peripheral IV fluids?
    a. "Be sure to put the infusion pumps on hold before taking blood pressures."
    b. "Have the patients sit up at the side of the bed before taking blood pressures."
    c. "Check blood pressures by placing the cuff at least 12 inches above the IV site."
    d. "Do the blood pressure checks on the arm that doesn't have the IV fluids infusing."

55. A patient has a local complication from a peripheral IV access with 0.9% normal saline infusing at 100 mL/hour. What does the nurse assess at the insertion site? **Select all that apply.**
    a. Blood returns in the catheter when nurse draws back on the IV access.
    b. A red streak is present proximal to the site.
    c. Edema is present proximal to the site.
    d. A scant amount of blood is noted beneath the clear dressing at the site.
    e. The IV fluids are not infusing.
    f. The patient reports numbness and tingling at the site.

56. The nurse is caring for the patient receiving arterial therapy via the carotid artery. What important nursing action is **specific** to this therapy?
    a. Assess the extremities for sensation and pulses.
    b. Monitor respirations for rate and regularity.
    c. Perform frequent neurologic assessments.
    d. Place antiembolic stockings on the patient's lower extremities.

57. Which statements are correct about intraperitoneal (IP) infusions? **Select all that apply.**
    a. Clean technique is used with IP access and supplies.
    b. IP can be accomplished by a catheter with an implanted port and large internal lumens.
    c. Strict aseptic technique is used with IP access and supplies.
    d. IP is used for patients who are receiving medications for diagnostic tests.
    e. IP can be accomplished by a tunneled catheter with capped ports and large internal lumens.
    f. IP is used for patients who are receiving chemotherapy agents.

58. During intraperitoneal therapy, a patient reports nausea and vomiting. What does the nurse do **next**?
    a. Help the patient move from side to side.
    b. Flush the catheter with normal saline.
    c. Reduce the flow rate and give antiemetics.
    d. Obtain an order for an abdominal x-ray.

59. In what position does the nurse place a patient before starting intraperitoneal therapy?
    a. Semi-Fowler's
    b. Prone
    c. Supine
    d. Side-lying

60. Which task would the nurse delegate to an unlicensed assistive personnel (UAP) for a patient receiving intraperitoneal therapy?
    a. Place the patient in a high Fowler's position for nausea.
    b. Assist the patient to move from side to side to distribute fluid evenly.
    c. Assess the patient for side effects of the therapy.
    d. Flush the catheter with normal saline when the therapy is completed.

61. Hypodermoclysis can be used for a patient under which types of circumstances? **Select all that apply.**
    a. If the patient requires palliative care
    b. For IV fluid replacement that is less than 2000 mL
    c. When a subcutaneous IV infusion is warranted
    d. If the patient requires acute care
    e. When short-term fluid volume replacement is warranted
    f. When a patient requires emergency resuscitation

62. The nurse is preparing to start a hypodermoclysis treatment on a patient. What is a **preferred** insertion site?
    a. Anterior forearm
    b. Anterior tibial area
    c. Lateral aspect of the upper arm
    d. Area under the clavicle

63. The home health nurse is adjusting the rate for a hypodermoclysis treatment. What is the usual **maximum** rate for this therapy?
    a. 20 mL/hr
    b. 30 mL/hr
    c. 80 mL/hr
    d. 120 mL/hr

64. The home health nurse is caring for a patient receiving hypodermoclysis therapy. How often are the subcutaneous sites rotated?
    a. Every 4 hours
    b. Every 24 hours
    c. At least every 3 days
    d. At least once a week

65. Which illnesses can be treated by an intrathecal infusion? **Select all that apply.**
    a. Cancer of the central nervous system
    b. Reflex sympathetic dystrophy
    c. Irritable bowel syndrome
    d. Multiple sclerosis
    e. Leukemia
    f. Anoxic acquired brain injury

66. A patient is receiving epidural medication therapy. The nurse assesses for which potential problem specific to this type of therapy?
    a. Meningitis
    b. Loss of bowel function
    c. Allergic reactions
    d. Cardiac dysrhythmias

67. A patient is brought to the emergency department (ED) after a serious motor vehicle accident. Which factor makes the patient a candidate for intraosseous (IO) therapy?
    a. Patient has a history of chronic renal failure.
    b. Endotracheal intubation is difficult to accomplish.
    c. Patient is an older adult and very thin.
    d. IV access cannot be achieved within a few minutes.

68. A patient has an intraosseous (IO) needle in place. Why does the nurse advocate for removal of the device within 24 hours after insertion?
    a. There is an increased risk for osteomyelitis.
    b. There is an increased risk for arterial insufficiency.
    c. The device hinders patient mobility.
    d. The device is unstable and easily dislodged.

69. The patient has an order for one unit of packed red blood cells (PRBCs). Which **priority** action must the nurse complete before starting this infusion?
    a. Place a new IV line designated only for blood product infusion.
    b. Ensure that the IV line to be used for infusion is larger than 22-gauge.
    c. Check patient identification with another RN using two identifiers.
    d. Ensure that the unit of PRBCs has been warmed to body temperature.

70. Which site is most commonly used for intraosseous (IO) therapy?
    a. Distal femur
    b. Proximal humerus
    c. Iliac crest
    d. Proximal tibia

71. The patient has an order for 0.45% normal saline 1000 mL to infuse over 15 hours. At what rate in mL/hr would the nurse set the infusion pump?
    a. 50 mL/hr
    b. 67 mL/hr
    c. 75 mL/hr
    d. 83 mL/hr

72. Which **priority** concept is of concern to the nurse when performing infusion therapy?
    a. Acid-base imbalance
    b. Tissue integrity
    c. Fluid and electrolyte balance
    d. Perfusion

14

CHAPTER

Care of Preoperative Patients

1. Which is the top priority for nurses during the perioperative period?
   a. Patient teaching
   b. Patient diagnostic testing
   c. Patient safety
   d. Patient care documentation

2. During the perioperative period a patient receives surgery on the wrong extremity. To which agency must this occurrence be reported?
   a. Association of periOperative Registered Nurses (AORN)
   b. Centers for Medicare and Medicaid Services (CMS)
   c. The Joint Commission (TJC)
   d. American Society of Anesthesiologists (ASA)

3. Which statements best describe the preoperative period? **Select all that apply.**
   a. It begins when the patient makes the appointment with the surgeon to discuss the need for surgery.
   b. It ends at the time of transfer to the surgical suite.
   c. It is a time during which the patient's need for surgery is established.
   d. It begins when the patient is scheduled for surgery.
   e. It is a time during which the patient receives testing and education related to impending surgery.
   f. It is a time when patients and families receive discharge instructions.

4. Which are the focus areas for the Surgical Care Improvement Project (SCIP)? **Select all that apply.**
   a. Prevention of infection
   b. Prevention of respiratory complications
   c. Prevention of serious cardiac events
   d. Prevention of venous thromboembolism
   e. Prevention of acute kidney injury
   f. Maintenance of normothermia

5. A female patient is having a biopsy of a nodule found in the right breast. Which classification identifies this surgery?
   a. Urgent
   b. Minor
   c. Cosmetic
   d. Diagnostic

6. A patient who can barely ambulate with a walker at home is having a left total knee replacement. What is the **most** appropriate category for this surgery?
   a. Urgent
   b. Restorative
   c. Simple
   d. Palliative

7. A colostomy is scheduled to be done on a patient who has severe Crohn's disease. What is the correct classification for this surgery?
   a. Palliative
   b. Minor
   c. Restorative
   d. Curative

8. A male patient is having revision of a scar on his forehead from a third-degree burn. What is the correct classification for this surgery?
   a. Major
   b. Restorative
   c. Cosmetic
   d. Curative

9. An appendectomy is being performed on a patient with appendicitis. What is the correct classification for this surgery?
   a. Curative
   b. Diagnostic
   c. Urgent
   d. Radical

10. A patient with an abdominal aortic aneurysm is having surgical repair. What is the correct classification for this surgery?
    a. Restorative
    b. Emergent
    c. Urgent
    d. Minor

11. A 76-year-old patient is having a bilateral cataract removal. What is the correct classification for this surgery?
    a. Major
    b. Cosmetic
    c. Elective
    d. Emergent

12. A 47-year-old patient is having surgery to remove kidney stones. What is the correct classification for this surgery?
    a. Restorative
    b. Emergent
    c. Palliative
    d. Urgent

13. The patient is scheduled for same-day surgery for an uncomplicated cholecystectomy. Which surgical approach will **most likely** be used?
    a. Simple
    b. Minimally invasive
    c. Open
    d. Radical

14. The nurse screens a preoperative patient for conditions that may increase the risk for complications during the perioperative period. Which conditions are possible risk factors? **Select all that apply.**
    a. Emotionally stable
    b. Age 67
    c. Obesity
    d. Marathon runner
    e. Pulmonary disease
    f. Hypertension

15. A patient scheduled for surgery has a history of myocardial infarction 6 weeks ago. Which classification will this patient meet preoperatively based on the ASA Physical Status Classification system?
    a. ASA class I
    b. ASA class II
    c. ASA class III
    d. ASA class IV

16. A 75-year-old patient is having an exploratory laparotomy tomorrow. The wife tells the nurse that at night the patient gets up and walks around his room. What **priority** action does the nurse take after hearing this information?
    a. Notifies the provider
    b. Develops a plan to keep the patient safe
    c. Obtains an order for sleep medication
    d. Tells the patient not to get out of bed at night

17. The nurse has received a patient in the holding area who is scheduled for a left femoral-popliteal bypass. What are the **priority** safety measures for this patient before surgery? **Select all that apply.**
    a. The operative limb is marked by the surgeon.
    b. The patient is positively identified by checking the name and date of birth.
    c. The patient is asked to confirm the marked operative limb.
    d. The patient is identified by checking the name and room number.
    e. The patient is instructed to verify any family members waiting.
    f. The patient is kept on NPO status.

18. The 79-year-old patient with type 2 diabetes is scheduled for surgery to remove his left great toe. Which risk factors for complications of surgery does the nurse assess in this patient? **Select all that apply.**
    a. Presence of chronic illnesses
    b. Problems with healing
    c. Absence of smoking history
    d. Dehydration
    e. Electrolyte imbalances
    f. Daily exercise routine

19. During preoperative screening, the nurse discovers that the patient is allergic to shellfish. What is the nurse's **best first** action?
    a. Notifies the surgeon
    b. Develops a plan to keep the patient safe
    c. Obtains an order for a shellfish-free diet
    d. Asks the patient if any other family members have the same allergy

20. The preoperative patient tells the nurse that she is afraid that she may experience a reaction if she must receive blood during or after her surgery. What is the nurse's **best** response to the patient's concern?
    a. "The likelihood that you will need a blood transfusion for your surgery is minimal, so do not worry about this."
    b. "You could donate some of your own blood (autologous donation) a few weeks before your surgery."
    c. "With today's technology and procedures, it is very unlikely that you would have a reaction to donated blood."
    d. "The nursing staff follows strict procedures to prevent such an event from ever happening."

21. The nurse is preparing the patient for surgery. Which common laboratory tests does the nurse anticipate being ordered? **Select all that apply.**
    a. Total cholesterol
    b. Urinalysis
    c. Electrolyte levels
    d. Uric acid
    e. Clotting studies
    f. Serum creatinine

22. Which statement is true regarding the patient who has given consent for a surgical procedure?
    a. Information necessary to understand the nature of and reason for the surgery has been provided.
    b. The length of stay in the hospital has been preapproved by the managed care provider.
    c. Information about the surgeon's experience has been provided.
    d. The nurse has provided detailed information about the surgical procedure.

23. Which statement best describes the collaborative roles of the nurse and surgeon when obtaining the informed consent?
    a. The nurse is responsible for having the informed consent form on the chart for the health care provider (HCP) to witness.
    b. The nurse may serve as a witness that the patient has been informed by the HCP before surgery is performed.
    c. The nurse may serve as witness to the patient's signature after the HCP has the consent form signed before preoperative sedation is given and before surgery is performed.
    d. The nurse has no duties regarding the consent form if the patient has signed the informed consent form for the HCP, even if the patient then asks additional questions about the surgery.

24. A patient with type 1 diabetes mellitus is scheduled for surgery at 0700. Which actions must the nurse perform for this patient before he goes to the operating room? **Select all that apply**
    a. Modify the dose of insulin given based on the patient's blood glucose as ordered.
    b. Complete the preoperative checklist before transfer to the surgical suite.
    c. Teach the patient about foot care and properly fitted shoes.
    d. Delegate obtaining the patient's fingerstick blood glucose and vital signs to the unlicensed assistive personnel (UAP).
    e. Check if the patient is wearing any jewelry and call security to secure valuables if necessary.
    f. Place the patient on NPO status for the period ordered by the surgeon.

25. After a patient is prepared for surgery and before preoperative drugs are given and the patient is transported to surgery, which essential intervention can the nurse delegate to the unlicensed assistive personnel (UAP) at this time?
    a. Assist the patient to empty his or her bladder.
    b. Help the patient to remove all clothing.
    c. Ask the patient if he or she wants to brush teeth.
    d. Recheck the patient's identity.

26. The nurse has given the ordered preoperative medications to the patient. What actions must the nurse take after administering these drugs? **Select all that apply.**
    a. Raise the side rails.
    b. Place the call light within the patient's reach.
    c. Ask the patient to sign the consent form.
    d. Instruct the patient not to get out of bed.
    e. Place the bed in its lowest position.
    f. Tell the patient that he or she may become drowsy.

27. Which postoperative interventions will the nurse typically teach a patient to prevent complications following surgery? **Select all that apply.**
    a. Range-of-motion exercises
    b. Massaging of lower extremities
    c. Taking pain medication only when experiencing severe pain
    d. Incision splinting
    e. Deep-breathing exercises
    f. Use of incentive spirometry

28. Which drug may the surgeon allow the patient to take prior to surgery?
    a. Daily vitamin
    b. Stool softener
    c. Antiseizure drug
    d. Daily baby aspirin

29. A blind patient is to have a surgical procedure. She asks the nurse whether she will be able to sign her own consent form. What is the nurse's **best** response?
    a. "Yes, but your signature will need to have two witnesses."
    b. "No, but your next of kin can sign the consent form for you."
    c. "Yes, but you will need to make an X instead of signing your name."
    d. "No, but you can give instructions to sign for you to any responsible adult."

30. An older adult is scheduled for an elective surgical procedure. On assessment the nurse notes brittle nails, dry flaky skin, muscle wasting, and dry sparse hair. The patient's BP is 82/48 and heart rate is 112/minute. How does the nurse interpret this assessment data?
    a. Poor fluid and nutrition status
    b. Improper care in the home
    c. Expected physiological changes of aging
    d. Depression related to aging processes

31. A preoperative patient is scheduled for surgery at 7:30 am. At 0600, the patient's vital signs are BP 90/60, HR 110 and irregular, respirations 22/minute, and oral temperature 100.9°F (38.3 °C). The patient's oxygen saturation is 92% and he has a productive cough. What is the nurse's **priority** action at this time?
    a. Administer acetaminophen (Tylenol) with just a sip of water.
    b. Recheck the vital signs at 7:00 am.
    c. Call and notify the surgeon immediately.
    d. Have the patient cough and take some deep breaths.

32. Which are implied with informed consent? **Select all that apply.**
    a. The patient understands the nature of and the reason for surgery.
    b. The patient is informed of what type of anesthesia drugs will be used.
    c. The patient understands who will do the surgery and who will be present during surgery.
    d. The patient understands the risks associated with the surgical procedure and its potential outcomes.
    e. The patient understands that blood and blood products must be available during surgery.
    f. The patient is informed of all available options and the benefits and risks associated with each option.

15
CHAPTER

Care of Intraoperative Patients

1. Which nursing intervention is **most** appropriate for the patient in the operative setting?
   a. Provide a climate of privacy, comfort, and confidentiality when caring for the patient.
   b. Instruct the patient that after the preoperative medication has taken effect, he or she will be drowsy.
   c. Avoid discussing the activities taking place around the patient while in the holding area.
   d. Assist members of the surgical team readying the operating room suite.

2. Which interventions must the operating room (OR) nurses provide for patient physiological integrity during the intraoperative period? **Select all that apply.**
   a. Apply padding to the OR bed to protect skin integrity.
   b. Communicate patient's fears about anesthesia to the nurse anesthetist.
   c. Monitor patient's airway, vital signs, electrocardiogram (ECG), and oxygen saturation during and after sedation.
   d. Assess and document skin condition before transferring patient to the postanesthesia care unit (PACU).
   e. Ensure that patient's wishes about advance directives are respected.
   f. Reposition the patient every 2 hours, especially for very long surgeries.

3. A patient with breast cancer is scheduled for a left mastectomy. The patient has informed the surgeon and nurse that she is a Jehovah's Witness and does not want any blood transfusions. In preparation for intraoperative care of this patient, what measures does the nurse take? **Select all that apply.**
   a. Obtain two units of packed red blood cells, typed and cross-matched.
   b. Make provider aware of patient's request for no blood transfusions.
   c. Ensure autotransfusion device is in place intraoperatively.
   d. Ensure patient has a medical necessity order for emergency blood transfusion.
   e. Inform the patient of potential risks if blood transfusion is not given.
   f. Tell the patient that in case of emergency she may receive blood to save her life.

4. To reduce the incidence of patients with a known history or risk of malignant hyperthermia (MH), what **best** practices are put in place in the operating room? **Select all that apply.**
   a. List of medications available for emergency treatment of MH
   b. Genetic counseling after each episode of MH
   c. Dedicated MH cart with treatment medications
   d. Treatment before, during, and after surgery if the patient has a known history or risk
   e. Additional nursing support on call if MH develops
   f. Available MH hotline number

5. A patient has an malignant hyperthermia (MH) incident during surgery. To whom does the nurse report this incident?
   a. North American Malignant Hyperthermia Registry
   b. The Joint Commission
   c. Centers for Disease Control
   d. Occupational Safety and Health Administration

6. Which duties are within the scope of practice of the circulating nurse in the operative setting?
   a. Manages the patient's care while the patient is in this area and initiates documentation on a perioperative nursing record
   b. Sets up the sterile field; assists with the draping of the patient; and hands sterile supplies, equipment, and instruments to the surgeon
   c. Assumes responsibility for the surgical procedure and any surgical judgments about the patient
   d. Coordinates, oversees, and participates in the patient's nursing care while the patient is in the operating room

7. During surgery, what things do anesthesia personnel monitor, measure, and assess?
   Select all that apply.
   a. Intake and output
   b. Room temperature
   c. Cardiopulmonary function
   d. Level of anesthesia
   e. Family concerns
   f. Vital signs

8. Which nursing interventions are appropriate during stage 2 of anesthesia?
   a. Prepare for and assist in treatment of cardiovascular and/or pulmonary arrest. Document in record.
   b. Shield patient from extra noise and physical stimuli. Protect the patient's extremities. Assist anesthesia personnel as needed. Stay with patient.
   c. Close operating room doors and control traffic in and out of room. Position patient securely with safety belts. Maintain minimal discussion in operating room.
   d. Assist anesthesia personnel with intubation of patient. Place the patient in position for surgery. Prep the patient's skin in area of operative site.

9. The acute, life-threatening complication of malignant hyperthermia (MH) results from the use of which agents?
   a. Hypnotics and neuromuscular blocking agents
   b. Succinylcholine and inhalation agents
   c. Nitrous oxide and pancuronium for muscle relaxation
   d. Fentanyl and regional anesthesia for spinal block

10. Which clinical features are found in a malignant hyperthermia (MH) crisis?
    Select all that apply.
    a. Sinus tachycardia
    b. Jaw muscle rigidity
    c. Hypotension
    d. A decrease in end-tidal carbon dioxide level
    e. Skin mottling and cyanosis
    f. An extremely elevated temperature at onset

11. The surgical team understands that time is crucial in recognizing and treating a malignant hyperthermia (MH) crisis. Once recognized, what is the treatment of choice?
    a. Danazol gluconate
    b. Phenytoin sodium
    c. Diazepam sulfate
    d. Dantrolene sodium

12. Which factors may lead to an anesthetic overdose in a patient? **Select all that apply.**
    a. Amount of anesthesia retained by fat cells
    b. Older age of patient
    c. Slowed metabolism and drug elimination
    d. An uncooperative patient
    e. Liver or kidney disease
    f. Drugs that alter metabolism

13. A patient experiences malignant hyperthermia (MH) immediately after induction of anesthesia. What is the nurse anesthetist's **priority** action?
    a. Administer IV dantrolene sodium (Dantrium) 2-3 mg/kg.
    b. Apply a cooling blanket over the torso.
    c. Assess arterial blood gases (ABGs) and serum chemistries.
    d. Stop all inhalation anesthetic agents and succinylcholine.

14. What techniques are essential to performing a proper surgical scrub of the hands by the surgeon, assistants, and scrub nurse? **Select all that apply.**
    a. Use a broad-spectrum, surgical antimicrobial solution.
    b. Scrub for 2 minutes, followed by a rinse with water.
    c. Use an alcohol-based antimicrobial solution.
    d. Hold hands and arms so that water runs off, not up or down the arms.
    e. Scrub for 3-5 minutes, followed by a rinse with water.
    f. Keep hands below the elbows during the scrub and rinse.

15. Which nursing interventions will prevent the potential intraoperative complication of radial nerve complications (wrist drop)?
    a. Support the wrist with padding; do not overtighten wrist straps.
    b. Place pillows or foam padding under bony prominences, maintain good body alignment, and slightly flex joints and support with pillows and pads.
    c. Pad the elbow, avoid excessive abduction, and secure the arm firmly on an arm board positioned at shoulder level.
    d. Place a safety strap above or below the area. Place a pillow or padding under the knees.

16. In which situations is regional anesthesia used instead of general anesthesia? **Select all that apply.**
    a. For an endoscopy or cardiac catheterization
    b. In patients who have had an adverse reaction to general anesthesia
    c. In some cases when pain management after surgery is enhanced by regional anesthesia
    d. In patients with serious medical problems
    e. When the patient has a preference and a choice is possible
    f. When the patient is having surgery of the head, neck, upper torso, and abdomen

17. Which characteristics are appropriate to moderate sedation drugs? **Select all that apply.**
    a. Reduce sensory perception.
    b. Require placement of an artificial airway.
    c. Amnesia action is short.
    d. Return to normal function is rapid.
    e. Increase level of consciousness.
    f. May be administered only by a physician.

18. To avoid electrical safety problems during surgery, what does the nurse do?
    a. Observes for breaks in sterile technique
    b. Continuously assists the anesthesia provider
    c. Ensures proper placement of the grounding pads
    d. Monitors the operating room with available cameras

19. Which medical condition **increases** a patient's risk for surgical wound infection?
    a. Anxiety
    b. Hiatal hernia
    c. Diabetes mellitus
    d. Amnesia

20. Which definition is appropriate for local anesthesia?
    a. Injection of anesthetic agent into or around a nerve or group of nerves, resulting in blocked sensation and motor impulse transmission.
    b. Injection of the anesthetic agent into the epidural space; the spinal cord areas are never entered.
    c. Injection of an anesthetic agent directly into the tissue around an incision, wound, or lesion.
    d. Injection of anesthetic agent that blocks multiple peripheral nerves and reduces sensation in a specific body region.

21. Which patient would be a candidate for moderate sedation? **Select all that apply.**
    a. Endoscopy
    b. Cesarean section delivery
    c. Closed fracture reduction
    d. Cardiac catheterization
    e. Abdominal surgery
    f. Cardioversion

22. A patient is requesting moderate sedation for repair of a torn meniscus and has no medical contraindications. How does the nurse respond to this patient's request?
    a. "Your surgeon will decide if you will receive moderate sedation or general anesthesia."
    b. "You can discuss your request for moderate sedation with your surgeon and anesthesiologist."
    c. "Most patients prefer general anesthesia. Can you tell me why you want moderate sedation?"
    d. "It can be frightening to see surgery done on yourself. You need to think about that."

23. The patient is scheduled to have minimally invasive surgery (MIS) for a laparoscopic cholecystectomy. Part of this surgery is the injection of air (insufflation) into the abdomen to separate and better see the organs. What patient teaching must the nurse do about the insufflation?
    a. "Your surgeon will make several small incisions instead of a large one."
    b. "You will be able to go home once your surgery is completed and you are awake."
    c. "You may experience some abdominal discomfort from the air injected with the surgery."
    d. "You will have a tube for drainage for a few days after your surgery is completed."

24. The patient in the OR holding area tells the nurse that his surgery is for the right foot. The patient's chart states that the surgery is for his left foot. What is the nurse's **best** action?
    a. Do nothing because the patient is confused after receiving premedications.
    b. Make a note about this in the nursing notes of the patient's chart.
    c. Call the nurse anesthetist to check whether the chart or patient is correct.
    d. Notify the surgeon immediately before the patient goes into the OR about this discrepancy.

25. The patient received moderate sedation (conscious sedation) intravenously prior to a bronchoscopy procedure. Before allowing the patient to have oral liquids, what must the nurse assess in this patient?
    a. The patient is arousable.
    b. The patient is able to speak.
    c. The patient's gag reflex is working.
    d. The patient is able to rotate his head.

26. The older overweight patient is being placed on the operating table for an appendectomy. What is the **priority** medical-surgical concept for this patient?
    a. Safety
    b. Tissue integrity
    c. Immunity
    d. Gas exchange

27. Which intervention takes priority when a patient is emerging and recovering from general anesthesia?
    a. Check vital signs every 5 minutes.
    b. Be prepared to suction the patient.
    c. Increase the rate of IV fluid administration.
    d. Check the patient's pupil sizes.

28. Which member of the operating room team is responsible for setting up the sterile field?
    a. Nurse anesthetist (CRNA)
    b. Surgical assistant
    c. Circulating nurse
    d. Scrub nurse

29. The patient is to receive regional anesthesia for injured knee repair surgery. Which type of regional anesthesia is this patient likely to receive?
    a. Field block
    b. Nerve block
    c. Spinal anesthesia
    d. Epidural anesthesia

30. The patient is transferred to the operating room for right foot surgery. How does the nurse safely assure the patient's identification?
    a. Ask the patient what type of surgery is scheduled.
    b. State the patient's name and ask the patient if he or she is that person.
    c. Check the patient's armband and ask the patient to state his or her name and birth date.
    b. Check the patient's chart and armband to assure that these match.

16 CHAPTER

Care of Postoperative Patients

1. Which description illustrates the beginning of the postoperative period?
   a. Completion of the surgical procedure and arousal of the patient from anesthesia in the operating room (OR)
   b. Providing care before, during, and after surgery
   c. Closure of the patient's surgical incision with sutures
   d. Completion of the surgical procedure and transfer of the patient to the postanesthesia care unit (PACU)

2. What is the primary purpose of a postanesthesia care unit (PACU)?
   a. Follow-through on the surgeon's postoperative orders
   b. Ongoing critical evaluation and stabilization of the patient
   c. Prevention of lengthened hospital stay
   d. Arousal of patient following the use of conscious sedation

3. A patient develops respiratory distress after having a left total hip replacement. The patient develops labored breathing, and a pulse oximetry reading is 83% on 2 L oxygen via nasal cannula. Which intervention is appropriate for the nurse to delegate to unlicensed assistive personnel (UAP)?
   a. Assess change in patient's respiratory status.
   b. Order necessary medications to be administered.
   c. Insert oral airway to maintain open airway.
   d. Check the patient's vital signs.

4. Which statement best describes phase I care after surgery?
   a. Phase I care occurs immediately after surgery, most often in a postanesthesia care unit (PACU).
   b. Phase I care focuses on preparing the patient for care in an extended care environment.
   c. Phase I care discharge occurs when presurgery level of consciousness has returned, oxygen saturation is at baseline, and vital signs are stable.
   d. Phase I care most often occurs on a hospital unit, in an extended care facility, or in the home.

5. The patient is recovering in a postanesthesia care unit (PACU) environment that advances the patient quickly from a Phase I care level to a Phase III care level, preparing for discharge to home. What type of surgery is this patient **most** likely having?
   a. Elective surgery
   b. Emergency surgery
   c. Same-day surgery
   d. Urgent surgery

6. Which signs/symptoms are considered postoperative complications? **Select all that apply.**
   a. Sedation
   b. Pain at the surgical site
   c. Pulmonary embolism
   d. Hypothermia
   e. Wound evisceration
   f. Postoperative ileus

7. If a patient experiences a wound dehiscence, which description best characterizes what is happening with the wound?
   a. Purulent drainage is present at incision site because of infection.
   b. Extreme pain is present at incision site.
   c. A partial or complete separation of outer layers is present at incision site.
   d. The inner and outer layers of the incision are separated.

8. A patient who is 2 days postoperative for abdominal surgery states, "I coughed and heard something pop." The nurse's immediate assessment reveals an opened incision with a portion of large intestine protruding. Which statements apply to this clinical situation? **Select all that apply.**
   a. Incision dehiscence has occurred.
   b. This is an emergency.
   c. The wound must be kept moist with normal saline-soaked sterile dressings.
   d. This is an urgent situation.
   e. Incision evisceration has occurred.
   f. A nasogastric (NG) tube may be ordered to decompress the stomach.

9. In the postanesthesia care unit (PACU), the nurse assesses that a patient is bleeding profusely from an abdominal incision. What is the nurse's **best first** action?
   a. Notify the surgeon.
   b. Apply pressure to the wound dressing.
   c. Instruct the unlicensed assistive personnel (UAP) to get additional dressing supplies.
   d. Request and draw a complete blood count.

10. Which members of the surgical team usually accompany a postoperative patient to the postanesthesia care unit (PACU)?
    a. Anesthesia provider and circulating nurse
    b. Circulating nurse and surgeon
    c. Surgeon and anesthesia provider
    d. Surgical assistant and surgeon

11. The nurse transfers a patient to the postanesthesia care unit (PACU) with an incision and drainage of an abscess in the right groin under general anesthesia. Blood pressure is 80/47 mm Hg, heart rate 117/min in sinus tachycardia, respiratory rate 28/min, pulse oximetry reading 93% on oxygen at 3 L per nasal cannula, and temp 101.3°F (38.5°C). The Jackson-Pratt drain has 70 mL of a cream-colored output. Normal saline is infusing at 150 mL/hr. The surgeon orders a bolus of 500 mL IV normal saline over 1 hour, two sets of blood cultures, and culture drainage from the Jackson-Pratt drain. The patient's history includes vulvar cancer with a needle biopsy of the right groin, hypertension treated with lisinopril 5 mg PO daily, and no known drug allergies. The patient is designated as a full code. Using the Situation, Background, Assessment, Recommendation (SBAR) charting format, which information should be included in assessment?
    a. Nurse transfers patient to the PACU with an incision and drainage of an abscess in the right groin with general anesthesia.
    b. Surgeon sends orders to bolus the patient with 500 mL normal saline over an hour, draw two sets of blood cultures, and send a culture of drainage from the Jackson-Pratt drain.
    c. Blood pressure is 80/47 mm Hg, heart rate 117/min in sinus tachycardia, respirations 28/min, pulse oximetry 93% on O_2 at 3 L nasal cannula, and temp 101.3°F (38.5°C); Jackson-Pratt drain with 70 mL cream-colored output.
    d. Patient had a right groin abscess. History of vulvar cancer. Needle biopsy of right groin completed 1 week ago. History of hypertension treated with lisinopril (Zestril) 5 mg. No known drug allergies. Full code.

12. A postoperative patient in the postanesthesia care unit (PACU) has had an open reduction internal fixation of a left fractured femur. Vital signs are blood pressure 87/49 mm Hg, heart rate 100/min sinus rhythm, respirations 22/min, and temperature 98.3°F (36.8°C). The Foley catheter has a total of 110 mL of clear yellow urine in the last 4 hours. Which body systems have been assessed by the nurse? **Select all that apply.**
    a. Respiratory
    b. Cardiovascular
    c. Neurovascular
    d. Integumentary
    e. Renal/urinary
    f. Gastrointestinal

13. A patient cared for in the postanesthesia care unit (PACU) had a colostomy placed for treatment of Crohn's disease. The nurse assesses that an abdominal dressing is 25% saturated with serosanguineous drainage and the incision is intact. An IV is infusing with D_5/lactated Ringer's at 100 mL/hr through a 20-g peripheral IV access. Auscultation of abdomen reveals hypoactive bowel sounds in all four quadrants, abdomen soft, and no distention. Foley catheter is in place and draining yellow urine with sediment, 375 mL output in Foley bag. Which body systems have been assessed by the nurse? **Select all that apply.**
    a. Renal/urinary
    b. Gastrointestinal
    c. Respiratory
    d. Musculoskeletal
    e. Integumentary
    f. Cardiovascular

14. A 49-year-old patient is in the postanesthesia care unit (PACU) following a frontal craniotomy for repair of a ruptured cerebral aneurysm. The nurse assesses that the patient's eyes open on verbal stimulation. Pupils are equal and reactive to light, and diameter is 3 mm. The patient's hand grasps are equal and strong. The patient is able to state name correctly. The patient has had one episode of nausea and vomiting. Incision edges are dry and approximated with sutures. Lung sounds are slightly diminished on auscultation, and the nurse observes the patient is using abdominal accessory muscles to breathe. Which body systems has the nurse assessed? **Select all that apply.**
    a. Cardiovascular
    b. Gastrointestinal
    c. Neurologic
    d. Integumentary
    e. Respiratory
    f. Renal/urinary

15. The postanesthesia care unit (PACU) nurse is assessing a patient transferred in from the OR. Which assessment findings apply to assessment of the cardiovascular system? **Select all that apply.**
    a. Opens eyes on command.
    b. Absent dorsalis pedis pulse in left foot.
    c. Foley catheter in place with clear yellow drainage.
    d. Monitor shows normal sinus rhythm.
    e. States name correctly when asked.
    f. Apical pulse 85 beats/minute.

16. The postanesthesia care unit (PACU) nurse is receiving the "handoff" report for a patient transferred in from the OR. Which statements about this report are accurate? **Select all that apply.**
    a. A handoff report requires clear, concise language.
    b. A handoff report is a two-way verbal interaction between the health care professional giving the report and the nurse receiving it.
    c. A handoff report should be individualized based on the patient and his or her surgery.
    d. The receiving nurse takes the time to restate (report back) the information to verify what was said.
    e. The receiving nurse takes the time to ask questions, and the reporting professional must respond to the questions until a common understanding is established.
    f. The receiving nurse continues assessing other patients while the handoff report is being given.

17. A patient arrives in the postanesthesia care unit (PACU). Which action does the nurse perform **first**?
    a. Assess for a patent airway and adequate gas exchange.
    b. Assess the patient's pain level using the 0-10 pain assessment scale.
    c. Position the patient in a supine position to prevent aspiration.
    d. Calculate the patient-controlled analgesia (PCA) pump maximum dose per hour to avoid an overdose.

18. A patient arrives at the postanesthesia care unit (PACU), and the nurse notes a respiratory rate of 10 with sternal retractions. The report from the anesthesia provider indicates that the patient received fentanyl during surgery. What is the nurse's **best first** action?
    a. Monitor the patient for effects of anesthetic for at least 1 hour.
    b. Closely monitor vital signs and pulse oximetry readings until the patient is responsive.
    c. Administer oxygen as ordered, monitoring pulse oximetry.
    d. Maintain an open airway through positioning and suction if needed.

19. The nurse is teaching incisional care to a patient who is being discharged after abdominal surgery. Which **priority** instruction must the nurse include?
    a. Do not rub or touch the incision site.
    b. Practice proper handwashing.
    c. Clean the incision site two times a day with soap and water.
    d. Splint the incision site as often as needed for comfort.

20. The health care team determines a patient's readiness for discharge from the postanesthesia care unit (PACU) by noting a postanesthesia recovery score of at least 10. After determining that all criteria have been met, the patient is discharged to the hospital unit or home. Review the patient profiles after 1 hour in the PACU listed below. Which patient should the nurse expect to be discharged from the PACU **first**?
    a. 10-year-old female, tonsillectomy, general anesthesia. Duration of surgery 30 minutes. Immediate response to voice. Alert to place and person. Able to move all extremities. Respirations even, deep, rate of 20. Vital signs (VS) are within normal limits. IV solution is D_5RL. Has voided on bedpan. Eating ice chips. Complaining of sore throat.
    b. 55-year-old male, repair of fractured lower left leg. General anesthesia. Duration of surgery 1 hour, 30 minutes. Drowsy, but responds to voice. Nausea and vomiting twice in PACU. No urge to void at this time. IV infusing D_5NS. Pedal pulses noted in both lower extremities. VS: temperature 98.6° F (37°C); pulse 130 beats/min; respiratory rate 24/min; blood pressure 124/76 mm Hg.
    c. 24-year-old male, reconstruction of facial scar. General anesthesia. Duration of surgery 2 hours. Sleeping, groans to voice command. VS are within normal limits. Respirations 10 breaths/min. No urge to void. IV of D_5RL infusing. Complains of pain in surgical area.
    d. 42-year-old female, colonoscopy. IV conscious sedation. Awake and alert. Up to bathroom to void. IV discontinued. Resting quietly in chair. VS are within normal limits.

21. The nurse is caring for a patient who has had abdominal surgery. After a hard sneeze, the patient reports pain in the surgical area, and the nurse immediately sees that the patient has a wound evisceration. What priority action must the nurse do **first**?
    a. Call for help and stay with the patient.
    b. Leave the patient to immediately call the surgeon.
    c. Cover the wound with a nonadherent dressing moistened with normal saline.
    d. Take the patient's vital signs.

22. Which intervention for postsurgical care of a patient is correct?
    a. When positioning the patient, use the knee gatch of the bed to bend the knees and relieve pressure.
    b. Gently massage the lower legs and calves to promote venous blood return to the heart.
    c. Encourage bedrest for 3 days after surgery to prevent complications.
    d. Teach the patient to splint the surgical wound for support and comfort when getting out of bed.

23. The morning after a patient's lower leg surgery, the nurse notes that the dressing is wet from drainage. The surgeon has not yet been in to see the patient on rounds. What does the nurse do about the dressing?
    a. Removes the dressing and puts on a dry, sterile dressing.
    b. Reinforces the dressing by adding dry, sterile dressing material on top of the existing dressing.
    c. Applies dry, sterile dressing material directly to the wound and then retapes the original dressing.
    d. Does nothing to the dressing but calls the surgeon to evaluate the patient immediately.

24. The postanesthesia care unit (PACU) nurse is caring for a postoperative patient. The patient's oxygen saturation drops from 98% to 88%. What is the nurse's **priority** action?
    a. Call the anesthesia provider.
    b. Call the surgeon.
    c. Call the Rapid Response Team.
    d. Call the respiratory therapist.

25. What information should be included in the handoff report when a patient is transferred from the OR to the postanesthesia care unit (PACU) staff? **Select all that apply.**
    a. Type and extent of surgical procedure.
    b. Intraoperative complications and how they were handled.
    c. List of usual daily medications.
    d. Type and amount of IV fluids and blood products given.
    e. Location and type of incisions, dressings, catheters, tubes, drains, or packing.
    f. Name, address, and phone number of next of kin.

26. The nurse on the medical-surgical unit is caring for a postoperative patient. Which assessment criteria indicate to the nurse that the patient is experiencing respiratory difficulty? **Select all that apply.**
    a. The patient's oxygen saturation drops from 98% to 94%.
    b. The patient is using accessory muscles to breathe.
    c. The patient makes a high-pitched crowing sound when breathing.
    d. The patient's blood pressure drops from 120/80 to 110/78 mm Hg.
    e. The patient's respiratory rate is 29/min.
    f. The patient's urine output drops from 50 mL/hr to 30 mL/hr.

27. When assessing the hydration status of an older postoperative patient, where must the nurse assess for tenting of the skin? **Select all that apply.**
    a. On the back of the hand
    b. On the forehead
    c. On the forearm
    d. On the sternum
    e. On the abdomen
    f. On the thigh

28. Which patient is most at risk for postoperative nausea and vomiting (PONV)?
    a. The patient with a history of motion sickness
    b. The patient with a nasogastric tube
    c. The patient who recently experienced a weight loss of 50 pounds
    d. The patient who had minimally invasive surgery (MIS)

29. The nurse is assessing a postoperative patient's gastrointestinal system. What is the **best** indicator that peristaltic activity has resumed?
    a. Presence of bowel sounds
    b. Patient states he is hungry
    c. Passing of flatus or stool
    d. Presence of abdominal cramping

30. The postanesthesia care unit (PACU) nurse is assessing an older adult patient for postoperative pain. Which nonverbal manifestations by the patient suggest pain to the nurse? **Select all that apply.**
    a. Restlessness
    b. Profuse sweating
    c. Difficult to arouse
    d. Confusion
    e. Increased blood pressure
    f. Decreased heart rate

31. Which indicator of return to consciousness occurs **first** as a patient recovers from general anesthesia?
    a. Muscular irritability
    b. Restlessness and delirium
    c. Recognition of pain
    d. Ability to reason and control behavior

32. The medical-surgical nurse is caring for a postoperative patient whose lab values reveal an increase in band cells (immature neutrophils). What is the nurse's **best** interpretation of this value?
    a. The patient may need a transfusion.
    b. The patient is using up clotting factors.
    c. The patient is developing an infection.
    d. The patient's result is expected postoperatively.

33. Which are interventions for the medical-surgical nurse to use in preventing hypoxemia for the postoperative patient? **Select all that apply.**
    a. Monitor the patient's oxygen saturation.
    b. Position the patient supine.
    c. Encourage the patient to cough and breathe deeply.
    d. Get the patient ambulating as soon as possible.
    e. Instruct the patient to rest as much as possible.
    f. Remind the patient to use incentive spirometry every hour while awake.

34. The health care provider removed a patient's original surgical dressing 2 days after surgery and is discharging the patient home with daily dressing changes. Which actions will the nurse take for this patient's discharge teaching? **Select all that apply.**
    a. Ask the patient's family or significant other to observe the dressing change.
    b. Ask the UAP to get dressing supplies for the patient.
    c. Instruct that the drainage will appear serosanguineous.
    d. Instruct the patient to go to the emergency department (ED) for problems related to dressing changes.
    e. Have the case manager arrange for a home health nurse to ensure that dressing changes are done and there are no complications or infection.
    f. Teach the patient and family the signs and symptoms of infection.

35. The patient who received moderate sedation with midazolam appears to be overly sedated and has respiratory depression. Which drug does the nurse prepare to administer to this patient?
    a. Lorazepam
    b. Naloxone
    c. Flumazenil
    d. Butorphanol tartrate

36. Which are criteria used by the health care team to determine when a patient is ready to be discharged from the PACU? **Select all that apply.**
    a. Recovery rating score of 7 to 10 on rating scale
    b. Stable vital signs with normal body temperature
    c. Ability to swallow but remains NPO for at least 4 hours
    d. Intact cough and swallow reflexes
    e. Adequate urine output
    f. Return of gag reflex

37. Which intervention by the nurse will help a postoperative patient with compliance in getting up to ambulate?
    a. Offer the patient pain medication 30-45 minutes before ambulation.
    b. Assist the patient to turn from side to side every 2 hours.
    c. Remind the patient to perform extremity exercises every 4 hours.
    d. Teach the patient that activity helps prevent postoperative complications.

38. The postoperative patient has a Penrose drain in place. Which action does the nurse take to prevent skin irritation, wound contamination, and infection?
    a. Keeps a sterile safety pin in place at the end of the drain
    b. Places absorbent pads under and around the exposed drain
    c. Uses minimal tape; when tape is needed, uses hypoallergenic tape
    d. Shortens the drain by pulling it out a short distance and trimming off the excess external portion

17

CHAPTER

Principles of Inflammation and Immunity

1. The nurse is performing a physical assessment on an adult with no known health problems. Which assessment finding poses the **greatest** potential threat to the patient's immune system?
   a. Has old scar formation related to an appendectomy
   b. Has poor oral hygiene and numerous dental caries
   c. Displays occasional skipped heartbeats during auscultation
   d. Displays orthostatic hypotension and is mildly dehydrated

2. Which patients have factors that may affect the function of the immune system?
   Select all that apply.
   a. Patient has been on a severely limited diet for several weeks to quickly lose weight.
   b. Patient is homeless and is continuously seeking shelter for cold weather conditions.
   c. Patient is on multiple medications, including corticosteroids and a nonsteroidal anti-inflammatory.
   d. Patient is a 30-year-old adult with a family history of hypertension and high cholesterol.
   e. Patient is 84 years old and lives alone in her own house.
   f. Patient has type 2 diabetes mellitus that is well controlled with oral antidiabetic medication.

3. Based on the nurse's knowledge of the concept of immunity, what is an example of self-tolerance?
   a. Patient is given chemotherapy to eradicate the cancer cells.
   b. Antibiotic medication cures the patient's urinary tract infection.
   c. Skin from the patient's thigh is successfully grafted to a burn wound.
   d. Patient receives an uneventful blood transfusion during surgery.

4. Production of immune cells will be **most jeopardized** by which event?
   a. Patient's thymus gland atrophies because of the aging process.
   b. Patient's spleen is removed because of a serious car accident.
   c. Patient has liver failure secondary to alcohol abuse.
   d. Patient develops a bone marrow disorder.

5. Which person is **most likely** to be immuno-competent?
   a. 79-year-old male who lives independently, exercises daily, and eats balanced meals
   b. 25-year-old female who drinks alcohol and who stays out late every night with her friends
   c. 6-year-old male who is energetic but frequently has minor upper respiratory infections
   d. 45-year-old female who works daily in her garden and eats a vegetarian diet

6. A patient has sustained a severe right ankle sprain, and the nurse is explaining the process of inflammation to the patient and family. Which information does the nurse include in this teaching?
   a. Because inflammation is present, treatment for infection is advised.
   b. The inflammation response is painful but provides long-term protection.
   c. Inflammation is a specific body defense in response to the ankle injury.
   d. Symptoms of inflammation depend on the intensity and severity of the injury.

7. Which circumstance poses the **greatest** risk to good health via exposure to living organisms?
   a. A healthy adult nurse takes care of a patient with a bacterial infection of the leg.
   b. A sanitation worker forgets to wear gloves when picking up a garbage can.
   c. Infant children in a daycare play together and share toys and food.
   d. An animal care technician gives vaccinations and draws blood from cats and dogs.

8. The actions of leukocytes provide the body protection against invading organisms. What are actions of leukocytes? **Select all that apply.**
   a. Phagocytic destruction of foreign invaders and unhealthy or abnormal cells
   b. Lytic destruction of foreign invaders and unhealthy cells
   c. Stimulate maturational pathway of stem cells
   d. Production of antibodies directed against invaders
   e. Production of cytokines that decrease specific leukocyte growth and activity
   f. Increase growth and differentiation of platelets

9. Which patient would benefit **most** from receiving a detailed explanation about human leukocyte antigens (HLAs)?
   a. Patient has anorexia nervosa and is refusing to eat.
   b. Patient has an identical twin who needs a kidney transplant.
   c. Patient has strong family history of breast cancer.
   d. Patient is refusing to take antibiotics because of the side effects.

10. In which conditions is the inflammatory response present? **Select all that apply.**
    a. Sprain injuries to joints
    b. Appendicitis
    c. Hypothyroidism
    d. Myocardial infarction
    e. Contact dermatitis
    f. Allergic rhinitis

11. Which cell types associated with the inflammatory response participate in phagocytosis?
    a. Neutrophils and eosinophils
    b. Macrophages and neutrophils
    c. Macrophages and eosinophils
    d. Eosinophils and basophils

12. Which type of white blood cell does the body produce most?
    a. Macrophages
    b. Eosinophils
    c. Neutrophils
    d. Band neutrophils

13. The nurse is reviewing the patient's laboratory results and sees that there is a left shift (bandemia). Which assessment is the nurse **most likely** to perform?
    a. Look for signs of bleeding, such as petechiae.
    b. Look for signs of infection and check temperature and pulse.
    c. Check for signs of anemia, such as pallor or tachycardia.
    d. Check for signs and symptoms of inflammatory response.

14. What is the significance of toll-like receptors (TLRs) in helping the body to fight infection?
    a. Research shows that diseases are spread by flies through TLRs.
    b. TLRs interact with the surface of an organism and allow recognition of nonself.
    c. Persons who have more TLRs are more likely to develop infections.
    d. Older people and immunocompromised persons will not produce TLRs.

15. When an injury or invasion occurs, phagocytosis involves seven steps. Degradation is the final (7th) step. **Place the first six steps that precede degradation in the correct order.**

    _____ a. Adherence

    _____ b. Exposure and invasion

    _____ c. Phagosome formation

    _____ d. Cellular ingestion

    _____ e. Attraction

    _____ f. Recognition

16. What feature of stem cells has made them valuable to research and therapy?
    a. Found only in fetus tissue
    b. Possess long life span
    c. Resistant to cancer
    d. Pluripotency

17. The nurse assesses a patient who sustained a scalding burn to the left dorsal surface of the hands and fingers that occurred one day ago. There is redness, swelling, and warmth. The patient has pain, decreased fine motor movements, and limited range of motion. What do these findings indicate?
    a. Stage II of inflammation
    b. Serious infection that should be reported
    c. Cardinal signs of inflammation
    d. Probable inappropriate first-aid treatment

18. The nurse is caring for a patient prescribed a new oral antibiotic. Eosinophil and basophil levels are elevated. What is the nurse's **best** interpretation of this laboratory report?
    a. The patient may be having an allergic reaction to the antibiotic.
    b. The patient's body is fighting off an infection.
    c. The patient's white blood cells are phagocytizing the invasive organisms.
    d. The patient is at high risk for pneumonia and other respiratory infections.

19. The patient's leg wound has increased blood flow (hyperemia) and swelling. The nurse recognizes this as Stage 1 in the sequence of inflammation process. What would be considered a normal outcome for this stage?
    a. Symptoms usually subside within 24 to 72 hours.
    b. Symptoms will resolve after antibiotic therapy.
    c. Symptoms are not normal and should be reported.
    d. Symptoms will disappear if the leg is elevated.

20. The patient reports a sore throat. The nurse notes that the throat is red and the tissues look swollen and inflamed. Based on the concepts of general immunity and inflammatory response, what should the nurse tell the patient about immune protection?
    a. Protection is immediate but short term and does not provide true immunity.
    b. Protection will occur with any future exposure to the same organisms.
    c. Inflammation is a specific response that protects only the throat area.
    d. Inflammation provides some protection against passing the infection to others.

21. The patient is receiving erythropoietin. If the therapy is successful in correctly stimulating stem cells, which laboratory results would the nurse expect to see?
    a. Increase in T-lymphocytes
    b. Increase in leukocytes
    c. Increase in erythrocytes
    d. Increase in platelets

22. Which type of infection is **most likely** to result in a left shift (bandemia) that indicates an increased number of immature neutrophils?
    a. Viral infection
    b. Parasitic infection
    c. Fungal infection
    d. Bacterial infection

23. In which conditions might the nurse observe inflammation **without** infection? **Select all that apply.**
    a. Joint sprains
    b. Myocardial infarction
    c. Otitis media
    d. Blister formation
    e. Allergic rhinitis
    f. Contact dermatitis

24. What is the clinical significance of the absolute neutrophil count (ANC)?
    a. High numbers of mature neutrophils are seen only in patients with severe sepsis.
    b. The higher the number of mature circulating neutrophils, the greater the resistance to infection.
    c. Low ANC suggests that the infection is resolving because total number is depleted.
    d. Low ANC occurs when antibiotic therapy successfully takes over for the neutrophils.

25. Which cells interact in the presence of an antigen to start antibody production? **Select all that apply.**
    a. B-lymphocytes
    b. Macrophages
    c. Neutrophils
    d. T-helper/inducer cells
    e. T-suppressor cells
    f. Red blood cells

26. Which findings are the **most likely** to manifest in a patient who is experiencing the release of histamine and kinins by basophils?
    a. Fever and tachycardia
    b. Foul odor and pus
    c. Shortness of breath
    d. Swelling and edema

27. In what way is antibody-mediated immunity (AMI) different from cell-mediated immunity (CMI)?
    a. AMI is more powerful than CMI.
    b. AMI can be transferred from one person to another; CMI cannot.
    c. CMI requires constant re-exposure for "boosting"; AMI does not.
    d. CMI requires inflammatory actions; AMI is independent of inflammatory actions.

28. What is an example of the clinical significance of the anamnestic response?
    a. Person who had childhood measles is re-exposed as an adult but does not develop measles.
    b. Person had influenza last year and therefore decides that this year's immunization is unnecessary.
    c. Person had cancer that is in remission; response to therapy was better than expected.
    d. Person is very healthy, has few infectious illnesses, and always recovers quickly.

29. What is an example of innate-native immunity?
    a. Nurse obtains hepatitis B series before starting a new job abroad.
    b. Patient, bitten by wild rabid animal, receives four doses of rabies vaccine.
    c. New mother decides to breastfeed her infant for first several months.
    d. Nurse has intact healthy skin on hands and healthy mucous membranes.

30. An older resident living in a long-term care facility asks for help to go to the bathroom more frequently than usual. The nurse suspects a urinary tract infection. What changes in the immune system of an older adult should the nurse keep in mind? **Select all that apply.**
    a. Older adults are more at risk for bacterial and fungal infections in the genitourinary tract.
    b. Older adults may have an infection but not show expected changes in white blood cell counts.
    c. Older adults may not have a fever during inflammatory or infectious episodes.
    d. Urinalysis results for older patients are more likely to show false negative results.
    e. Older patients are less likely to become septic because of history of antibody-antigen activity.
    f. Neutrophil counts may be normal, but activity is reduced, increasing the risk for infection.

31. Why do older adults have an increased risk for autoimmune diseases?
    a. The number of neutrophils and macrophages are increased, as are their functions.
    b. Memory cells are damaged by age and they fail to react to antigens.
    c. There is loss of recognition of self and an increase in circulating autoantibodies.
    d. The white blood cell count is markedly decreased or absent.

32. An older patient reports that he has been treated for tuberculosis in the distant past. He currently has a negative tuberculosis skin test. How does the nurse interpret the test results?
    a. Patient does not currently have tuberculosis.
    b. Patient has incorrectly remembered being treated for tuberculosis.
    c. In older patients, false negative tuberculosis results are a possibility.
    d. Test results are documented, and patient is to be retested annually.

33. A nurse is exposed to a viral infection at work. After several days, the nurse fully recovers and returns to work. What is the role of the memory cell in relation to the nurse's viral illness?
    a. The memory cell reminds the nurse's healthy cells to function after recovery.
    b. If the nurse develops other viral infections, the memory cell seeks out an antigen match.
    c. The memory cell prevents viral shedding from the nurse to patients who are immunocompromised.
    d. When the nurse is reexposed to the same antigen, the memory cell will produce antibodies.

34. A patient who is in good health is naturally assisted in cancer prevention by which type of immunity?
    a. Cell-mediated
    b. Innate
    c. Lymphokine
    d. Humoral

35. A babysitter is caring for a child who is in the presymptomatic stage of *influenza A*. The babysitter has never had *influenza A* and develops symptoms several days after caring for the child. What type of immunity will the babysitter have as a result of antibody-antigen actions?
    a. B cells will be sensitized to *influenza A and B*.
    b. B cells will be sensitized only to *influenza A*.
    c. Immunity is short term because B-cell sensitization is not adaptive.
    d. Antibody-antigen B-cell action is nontransferable from child to adult.

36. The action of which cell types must be suppressed to prevent acute rejection of transplanted organs? **Select all that apply.**
    a. Eosinophils
    b. Suppressor T-cells
    c. Natural killer cells
    d. Cytotoxic/cytolytic T-cells
    e. Helper/inducer T-cells
    f. Neutrophils

37. During surgery, a patient undergoing a heart transplant experiences rejection of the organ. What type of rejection is this?
    a. Acute
    b. Chronic
    c. Hyperacute
    d. Transplant

38. A patient who had a kidney transplant 5 years ago is experiencing progressively reduced function of the organ. Which intervention is appropriate for this patient?
    a. Patient should be admitted to intensive care for observation and possible dialysis.
    b. Patient should be educated about retransplantation; related living donor should be sought.
    c. Drug management may limit the damage and allow the graft to be maintained.
    d. Patient should be immediately prepped for surgical removal of the organ.

39. The nurse is caring for a patient after a kidney transplant. Which finding prompts the nurse to quickly alert the health care provider about a probable hyperacute rejection?
    a. There is no urine output and problems occur immediately.
    b. Blood urea nitrogen and creatinine show trend for elevation.
    c. Patient reports some tenderness at the incision site.
    d. Patient has an allergic reaction to the transplant medications.

40. A patient is admitted to the hospital for acute rejection of a kidney transplant that was preformed 2 months ago. Which intervention is appropriate for this patient?
    a. Immediate removal of the transplanted kidney
    b. Grief and loss counseling to prepare for loss of organ
    c. Magnetic resonance imaging of organ
    d. Organ biopsy to diagnose impaired function

41. How does the immune system respond to a graft when a transplant rejection occurs?
    a. Collateral circulation develops and the transplanted organ becomes engorged.
    b. Opportunistic infections develop because the body is immunosuppressed.
    c. Host's immune system starts inflammation and immunologic actions to destroy nonself cells.
    d. Systemic tissue destruction occurs because of inability to differentiate self from nonself cells.

42. What precaution or intervention has the **highest priority** for a patient going home on maintenance drugs after receiving a kidney transplant?
    a. Monitoring for bacterial and fungal infections
    b. Avoiding the use of table salt
    c. Measuring abdominal girth daily
    d. Avoiding blood donation

43. Under what circumstance are the tissue mast cells **most likely** to be involved in the immune response?
    a. Person has an allergic reaction to peanuts.
    b. Person cuts hand while chopping vegetables.
    c. Person is sitting by someone who is coughing.
    d. Person has a flare-up of rheumatoid arthritis.

44. The nurse is instructing a patient who has undergone an organ transplant about immunosuppressant medications. What information does the nurse include?
    a. All immunosuppressive medications increase the risk of infection and cancer.
    b. These medications will be gradually discontinued.
    c. These medications prevent infection in the transplanted organ.
    d. Intravenous forms are more effective than oral medications.

45. To combat rejection of a transplanted kidney, the patient is prescribed intravenous daclizumab. Which question is the nurse **most likely** to ask to assess for side effects of this medication?
    a. "Are you having any nausea, vomiting, or abdominal discomfort?"
    b. "Have you noticed bruising or bleeding when brushing your teeth?"
    c. "Do you notice unusual fatigue or feelings of lightheadedness?"
    d. "Have you experienced any tremors or muscular weakness?"

46. The nurse is reviewing the patient's medication administration record and sees that the patient takes muromonab-CD3. What question is the nurse **most likely** to ask?
    a. "When were you first diagnosed with cancer?"
    b. "When was your organ transplant performed?"
    c. "Is the medication controlling your allergy symptoms?"
    d. "Are you still having symptoms of infection?"

47. A patient is admitted with pneumonia and has developed sepsis. What can the findings from a differential white blood cell count reveal about this patient?
    a. Whether an infection is bacterial or viral
    b. Whether the patient has active immunity
    c. The tissue type from the human leukocyte antigen
    d. The type of antibody response occurring

48. The patient experienced a myocardial infarction 6 months ago during which 25% of his left ventricle was damaged and replaced by scar tissue. Which is the **most likely** outcome?
    a. The patient will lose 25% of the effectiveness of his left ventricular contraction.
    b. The patient will lose 50% of his ejection fraction.
    c. The patient will regain 25% of the effectiveness of his left ventricle after healing.
    d. The patient will lose 75% of his activity tolerance.

49. The health care provider writes a prescription for the patient to be immunized with the flu vaccine. Which type of immunity does the nurse provide the patient by injecting this vaccine?
    a. Natural active immunity
    b. Artificial active immunity
    c. Adaptive immunity
    d. Passive immunity

18 CHAPTER

Care of Patients with Arthritis and Other Connective Tissue Diseases

1. A rheumatic disease is any condition or disease of which body system?
   a. Cardiovascular
   b. Hematopoietic
   c. Integumentary
   d. Musculoskeletal

2. Which patient is manifesting signs/symptoms that are likely to be associated with connective tissue disease?
   a. Patient has chronic pain, decreased function, and joint deterioration.
   b. Patient has cardiac dysthymias and occasional chest pain.
   c. Patient has acute back pain after exercise and exertion.
   d. Patient has poor skin turgor and sluggish capillary refill.

3. The nurse is working in an ambulatory clinic. Which statement represents the **most typical** reason for a patient with osteoarthritis (OA) to seek medical care at a clinic?
   a. "I think that being overweight is putting too much stress on my joints."
   b. "I am having a lot of joint pain, and I'm frequently taking over-the-counter pain medicine."
   c. "I noticed that my third finger joint seems to be tilting inward toward my index finger."
   d. "I have a family history of OA, and I wondered if there is anything I can do to prevent it."

4. The nurse is interviewing a middle-aged woman who reports chronic joint pain and stiffness. Which patient statement is indicative of **early** osteoarthritis?
   a. "My joint pain diminishes after rest and worsens after activity."
   b. "I have discomfort with slight motion or even when at rest."
   c. "I have a tingling sensation and sometimes numbness in my joints."
   d. "There are bony lumps in some of my finger joints."

5. The nurse is caring for an obese patient with osteoarthritis (OA). What is the **best** rationale for encouraging this patient to lose weight?
   a. An obese person with OA has an increased risk of also developing rheumatoid arthritis.
   b. Obesity interferes with the metabolism of drugs that are usually prescribed to manage OA.
   c. Extra weight of obesity increases the degeneration rate of hip and knee joints.
   d. Obesity has a negative effect on self-esteem and body image of patients with OA.

6. Which patients are at risk for developing osteoarthritis? **Select all that apply.**
   a. Obese older woman living alone
   b. Slender, nonsmoking, middle-aged man
   c. Middle-aged man who worked construction for 25 years
   d. Young woman with family history of rheumatoid arthritis
   e. Middle-aged adult with multiple knee injuries from playing soccer in high school
   f. Overweight lesbian woman who has experienced discrimination when seeking health care

7. The nurse reads in the documentation that the patient has crepitus associated with osteoarthritis of the right hand. Which assessment would the nurse perform to validate this finding?
   a. Observe the finger joints for redness and swelling.
   b. Ask the patient to flex and extend fingers and listen for a grating sound.
   c. Gently palpate for protruding bony lumps in the finger joints.
   d. Ask the patient to demonstrate full range of motion of finger joints.

8. The nurse is preparing an educational session for a group of patients newly diagnosed with osteoarthritis. What lifestyle changes does the nurse suggest to help slow joint degeneration? **Select all that apply.**
   a. Keep body weight within normal limits.
   b. Quit smoking.
   c. Do not participate in outdoor activities.
   d. Avoid risk-taking behaviors that may result in trauma.
   e. Avoid high-intensity exercise.
   f. Avoid direct sunlight and any other type of ultraviolet lighting.

9. The health care provider informs the nurse that the patient has a joint effusion of the right knee. What is the nurse **most likely** to find during physical assessment of the knee?
   a. Hard bony protrusion palpated at the joint space
   b. Tightness during flexion and extension of knee
   c. Inability to independently stand or walk
   d. Dry, red, scaly skin over the knee that itches and flakes

10. Patients with osteoarthritis that affects the spine are **most likely** to have what types of symptoms?
    a. Localized pain at L3-4, bone spurs, stiffness, and muscle atrophy
    b. Radiating pain at L3-4 and C4-6, stiffness, muscle spasms, and bone spurs
    c. Localized pain at T6-12, inflexibility, and muscle asymmetry
    d. Radiating pain throughout the spine, stiffness, and muscle weakness

11. Which response, from a patient with advanced osteoarthritis, alerts the nurse that the patient is having a problem coping with the image and role changes related to disease progression?
    a. "I used to be a playground assistant; now I work with children who need help with reading."
    b. "I'm a musician and my instrument is the piano, so I get a lot of enjoyment going to concerts."
    c. "I used to work in the garden, but my joints are so stiff; I mostly sit and look out the window."
    d. "I must be getting younger. I used to tie my shoes; now I am using Velcro closures just like my kids."

12. The patient tells the nurse that he has been taking glucosamine for joint pain. Which physical finding is cause for **greatest** concern?
    a. Patient is 15 lbs overweight
    b. Blood pressure is 150/80
    c. Resting pulse is 90/min
    d. Patient has a light red rash

13. The nurse is evaluating laboratory results from a patient with osteoarthritis. Which lab results could the nurse expect to find elevated?
    a. White blood cells, including neutrophils, basophils, macrophages, and eosinophils
    b. Erythrocyte sedimentation rate and high-sensitivity C-reactive protein
    c. Electrolytes such as potassium, calcium, magnesium, phosphorus, and sodium
    d. Partial thromboplastin time and International Normalized Ratio

14. Which patient statement indicates that the patient knows to take the primary drug of choice for osteoarthritis as recommended by the American Pain Society, American Geriatrics Society, and Osteoarthritis Research Society International?
    a. "I buy the generic form of ibuprofen because it saves me a lot of money."
    b. "My daughter is trying to get me a prescription for celecoxib."
    c. "Usually acetaminophen is sufficient for most painful episodes."
    d. "I got some of those over-the-counter patches that create a warm sensation."

15. Which treatment modalities might the nurse expect for a patient who is undergoing nonsurgical management of chronic joint pain? **Select all that apply.**
    a. Immobilization to promote rest
    b. Weight control
    c. Exercise balanced with rest
    d. Thermal modalities
    e. Limit foods and liquids that contain calcium
    f. Home traction

16. When educating a patient about total joint arthroplasty (TJA), what does the nurse do **first**?
    a. Ensure that the patient wants the procedure.
    b. Review instructions and ask the patient to repeat back.
    c. Assess the patient's knowledge about TJA.
    d. Ask if the provider has explained the procedure.

17. For preoperative care of a patient scheduled for total joint arthroplasty, what does the nurse plan to do? **Select all that apply.**
    a. Provide written or videotaped information about the procedure.
    b. Assess the patient's understanding of the procedure.
    c. Assess and include the patient's support people or family.
    d. Obtain the patient's signature on the consent form.
    e. Assist in scheduling needed dental procedures after the surgery.
    f. Include interdisciplinary team members, if possible.

18. Which patient circumstance would be considered a contraindication for total joint arthroplasty?
    a. Patient is currently being treated for a persistent urinary tract infection.
    b. Patient reports pain and loss of mobility related to joint dysfunction.
    c. Patient reports her osteopenia is now considered to be osteoporosis.
    d. Patient is elderly and has no one to provide postoperative care.

19. A patient with rheumatoid arthritis (RA) may need to undergo general anesthesia for a hip replacement. Which information needs to be brought to the immediate attention of the surgeon before the procedure is scheduled?
    a. Patient has a previous history of joint surgery on the affected side.
    b. Patient has been taking vitamin C and nonsteroidal anti-inflammatory drugs for years.
    c. Patient has cervical spine disease and has not had any recent spinal x-rays.
    d. Patient fears that the procedure will cause complications because of the RA.

20. The nurse is caring for a patient who had a total hip replacement. On assessment, the nurse observes shortening of the affected leg and internal rotation. The patient reports increased pain that is not relieved with medication. What should the nurse do?
    a. Conduct additional pain assessment and obtain new medication orders.
    b. Position the leg in an anatomical position and place pillows for support.
    c. Compare the length of the affected leg to the unaffected leg.
    d. Keep the patient in bed and immediately notify the surgeon.

21. Which interventions can the nurse use to prevent or manage infections in patients who have undergone total joint replacement? **Select all that apply.**
    a. Use aseptic technique for wound care and emptying of drains.
    b. Wash hands thoroughly when caring for patients.
    c. Culture drainage fluid if a change is observed.
    d. Encourage early ambulation along with leg exercises.
    e. Monitor the incision every 4 hours for the first 24 and every 8 to 12 hours thereafter.
    f. Advocate that the patient be placed in a private isolation room.

22. The nurse is caring for a patient who had a total joint replacement and administers subcutaneous enoxaparin as ordered. Which outcome statement indicates that the intended goal of the enoxaparin therapy is being met?
    a. Patient does not show signs or symptoms of venous thromboembolism.
    b. Prothrombin time and International Normalized Ratio are within normal range.
    c. Pain is rated at 3/10 within 30 minutes after receiving the medication.
    d. Wound site is free of infection signs and oral temperature is 98.8°F (37.1°C).

23. A patient is reluctant to consider hip surgery because of a fear of blood transfusion reaction. What is the nurse's **best** response?
    a. "No one will force you to receive blood if you don't want it."
    b. "A cell saver can be used to collect your own red blood cells during surgery."
    c. "It's unlikely that you will need a blood transfusion; please don't worry."
    d. "Blood products are very safe these days and there are numerous safety protocols."

24. Which routine interventions would the nurse perform to prevent the life-threatening complication of venous thromboembolism? **Select all that apply.**
    a. Ensure that sequential compression device is in place and functional.
    b. Administer anticoagulant therapy as ordered.
    c. Roll and secure top of antiembolic stockings to midcalf area.
    d. Encourage early ambulation.
    e. Teach patient about leg exercises.
    f. Encourage foods that are rich in iron and protein.

25. The nurse is providing care for a patient scheduled for a total hip arthroplasty. Which medication should the patient receive one hour before the surgical incision in accordance with the Surgical Care Improvement Project Core Measures?
    a. Low-molecular-weight heparin, such as subcutaneous enoxaparin
    b. Fast-acting opioid, such as IV morphine
    c. Broad-spectrum antibiotic, such as IV cefazolin
    d. Routine daily dose of oral antihypertensive

26. The nurse assesses the patient's surgical hip site and measures the drainage every 4 hours. At 7:00 am there is 30 mL in the drainage container; at 11:00 am there is 10 mL; at 3:00 pm there is 5 mL, and at 7:00 pm there is 20 mL. What should the nurse do?
    a. Document the drainage and continue to observe the site and drainage every 4 hours.
    b. Take vital signs, observe the site for signs of hemorrhage, and notify the surgeon.
    c. Document the findings but change the assessment frequency to every 2 hours.
    d. Ask the patient if there is increased pain or decreased sensation on the affected side.

27. A patient is postoperative for a total hip arthroplasty and needs to get out of bed for the **first** time. What should the nurse do?
    a. Schedule an appointment with physical therapy and wait for the therapist to assist the patient.
    b. Caution unlicensed assistive personnel about fall prevention and instruct to observe for dizziness.
    c. Put a gait belt on the patient and stand on the same side of the bed as the affected leg.
    d. Ask the patient how much assistance is needed to stand and pivot into the chair.

28. Following a total joint arthroplasty, which patients have a **higher** risk of venous thromboembolism (VTE)? **Select all that apply.**
    a. Older patient who has trouble with mobility at baseline
    b. Obese patient with chronic pain associated with rheumatoid arthritis
    c. Patient with a previous history of VTE related to job as a truck driver
    d. Thin patient who needs medication for hyperthyroidism
    e. Patient with compromised circulation secondary to sickle cell disorder
    f. Patient with a history of osteoarthritis pain that is treated with acetaminophen

29. To prevent venous thromboembolism, several types of anticoagulant medications can be ordered. Which drug is **most commonly** used during hospitalization?
    a. Oral or parenteral aspirin
    b. Oral warfarin
    c. Intravenous tissue plasminogen activator (tPA)
    d. Subcutaneous low-molecular-weight heparin (LMWH)

30. A patient is on anticoagulant therapy with dalteparin after total joint arthroplasty. Which laboratory test should the nurse monitor?
    a. Prothrombin time and International Normalized Ratio
    b. Oxygen saturation and liver enzymes
    c. Complete blood count and platelet count
    d. Erythrocyte sedimentation rate and C-reactive protein

31. Every 2 to 4 hours, the nurse assesses a patient who has a continuous femoral nerve blockade for postoperative pain management following a knee joint replacement. What findings prompt the nurse to alert the surgeon about untoward systemic effects of the local anesthesia?
    a. Patient is unable to detect pain with plantar flexion of the affected foot.
    b. Patient reports a metallic taste, tinnitus, and a nervous feeling.
    c. Patient says that the affected foot feels warmer than the unaffected foot.
    d. Patient reports nausea and mild abdominal discomfort.

32. Which outcome statement indicates that the therapeutic goal of continuous passive motion (CPM) therapy is being met?
    a. Patient has no signs or symptoms of venous thromboembolism.
    b. Stress and strain on the knee joint are reduced.
    c. Mobility of the patient's prosthetic knee is maintained.
    d. Patient uses the CPM device while ambulating.

33. The nurse is supervising a nursing student in the postoperative care of a patient who had total knee replacement and has a continuous passive motion (CPM) device. When would the nurse intervene?
    a. Student applies hot moist compresses to the incisional area.
    b. Student turns off the CPM while the patient is having a meal in bed.
    c. Student places a cloth between skin of incisional area and ice packs.
    d. Student checks to see that the CPM is well padded to protect the skin.

34. Which intervention does the nurse implement to improve mobility for a patient who has undergone a total hip replacement?
    a. Encourage use of assistive devices such as a walker when ambulating.
    b. Recommend to quickly decrease rest periods between activities.
    c. Instruct to flex and extend the hips at least 90 degrees when doing leg exercises.
    d. Advise to progressively put more weight on the affected side.

35. What is an important health teaching point for a patient with total joint arthroplasty?
    a. "Do not use the joint."
    b. "Stress the joint."
    c. "Protect the joint."
    d. "Guard the muscles."

36. Although arthritis is not curable, many "cures" are marketed to patients with the disease. What does the nurse encourage the patient to do?
    a. Avoid alternative and complementary therapies because they are invalid.
    b. Check with the Arthritis Foundation for appropriate modalities.
    c. Apply liniments and creams freely, because they are harmless.
    d. Use herbals and vitamins if they provide subjective relief.

37. The nurse assesses a postoperative patient who had a total knee replacement for neurovascular compromise. Which assessments must the nurse document? **Select all that apply.**
    a. Skin color and temperature
    b. Presence or absence of distal peripheral pulses
    c. Full range of motion for operative and nonoperative legs
    d. Capillary refill of operative leg
    e. Comparison of operative leg to nonoperative leg
    f. Ability to use extremity compared to baseline

38. The nurse is caring for a patient who underwent a hemiarthroplasty of the right shoulder. The patient arrives on the unit with an abduction immobilizer in place. Which nursing action is correct in the care of this patient?
    a. Remove the immobilizer and observe the incision site for infection and inflammation.
    b. Assess patient's comfort and adjust the position of the immobilizer accordingly.
    c. Leave the immobilizer in place and perform neurovascular assessments every 4 hours.
    d. Call the surgeon and ask for an order that specifies when the immobilizer can be removed.

39. What musculoskeletal health problem is often associated with rheumatoid arthritis?
    a. Paget's disease
    b. Lyme disease
    c. Marfan syndrome
    d. Osteoporosis

40. Although the etiology of rheumatoid arthritis is unknown, it is considered to be what type of disorder?
    a. Autoimmune disease
    b. Disease associated with aging
    c. Genetic disorder
    d. Trauma disorder

41. Which assessment finding indicates to the nurse that the patient is experiencing **early** rheumatoid arthritis?
    a. Joint deformities
    b. Joint inflammation
    c. Weight loss
    d. Subcutaneous nodules

42. Which patient-reported symptom(s) would typify **early** rheumatoid arthritis?
    a. "I feel tired and weak."
    b. "I feel like my hands are burning."
    c. "I have severe stiffness in the morning."
    d. "I have gained a lot of weight."

43. The nurse reads in the documentation that the patient has a Baker's cyst. Which assessment will the nurse perform to validate this finding?
    a. Check distal lateral ankles for deformities or lumps.
    b. Observe the wrists bilaterally for abduction.
    c. Gently palpate the popliteal area behind the knee.
    d. Ask the patient to flex and extend the Achilles tendon.

44. What is the **most common** area of involvement of rheumatoid arthritis in the spine?
    a. Lumbar spine
    b. Sacral spine
    c. Cervical spine
    d. Thoracic spine

45. The patient with rheumatoid arthritis suffers a subluxation of the first and second vertebrae. What should the nurse do **first**, before immediately notifying the health care provider?
    a. Assess respiratory status, and apply oxygen as needed.
    b. Assess for loss of sensation or loss of movement in the extremities.
    c. Assess for pain that radiates down the arm and check pulses.
    d. Assess for change in mental status and orient the patient.

46. When a patient has rheumatoid arthritis of the temporomandibular joint, what is the major complaint?
    a. Toothache on the affected side
    b. Headache in the temple area
    c. Pain on chewing and opening the mouth
    d. Earache on the affected side

47. The nurse reads in the documentation that the patient with rheumatoid arthritis may have Sjögren's syndrome. Which assessment is the nurse **most likely** to perform to validate this documentation?
    a. Weigh the patient and compare weight to baseline.
    b. Take the temperature and assess for signs of infection.
    c. Inspect mouth for dry, sticky membranes and eyes for redness.
    d. Observe for joint contractures and loss of range of motion.

48. The patient with rheumatoid arthritis (RA) expresses uncertainty about the disease process and fear of becoming dependent. What is the nurse's **best** response?
    a. "You'll be okay. Very few people with RA actually become wheelchair bound."
    b. "Do you have anyone to help you when you can't take care of yourself?"
    c. "Tell me what you know about living with RA and the treatment options."
    d. "So, you are feeling afraid and uncertain. That seems normal to me."

49. In rheumatoid arthritis, autoantibodies (rheumatoid factors) are formed that attack healthy tissue, especially synovium, causing which condition?
    a. Nerve pain
    b. Bone porosity
    c. Ischemia
    d. Inflammation

50. The nurse is providing teaching for a patient with rheumatoid arthritis who is receiving methotrexate. Which teaching point must the nurse include?
    a. Medication is taken every morning on an empty stomach.
    b. Avoid driving or operating heavy machinery.
    c. Expect some increase in swelling while taking this medication.
    d. Avoid crowds of people and people who are ill.

51. What is the **best** laboratory test to detect **early** rheumatoid arthritis?
    a. Rheumatoid factor
    b. Erythrocyte sedimentation rate
    c. Complete blood cell count
    d. Anti-cyclic citrullinated peptide

52. The nurse sees an increased number of periungual lesions on a patient with rheumatoid arthritis and reports this vascular change to the health care provider. What is the **best** rationale for reporting this finding?
    a. The nurse should always report any unusual findings to the health care provider.
    b. If arterial involvement is occurring, major organs can become ischemic.
    c. The brownish spots affect body image but will readily resolve with treatment.
    d. The lesions will eventually ulcerate and become infected.

53. The nurse is teaching a patient about the common side effects of long-term salicylate and nonsteroidal anti-inflammatory therapy. Which body system side effects does the nurse focus on in the teaching plan?
    a. Central nervous system
    b. Skin
    c. Gastrointestinal
    d. Cardiovascular

54. The nurse is reviewing the complete blood count results of a patient with rheumatoid arthritis. The results show a low hemoglobin, hematocrit, and red blood cell count. Based on these laboratory results, which intervention is the nurse **most likely** to implement?
    a. Encourage rest and ensure rest periods between activities and therapies.
    b. Instruct the patient to drink extra fluids and to fully consume meals and snacks.
    c. Instruct unlicensed assistive personnel to handle the patient carefully to prevent bruising.
    d. Encourage the patient to ambulate in the hall at least three times during the shift.

55. The nurse is caring for a patient with rheumatoid arthritis who just had an arthrocentesis. What is the **priority** intervention?
    a. Assess frequently for post procedural pain and ensure optimal pain relief.
    b. Place the patient in a prone position and elevate the extremity.
    c. Monitor the insertion site for bleeding or leakage of synovial fluid.
    d. Teach and encourage leg-, gluteal-, and quadriceps-setting exercises.

56. The patient is taking hydroxychloroquine for rheumatoid arthritis. Which patient statement is cause for **greatest** concern?
    a. "I seem to have a mild stomach discomfort when I take this medication."
    b. "I get kind of light headed. I suppose I should stand up a little slowly."
    c. "Could you give me a Tylenol or something mild? I have some muscle pain."
    d. "I think I must need new glasses. Lately, my vision is really blurry."

57. The unlicensed assistive personnel (UAP) tells the nurse that the patient with rheumatoid arthritis is increasingly manipulative and demanding and trying to meet the patient's requests is interfering with the care of other patients. What is the **best** action for the nurse to take?
    a. Tell the UAP to ignore the demands, complete assigned tasks, and go on to other patients.
    b. Inform the patient that the UAP has additional duties and has a fixed amount of time per patient.
    c. Assess patient behaviors and help the patient to focus on realistic goals and coping strategies.
    d. Temporarily perform the UAP duties until boundaries and expectations are established.

58. What can be expected for a patient with recently diagnosed systemic lupus erythematosus?
    a. Frequent acute inflammatory episodes
    b. Spontaneous remissions and exacerbations
    c. Symptoms similar to osteoarthritis
    d. Frequent infections and reduced immune response

59. Based on the nurse's knowledge of the **most common** cause of death for patients with systemic lupus erythematosus, which laboratory tests will the nurse closely monitor when caring for these patients?
    a. Cardiac enzymes and sedimentation rate
    b. Blood urea nitrogen and creatinine
    c. Complete blood count and platelet count
    d. Liver enzymes and cholesterol levels

60. The nurse is assessing the skin of a patient with systemic lupus erythematosus. What is the nurse **most likely** to notice about the skin?
    a. Small, brownish spots around the nail bed
    b. Generalized hardening of the skin
    c. Dry, scaly, raised rash on the face
    d. Raynaud's phenomenon

61. Which laboratory test is the **only** significant test for diagnosing a patient with discoid lupus?
    a. Antinuclear antibody
    b. Serum complement
    c. Complete blood count
    d. Skin biopsy

62. The nurse is caring for a patient with systemic lupus erythematosus who is having a flare-up of the condition. Which abnormal vital sign is a **classic** sign for an exacerbation?
    a. Increased blood pressure
    b. Decreased pulse
    c. Increased temperature
    d. Decreased respirations

63. The nurse is reviewing the laboratory results of a patient with systemic lupus erythematosus. Which test result is **most likely** to be a false positive?
    a. Elevated erythrocyte sedimentation rate
    b. Positive syphilis test
    c. Positive tuberculosis test
    d. Increase in components of complete blood count

64. A patient with systemic lupus erythematosus is prescribed a relatively new drug, belimumab. Which concept will the nurse use to emphasize important teaching points about this medication?
    a. Comfort
    b. Immunity
    c. Mobility
    d. Oxygenation

65. For a patient in the **early** phase of scleroderma, the nurse is **most likely** to observe which signs/symptoms during the physical examination?
    a. Digit necrosis with severe pain
    b. Localized hardening of the skin
    c. Arthralgia and joint stiffness
    d. Dysphagia and esophagitis

66. For a patient who is experiencing gout, what is the **most likely** reason that the patient will seek medical attention?
    a. Dry, red, scaly rash with butterfly pattern on face
    b. Trouble passing urine because of uric acid formation
    c. Presence of hard irregular tophi in the outer ear
    d. Severe pain in the joint of the great toe

67. A patient was prescribed the combination drug of probenecid and colchicine for the treatment of gout. How does the health care team evaluate the effectiveness of the therapy?
    a. Monitor serum uric acid level.
    b. Check results of urinalysis.
    c. Review compliance with a low-purine diet.
    d. Assess mobility of affected joints.

68. A patient comes to the clinic because he thinks he may have Lyme disease. What is the **most important** question to ask to assist the health care provider in determining if Lyme disease is the correct diagnosis?
    a. "Have you had flu like symptoms?"
    b. "Do you notice stiffness in your joints?"
    c. "Did you notice a bull's-eye-shaped lesion?"
    d. "Have you had any facial drooping?"

69. Patients with ankylosing spondylitis have risk for which condition?
    a. Compromised respiratory function
    b. Cardiac arrhythmias
    c. Hip pain with osteonecrosis
    d. Dysphagia and decreased gag reflex

70. For a patient with Reiter's syndrome, besides asking about joint pain, which additional question would the nurse ask?
    a. "Is there any chance that you were bitten by an insect?"
    b. "Are you having pain or burning with urination?"
    c. "Do you have a family history of arthritis?"
    d. "Do you get short of breath after minor exertion?"

71. The nurse is interviewing a young patient who seems to be excessively tall, and his hands and feet are elongated. The nurse suspects Marfan syndrome. What is the **best** rationale for the nurse to alert the health care provider of these findings?
    a. Patient has a growth disorder that should be monitored.
    b. In Marfan syndrome, death often occurs in the 30s.
    c. Patient is likely to experience joint deformity and dysfunction.
    d. Marfan syndrome is reversible if detected at an early stage.

72. The nurse is assessing a patient with fibromyalgia and identifies the trigger points by palpation. In which specific areas does the nurse expect to elicit pain and tenderness? **Select all that apply.**
    a. Neck
    b. Lips
    c. Trunk
    d. Lower back
    e. Upper abdomen
    f. Extremities

73. A patient is prescribed amitriptyline for the diagnosis of fibromyalgia. What is the classification of this medication?
    a. Anti-inflammatory
    b. Antirheumatic
    c. Antidepressant
    d. Antipsychotic

19
CHAPTER

Care of Patients with HIV Disease

1. What is the **best** rationale for the nurse to be familiar with the HIV infectious viral particle process?
   a. To help patients to identify the timeframe of greatest risk for infection
   b. To teach HIV-positive patients about how they became infected with the virus
   c. To assist in identifying nonprogressors from those who will progress to AIDS
   d. To educate HIV patients about the importance of adhering to a medication schedule

2. The nurse is assessing a patient whose lifestyle creates a high risk for HIV/AIDS. Which assessment is the nurse **most likely** to perform to differentiate HIV from AIDS?
   a. History of substance or alcohol abuse
   b. History of any occupational exposure to HIV
   c. Signs/symptoms of opportunistic infections
   d. Practice of safe versus risky sexual behaviors

3. A young male has just been diagnosed as HIV positive. He tells the nurse that he suspects contracting the virus from a female several weeks ago and that he had sex with his girlfriend several days ago. What is the nurse's **best** response?
   a. "The virus needs time to replicate, so your girlfriend is probably okay, but she should get tested."
   b. "Even in the early phase, it is possible to pass the HIV virus; both women should be notified."
   c. "HIV always progresses to AIDS. You and your girlfriend need to start medication right away."
   d. "You should tell your girlfriend about being HIV positive; the health department will contact the other woman."

4. A patient who is HIV positive has been taking combination antiretroviral therapy (cART) for several years. Today the nurse sees that test results now show a CD4+ T-cell count of less than 200 cells/mm^3. Which intervention is the nurse most likely to perform?
   a. Reinforce patient's successful compliance with medication regimen.
   b. Assess patient's understanding of the importance of medication schedule.
   c. Provide emotional support when patient is informed about AIDS diagnosis.
   d. Emphasize need to practice safe sex because risk of transmission is high.

5. The health care provider prescribed an integrase inhibitor drug for the patient with HIV. The patient asks the nurse how this drug works. What is the nurse's **best** response?
   a. "It reduces efficiency of converting human genetic material into HIV genetic material."
   b. "It reinforces your immune system's ability to fight off an HIV infection."
   c. "It prevents viral deoxyribonucleic acid (DNA) from integrating into your DNA."
   d. "It will prevent your HIV infection from progressing to AIDS."

6. Which groups are experiencing increased numbers of new HIV infections in the United States and Canada?
   a. White homosexual men and women
   b. Older heterosexual men and women
   c. Asian women who have sex with men
   d. Persons of color: African and Hispanic

7. The health care provider tells the nurse that the patient is considered Stage 1 according to the Centers for Disease Control and Prevention case definition for HIV disease. What would the nurse expect to find when assessing the patient?
   a. Signs/symptoms associated with Kaposi's sarcoma
   b. No signs/symptoms of AIDS-defining illness
   c. Respiratory symptoms due to pneumonia
   d. Symptoms of AIDS wasting syndrome

8. Which statements about the transmission of HIV are true? **Select all that apply.**
   a. HIV may be transmitted only during the end stages of the disease.
   b. Those with recent HIV infection and high viral load are very infectious.
   c. Those with end-stage HIV and no drug therapy are very infectious.
   d. HIV is transmitted through touching an infected person.
   e. All people infected with HIV can easily infect others with AIDS.
   f. An undetectable viral load requires greater or multiple exposures.

9. Which conditions may be the **first** signs of HIV in women? **Select all that apply.**
   a. Vaginal candidiasis
   b. Bladder infection
   c. Spontaneous abortion
   d. Pelvic inflammatory disease
   e. Mononucleosis
   f. Genital herpes

10. Although there is a wide range of time from the beginning of HIV infection to the development of AIDS, which patient is **most likely** to develop AIDS very quickly?
    a. Adult female who has one-time sex with an HIV-positive partner
    b. Older male who has vaginal sex with an HIV-positive female
    c. Adult male who is transfused with HIV-contaminated blood
    d. Older nurse who is stuck by HIV-contaminated needle at work

11. What is the **most important** means of preventing HIV spread or transmission?
    a. Genetic research
    b. Education
    c. Medication therapy
    d. Standard precautions

12. HIV is **most commonly** transmitted by which routes? **Select all that apply.**
    a. Oral
    b. Sexual
    c. Parenteral
    d. Airborne
    e. Perinatal
    f. Enteral

13. What is a clinically significant feature for patients who are identified as nonprogressors?
    a. They rarely ever convert to full-blown AIDS.
    b. They do not transmit virus to sexual partners.
    c. Viral load is either undetectable or very low.
    d. Opportunistic infections never manifest.

14. The HIV-positive patient tells the nurse that his HIV-negative partner will be using preexposure prophylaxis (PrEP) emtricitab. Which statement indicates to the nurse the need for additional teaching about this drug?
    a. "My partner will need to be tested for HIV every 3 months."
    b. "This drug will decrease the chances of my partner becoming HIV positive."
    c. "Once we start using emtricitab I will no longer need to use a condom."
    d. "My partner will need to be monitored for any side effects of this drug."

15. A patient is an IV drug user who regularly shares needles and syringes with friends. What information does the nurse provide to decrease the patient's risk of HIV through shared needles and syringes after each use?
    a. Fill and flush needle and syringe with water, then fill syringe with bleach, shake approximately 30-60 seconds, and rinse with water.
    b. Fill and flush needle and syringe with water, then fill syringe with soap and hot water, shake 2 minutes, and rinse with cold water.
    c. Soak needles and syringes after each use in a bleach and hot water solution overnight, then allow to air dry.
    d. Never reuse needles; rinse syringes after each use with rubbing alcohol or bleach solution, and then rinse them with hot water.

16. Which practices are generally recommended to prevent sexual transmission of HIV?
    Select all that apply.
    a. Use of latex or polyurethane condoms for genital and anal intercourse
    b. Use of natural-membrane condoms for genital and anal intercourse
    c. Use of an appropriate water-based lubricant with a latex condom
    d. Use of antiviral medications taken on a precise schedule
    e. Use of a latex barrier for genital and anal intercourse
    f. Use of latex gloves for finger or hand contact with the vagina or rectum

17. A pregnant woman who is HIV positive arrives at the labor and delivery unit in active labor. The patient tells the nurse that she has been consistently taking her antiretroviral therapy but did not have access to prenatal care. Which situation is the labor and delivery team **most likely** to prepare for?
    a. Birth of a distressed infant who is likely to manifest opportunistic infections
    b. Birth of a premature infant who is likely to have a low birth weight
    c. Excessive bleeding and high risk for septicemia in the mother
    d. A vaginal delivery with isolation precautions for the infant

18. What is the **most common** route for health care providers to be exposed to the HIV virus?
    a. Getting blood on exposed skin of hands or arms
    b. Touching infected body fluids with bare hands
    c. Having body fluid splashed on mucous membranes
    d. Getting stuck with a contaminated needle

19. The nurse is orienting a newly graduated RN to the medical unit. Which point should be included about protecting self from HIV exposure when caring for patients?
    a. Wear gloves when in contact with patients' mucous membranes or nonintact skin.
    b. Wear full protective gear when providing any care to HIV-positive patients.
    c. Always wear a mask when entering an HIV-positive patient's room.
    d. Talk to the employee health nurse about starting preexposure prophylaxis.

20. Which age-related change increases the likelihood that the older adult will develop the infection after an HIV exposure?
    a. Decline in the overall efficiency of the immune system
    b. Belief that HIV is not an issue for older people
    c. Reluctance to seek treatment for sexual problems
    d. Mistaking signs/symptoms as normal part of aging

21. A patient is diagnosed with *Pneumocystis jiroveci* pneumonia. Which signs/symptoms does the nurse expect to find when assessing the patient?
    a. Dyspnea, tachypnea, persistent dry cough, and fever
    b. Cough with copious thick sputum, fever, and dyspnea
    c. Substernal chest pain and difficulty swallowing
    d. Fever, persistent cough, and vomiting blood

22. Based on the concept of Treatment as Prevention, which outcome statement indicates that the goal of combination antiretroviral therapy is being met?
    a. Patient states understanding of medication regimen.
    b. Patient's viral load is at an undetectable level.
    c. Patient is classified as Stage Unknown.
    d. Patient has no signs of opportunistic infection.

23. The nurse is caring for a patient with AIDS who has been admitted for treatment of exacerbation of cryptosporidiosis. What is the **priority** assessment for this patient?
    a. Assess breath sounds and monitor respiratory status.
    b. Assess neurologic status and monitor for headaches.
    c. Assess for difficulty in swallowing and pain behind the sternum.
    d. Assess for signs of dehydration and monitor electrolytes.

24. Which nursing actions can the nurse delegate to unlicensed assistive personnel who will be giving mouth care to a patient with HIV/AIDS? **Select all that apply.**
    a. Offer the patient mouth rinses with sodium bicarbonate and sterile water several times a day.
    b. Assess the patient's mouth for increased presence of sores or white plaques.
    c. Encourage the patient to drink plenty of fluids.
    d. Assist the patient to brush teeth with a soft toothbrush.
    e. Apply an oral analgesic gel to gums as needed.
    f. Offer an alcohol-based mouthwash if patient reports "funny" taste in mouth.

25. Which person should be advised to have periodic screening for HIV?
    a. An 18-year-old college student who recently started dating a new person
    b. A 65-year-old widower who may be moving in with a homosexual friend
    c. A 28-year-old woman who plans to get pregnant in a few years
    d. A 23-year-old man who plans to enjoy serial monogamy for a few years

26. Rank the safety of sexual practices, **with 1 being the safest practice and 6 being the least safe.**

    _____ a. Mutual masturbation with latex gloves

    _____ b. Oral sex without condom

    _____ c. Abstinence

    _____ d. Vaginal sex with male condom use

    _____ e. Monogamy

    _____ f. Unprotected anal sex

27. The patient with HIV/AIDS develops manifestations of tuberculosis. What type of precautions does the nurse institute at this time?
    a. Standard precautions
    b. Airborne precautions
    c. Enteric precautions
    d. Neutropenic precautions

28. The nurse hears in shift report that the patient has toxoplasmosis encephalitis. The nurse is **most likely** to perform which types of focused assessments?
    a. Perform a mental status examination and assess for headache.
    b. Auscultate heart sounds and monitor for cardiac arrhythmias.
    c. Palpate the abdomen for tenderness and listen for bowel sounds.
    d. Monitor intake and urine output and palpate the bladder.

29. The patient reports numbness or tingling on the lip that occurred 24 hours ago, and now there is a painful lesion. Which action is the nurse **most likely** to take?
    a. Ask patient if he ate undercooked meat because of potential exposure to *Toxoplasma gondii.*
    b. Obtain an order for ketoconazole because patient is developing candidal esophagitis.
    c. Check for fever and palpate lymph nodes because the patient may have histoplasmosis.
    d. Instruct caregiver to wear gloves during oral hygiene because of suspected herpes simplex virus.

30. The patient with HIV has pain and burning along sensory nerve tracts, and the nurse observes fluid-filled blisters with crusts. Which question is the nurse **most likely** to ask to assist the health care provider in making the diagnosis of shingles caused by the varicella zoster virus?
    a. "Are you allergic to any types of antibiotics?"
    b. "Did you have chickenpox during childhood?"
    c. "Are you having any trouble with your vision?"
    d. "Did you notice any pruritus or perineal irritation?"

31. Which malignancy is **most** common in patients with HIV/AIDS?
    a. Non-Hodgkin's B-cell lymphoma
    b. Anal cancer
    c. Primary brain cancer
    d. Kaposi's sarcoma

32. Which person is the **most likely** candidate for combination antiretroviral therapy as post-exposure prophylaxis?
    a. Person who routinely injects recreational drugs with friends
    b. Nursing student who was stuck with a needle from a known HIV-negative source
    c. College student who had consensual sex with an HIV-negative partner
    d. Woman who was raped by an assailant with unknown HIV status

33. The patient with HIV/AIDS appears emaciated and has diarrhea, anorexia, mouth lesions, and persistent weight loss. What condition does the nurse suspect this patient is developing?
    a. AIDS dementia complex
    b. AIDS wasting syndrome
    c. AIDS gastrointestinal opportunistic infection
    d. AIDS candidiasis opportunistic infection

34. The unlicensed assistive personnel comes to the nurse crying and upset because "Some of the patient's spit got on my arm when I was helping him with oral hygiene, and he is HIV positive." What is the nurse's **best** response?
    a. "You'll be okay; don't worry about it. A little bit of saliva is no big deal."
    b. "Wash your arm; saliva is not infectious with HIV unless it is bloody."
    c. "Let's use chlorhexidine to wash your arm and send you for HIV testing."
    d. "Did you wash your arm? Next time, stand back during the swish and spit."

35. A nursing student sustains a needlestick from a hollow-bore needle while attempting to establish a peripheral intravenous (IV) catheter. What should the student do **first**?
    a. Finish the procedure and establish the IV.
    b. Go to the employee clinic for postexposure prophylaxis.
    c. Inform the nursing instructor or charge nurse.
    d. Thoroughly scrub and flush the puncture site.

36. The nurse reads in the chart that the patient has *Candida* stomatitis. Which concept is the nurse **most likely** to consider in planning interventions for this patient?
    a. Gas exchange
    b. Cellular regulation
    c. Comfort
    d. Elimination

37. The patient with AIDS comes to the emergency department and reports a cough, dyspnea, chest pain, fever, chills, night sweats, weight loss, and anorexia. He tells that nurse that he recently had a tuberculosis (TB) skin test (purified protein derivative [PPD]), which was negative. What should the nurse do **first**?
    a. Complete the assessment and notify the health care provider.
    b. Initiate airborne precautions and assess respiratory status.
    c. Seek out validation of the patient's negative PPD test results.
    d. Obtain order for automated nucleic acid amplification test for TB.

38. The patient with HIV/AIDS tells the nurse that food tastes funny and it is difficult to swallow. What is the nurse's **priority** action at this time?
    a. Instruct unlicensed assistive personnel to assist patient with oral hygiene.
    b. Place the patient in a high Fowler's and restrict oral intake.
    c. Examine mouth and throat for white plaques or inflammation.
    d. Collaborate with the dietitian to provide a soft diet.

39. The HIV-positive patient is receiving combination antiretroviral therapy drugs. Why is it essential that the drugs be taken every day at the same time?
    a. Missing or delaying doses decreases the blood concentration needed to inhibit viral replication.
    b. Missing or delaying doses decreases the risk of developing opportunistic mutations.
    c. Missing or delaying doses decreases the effectiveness of the viral replication.
    d. Missing or delaying doses decreases the risk of developing HIV-resistant mutations.

40. A patient who has HIV/AIDS and tuberculosis (TB) was recently started on the combination antiretroviral therapy (cART) regimen. The TB symptoms worsen and the nurse informs the health care provider, who makes the diagnosis of immune reconstitution inflammatory syndrome (IRIS). Which therapy is the provider **most likely** to order to treat IRIS?
    a. Bronchodilators
    b. Adjustment of cART
    c. Corticosteroids
    d. Antitubercular drugs

41. The home health nurse is assisting a family who lives with and cares for a member who is HIV positive. Which item would the nurse instruct the family not to share in order to decrease the risk of accidental exposure to HIV?
    a. Safety razor
    b. Household utensils
    c. Towels
    d. Toilet

42. The nurse is teaching a group of college students about preventing HIV infection through sexual contact. Which statement made by one of the students indicates **effective** teaching?
    a. "A latex condom with spermicide provides the best protection against getting infected with HIV."
    b. "Mutually monogamous sex with a noninfected partner is the best method to prevent HIV infection."
    c. "Contraceptive methods like implants and injections are recommended to prevent HIV transmission."
    d. "If my same sex partner and I are both HIV positive, then there is no point in using a condom."

43. Which laboratory results are expected to **decrease** in a patient who has untreated HIV/AIDS? **Select all that apply.**
    a. CD4+
    b. CD8+
    c. White blood cell count
    d. Lymphocytes
    e. HIV antibodies
    f. Viral load

44. A patient diagnosed with HIV is receiving combination antiretroviral therapy. Which laboratory test is the **best** for determining the effectiveness of the therapy?
    a. Western blot analysis
    b. Viral load testing
    c. Enzyme-linked immunosorbent assay
    d. 4th generation testing

20

CHAPTER

Care of Patients with Hypersensitivity (Allergy) and Autoimmunity

1. Which type I hypersensitivity reaction requires **immediate** intervention by the nurse?
   a. Rhinosinusitis
   b. Bronchoconstriction
   c. Urticaria
   d. Pruritus

2. The nurse is taking a history on a patient who is scheduled to undergo diagnostic testing with use of contrast dye. Which patient statement is cause for **greatest** concern?
   a. "My sister is allergic to the dye that they use for x-ray procedures."
   b. "I have a lot of seasonal allergies, and they make me pretty miserable."
   c. "My doctor thinks I might be at risk for diabetes and high blood pressure."
   d. "Last year I had a procedure and my face got so swollen I could not see."

3. Which statement **best** describes allergy or hypersensitivity?
   a. Excessive response to the presence of an antigen
   b. Excessive response against self-cells and cell products
   c. Failure of the immune system to recognize self-cells as normal
   d. Failure of the immune system to recognize foreign cells and microbial invaders

4. Which clinical examples are type I immediate hypersensitivities? **Select all that apply.**
   a. Goodpasture's syndrome
   b. Hay fever
   c. Serum sickness
   d. Anaphylaxis
   e. Autoimmune hemolytic anemia
   f. Allergic asthma

5. Which clinical condition **best** represents a type IV stimulated hypersensitivity?
   a. Poison ivy
   b. Graves' disease
   c. Myasthenia gravis
   d. Vasculitis

6. Which patient is **most likely** to be the **best** candidate for desensitization therapy for allergies?
   a. Patient lives on a farm in a remote area and suffers from hay fever.
   b. Patient lives in an urban area and has allergies to animal dander.
   c. Patient travels frequently outside the United States and has seasonal allergies.
   d. Patient lives on the street and is allergic to dust and has no health insurance.

7. During assessment of a newly admitted patient, the nurse notes that the patient has a runny nose with clear drainage; pink, swollen mucosa; itchy, watery eyes; and a nasal-sounding voice. What does the nurse expect is the patient's diagnosis?
   a. Hypersensitivity
   b. Allergic response
   c. Allergic rhinitis
   d. Autoimmune response

8. Which allergy management strategy is the **best** for a patient who has a history of allergic asthma?
   a. Practicing avoidance
   b. Undergoing desensitization
   c. Taking corticosteroids
   d. Carrying an automatic epinephrine injector

9. Which method of testing for allergies would be used if the patient wants to undergo "allergy shots"?
   a. T-lymphocyte count
   b. Blood test for C1-INH
   c. Skin biopsy
   d. Intradermal testing

10. The nurse has just received handoff reports on several patients who are being treated for hypersensitivity or autoimmune responses. Which patient is the nurse **most likely** to check on **first**?
    a. Patient who was treated for angioedema with epinephrine and oxygen
    b. Patient who has serum sickness and received a dose of oral diphenhydramine
    c. Patient who had hemolytic transfusion reaction and infusion was discontinued
    d. Patient with tissue transplant rejection awaiting transplant surgeon consult

11. The nursing instructor is quizzing a nursing student about the pharmacologic action of a decongestant drug that is prescribed for the patient. What is the **best** response to the instructor's query?
    a. "This drug will prevent vasodilation and decrease secretions."
    b. "This drug causes vasoconstriction and reduces the swelling."
    c. "This drug will decrease allergens and allergic response."
    d. "This drug will desensitize any allergic reactions."

12. The nurse has just given an African-American patient a **first-time** dose of an angiotensin converting enzyme inhibitor (ACEI). Which assessment is **most** important for this patient?
    a. Observes for any untoward effects of any medication
    b. Watches for angioedema and laryngeal edema
    c. Checks pulse and blood pressure before and after medication
    d. Monitors for excessive drowsiness and confusion

13. For a patient who is having an anaphylactic reaction, which common symptoms will manifest **almost immediately** after being exposed to an allergen? **Select all that apply.**
    a. Erythema of the eyes and lips
    b. Apprehension
    c. Chills
    d. Fever
    e. Urticaria
    f. Confusion

14. A patient in anaphylaxis is at risk for respiratory failure. Which assessment finding prompts the nurse to prepare equipment to assist the health care provider to intubate the patient?
    a. Crackles
    b. Hypoxemia
    c. Wheezing
    d. Stridor

15. The patient has a documented allergy to latex. Which piece of common medical equipment could trigger the patient's latex allergy if special precautions are not taken to ensure a latex-free product?
    a. Indwelling urinary catheter
    b. 4 × 4 gauze sponge
    c. Blood pressure cuff
    d. Hospital meal tray

16. The nurse is caring for a patient and suspects anaphylaxis. What **priority** action does the nurse perform?
    a. Place the patient on a cardiac monitor and observe for arrhythmias.
    b. Insert a large-bore intravenous (IV) line with normal saline.
    c. Ask the patient to describe previous responses to various types of allergens.
    d. Apply oxygen using a high-flow, nonrebreather mask at 90%-100%.

17. For a patient with anaphylaxis, which **priority** treatment does the nurse expect to administer?
    a. Oral diphenhydramine
    b. Intravenous epinephrine
    c. Albuterol via high-flow nebulizer
    d. Intravenous corticosteroids

18. The nurse is assessing a patient experiencing a cytotoxic reaction to IV drugs. What is the nurse's **first** action?
    a. Discontinue drug administration.
    b. Decrease the infusion rate.
    c. Change the IV tubing.
    d. Call the Rapid Response Team.

19. What are the clinical manifestations of systemic lupus erythematosus that are caused by an immune complex reaction?
    a. Vasculitis, glomerulonephritis, nephritis
    b. Hypertension, hyperlipidemia
    c. Excessive mucus and secretions
    d. Angioedema, urticaria, stridor

20. The patient comes to the clinic with symptoms of achy joints, rash, and malaise. Which question would be the **most** useful in helping the health care provider to make the diagnosis of serum sickness?
    a. "Have you had fever over 101°F (38.3°C) or chills?"
    b. "Did you recently get bitten or stung by an insect or spider?"
    c. "Have you been exposed to any poisonous plants, such as poison ivy?"
    d. "Have you taken or received any new drugs within the past 7-12 days?"

21. Which responses are characterized as type IV delayed hypersensitivity reactions? **Select all that apply.**
    a. Positive purified protein derivative test for tuberculosis
    b. Systemic lupus erythematosus
    c. Immune thrombocytopenic purpura
    d. Contact dermatitis
    e. Graft rejection
    f. Local response to insect stings

22. The nurse is reviewing the laboratory results of a patient who has had more than one episode of angioedema. Which intervention would be the **most** appropriate follow-up for a positive result of a C1-INH blood test?
    a. Assessing for angiotensin converting enzyme inhibitors that can cause angioedema
    b. Arranging for genetic counseling related to genetic deficiency and angioedema
    c. Ensuring that the patient knows to take corticosteroid as prescribed for angioedema
    d. Advising the patient to have annual allergy testing to predict potential triggers of angioedema

23. Which nursing intervention is the **most** important for the nurse to perform before administering any drug or therapeutic agent to an adult patient?
    a. Ask the patient about allergies to drugs or other substances.
    b. Check the medication administration record for allergic response to drugs.
    c. Make sure that emergency medications are readily available.
    d. Be aware of types of drugs that are likely to cause allergic reactions.

24. A patient who had a positive purified protein derivative (PPD) test for tuberculosis has redness and a 9-mm induration at the injection site. The nurse suspects which type of hypersensitivity reaction?
    a. Type I, immediate
    b. Type II, cytotoxic
    c. Type III, immune complex-mediated
    d. Type IV, delayed

25. A patient reports a runny nose with clear drainage, watery eyes, and a scratchy throat and being in close contact with several cats. Which therapy does the nurse anticipate?
    a. Intramuscular epinephrine and oxygen
    b. Oral corticosteroids and avoidance education
    c. Observation for worsening symptoms
    d. Decongestants and intranasal steroid spray

26. The nurse is preparing a teaching plan for the patient and family on how to use and care for an automatic epinephrine injector. Which essential points must the nurse include? **Select all that apply.**
    a. "Keep the device with you at all times."
    b. "You can inject the drug right through your pants."
    c. "When you use the device, call your doctor and rest in bed for 24 hours."
    d. "Protect the device from light and avoid temperature extremes."
    e. "Keep the safety cap in place until you are ready to use the device."
    f. "Inject yourself when you get short of breath."

27. The patient was treated in the emergency department for angioedema and now reports "feeling fine" and wants to go home. What is the nurse's **best** response?
    a. "Sir, the doctor has not discharged you yet, so you have to stay, but we'll take good care of you."
    b. "Let me check your vital signs one more time; then I'll get the doctor to write a discharge order."
    c. "Your symptoms are gone, but they could reoccur, so we have to observe you for a few more hours."
    d. "Oh, you are not finished yet. There is a lot of patient education that we need to review."

28. In caring for a patient with severe hypersensitivity response, under what circumstances would the nurse prepare to assist the health care provider with a tracheostomy?
    a. Patient has excessive laryngeal edema and intubation is impossible.
    b. Patient with anaphylaxis has a previous history of angioedema.
    c. Patient has wheezing, dypsnea, hypoxia, and cyanosis.
    d. Patient is unable to give a clear history but has respiratory distress.

29. The patient has anaphylaxis. What is the major factor that is **most likely** to result in the patient's death?
    a. Delay in locating intubation equipment
    b. Delay in administering epinephrine
    c. Inappropriately discharging the patient
    d. Administering the wrong rescue medication

30. The nurse is reviewing the patient's medication orders and knows that the patient has an allergy to penicillin. Which prescribed medication is the nurse **most likely** to question?
    a. Analgesic for pain as needed
    b. Cephalosporin on call to surgery
    c. Decongestant as needed for rhinorrhea
    d. Angiotensin converting enzyme inhibitor daily

31. Which description **best** characterizes autoimmunity?
    a. Cell-mediated immune response that does not cause an antibody-mediated response
    b. The synthetic substances used to stimulate or suppress the response of the immune system
    c. Inappropriate immune response to one's own healthy cells and tissues
    d. An altered immune response that results in an immediate hypersensitivity reaction

32. Which disorders have an autoimmune basis? **Select all that apply.**
    a. Type 2 diabetes
    b. Systemic lupus erythematosus
    c. Hypothyroidism
    d. Ulcerative colitis
    e. Rheumatoid arthritis
    f. Irritable bowel disease

33. Which management strategy does the nurse expect when caring for a patient with an autoimmune disease?
    a. Antibiotic drugs
    b. Antihistamine drugs
    c. Anti-inflammatory drugs
    d. Bronchodilator drugs

34. Which patient is **most likely** to undergo and benefit from plasmapheresis therapy?
    a. Patient with drug-induced hemolytic anemia who has a high risk for kidney failure
    b. Patient with scleroderma who is not responding to first-line treatments
    c. Patient with tissue transplant who is experiencing organ rejection
    d. Patient who has angioedema with an offending agent that has a long half-life.

35. For which patient circumstance would it be safe to prescribe a disease-modifying antirheumatic drug, such as adalimumab?
    a. Patient has been in remission of cancer for 5 years.
    b. Patient is breastfeeding a newborn infant.
    c. Patient was treated for tuberculosis 15 years ago.
    d. Patient is currently being treated for early heart failure.

36. Which outcome statement reflects one of the goals of drug therapy for autoimmune disease?
    a. The patient lists steps to take in case of a hypersensitivity response.
    b. The patient demonstrates a respiratory rate within the normal range.
    c. The patient verbalizes feelings of reduced anxiety and apprehension.
    d. The patient retains enough immunity to prevent serious infections.

37. The nurse is working in a clinic that serves a patient population that is frequently treated with selective immunosuppressive therapy. Which questions is the nurse **most likely** to ask when initially interviewing new patients? **Select all that apply.**
    a. "Are you currently pregnant or planning to try to get pregnant in the near future?"
    b. "Are you currently being treated for any infections?"
    c. "Have you ever had an anaphylactic reaction to prescribed medication?"
    d. "Have you ever had any genetic testing or counseling related to allergies?"
    e. "Would you be willing to learn how to self-inject medication?"
    f. "Have you ever been treated or diagnosed with tuberculosis?"

38. The nurse is preparing the 9:00 am medication and sees that the patient is due for a morning dose of thalidomide. The nurse has heard of the medication but is not exactly sure why it has been prescribed for this patient. What should the nurse do?
    a. Give the 9:00 am dose so it is not delayed and look up the drug when there is more time.
    b. Ask the patient if the medication looks familiar and why it was prescribed.
    c. Call the health care provider and ask for clarification of the order and the purpose of the drug.
    d. Use a drug resource to look up information and cross-check the patient's medical history.

21
CHAPTER

Principles of Cancer Development

1. Which task is the nurse **most likely** to perform when caring for a patient with cancer?
   a. Informs a 36-year-old woman about the initial diagnosis of breast cancer
   b. Explains recommendations for yearly mammograms to a 50-year-old woman
   c. Suggests treatments based on staging of breast tumor to a 65-year-old woman
   d. Advises a 23-year-old woman to have surgery for breast cancer

2. Which patient has benign tumor cells that are the result of a small problem with cellular regulation?
   a. Patient is diagnosed with uterine fibroids.
   b. Patient is advised that she has melanoma.
   c. Patient is advised that he has a G_1 tumor.
   d. Patient is diagnosed with hairy cell leukemia.

3. African Americans have the highest rate of cancer and the highest death rate from cancer. Which intervention targets the **most likely** explanation for this disparity?
   a. Increase local efforts to dispense cancer information to this vulnerable group.
   b. Develop educational materials that are culturally sensitive toward African Americans.
   c. Provide referral information to health care facilities that are affordable and accessible.
   d. Continue research that further clarifies the genetic or racial risk for cancer.

4. Which patient circumstance represents the normal physiologic progress of mitosis and cellular regulation?
   a. A 25-year-old woman is diagnosed with endometriosis.
   b. A 45-year-old woman notices several skin tags on her neck.
   c. A 35-year-old male has ulcer disease that is slowly resolving.
   d. A 65-year-old man has a benign tumor that seems to be enlarging.

5. The nurse reads a laboratory report indicating that the tissue sample of a patient is essentially neoplastic. How does the nurse interpret this report?
   a. Cell growth is abnormal and not needed for tissue replacement.
   b. The tissue specimen shows malignant cell growth.
   c. The parent cell was abnormal, but new growth is benign.
   d. Early cell death is inevitable because the morphology is abnormal.

6. Which cells would normally not produce fibronectin?
   a. Normal nerve cells
   b. Normal cardiac muscle cells
   c. Normal red blood cells
   d. Cells that are undergoing normal mitosis

7. Which areas of the body contain cells that grow throughout the life span? **Select all that apply.**
   a. Heart
   b. Hair
   c. Brain
   d. Bone marrow
   e. Skin
   f. Lining of intestines

8. Which biologic process demonstrates the differentiated function of red blood cells (RBCs)?
   a. RBCs float freely through the circulatory system.
   b. RBCs die according to programmed cell death.
   c. RBCs make hemoglobin, which carries oxygen.
   d. RBCs are formed with 23 pairs of chromosomes.

9. Which biologic process demonstrates that there is a problem with cellular regulation?
   a. Living cells spend most of their time in G_0 state.
   b. Mitosis occurs to replace damaged tissue.
   c. Cyclin activity is balanced by suppressor genes.
   d. Cells continue to divide without contact inhibition.

10. The nurse is aware that the **most** common way for cancer to spread is bloodborne metastasis. In caring for a patient with cancer, what type of precautions would the nurse use?
    a. Contact isolation precautions
    b. Standard precautions
    c. Neutropenic precautions
    d. Droplet precautions

11. If apoptosis is occurring within a patient's body, what is the expected outcome of this physiologic process?
    a. Rapid growth of malignant tumors metastasizing through the body.
    b. Organs have an adequate number of cells at their functional peak.
    c. Normal tissue continues to function in an abnormal place.
    d. Cells will initially resemble parent cells but will rapidly mutate.

12. Benign cells have which characteristics? **Select all that apply.**
    a. Contain few pairs of chromosomes.
    b. Resemble the parent tissue.
    c. Growth is orderly with normal growth patterns.
    d. Perform their differentiated function.
    e. Invade other tissues.
    f. Continue to make fibronectin.

13. Which features are specific to cancer cells?
    a. They grow very slowly but eventually harm the body.
    b. They have a small, fragile nucleus that is easily damaged.
    c. They produce fibronectin, which strengthens the cell wall.
    d. They have an unlimited life span and spread easily.

14. What is an action of carcinogens?
    a. Damage the DNA.
    b. Increase migration of cells.
    c. Turn off oncogenes.
    d. Stimulate viral activity.

15. Why do cancer cells spread throughout the body? **Select all that apply.**
    a. They enrich nutrients at the original site.
    b. They have loose adherence.
    c. They readily slip through blood vessel walls and tissue.
    d. They do not respond to contact inhibition.
    e. They are fragile and easily break apart.
    f. They readily respond to signals for apoptosis.

16. Ideally, the health care team should encourage primary prevention measures to target which step of carcinogenesis?
    a. Initiation
    b. Promotion
    c. Progression
    d. Metastasis

17. What role do normal hormones and proteins such as insulin and estrogen play in the development of cancer?
    a. They prolong or delay the growth of cancer cells.
    b. They can promote frequent division of cells.
    c. They act like carcinogens under certain conditions.
    d. They turn off the suppressor genes.

18. What is the minimum size for a detectable tumor?
    a. 1 millimeter
    b. 1 centimeter
    c. Depends on type of tumor
    d. Depends on site of tumor

19. If a primary tumor is located in a vital organ, what happens?
    a. Cancer is more likely to spread to other sites.
    b. The organ stops producing normal cells.
    c. There is interference with organ function.
    d. Function of the organ is initially increased.

20. Which statement correctly describes metastatic tumors?
    a. They are caused by cells breaking off from the primary tumor.
    b. They become less malignant over time.
    c. They are usually less harmful than a primary tumor.
    d. They become the tissue of the organ where they spread.

21. What role does vascular endothelial growth factor (VEGF) have in the metastasis of cancer?
    a. VEGF triggers capillary growth to ensure blood supply to the tumor.
    b. Use of VEGF helps to stop the growth and spread of the primary tumor.
    c. VEGF is a carcinogen that activates when cancer cells reach the vascular system.
    d. For cancers with a genetic link, VEGF must be present before metastasis occurs.

22. Which information can be obtained from grading a tumor?
    a. Genetic linkage to the cancer
    b. Location and origin of metastasis
    c. Evaluating prognosis and appropriate therapy
    d. How long the cancer has been present

23. What information can be obtained by surgical staging? **Select all that apply.**
    a. Assessment of tumor size
    b. Number of tumors
    c. Sites of tumors
    d. Types of tumors
    e. Pattern of spread of tumors
    f. Pain related to tumors

24. Why would the nurse encourage a patient to get a vaccine such as Gardasil or Cervarix?
    a. Protects against human papillomaviruses, which are associated with genital cancers.
    b. Protects against Epstein-Barr virus, which may contribute to Burkitt's lymphoma.
    c. Protects against hepatitis B virus, which may contribute to primary liver cancer.
    d. Protects against human lymphotrophic virus, which may contribute to T-cell leukemia.

25. From a primary prevention perspective, what is the **most** important information that the nurse should emphasize when teaching patients about tobacco and cancer risk?
    a. Risk for cancer increases when tobacco and alcohol are both used.
    b. Tobacco use is linked to many different types of cancer.
    c. Risk for cancer depends on the amount of tobacco used.
    d. Tobacco is the single most preventable source of carcinogenesis.

26. The nurse is talking to a young woman who "is using a tanning salon, because it is a safer way to get a tan than lying in the sun." What is the **best** response?
    a. "Even if you use a tanning salon, you should still use a sunscreen."
    b. "Tanning salons are safer because exposure to radiation is very controlled."
    c. "Ultraviolet radiation from sun exposure or tanning salons can cause skin cancer."
    d. "Ionizing radiation is dangerous, but tanning salons use ultraviolet radiation."

27. Which person has the **greatest** risk for developing cancer?
    a. 10-year-old African American with allergic asthma
    b. 32-year-old Asian immigrant with low income
    c. 23-year-old white American who has type 1 diabetes
    d. 62-year-old African American who had an organ transplant

28. The nurse is assessing a patient who is undergoing outpatient therapy for breast cancer. Which patient report causes the **greatest** concern because of possible metastasis to a common site?
    a. "I don't seem to have a very good appetite."
    b. "My ribs hurt but I haven't had any injuries."
    c. "My skin is dry and it feels itchy and irritated."
    d. "I feel like I need to urinate all of the time."

29. The nurse hears in report that the patient is diagnosed with glioblastoma. Which question is the **most** important to ask the off-going nurse?
    a. "What is the patient's current mental status?"
    b. "Does the patient have leg pain during ambulation?"
    c. "Is the patient able to eat a normal diet?"
    d. "Does the patient have trouble passing urine?"

30. Which tumor, node, metastasis (TNM) staging classification would indicate the **best** prognosis for the patient's survival?
    a. $T_{IS}N_0M_0$
    b. $T_xN_xM_x$
    c. $T_2N_1M_0$
    d. $T_2N_3M_1$

31. Which patient report should be investigated as one of the seven warning signs of cancer?
    a. Soreness and stiffness to joints in the morning
    b. Abdominal pain related to irregular meals
    c. Redness to skin with pain after sun exposure
    d. Sore on nipple present for several months

32. Which patient circumstance would prompt the nurse to create a three-generation pedigree to more fully explore the possibility of genetic risk?
    a. Smoked for 20 years but quit 5 years ago
    b. Strong family history of colorectal cancer
    c. Male relatives with prostate problems
    d. Personal history of excessive sun exposure

33. The American Cancer Society reports that the cancer incidence and survival rate are related to which factors?
    a. Gender of patient and gender of family caregiver
    b. Availability of and access to health care services
    c. Belief that cancer is a chronic disorder
    d. Age at initiation of lifestyle modification

34. Which lunch tray represents a diet that would decrease the risk of cancer?
    a. Plain chicken breast on white bread
    b. Vegetable plate with a bran muffin
    c. Grilled cheese sandwich with fruit salad
    d. Bacon cheeseburger with French fries

35. The nurse is preparing a brochure to inform patients about secondary prevention of cancer. Which information would be included?
    a. Yearly mammography for women starting at the age of 45
    b. Chemoprevention with vitamin therapy
    c. Removing colon polyps for cancer prophylaxis
    d. Using sunscreen and hat when outdoors

36. Which woman would be the **most likely** candidate to consider removal of "at-risk" breast tissue?
    a. Has a family history of breast and colon cancer and eats a high-fat diet
    b. Has large breasts that make self-examination difficult and smokes cigarettes
    c. Has mutations in the BRCA1 and BRCA2 genes and sister had breast cancer
    d. Has mammogram results that suggest an immediate biopsy is needed

22 CHAPTER

Care of Patients with Cancer

1. Which patient with cancer has the **greatest** risk for infection?
   a. Recently diagnosed with breast cancer
   b. With neutropenia from leukemia
   c. With lung cancer who has a persistent cough
   d. Diagnosed with prostate cancer 3 years ago

2. The health care provider informs the nurse that it is likely that the patient's cancer has invaded the bone marrow. Based on this information, the nurse will be vigilant for which signs and symptoms? **Select all that apply.**
   a. Nausea and vomiting
   b. Fatigue and weakness
   c. Decreasing white blood cell counts
   d. Confusion with memory loss
   e. Bruises or other bleeding signs
   f. Tachycardia and shortness of breath

3. A patient with colon cancer asks, "Why does everyone keep insisting that I eat so much? I'm not hungry and I have been overweight my whole life." Which response is the **most** appropriate?
   a. "What would you like to eat? I can get you something that you will really enjoy."
   b. "The cancer may spread to your stomach; you should eat while you still can."
   c. "Cancer in the intestinal tract may increase metabolic rate and needs for nutrients."
   d. "Well, you don't have to eat if you don't want to, but eating will help your body to heal."

4. The nurse hears in report that the patient has cachexia. Which assessment will the nurse plan to perform?
   a. Ability to ambulate independently
   b. Appetite and nutritional intake
   c. Mental status and cognition
   d. Sensation and pulses in extremities

5. The patient has breast cancer with bone metastasis. Based on this information, which laboratory result would the nurse carefully monitor?
   a. Serum calcium level
   b. Serum blood glucose
   c. Serum potassium level
   d. Serum sodium level

6. Which factors determine the type of therapy for cancer? **Select all that apply.**
   a. Type and location of cancer
   b. Overall health of the patient
   c. Whether the cancer has metastasized
   d. Previous lymph node biopsy
   e. Patient's gender
   f. Family history and genetics

7. Which example **best** illustrates appropriate prophylactic cancer surgery?
   a. Removal of polyp from the colon to prevent colon cancer
   b. Biopsy of lymph node at a site distal to the primary tumor
   c. Breast reconstruction after a mastectomy
   d. Partial removal of a tumor to provide pain relief

8. Which patient circumstance would prompt the health care team to use the National Comprehensive Cancer Network Distress Thermometer?
   a. Patient was recently diagnosed with breast cancer and is refusing to discuss treatment options.
   b. Family member of dying cancer patient is overwhelmed by anticipatory grief and loss.
   c. Patient is having multiple physical symptoms and emotional problems related to cancer therapy.
   d. Patient and family are distressed because cancer therapy has not induced remission.

9. Which outcome statement indicates that the goal of cytoreductive surgery for cancer has been met?
   a. Tumor size has been decreased and chemotherapy is pending.
   b. The noninvasive skin cancer was completely removed during surgery.
   c. Subjective back pain has decreased since the removal of the tumor.
   d. Incisional site of breast reconstruction shows no signs of infection.

10. Which cancer patient is the **most likely** candidate for palliative surgery?
    a. Needs extensive cosmetic repair after treatment of neck cancer
    b. Has continuous vomiting because tumor is obstructing the intestines
    c. Has a suspicious skin lesion that requires further investigation
    d. Has been treated for cancer and is currently asymptomatic

11. Which cancer patient is the **most likely** candidate for reconstructive surgery?
    a. Has severe back pain and decreased sensation in the lower extremities
    b. Has significant scarring of the face and neck after completing treatments
    c. Requires lymph node removal for possible metastasis of primary tumor
    d. Has leukemia that is not responding to transfusion therapy

12. The nurse is talking to a young athlete who needs lung removal for treatment of lung cancer. Which statement **best** indicates that the patient is coping with the uncertainty of cancer and long-term impact on his physical activities?
    a. "If I delay the surgery, I could still compete for a couple of months."
    b. "My coach says I might be able to compete even with one lung."
    c. "Competing in sports is important to me, and eventually I will recover."
    d. "I love to compete in sports, but I like to do a lot of other things too."

13. The nurse is caring for a 56-year-old woman who had a modified mastectomy for breast cancer. The woman jokes, "That breast was too saggy anyway. Good riddance to it." Later, the nurse sees the woman crying. What should the nurse do **first**?
    a. Encourage the woman to accept body changes by looking at the surgical site.
    b. Suggest participation in a support group sponsored by the American Cancer Society.
    c. Invite a breast cancer survivor who successfully coped with mastectomy.
    d. Sit with the woman and encourage her to express her feelings and concerns.

14. Which factors are used to determine a cancer patient's absorbed radiation dose? **Select all that apply.**
    a. Intensity of radiation exposure
    b. Proximity of radiation source to body
    c. Type of radiation particle
    d. Age of the patient during radiation therapy
    e. Overall health at time of radiation therapy
    f. Duration of radiation exposure

15. Based on the "inverse square law" for radiation exposure, which patient received the smallest radiation dose?
    a. Received radiation dose at a distance of 0.5 meter
    b. Received radiation dose at a distance of 1 meter
    c. Received radiation dose at a distance of 2.5 meters
    d. Received radiation dose at a distance of 3 meters

16. What is the **most** typical schedule for radiation therapy?
    a. Small doses of radiation given on a daily basis for a set time period
    b. Large one-time dose of radiation given after completing chemotherapy
    c. Small doses of radiation given several days apart to minimize side effects
    d. Large doses administered monthly for a set period of months

17. What instructions will the nurse give to unlicensed assistive personnel regarding the hygienic care of a patient with neutropenia?
    a. Do not enter the room unless absolutely necessary and then minimize time spent in the room.
    b. Mouth care and washing of the axillary and perianal regions must be done during the shift.
    c. If the patient seems very tired, assist with toileting but defer all other aspects of hygienic care.
    d. Assist the patient to perform hygienic care according to the standard routine for all patients.

18. The nurse in the radiation department is caring for a patient who will receive stereotactic body radiotherapy. Which intervention is the nurse **most likely** to use in the care of this patient?
    a. Remind the patient that no pregnant visitors should come for several days.
    b. Dispose of radioactive urine and stool so that self and others are not exposed.
    c. Teach the patient about the need for exact positioning during the treatment.
    d. Assess the patient for history of allergies to iodine or contrast media.

19. A patient is receiving radiation treatment by teletherapy. When does exposure to the patient create a risk for harmful radiation?
    a. The patient is never radioactive
    b. During the mechanical delivery of gamma rays
    c. For the first 24 to 48 hours after treatment
    d. Until the radiation source has decayed by one half-life

20. What is the **most** common side effect of radiation?
    a. Altered taste sensation
    b. Radiodermatitis
    c. Nausea
    d. Fatigue

21. For a patient undergoing external radiation therapy, what do the nurse's instructions include? **Select all that apply.**
    a. Do not remove the markings.
    b. Use lotions liberally to keep skin soft and moist.
    c. Avoid direct skin exposure to sunlight for up to a year.
    d. Use mild soap and water on the affected skin.
    e. Gently rub treated areas to stimulate circulation.
    f. Avoid wearing belts or clothing that binds the irradiated area.

22. Why does the nurse wear a dosimeter when providing care to a patient receiving brachytherapy?
    a. Indicates special expertise in radiation therapy.
    b. Protects the nurse from absorbing radiation.
    c. Measures the nurse's exposure to radiation.
    d. Ensures that the radiation dosage is accurate.

23. The patient has thyroid cancer and will be treated with injection of the radionuclide iodine-131 (brachytherapy). Which guideline is the **most** relevant when instructing unlicensed assistive personnel on how to assist the patient with hygiene and activities of daily living?
    a. Oncology Nursing Society practice guidelines
    b. American Cancer Society treatment guidelines
    c. Institutional evidence-based policies for infection control
    d. Institutional policies for handling body fluids and wastes

24. The nurse is supervising a nursing student who is giving care to a patient with a sealed implant. The nurse would intervene if the student performed which action?
    a. Places a "Caution: Radioactive Material" sign on the door of the patient's room.
    b. Wears a dosimeter film badge at all times while caring for the patient.
    c. Wears a lead apron while providing care and turns away from the patient.
    d. Saves all dressings and bed linens in the patient's room.

25. The nurse hears in report that the patient has xerostomia. Which teaching point does the nurse plan to review with the patient?
    a. Regular dental visits are essential because of increased risk for dental caries.
    b. Use mild soap and apply unscented moisturizers to reduce itching sensation.
    c. Avoid rigorous sports because bones are more prone to pathologic fractures.
    d. Avoid direct sun exposure for at least 1 year because skin will be sensitive.

26. According to Quality and Safety Education for Nurses (QSEN), what is the **priority** nursing assessment that the nurse should perform every 8 hours to protect a patient who has neutropenia?
    a. Assess patient's concerns first and then follow up by addressing each concern and problem.
    b. Monitor for complications that are associated with the type of therapy that patient is receiving.
    c. Perform focused assessment that includes pain and body system most affected by cancer.
    d. Perform total patient assessment and check for common symptoms associated with infection.

27. The nurse works at an institution where pharmacogenomics is incorporated into the care of cancer patients. How does this newer approach impact nursing care?
    a. Nurse is likely to see fewer cancers that are linked to a genetic etiology.
    b. Targeted chemotherapy selection will eliminate side effects.
    c. Prophylactic treatment of first-degree family members is likely to increase.
    d. Patients' risk for the more dangerous side effects is decreased.

28. Which laboratory result is the **most** important in relation to the nadir for a chemotherapeutic agent?
    a. Red blood cell count
    b. White blood cell count
    c. Platelet count
    d. Serum calcium level

29. Each chemotherapeutic agent has a specific nadir. What is important for the nurse to do when giving combination therapy?
    a. Give two agents with similar nadirs.
    b. Avoid giving agents with similar nadirs at the same time.
    c. Watch for first agent's nadir and then give second agent.
    d. Give two agents from different drug classes.

30. Because chemotherapy drug dosage is based on total body surface area, the nurse should perform what assessment?
    a. Measure the patient's height and weight.
    b. Compare the patient's weight to a nomogram.
    c. Calculate body mass index.
    d. Measure abdominal girth.

31. Which patient has a condition that is a significant contraindication for photodynamic therapy?
    a. Patient has a history of frequent sunburn and is at risk for skin cancer.
    b. Patient has known tumor involvement of a major blood vessel.
    c. Patient needs treatments that would involve the upper airways.
    d. Patient had surgery for breast cancer several years ago.

32. A patient is on a newer protocol, dose-dense chemotherapy. Which factor is **most likely** to contribute to patient noncompliance if the nurse fails to educate the patient and the family?
    a. Treatment is expensive and less likely to be covered by insurance.
    b. Length of therapy is prolonged and progress is slow to manifest.
    c. Side effects are likely to be more intense and unpleasant.
    d. Medication administration is painful and pain does not respond to medications.

33. The charge nurse sees an order for intravenous (IV) chemotherapy. According to the Oncology Nursing Society, who should the charge nurse assign to administer the medication?
    a. Any nurse who studied pharmacology and has IV therapy training
    b. Advanced-practice nurse who specializes in oncology education
    c. Registered nurse who completed an approved chemotherapy course
    d. Licensed practical nurse with years of experience in giving medications

34. The nurse is caring for a patient who must receive a chemotherapy infusion. What is the **most** important intervention related to extravasation?
    a. Identify the specific antidote and make sure it is readily available.
    b. Frequently monitor the access site to prevent leakage of large volumes.
    c. Advocate that an implanted port be established prior to administration.
    d. Avoid administering any drugs or fluids that are vesicants to tissue.

35. What is the **major** side effect that limits the dose of chemotherapy?
    a. Nausea and vomiting
    b. Peripheral neuropathy
    c. Bone marrow suppression
    d. "Chemo brain"

36. A patient is being discharged with a prescription for an oral cancer agent. Which teaching point will the nurse emphasize?
    a. Oral anticancer medications are less toxic and can be handled like regular medications.
    b. Oral forms are more convenient and portable and cost less than IV medications.
    c. Crushing the medication and mixing it with pudding or juice will mask the unpleasant taste.
    d. Skipping or reducing doses may seem unimportant but can lead to disease progression.

37. The nurse hears in report that the patient is distressed by the prospect of developing alopecia. Which question is the nurse **most likely** to ask to assess the patient's concerns?
    a. "Would you like additional information about side effects of chemotherapy?"
    b. "What questions do you have about hair and skin care products?"
    c. "How would losing your hair affect your life and activities?"
    d. "How would you feel about talking to someone who experienced hair loss?"

38. The nurse reads in the patient's chart that the health care provider is concerned about myelosuppression. Which laboratory results will the nurse closely monitor and report to the provider? **Select all that apply.**
    a. White blood cell count
    b. Serum potassium level
    c. Red blood cell count
    d. Platelet count
    e. Serum sodium level
    f. Serum calcium level

39. The nurse is caring for an older patient who is getting chemotherapy and filgrastim. Which intervention is the nurse **most likely** to use to facilitate the purpose of the filgrastim?
    a. Teach patient, family, and all visitors about meticulous hand hygiene.
    b. Administer the filgrastim prior to chemotherapy to prevent nausea.
    c. Teach and assess for bleeding signs such as bruising or bleeding gums.
    d. Assess the patient for fatigue and plan for periods of uninterrupted rest.

40. How does the nurse apply the "inverse square law" in caring for a patient with cancer who is treated with a radiation implant?
    a. Assists the health care provider to calculate the radiation dose
    b. Reminds all care staff to wear a dosimeter film badge for protection
    c. Stands at a distance from the patient as much as possible
    d. Monitors condition of skin after therapy with gamma rays

41. A patient is taking oprelvekin. Which assessment data finding indicates that the therapy is working?
    a. Weight has increased by 2 lbs.
    b. Nausea and vomiting are relieved.
    c. Platelet count is increasing.
    d. Hemoglobin level is normalizing.

42. The patient is having nausea and vomiting, so the nurse checks the medication orders for an antiemetic. The orders indicate to give rosiglitazone maleate and metformin hydrochloride as needed for nausea and vomiting. What should the nurse do?
    a. Give the medication as ordered and observe for symptom relief.
    b. Contact the provider for clarification, because the medication is not an antiemetic.
    c. Check the medication administration record for time of last dose of medication.
    d. Assess the patient for delayed nausea before giving the medication.

43. An older adult is having frequent and severe chemotherapy-induced nausea and vomiting that seems to be anticipatory and acute. Which assessment is the **most** important to make?
    a. Fears and feelings associated with chemotherapy
    b. Patient's self-management of distressing symptoms
    c. Signs of dehydration or electrolyte imbalance
    d. Willingness to try complementary or alternative therapies

44. What technique is used in oral care for a patient with mucositis?
    a. Apply petrolatum jelly to lips after each mouth care.
    b. Brush teeth and tongue rigorously with a toothbrush every 8 hours.
    c. "Swish and spit" room-temperature tap water every 1-2 hours for comfort.
    d. Use commercial mouthwashes and glycerin swabs to refresh mouth.

45. The nurse is responsible for teaching the immunosuppressed patient and the family about health-promoting activities. Which information is correct?
    a. Wash hands thoroughly with an antimicrobial soap.
    b. Do not drink water, milk, juice, or other cold liquids.
    c. Boil dishes or use disposables whenever possible.
    d. Don a mask before entering the patient's personal space.

46. The patient is prescribed a biologic response modifier, leukine. Which outcome statement about the medication therapy reflects the concept of immunity?
    a. Electrolyte levels are improving and there is no edema.
    b. Erythrocytes are increased and fatigue is resolving.
    c. Platelet count is normalizing and there are no signs of bleeding.
    d. White cell count is improving and there are no signs of infection.

47. The nurse is caring for several patients who are receiving chemotherapy. Which patient is the **most likely** to need transfer to the intensive care unit?
    a. Patient receiving interleukin therapy for renal cell carcinoma develops widespread edema.
    b. Patient receiving estrogen therapy develops calf pain with redness and swelling.
    c. Patient receiving vascular endothelial growth factor/receptor inhibitor has high blood pressure.
    d. Patient receiving an antiandrogen receptor develops gynecomastia.

48. A patient with advanced breast cancer tells the nurse she has pain in the back. Which assessment will the nurse perform to detect the complication of spinal cord compression?
    a. Assess for muscle weakness and/or decreased sensation in the lower extremities.
    b. Auscultate bowel sounds and gently palpate for abdominal pain and distention.
    c. Auscultate breath sounds, observe for dyspnea, and check for edema in the arms and hands.
    d. Assess for dehydration and monitor for signs of hyperkalemia or hyperuricemia.

49. Which outcome statement supports the **priority** goal in the care of a patient who has chemotherapy-induced peripheral neuropathy?
    a. Patient did not sustain falls or injury during the shift.
    b. Patient's electrolyte values are within normal limits.
    c. Patient verbalized understanding of when to take medication.
    d. Patient and family demonstrate good hand hygiene.

50. A patient with lymphoma wakes up from a night's sleep with severe facial swelling and tightness of the gown collar. Which emergency complication does the nurse suspect?
    a. Tumor lysis syndrome
    b. Cancer-induced hypercalcemia
    c. Superior vena cava syndrome
    d. Left-sided heart failure

51. A patient has a diagnosis of cancer with a gram-negative infection. Which assessment finding alerts the nurse that the patient may have developed the life-threatening complication of disseminated intravascular coagulation?
    a. Altered cognition and reports of skeletal pain
    b. Irregular heart rate and with elevated potassium level
    c. Bleeding from multiple sites throughout the body
    d. 2+ pitting edema and weight gain

52. A patient diagnosed with bone cancer reports fatigue, loss of appetite, and constipation. Which laboratory result does the nurse report **immediately**?
    a. Potassium level of 4.2 mEq/L
    b. Magnesium level of 2.0 mg/dL
    c. Sodium level of 140 mEq/L
    d. Calcium level of 10.5 mEq/dL

53. Which cancer patient has the **highest** risk to develop sepsis?
    a. 34-year-old patient who has received high-dose radiation to the upper chest area
    b. 66-year-old patient with hypercalcemia and dehydration
    c. 53-year-old patient with small cell lung cancer and hyponatremia
    d. 82-year-old patient with neutropenia and a low-grade fever

54. The nurse sees that the patient's platelet count is 18,000/mm^3 (18 × 10^9/L). What is the nurse's **greatest** concern related to this laboratory result?
    a. There is great risk that spontaneous and uncontrollable bleeding may occur.
    b. Patient should be immediately placed in isolation to prevent sepsis or septicemia.
    c. Oxygen-carrying capacity is decreased and patient is likely to experience dyspnea.
    d. Fluid retention increases the risk for heart failure and pulmonary edema.

55. An older patient is receiving epoetin alfa. Based on the knowledge that this medication increases erythrocytes and many other types of blood cells, which abnormal assessment finding suggests the patient is experiencing an adverse effect of the medication?
    a. Temperature is 100.5°F (38.6°C).
    b. Blood pressure is 160/90 mm Hg.
    c. Patient has hemorrhagic cystitis.
    d. Mucous membranes are dry.

23 CHAPTER

Care of Patients with Infection

1. Which circumstance is an example of colonization?
   a. Health care provider contacts the Centers for Disease Control and Prevention because patient has symptoms of smallpox.
   b. Unlicensed assistive personnel is positive for methicillin-resistant *Staphylococcus aureus* (MRSA) but is asymptomatic.
   c. Elderly person with multiple chronic health problems lives in a long-term care facility and has an increased risk for infection.
   d. Nurse instructs unlicensed assistive personnel not to use alcohol-based hand rub after caring for a patient with *Clostridium difficile.*

2. Which health behavior is intended to prevent normal flora from improperly entering the body and causing disease?
   a. Washing fruit and vegetables first before eating them raw.
   b. Wiping perineal area from front to back after toileting for females.
   c. Wearing insect repellent or long sleeves to avoid mosquito bites.
   d. Getting yearly influenza vaccine to prevent infection from common strains.

3. What is an example of an animate reservoir?
   a. It is probable that Ebola virus originated from contaminated bats or primates.
   b. Foodborne infections have been associated with contaminated fresh spinach.
   c. A stethoscope can carry *Staphylococcus aureus* from one patient to another.
   d. During a city-wide disaster, contaminated water can be a source of infection.

4. To meet The Joint Commission's National Patient Safety Goals related to hand hygiene, what is the **best** action for the charge nurse to perform?
   a. Educate all health care staff about effective hand hygiene and use of alcohol-based hand rubs.
   b. Ensure that visitors perform hand hygiene before and after visiting immunocompromised patients.
   c. Participate in committee meetings to ensure that any redesign of facility includes access to sinks.
   d. Track and record episodes of person-to-person infection to improve infection control protocols.

5. What instruction should the nurse give to unlicensed assistive personnel about disinfecting equipment?
   a. "Discard anything with a narrow lumen, because debris can't be removed or disinfected."
   b. "Rinsing items such as bedpans or urinals with clean water is adequate for disinfection."
   c. "Debris such as dried blood or feces must be scrubbed off before using disinfectant."
   d. "We want to protect our patients, so disinfect any items that come into contact with patients."

6. Which patients have factors that increase susceptibility to infection? **Select all that apply.**
   a. Patient consumes 2 to 3 alcoholic drinks daily.
   b. Patient has poorly controlled type 2 diabetes mellitus.
   c. Patient smokes a pack of cigarettes every day.
   d. Patient is 3 months pregnant with her second child.
   e. Patient is thin and has eaten a vegetarian diet for the past 10 years.
   f. Patient is elderly and lives in a long-term care facility.

7. From the list below, select **TWO** patients who would be the **most** appropriate for cohort placement.
   a. Elderly patient had hip replacement 2 days ago.
   b. Immunocompromised cancer patient recently had radiation therapy.
   c. Patient has a methicillin-resistant *Staphylococcus aureus* wound infection as a postoperative complication.
   d. Patient is HIV positive and is getting IV antibiotics for pneumonia.
   e. Elderly patient has watery diarrhea probably caused by *Clostridium difficile.*
   f. Patient has a boil that is draining and infected with methicillin-resistant *Staphylococcus aureus.*

8. Research indicates that biofilms are contributing to the rise of drug-resistant health care–related infections. Which nursing intervention will mechanically disrupt biofilms?
   a. Washing hands with chlorohexidine for 15 seconds
   b. Cleaning the skin with alcohol prior to venipuncture
   c. Using sterile technique when inserting a urinary catheter
   d. Assisting the patient to floss and to brush teeth

9. Which patient is the **most likely** candidate for directly observed therapy?
   a. College student needs to take antibiotics for a sexually transmitted disease.
   b. Toddler needs a liquid antibiotic and antipyretic for a recurrent ear infection.
   c. Homeless man has tuberculosis (TB) and needs multiregimen anti-TB therapy.
   d. Nursing student had an organ transplant and needs multiregimen drug therapy.

10. A patient has a postoperative abdominal wound infection caused by vancomycin-resistant *Enterococcus*. While performing a physical examination on this patient, which personal protective equipment must the nurse wear? **Select all that apply.**
    a. Gown
    b. Mask
    c. Gloves
    d. Shoe covers
    e. Face shield
    f. Double gloves

11. The nurse is preparing to hang an intravenous (IV) infusion of 1 g vancomycin in 250 mL of normal saline for a patient diagnosed with methicillin-resistant *Staphylococcus aureus* infection. The medication is to infuse over 1.5 hours. At what rate in mL per hour does the nurse set the IV pump?
    a. 109 mL/hr
    b. 127 mL/hr
    c. 153 mL/hr
    d. 167 mL/hr

12. Which patient is the **best** potential candidate for fecal microbiota transplantation?
    a. Patient has methicillin-resistant *Staphylococcus aureus* infection of the perineum.
    b. Patient has chronic constipation related to dietary patterns and history of laxative overuse.
    c. Patient has diarrhea caused by *Clostridium difficile* that is unresponsive to antibiotics.
    d. Patient has *Escherichia coli* food poisoning after eating raw vegetables at a restaurant.

13. The new nurse is discussing planned interventions to reduce a patient's isolation while on airborne precautions. Which statement by the new nurse requires that the preceptor intervene?
    a. "I have arranged to have the newspaper delivered to the room daily."
    b. "I will leave the door propped open to increase auditory and visual stimuli."
    c. "I have demonstrated the use of television and radio controls for the patient."
    d. "I will bundle nursing care so I have more time to talk to the patient while in the room."

14. Handwashing, rather than using alcohol-based hand rubs, must be performed during which situation?
    a. After setting up a basin and towels for a patient's morning care
    b. Before having direct contact with any patients
    c. Before donning and after removing sterile gloves
    d. After contact with a patient who has had diarrhea for 3 days

15. Appropriate methods for general infection control include which precautions? **Select all that apply.**
    a. Utilizing effective hand hygiene
    b. Using appropriate personal protective equipment
    c. Limiting time spent with patients
    d. Using standard precautions
    e. Administering prophylactic antibiotics
    f. Standing at least 3 feet away from patients

16. During the shift-to-shift handoff, the nurse is informed that a patient is experiencing a rash. What question does the nurse ask to clarify safety for **this patient**?
    a. "Were isolation precautions initiated?"
    b. "Did the patient receive an antibiotic before the onset?"
    c. "Was a culture specimen obtained from the site?"
    d. "Is there history of methicillin-resistant *Staphylococcus aureus*?"

17. The nurse is observing a new nurse perform hand hygiene. Which observation indicates a need for further instruction?
    a. Wetting hands before applying soap
    b. Using hot water and a scrub brush
    c. Using friction under running water
    d. Washing for at least 15 seconds

18. The patient's peripheral IV site is red and swollen. The insertion site is warmer than surrounding tissue and the patient reports mild discomfort. The nurse suspects localized infection; however, which action would the nurse take **first** to detect evidence of systemic infection?
    a. Remove the catheter and culture the tip.
    b. Obtain an order for blood cultures.
    c. Check the patient's temperature.
    d. Palpate cervical and axillary lymph nodes.

19. Which type of transmission-based precautions must the nurse use to prevent transmission by touch from a patient with or environment contaminated by methicillin-resistant *Staphylococcus aureus*?
    a. Contact precautions
    b. Droplet precautions
    c. Standard precautions
    d. Airborne precautions

20. Which type of transmission-based precautions must the nurse employ to prevent transmission from a patient with tuberculosis?
    a. Contact precautions
    b. Droplet precautions
    c. Standard precautions
    d. Airborne precautions

21. Which patient is at **most** risk for developing hospital-acquired methicillin-resistant *Staphylococcus aureus*?
    a. 78-year-old intensive care patient receiving IV antibiotics for pneumonia
    b. 45-year-old orthopedic patient with a total knee replacement
    c. 53-year-old medical patient with a venous thromboembolism
    d. 67-year-old gynecologic patient who had a hysterectomy

22. The unlicensed assistive personnel (UAP) tells the nurse that an 88-year-old patient has a temperature of 100.2°F (37.9°C). What should the nurse do **first**?
    a. Assess the patient for other signs/symptoms of infection.
    b. Administer two tablets of acetaminophen.
    c. Instruct the UAP to recheck the temperature in 4 hours.
    d. Report the elevated temperature to the health care provider.

23. Which situation requires that the nurse use soap and water for handwashing?
    a. Before a sterile dressing change
    b. After removing sterile gloves
    c. Hands feeling dry and chapped
    d. Hands feeling sticky or tacky

24. The nurse is reviewing a patient's laboratory results and sees that the patient has an elevated erythrocyte sedimentation rate (>20 mm/hr). How does the nurse interpret these findings?
    a. The patient is very sick and immunocompromised.
    b. There is inflammation or infection somewhere in the body.
    c. The infection is more likely to be bacterial rather than viral.
    d. The infection is resolving because of the immune response.

25. The health care provider orders a serum trough level of vancomycin. When must the blood be drawn for this level?
    a. At the halfway interval between two doses of vancomycin
    b. 30 minutes prior to the next ordered dose of vancomycin
    c. 60 minutes after the next ordered dose of vancomycin
    d. Immediately after giving a scheduled dose of vancomycin

26. The nurse is working in a facility that uses standing orders for prn acetaminophen 650 mg po for pain or discomfort. In which patient circumstance would the nurse consider withholding the prn antipyretic?
    a. Patient with chronic heart failure has fever of unknown origin.
    b. Patient has low-grade fever and is on third day of antibiotic therapy.
    c. Patient with a head injury seems restless and has low-grade fever.
    d. Patient has chills and has had two episodes of febrile seizures.

27. A patient has been prescribed gentamicin drug therapy. Which nursing intervention must be performed for the antimicrobial therapy to be effective?
    a. Evaluate culture results before and after drug therapy.
    b. Deliver a sufficient dosage and duration of therapy.
    c. Calculate dosage adjustments based on peak and trough.
    d. Closely monitor temperature and other signs of infection.

28. A patient is diagnosed with *Mycobacterium tuberculosis*. Which nursing intervention does the nurse implement for this patient?
    a. Wash hands before entering and after entering the room.
    b. Ensure the patient has a private room with negative airflow.
    c. Use contact and droplet precautions.
    d. Dispose of gown and shoe covers before leaving the room.

29. Which health care worker is at **greatest** risk for exposure to a bloodborne pathogen?
    a. Physical therapist who is helping a patient ambulate.
    b. Nurse who is changing the tubing on a patient's IV infusion.
    c. Provider who is injecting a patient with a local anesthetic.
    d. Janitorial worker who is mopping an area where a patient vomited.

30. A patient reports fever, chills, headache, and swollen glands in the groin and axillary areas. When the nurse assesses multiple reddened areas on both lower extremities, the patient states, "Those are flea bites from the refugee camp." What is the nurse's **first** action?
    a. Initiate droplet and contact precautions for suspicion of plague (*Yersinia pestis*).
    b. Immediately consult the Centers for Disease Control and Prevention and local health department.
    c. Obtain cultures and notify the health care provider for antibiotic orders.
    d. Move all patients and staff from the immediate area and arrange for decontamination.

31. What is a **major** factor that can contribute to mortality for a patient who has inhalation anthrax (*Bacillus anthracis*)?
    a. Initial symptoms may present as a common upper respiratory infection.
    b. Identifying the origin of the reservoir of the infectious agent may be very difficult.
    c. Bacillus anthracis is a multidrug-resistant organism; antibiotics do not always help.
    d. Most patients will have to be intubated with prolonged mechanical ventilation.

32. Three people traveling together come to the emergency department (ED) for severe vomiting and diarrhea. Two are also experiencing drooping eyelids and blurred vision, and one is having symmetrical flaccid paralysis. Which question would help the ED provider to determine if the patients have botulism?
    a. "Do the three of you work with animals or have you been recently exposed to animals?"
    b. "Over the past 36 hours, have the three of you eaten the same foods from the same source?"
    c. "Did any of you experience flu like symptoms before the diarrhea and vomiting started?"
    d. "Have any of you or your close friends or family recently traveled outside the United States?"

33. The nurse is caring for patients who are admitted to an infectious disease unit. Which patient has symptoms that indicate that all persons entering the patient's room should wear an N95 respirator as part of the personal protective equipment?
    a. Patient has high fever, headache, and vesicular and pustular rash on face, extremities, and palms.
    b. Patient has dysphasia, dry mouth, drooping eyelids, blurred vision, vomiting, and constipation.
    c. Patient has *Staphylococcus aureus* wound infection with redness, heat, pain, swelling, and drainage.
    d. Patient has copious fluid loss (diarrhea and vomiting) from *Escherichia coli* gastrointestinal infection.

34. Which interventions should be included when a patient is placed on droplet precautions? **Select all that apply.**
    a. Use chlorhexidine for handwashing.
    b. Wear a disposable gown whenever entering the patient's room.
    c. Use a mask when within 3 feet of the patient.
    d. Put a mask on the patient whenever transport is necessary.
    e. Double glove before entering the patient's room.
    f. Encourage visitors to email or phone instead of visiting.

35. Which physical factors increase the risk of infection in the older adult? **Select all that apply**.
    a. Increased antibody production
    b. Thin, delicate skin
    c. Decreased gag reflex
    d. Increased gastrointestinal motility
    e. Increased immobility
    f. Higher incidence of chronic disease

24 CHAPTER

Assessment of the Skin, Hair, and Nails

1. The patient has reddened scratch marks on the right forearm. Which is the **priority** medical surgical concept for this patient?
   a. Cellular regulation
   b. Perfusion
   c. Immunity
   d. Tissue integrity

2. A dark-skinned patient is admitted for pneumonia. What is the **most** accurate method to assess for cyanosis in this patient?
   a. Observe for shallow and rapid respirations.
   b. Check the tongue and lips for a gray color.
   c. Auscultate for decreased breath sounds in lung fields.
   d. Inspect the palms and soles for a yellow-tinged color.

3. A patient is at risk for hypovolemia. The nurse assesses this patient's skin using which assessment technique?
   a. Brush the skin surface and observe for flaking.
   b. Push on the skin and observe for blanching.
   c. Gently pinch the skin on the chest and observe for tenting.
   d. Push on the skin over the tibia and observe for depth of indentation.

4. A patient with a history of heart failure goes to the outpatient clinic for a follow-up appointment. How does the nurse assess for dependent edema in this patient?
   a. Palpate the dorsum of the foot or the medial ankle.
   b. Weigh the patient and compare to the baseline weight.
   c. Check the patient's buttocks or lower back.
   d. Ask the patient about intake and output.

5. The nurse is assessing the skin of an older adult patient who is at risk for dehydration as a result of excessive vomiting. The skin appears dry and loose. Where is the **best** site for the nurse to check skin turgor on this patient?
   a. Lower abdomen
   b. Forearm
   c. Forehead
   d. Midthigh

6. The nurse is preparing patient education material about healthy skin. What is the **single most** important preventive health behavior the nurse promotes?
   a. Limit continuous sun exposure.
   b. Drink plenty of water.
   c. Practice good skin hygiene.
   d. Eat a well-balanced diet.

7. The nursing student must perform a skin assessment on an older adult patient and observe for signs of skin breakdown. What does the student do to meet the clinical objective for effective time management?
   a. Examine the skin while bathing or assisting the patient with hygiene.
   b. Complete the assessment before the end of the clinical experience.
   c. Check to see if the primary nurse has already completed the assessment.
   d. Perform the examination when the patient willingly consents and agrees.

8. A patient is referred to a dermatologist for evaluation of a rash of unknown origin. The patient has trouble communicating specific information because of "nervousness." Which questions does the nurse use to help the patient prepare for the dermatologist's appointment? **Select all that apply.**
   a. "Have you received the flu vaccine?"
   b. "When did you first notice the rash?"
   c. "Where on the body did the rash first start?"
   d. "How do you feel about the skin rash?"
   e. "Are you having an itching or burning sensation?"
   f. "Have you been having fever or sore throat?"

9. In regulating body temperature, how much evaporative water loss can occur during hot weather or exercise?
   a. 500-600 mL/day
   b. 700-900 mL/day
   c. 2-4 L/day
   d. 10-12 L/day

10. The nurse is caring for a very dark-skinned patient who has high risk for thrombocytopenia. Which area of the patient's body is the **best** place to check for petechiae?
    a. Anterior chest
    b. Oral mucosa
    c. Palmar surface
    d. Periorbital area

11. The nurse is performing a skin assessment on a patient and notes an area on the forearm that feels hard or "woody." How does the nurse interpret this physical finding?
    a. Inflammation
    b. Subcutaneous fat
    c. Psoriasis
    d. Skin cancer

12. Age-related changes in the integumentary system include a **decrease** in which factors? **Select all that apply.**
    a. Vitamin D production
    b. Thickness of epidermis
    c. Thickness of dermis
    d. Epidermal permeability
    e. Dermal blood flow
    f. Size of nasal pores

13. During change of shift report, the nurse is informed that the patient has lichenified areas on both lower extremities. Based on this information, the nurse expects to observe which clinical finding on the lower extremities?
    a. Loss of hair
    b. Liver spots
    c. Thickened skin
    d. Yellow discoloration

14. A decreased number of active melanocytes in an older adult lead to which result?
    a. Decreased wound healing
    b. Decreased skin tone and elasticity
    c. Increased skin transparency
    d. Increased sensitivity to sun exposure

15. What is a key teaching point for an older patient with a decreased number of active melanocytes?
    a. Teach the patient to avoid applying tape to skin.
    b. Teach the patient to wear sunscreen and a large hat when outside.
    c. Teach the patient to keep track of pigmented lesions.
    d. Teach the patient to apply moisturizers to skin at least twice every day.

16. It is important for the nurse to avoid taping the skin of an older adult patient because of a decrease in which integumentary factor?
    a. Vitamin D production
    b. Thickness of epidermis
    c. Dermal blood flow
    d. Epidermal permeability

17. In an older adult, decreased vitamin D production increases the patient's susceptibility to which condition?
    a. Osteomalacia
    b. Osteodystrophy
    c. Hypothermia
    d. Dry skin

18. In caring for an older adult patient, the room may need to be kept warmer because of a decrease in which integumentary factor?
    a. Sebum production
    b. Subcutaneous fat layer
    c. Thickness of epidermis
    d. Number of active melanocytes

19. While obtaining a health history on a patient with a chronic skin condition, the nurse observes that the patient does not make eye contact and keeps the affected area covered with a scarf. What is the **most** appropriate nursing action?
    a. Explain all actions and procedures to the patient.
    b. Explain to the patient that it is normal to be embarrassed.
    c. Discuss the patient's behavior with another nurse for validation.
    d. Explore the patient's feelings about the condition.

20. The nurse is assessing the skin of an older patient. Which assessment finding needs follow-up?
    a. Multiple liver spots on the arms
    b. Dry, flaking skin on the lower extremities
    c. Presence of cherry hemangiomas
    d. Irregular light-brown macule (6.5 cm) on the right scapula

21. A patient reports a rash that itches but denies fever, shortness of breath, or other symptoms. Which questions does the nurse ask to help determine if the patient is having an allergic reaction? **Select all that apply.**
    a. "Are you taking any new medications?"
    b. "Have you been using any different soaps, cosmetics, or lotions?"
    c. "Is your skin unusually dry or flaky?"
    d. "Have you been exposed to any new cleaning solutions?"
    e. "Have you noticed any new bruises or brownish discolorations?"
    f. "Have you had any recent changes in your diet?"

22. Which factors are included in the ABCDE features associated with skin cancer? **Select all that apply.**
    a. Asymmetry of shape
    b. Border regularity
    c. Color variation within a lesion
    d. Crusting, bleeding, or itching
    e. Diameter greater than 5 mm
    f. Evolving or changing of any feature

23. The nurse is performing a physical exam on a patient and observes a dark asymmetrical lesion on the patient's back. The patient states, "I can't see back there and I don't know how long it has been there." What is the **most** important intervention for this patient?
    a. Encourage the patient to make an appointment with a dermatologist.
    b. Teach the patient how to do a total skin self-evaluation.
    c. Instruct the patient on self-care measures, such as use of sunscreen.
    d. Obtain an order for a fungal culture and take a fungal specimen.

24. To differentiate between color changes in the nail bed related to vascular supply and those from pigment disposition, what does the nurse do?
    a. Examine the nail plate under a Wood's light.
    b. Assess for thickness.
    c. Blanch the nail bed.
    d. Evaluate for lesions.

25. The nurse is taking a medication history of a patient and performing a physical assessment of the skin. During the assessment, the nurse notes the presence of ecchymoses (bruising). The nurse specifically asks if the patient is taking which types of medications? **Select all that apply.**
    a. Anticoagulants
    b. Oral hypoglycemics
    c. Long-term corticosteroids
    d. Herbal preparations
    e. Aspirin products
    f. Short-term loop diuretics

26. A young female patient reports an unusual increase in facial hair. Which question helps the nurse if an examination of the genitalia is required?
    a. "Have you noticed any bruising or unusual bleeding?"
    b. "Have you noticed any deepening of your voice quality?"
    c. "Are you having any trouble urinating?"
    d. "Does your skin seem unusually dry and flaky?"

27. What is the **best** rationale for encouraging the patient to follow through and seek treatment for dandruff?
    a. Dandruff flakes are caused by a dry scalp and suggest possible dehydration.
    b. Dandruff is merely a cosmetic problem, but appearance is important to self-esteem.
    c. Severe dandruff is caused by excessive oiliness and could cause hair loss.
    d. Brushing the hair every day prevents dandruff, but it weakens the hair follicle.

28. The nurse is assessing a patient who is African American with very dark skin. Which technique does the nurse use to assess the health of the nails?
    a. Gently squeeze the end of the finger, exert downward pressure, and then release the pressure.
    b. Obtain a color chart to identify the normal color of nails for the dark-skinned patient.
    c. Observe the nail bed for a pale pink color and a shiny, smooth surface.
    d. Soak the fingertips in warm water; then gently push back the cuticle.

29. A patient reports a subjective sensation of pain and tenderness "because my arthritis is flaring up." In order to assess for inflammation, what does the nurse do?
    a. Place the hand just above the area and feel for radiant warmth.
    b. Use fingertips to depress tissue area and then release and observe.
    c. Use the back of the hand to palpate the area for warmth.
    d. Use the palm and make a circular motion over the area.

30. A patient has a history of heart failure and demonstrates some mild shortness of breath, with crackles on auscultation. The skin is tight and shiny over the patient's lower extremities. How does the nurse interpret these findings?
    a. Fluid retention and edema
    b. Early signs of poor circulation
    c. Early stage of infection
    d. Normal for this patient

31. The nurse is caring for a patient who is several days postoperative. The unlicensed assistive personnel (UAP) reports that the patient's linens were changed but are wet again. The nurse notes that the patient's skin is excessively warm and moist. What is the nurse's **priority** action?
    a. Monitor intake and output.
    b. Check the patient's temperature.
    c. Direct the UAP to change the linens.
    d. Help the patient with hygiene.

32. The nurse is assessing a patient's skin and notes a slightly darkened area over the left ankle. The patient denies pain but reports a recent swelling in the area. Based on the skin appearance and the patient's report, what does the nurse do **next**?
    a. Ask the patient if there was a serious and deep burn to the area.
    b. Observe the area for scar tissue.
    c. Ask the patient if there was an inflammation to the area.
    d. Take a scraping of the skin for culture.

33. The nurse is caring for an older adult patient with very dark skin. The patient has a low hemoglobin and hematocrit. How does the nurse assess for pallor in this patient?
    a. Observe the mucous membranes for an ash-gray color.
    b. Use indirect, low fluorescent lighting.
    c. Gently push on the skin and watch for blanching.
    d. Inspect the conjunctivae for a yellowish color.

34. The nurse is interviewing a patient who has come to the walk-in clinic and observes the patient has matted hair, body odor, and soiled clothes. For which conditions will the nurse assess that could contribute to the patient's overall hygiene? **Select all that apply.**
    a. Range of motion and strength to perform self-care
    b. Access to shower facilities and a laundry
    c. Patient's knowledge (or memory) of how to perform hygiene care
    d. Patient's perception of how he or she appears to others
    e. Patient's current antihypertensive drug prescription
    f. Intactness of sensory functions (e.g., sight, smell)

35. The health care provider has ordered diagnostic testing to determine if a patient has a fungal infection of the skin. Which test does the nurse prepare the patient for?
    a. Shave biopsy
    b. Punch biopsy
    c. Wood's light examination
    d. KOH test

36. A fair-skinned patient has a history of chronic liver problems; liver enzyme tests and bilirubin results are pending. In order to assess for jaundice, where is the **best** place for the nurse to look for a yellowish discoloration?
    a. Hard palate
    b. Sclera
    c. Palms
    d. Conjunctivae

37. The nurse is collecting a superficial specimen for a suspected fungal infection from a patient's groin area. What is the correct technique to obtain this specimen?
    a. Obtain a small sample of tissue by using a biopsy needle.
    b. Express exudate from a lesion and use a sterile swab to collect the fluid.
    c. Gently scrape scales with a tongue blade into a clean container.
    d. Aspirate fluid from the lesion using sterile technique.

38. The nurse has collected several specimens from patients who have skin conditions. Which specimen must be **immediately** placed on ice?
    a. Punch biopsy performed with sterile technique for collection of a tissue piece.
    b. Exudate taken by sterile technique and swabbed on a bacterial culture medium.
    c. Aspirate taken by sterile technique and placed in a bacterial culture tube.
    d. Vesicle fluid taken by sterile technique and placed in a viral culture tube.

39. The unlicensed assistive personnel (UAP) is helping a patient with morning care. The patient has nonintact skin. What **priority** instruction does the nurse provide for the UAP when providing care for this patient?
    a. Wear gloves using universal precautions.
    b. Save any fingernail clippings or hair samples for testing.
    c. Have a second UAP assist you when getting this patient out of bed.
    d. Let the patient soak in the bathtub for 15 minutes before rinsing.

40. A patient is scheduled to have a punch biopsy for a lesion on the midback. What does the nurse tell the patient about the procedure?
    a. There will be a small scar similar to any surgical procedure.
    b. The surgeon uses a scalpel to punch through the lesion.
    c. A local anesthetic is used, and it causes a temporary burning sensation.
    d. The health care provider uses a lens that punches the skin to reveal the shape of the lesion.

41. The nurse is caring for a patient who is scheduled for a culture of a deep bacterial infection, and bacterial cellulitis is suspected. What preprocedural teaching should the nurse include for this patient?
    a. The health care provider will inject bacteriostatic saline, withdraw it, and send the return for culture.
    b. A cotton-tipped applicator is used to obtain vesicle fluid from intact lesions.
    c. A smear is obtained from the base of the lesion and examined under a microscope.
    d. The crusts will be removed with normal saline; then the underlying exudate is swabbed for a specimen.

42. The health care provider instructs the nurse to prepare a light-skinned patient for evaluation of skin pigment changes. Which piece of equipment does the nurse obtain to assist the provider with this examination?
    a. Wood's light
    b. Glass slide
    c. Biopsy tray
    d. Nonfluorescent light

43. The nurse is interviewing a patient who wants evaluation of a skin problem. When the nurse attempts to collect demographic data, the patient states, "My age, race, occupation, and hobbies should not affect my access to health care." What is the nurse's **best** response?
    a. "The information obtained has nothing to do with access to care."
    b. "I understand your concerns, but we will see you regardless of your answers."
    c. "Age, race, occupation, and hobbies can be contributing factors to skin problems."
    d. "We are happy to see you, but you have to answer these questions."

44. Which skin disorder is most associated with a familial disposition?
    a. Psoriasis
    b. Ringworm
    c. Cellulitis
    d. Paronychia

45. The nurse is caring for a patient who sustained trauma and blood loss. The patient is alert and anxious, blood pressure is decreased, and the heart rate is high. Which skin characteristics are most likely to manifest during impending shock?
    a. Dry, flushed appearance
    b. White or pale, cool skin
    c. Bluish color that blanches
    d. Poor turgor with a rough texture

46. The nurse is interviewing a patient with a red rash that itches and burns. Which question would the nurse ask to help identify a transmittable disorder?
    a. "When did you first notice the redness and itching?"
    b. "Is there a family history of chronic skin problems?"
    c. "Have you recently traveled outside of the United States?"
    d. "Have any of your family members had recent skin problems?"

47. An obese elderly patient who has been living alone presents with overall poor hygiene. Her clothes are dirty, and she has a strong body odor. The nurse systematically assesses the patient's skin surface and will give special attention to which area?
    a. Scalp
    b. Skinfolds
    c. Nails
    d. Mucous membranes

48. The health care provider tells the nurse that the patient is likely to have polycythemia vera. Based on this information, what skin discoloration does the nurse expect to observe?
    a. Localized café au lait spots
    b. Nonblanching pallor to nail beds
    c. Generalized reddish-blue tinge
    d. Yellowish tinge to sclera

49. The nurse is teaching the patient about total skin self-examination (TSSE). According to the American Cancer Society, when should the patient perform TSSE?
    a. After every bath or shower
    b. When a change of a lesion occurs
    c. On a monthly basis
    d. Depends on personal or family history

50. A home health nurse is visiting an older patient in January who lives alone in a small mobile home in the southwestern United States. The patient is recovering from a hip fracture. What is an expected finding for this patient?
    a. Wound healing is delayed.
    b. Skin is generally very dry.
    c. Affected leg has edema.
    d. Surgical site has petechiae.

51. The nurse observes that the patient has large areas of ecchymoses. Which laboratory result is the nurse **most** likely to check?
    a. Total serum bilirubin
    b. Platelet count
    c. Hemoglobin level
    d. White cell count

52. For which nursing action is the nurse **most** likely to don clean gloves?
    a. Inspecting for purpura, petechiae, or ecchymosis
    b. Comparing temperature between affected and nonaffected extremity
    c. Obtaining a bacterial culture from a primary lesion (vesicle)
    d. Gently pinching up the skin on the forehead to check for "tenting"

53. Which assessment finding is the **best** indicator of a healthy nail?
    a. Nail bed color is normal for the patient.
    b. Nail bed blanches with gentle pressure.
    c. Nails are well groomed and nicely shaped.
    d. Nail surface is smooth and transparent.

54. Which condition is **most** likely to result in clubbing of the fingernails?
    a. Chronic hypoxia
    b. Prolonged vitamin D deficiency
    c. Uncontrolled blood glucose
    d. Prolonged febrile state

55. Which individual has the **highest** risk for chronic paronychia?
    a. Construction worker
    b. Nurse
    c. Homeless veteran
    d. Immigrant from Southeast Asia

56. The nurse is assisting the health care provider to obtain specimens for diagnostic testing. For which test should the nurse obtain a vial of sterile nonbacteriostatic saline?
    a. Culture for a fungal infection
    b. Vesicle fluid to culture for viral infection
    c. Punch biopsy of a superficial skin lesion
    d. Biopsy for suspected deep cellulitis

57. The nurse and the unlicensed assistive personnel (UAP) are helping patients to move in bed. For which patient are they **most** likely to use a lift sheet?
    a. Elderly patient on steroids with thin, fragile skin
    b. Obese patient at risk for sacral pressure ulcer
    c. Child with a total body rash with vesicular oozing
    d. Patient with diabetes and delayed wound healing

58. Which instruction will the nurse emphasize with the older patient to address changes of the subcutaneous layer of the skin related to aging?
    a. Teach to wear sunscreen and hat and avoid direct sun exposure during midday.
    b. Urge use of a multivitamin or a calcium supplement with vitamin D.
    c. Encourage application of moisturizers while skin is still moist.
    d. Advise the patient to dress warmly in cold weather and change position every 2 hours.

59. Extensive destruction of the epidermis will result in the loss of the body's ability to perform which function?
    a. Cellular regeneration for wound healing and skin repair
    b. Photoconversion of 7-dehydrocholesterol to active vitamin D
    c. Cutaneous vascular promotion or inhibition of heat loss
    d. Storage of extra energy reserve for periods of decreased intake

60. The nurse is caring for a patient with a liver disorder. In addition to observing for a yellow-orange discoloration of the skin, which laboratory test is the nurse **most** likely to monitor?
    a. Hemoglobin level
    b. Vitamin D level
    c. Total serum bilirubin
    d. Serum calcium level

61. The nurse is caring for a postsurgical patient and observes that the patient's skin is red, moist, and hot to the touch. Which vital sign is of **primary** interest?
    a. Temperature
    b. Pulse
    c. Respirations
    d. Blood pressure

62. The nurse is caring for a patient with liver failure who has been unable to get out of bed for several days. In which area is the nurse most likely to find evidence of dependent edema?
    a. Dorsum of foot
    b. Medial ankle
    c. Buttocks and sacrum
    d. Lower abdomen

63. In which chronic health condition is the nurse most likely to observe **increased** moisture of the patient's skin?
    a. Kidney disease
    b. Diabetes mellitus
    c. Polycythemia vera
    d. Hyperthyroidism

64. The patient reports a red, raised, itchy rash over most of his body. What terms would the nurse use to document the patient's skin problem?
    a. Red, macular, lichenified
    b. Erythematous, diffuse, pruritic
    c. Cyanotic, annular, papular
    d. Red, universal, circinate

65. The home health nurse reads in the documentation that the patient has chronic venous stasis. Which assessment finding does the nurse expect to observe?
    a. Reddish-blue color to the hands
    b. Grayish-tan color in the lower legs
    c. Warmth and redness in the lower legs
    d. Yellowish tinge to soles of the feet

66. The nurse is caring for a patient with myxedema. Which area of the body is the nurse **most** likely to assess for evidence of nonpitting edema?
    a. Tibia
    b. Forehead
    c. Ankle
    d. Sacrum

67. What should the nurse notice in a patient with adequate tissue integrity and body protection related to skin function?
    a. Body temperature is normal after dose of antipyretic.
    b. Oral mucous membranes are moist and pink.
    c. Areas of uneven pigmentations are covered with clothing.
    d. Hair is patchy and brittle but clean and well groomed.

68. The nurse is examining a patient's skin and sees large, sore-looking, raised bumps with pustular heads. Which method does the nurse use to obtain a specimen to test for a bacterial infection?
    a. Take a culture swab of the purulent material.
    b. Take cells from the base of a lesion for a Tzanck smear.
    c. Scrape scales from the lesions and prepare a slide with KOH.
    d. Assist the health care provider with a skin biopsy.

69. The nurse is caring for a patient who had an excisional biopsy of a skin lesion. What does the postprocedural care for this patient include?
    a. Monitor the biopsy site for bleeding and infection.
    b. Keep the site clean and dry for at least 24 hours.
    c. Remove dried blood or crusts with diluted hydrogen peroxide.
    d. Return for suture removal in 2-3 days.

70. The patient has a superficial raised lesion. Which type of biopsy does the nurse prepare the patient for?
    a. Excisional biopsy
    b. Shave biopsy
    c. Punch biopsy
    d. Tzanck smear

25 CHAPTER

Care of Patients with Skin Problems

1. The patient has a diagnosis of acute pressure ulcers on both heels. Which medical-surgical concept has **highest priority** for this patient?
   a. Cellular regulation
   b. Fluid and electrolyte balance
   c. Immunity
   d. Tissue integrity

2. The nurse sees in the patient's record that the patient has a Braden score of 20. Which nursing action is the nurse **most** likely to perform in the care of this patient?
   a. Continue routine assessments.
   b. Turn patient every 2 hours.
   c. Consult with the nutritionist.
   d. Assist to keep skin clean and dry.

3. A patient weighs 110 pounds. The nurse knows that the patient must have an intake of 30 to 35 calories per kilogram of body weight in order to maintain a positive nitrogen balance. How many calories per day does the patient need to take in?
   a. 1200-1500
   b. 1500-1750
   c. 1800-2050
   d. 2100-2350

4. A thin, malnourished patient requires emergency abdominal surgery. After the operation, in order to promote wound healing, what does the nurse encourage?
   a. High-calorie diet
   b. Low-sodium and low-carbohydrate diet
   c. High-quality protein diet
   d. Low-fat diet with vitamin supplements

5. Which patients are at risk for pressure ulcers? **Select all that apply.**
   a. A confused patient who likes to wander through the halls
   b. A middle-aged quadriplegic patient who is alert and conversant
   c. A bedridden patient who is in the late stage of Alzheimer's
   d. A very overweight patient who must be assisted to move in the bed
   e. An ambulatory patient who has occasional urinary incontinence
   f. A thin patient who sits for long periods and refuses meals

6. The nurse is reviewing the results of a pressure mapping on a patient at high risk for pressure ulcers. The map shows a red area over the hips. How does the nurse interpret this evidence?
   a. Normal finding because there is always pressure on the hip area
   b. Greater heat production associated with greater pressure
   c. Validation of observable skin redness and breakdown
   d. Cool and well-hydrated skin associated with lower pressure

7. The nurse is irrigating a large pressure ulcer on a patient's hip and notes a small opening in the skin with purulent drainage. Which technique does the nurse use to check for tunneling?
   a. Ask the health care provider to order an ultrasound.
   b. Palpate the surface of the wound to identify spongy areas.
   c. Continue to flush the wound and watch the flow of the fluid.
   d. Use a sterile cotton-tipped applicator to probe gently for a tunnel.

8. The nurse is assessing a patient's skin and notes a 2" × 2" purplish-colored area on the coccyx with skin intact. These findings suggest which stage of a pressure ulcer?
   a. Suspected deep tissue injury
   b. Stage I pressure ulcer
   c. Stage II pressure ulcer
   d. Unstageable

9. A patient has a stage III pressure ulcer over the left trochanter area that has a thick exudate. The wound bed is visible and beefy red, and the edges are surrounded with swollen pink tissue. The exudate has an odor. How does the nurse determine which dressing is best for this wound?
   a. Selects a hydrophilic dressing for heavy exudate
   b. Obtains an order to consult certified wound care specialist
   c. Obtains an order for the type of dressing from health care provider
   d. Applies a dry dressing and observes for "strike through"

10. The nurse is caring for a patient in a prolonged coma after a serious head injury. The nurse uses which interventions to prevent the development of pressure ulcers for this patient? **Select all that apply.**
    a. Use pillows or padding devices to keep heels pressure free.
    b. Assess heel positioning every 8 hours.
    c. Delegate turning and positioning every 2 hours.
    d. Obtain an order for pressure-relief devices.
    e. Give special attention to fleshy or muscular areas.
    f. Provide adequate nutrition for positive nitrogen balance.

11. The nurse is instructing the unlicensed assistive personnel (UAP) about how to perform skin care for a patient who is at risk for pressure ulcers because of immobility and incontinence. What instructions would the nurse give?
    a. After cleaning, apply a commercial skin barrier to areas exposed to urine or feces.
    b. After cleaning, apply a light layer of powder or talc directly on the perineum.
    c. Scrub and vigorously rub the skin to completely remove soil or dried feces.
    d. Use an antibiotic soap and rinse with hot water to remove soap residue.

12. Which chronic health condition is most likely to contribute to delayed wound healing or recurrence of a pressure ulcer after healing has occurred?
    a. Osteoporosis
    b. Hypertension
    c. Psoriasis
    d. Diabetes mellitus

13. Using the Braden Scale to evaluate a patient for pressure ulcer risk, which factors are documented? **Select all that apply.**
    a. Incontinence
    b. Mental status
    c. Gas exchange
    d. Nutrition status
    e. Mobility
    f. Immunity

14. For which action must the nurse intervene when a nursing student is providing care for a patient with increased risk for pressure ulcer development?
    a. Student assists patient to consume most of lunch tray.
    b. Student provides assistance with bathing of back, lower legs, and feet.
    c. Student massages reddened area over the coccyx region.
    d. Student reminds patient to change positions every 2 hours.

15. The wound care specialist nurse is selecting a product to be used in caring for a patient with pressure ulcers. Which factors will the nurse consider? **Select all that apply.**
    a. Insurance reimbursement and cost
    b. Number and severity of pressure ulcers
    c. Patient's ability to reposition self
    d. Need to reduce shearing forces
    e. Risk for developing new pressure ulcers
    f. Wishes and concerns of family members

16. The nurse is assessing a patient's coccyx region and finds an area that is reddened but intact. When pressure is applied, the area does not blanch. What does this suggest to the nurse?
    a. Stage 1 pressure ulcer
    b. Stage 2 pressure ulcer
    c. Stage 3 pressure ulcer
    d. Stage 4 pressure ulcer

17. Which patients with pressure ulcers are at high risk for developing infection? **Select all that apply.**
    a. 39-year-old with rotator cuff injury
    b. 56-year-old with diabetes mellitus
    c. 62-year-old with COPD on steroid therapy
    d. 70-year-old with high cholesterol who walks 2 miles a day
    e. 76-year-old with low white blood cell count
    f. 80-year-old with right hip replacement who needs help repositioning

18. Which finding indicating infection does the nurse report to the health care provider immediately?
    a. Presence of granulation and re-epithelialization
    b. Changes in the quantity, color, or odor of exudate
    c. Progressive decrease in ulcer size or depth
    d. Beefy red color as it grows and fills the wound

19. The nurse is directing the home health unlicensed assistive personnel (UAP) in the care of an older adult patient. The patient wants to prevent dry skin. What does the nurse direct the UAP to do?
    a. Assist with a complete bath or shower only every other day (wash face, axillae, perineum, and any soiled areas with soap daily).
    b. Generously apply oil and leave it on for 20 minutes; then bathe the patient, especially the genital and axillary areas.
    c. Use an antimicrobial skin soap and wash the patient carefully; then apply alcohol-based astringent, especially to the legs and arms.
    d. Use hot water with a deodorant soap; then gently pat the patient dry and apply oil and cream to the skin.

20. The nurse is caring for an obese patient who has been on bedrest for several days. The nurse observes that the patient is beginning to develop redness on the sacral area. What intervention is used to **decrease** the shearing force?
    a. Place the patient in a high Fowler's position.
    b. Instruct the patient to use arms and legs to push when moving self in bed.
    c. Obtain an order for the patient to be up 3-4 times per day in a recliner chair.
    d. Place the patient in a side-lying position.

21. The nurse is assessing the nutritional status of a patient at risk for skin breakdown who has been refusing to eat the hospital food. Which indicator is the **most** sensitive in identifying inadequate nutrition for this patient?
    a. Serum albumin level of 3.5 mg/dL
    b. Prealbumin level of 17.5 mg/dL
    c. Lymphocyte count of 1900/mm³
    d. Weight loss of 10% of total body weight

22. Seeing a reddened area on a patient's skin, the nurse presses firmly with fingers at the center of the area and sees that the area blanches with pressure. The nurse interprets this finding as changes related to which factor?
    a. Inflammation
    b. Infection
    c. Blood vessel dilation
    d. Tissue damage

23. The nurse is assessing a wound on a patient's abdomen. What is the correct technique?
    a. Stand on the right side of the bed and lay a sterile cotton swab across the width and the length of the wound.
    b. Read the previous nursing documentation and follow the same pattern that other nurses are using for standardization.
    c. Assess the wound as a clock face with 12 o'clock toward the patient's head and 6 o'clock toward the patient's feet.
    d. Observe the wound after the dressing is removed and estimate the shape and record the appearance.

24. The nurse is assessing a patient's wound every day for signs of healing or infection. Which finding is a positive indication that healing is progressing as expected?
    a. Eschar starts to lift and separate from the tissue beneath, which appears dry and pale.
    b. Area appears pale pink, progressing to a spongy texture with a beefy red color.
    c. Tissue is softer and more yellow, and wound exudate increases substantially.
    d. Ulcer surface is excessively moist with a deep reddish-purple color.

25. When developing a plan of care for a patient who is at high risk for skin breakdown, what interventions does the nurse include in the plan of care? **Select all that apply.**
    a. Applying a pressure reduction overlay to the mattress
    b. Frequent repositioning of the patient
    c. Instructing UAP to assess the patient's skin daily
    d. Instructing UAP to massage reddened areas
    e. Using positioning devices to keep heels pressure free
    f. Applying a skin barrier to areas exposed to urine or stool

26. Which expected outcome is most appropriate for a patient with a 1" × 1" stage II sacral pressure ulcer?
    a. Wound will show healing and no infection.
    b. Patient will verbalize that wound is smaller.
    c. Wound will show granulation and decrease in size.
    d. Patient will rate pain at an acceptable level.

27. A patient receiving negative pressure wound therapy (NPWT) should be monitored closely for which potential complication?
    a. Bleeding
    b. Infection
    c. Pain
    d. Nausea

28. Which class of medication would exclude a patient from participating in negative pressure wound therapy (NPWT)?
    a. Antihypertensives
    b. Anticoagulants
    c. Nonsteroidal anti-inflammatory drugs
    d. Antidepressants

29. A patient on the unit has herpes zoster. Which staff members would be **best** to assign to the care of this patient?
    a. Any staff member, as long as personal protective equipment (PPE) is utilized
    b. Staff members who have had chickenpox
    c. Staff members who have completed training on herpes zoster
    d. Staff members with no small children at home

30. Which common complication should the nurse monitor for in an older patient diagnosed with herpes zoster?
    a. Nausea and vomiting
    b. Infections of the arms and legs
    c. Severe pain after the lesions have resolved
    d. Severe itching after the lesions have resolved

31. The nurse is caring for a patient admitted with a rash of white or red edematous papules or plaques of various sizes. The patient states that the rash developed after he ate seafood, and he thinks he is allergic to it. What does the nurse suspect?
    a. Urticaria
    b. Pruritus
    c. Eczema
    d. Psoriasis

32. The emergency department (ED) nurse is giving discharge instructions to the parents of a child who has been diagnosed with bedbug bites. What instructions does the nurse give to the parents?
    a. Washing linens in hot soapy water will eliminate the problem.
    b. Using a topical insecticide kills bedbugs on the body surface.
    c. Repeatedly vacuuming surfaces of furniture or mattresses will help.
    d. Hiring a pest control company with bedbug experience is an option.

33. A patient diagnosed with bedbug bites says to the nurse, "I am so embarrassed. I shower daily and do not live in an unclean environment." Which response by the nurse is **most** appropriate?
    a. "No need to be embarrassed. These things happen."
    b. "Showering will not kill bedbugs."
    c. "Have you been traveling or staying in a hotel?"
    d. "Have you seen bedbugs or their eggs on your clothing?"

34. The nurse reads in the chart that the patient has palmoplantar pustulosis (PPP). Which area of the patient's body will the nurse assess for this condition?
    a. Skinfold areas, such as axillae or beneath breasts
    b. Mouth area and oral mucous membranes
    c. Bony prominences such as heels, sacrum, or trochanters
    d. Palms of the hands and soles of the feet

35. A mother reports that her child has dry skin with itching that seems to worsen at night. What nonpharmacologic interventions does the nurse teach to the mother? **Select all that apply.**
    a. Keep the child's fingernails trimmed short and filed to reduce skin damage.
    b. Place mittens or splints on the child's hands at night if the scratching is causing skin tears.
    c. Ensure a warm and moderately humid sleeping environment.
    d. Read the child a relaxing and familiar story to reduce stress.
    e. Use antibacterial soap during bathing to decrease risk of infection.
    f. Provide adequate fluid intake to keep the child well hydrated.

36. The health care provider recommended over-the-counter diphenhydramine to treat the patient's hives. What does the nurse suggest to the patient for self-care?
    a. Avoid alcohol consumption, which can potentiate the sedative effect of diphenhydramine.
    b. Warm environments and warm showers will accelerate metabolism and recovery.
    c. Use an emollient cream or lotion after bathing to reduce the itching.
    d. Apply a topical antibiotic cream after bathing in the evening.

37. In order to assist the health care provider in determining if avoidance therapy is appropriate for a patient, which question would the nurse ask?
    a. Do you have a history of surgery for removal of skin growths?
    b. Have you noticed a change in appearance of a mole?
    c. Does anyone residing in your household have a similar skin problem?
    d. Have you used any new soaps, detergents, or personal care products?

38. The nurse is teaching a patient about self-care for a minor bacterial skin infection. What is the **most** important aspect the nurse emphasizes?
    a. Apply cool compresses twice a day.
    b. Do not squeeze any pustules or crusts.
    c. Apply astringent compresses.
    d. Bathe daily with an antibacterial soap.

39. A patient is diagnosed with psoriasis vulgaris. Which description of the characteristic lesions of psoriasis would the nurse expect to see in the patient's documentation?
    a. Plaques surmounted by silvery-white scales
    b. Circular areas of redness
    c. Multiple blisters with a yellowish crust
    d. Patches of tender, raised areas limited to extremities

40. What does the treatment for psoriasis include? **Select all that apply.**
    a. Ultraviolet light therapy
    b. Calcipotriene topical cream
    c. Topical methotrexate
    d. Oral ciprofloxacin
    e. Corticosteroids
    f. Light therapy with lasers

41. The health care provider informs the nurse that the patient is having severe pruritus. Based on this information, the nurse is **most** likely to observe which assessment finding?
    a. Fluid-filled, weeping blisters
    b. Excoriations from scratching
    c. Dry, flaking skin with peeling
    d. Signs or symptoms of infection

42. The nurse is teaching an older adult about how to deal with and prevent dry skin. What information does the nurse include? **Select all that apply.**
    a. Use a room humidifier during the winter months or whenever the furnace is in use.
    b. Take a complete bath or shower every day.
    c. Maintain a daily fluid intake of 1000 mL unless contraindicated.
    d. Avoid clothing that continuously rubs the skin, such as tight belts or pantyhose.
    e. Thoroughly rinse soap from the skin.
    f. Vigorously rub the skin until it is free of moisture.

43. The nurse is teaching a patient about treatment of pediculosis pubis. What information does the nurse include? **Select all that apply.**
    a. Proper use of topical sprays or creams, such as permethrin
    b. Abstinence from sexual intercourse with the infected person
    c. Treatment of the patient's social contacts
    d. Side effects of ciprofloxacin or doxycycline
    e. Washing clothing and bedding in hot water with detergent
    f. Pubic lice are found only in the genital regions

44. The school nurse is examining a child and observes linear ridges on the inner aspect of the wrists. The child reports intense itching, especially at night. The nurse scrapes the lesion and examines it under a microscope. Which condition does the nurse suspect?
    a. Head lice
    b. Scabies
    c. Body lice
    d. Dermatitis

45. The school nurse discovers a child has tinea capitis. What does the nurse instruct the parents to do?
    a. Treat the family pet and temporarily isolate the pet.
    b. Refrain from sharing items like combs or hats.
    c. Scrub the shower area and keep the feet dry.
    d. Ensure all family members carefully wash their hands.

46. The nurse is giving discharge instructions to a patient and family who must continue dressing changes and wound care at home. Which point does the nurse emphasize to help the family prevent infection and minimize cost?
    a. Scrupulous handwashing before and after wound care
    b. Use of sterile water for flushing and sterile dressing materials
    c. Use of clean gloves for performing dressing changes
    d. Careful disposal of contaminated dressings in a biohazard bag

47. A patient has been prescribed acitretin for psoriasis. What information does the nurse tell the patient about this drug?
    a. Wear dark glasses after taking a dose.
    b. It is the first choice for psoriasis.
    c. Strict birth control measures are necessary.
    d. Apply it to superficial lesions.

48. A patient is diagnosed with Stevens-Johnson syndrome. What is the **priority** action for the health care team?
    a. Treat the subjective symptoms of pain and itching.
    b. Closely observe for signs of renal failure.
    c. Protect against localized skin infection.
    d. Identify the offending drug and discontinue it.

49. A patient is prescribed a topical steroid for treatment of contact dermatitis. Which instruction does the nurse provide to the patient about this drug?
    a. Moisten dressings with warm tap water; place over topical steroids for short periods.
    b. Apply topical steroids and then cover with an occlusive dressing.
    c. Apply a topical corticosteroid sparingly on the face.
    d. Discontinue the use of topical steroids when symptoms subside.

50. Which statement is true about the application and use of topical preparations?
    a. Topical applications are generally much safer than oral medications.
    b. Using a water-soluble cream in the groin area could cause maceration.
    c. Using an oil-based ointment in the axillary area could cause folliculitis.
    d. An oil-based gel should be massaged into hairy areas.

51. A patient has a partial-thickness wound. How long does the nurse anticipate the healing by epithelialization will take?
    a. 24 hours
    b. 2-3 days
    c. 5-7 days
    d. 12-14 days

52. A toddler is miserable with itching from chickenpox. Which type of bath is the best to help relieve the toddler's discomfort?
    a. Sitz bath
    b. Bath with oil
    c. Sponge bath
    d. Colloidal oatmeal

53. The nurse is performing daily wound care and dressing changes on a patient with a full-thickness wound. The patient protests when the nurse attempts to debride the wound. What is the nurse's **best** response?
    a. "Reepithelialization, granulation, and contraction are natural body processes that will occur if this tissue is removed."
    b. "I know this is uncomfortable, but don't you want your wound to heal as fast as possible? This treatment allows the body to heal itself."
    c. "Harmful bacteria can grow in the dead tissue, and it also interferes with the body's attempt to fill in the wound with new cells and collagen."
    d. "I would never force a patient to do anything, but this really is the best treatment for the wound that you have."

54. The nurse is caring for a patient with arterial insufficiency in the lower right leg. In order to prevent leg ulcers, what does the nurse do?
    a. Elevates the leg frequently.
    b. Places the leg in a dependent position.
    c. Places a heel protector on the right foot.
    d. Encourages the patient to walk briskly.

55. Which are physiologic steps of healing of partial-thickness wounds? **Select all that apply.**
    a. Skin injury results in local inflammation and formation of a fibrin clot.
    b. New blood vessels form at the base of the wound and fibroblasts begin moving into the wound space.
    c. Fibrin clot acts as a frame or scaffold to guide cell movement.
    d. Regrowth is only one cell layer thick at first; then the cell layer thickens.
    e. Growth factors stimulate epidermal cell division and new skin cells move into open spaces.
    f. Thorough wound cleansing and debridement are essential for healing to occur.

56. The nurse is caring for several patients who are incontinent of stool and urine. Which task is delegated to the unlicensed assistive personnel (UAP)?
    a. Inspect the skin daily for any areas of redness.
    b. Massage the reddened areas after cleaning.
    c. Wash the skin with a pH-balanced soap to maintain normal acidity.
    d. Change the absorbent pads or garments every 4 hours.

57. The nurse is assessing a patient's skin and observes a superficial infection with a raised, red rash with small pustules. How does the nurse interpret this finding?
    a. Minor skin trauma
    b. Folliculitis
    c. Furuncles
    d. Cellulitis

58. An adolescent has a painful and unsightly herpes simplex blister on her lip and would like to have her school photo delayed until after the lesion has resolved. What does the nurse tell the patient about the duration of the outbreak?
    a. It should resolve completely in 2-3 days.
    b. Within 3-5 days the blister will be gone.
    c. Symptoms can last 3-10 days.
    d. It will begin to improve in 2 weeks.

59. The nurse is caring for a patient who needs frequent oral hygiene and endotracheal suctioning. In this particular circumstance, the nurse wears gloves to prevent contracting and spreading which organism?
    a. Herpetic whitlow
    b. Herpes zoster
    c. Methicillin-resistant *Staphylococcus aureus*
    d. Streptococcus

60. A patient is diagnosed with a primary herpetic infection. The nurse would **question** an order for which drug?
    a. Acyclovir
    b. Valacyclovir
    c. Ketoconazole
    d. Famciclovir

61. The nurse hears in report that a patient admitted for an elective surgery also has herpes zoster. The nurse initiates contact isolation for which factor?
    a. Fever and malaise are present as accompanying symptoms.
    b. Other patients or staff members have never had chickenpox.
    c. Lesions are present as fluid-filled blisters.
    d. Lesions are present and crusted over.

62. The public health nurse is reviewing case files of people who were exposed to and treated for cutaneous anthrax. Which patient who develops the disease warrants further investigation as a possible bioterrorism exposure?
    a. Farmer
    b. Veterinarian
    c. Tannery worker
    d. Construction worker

63. A patient reported painless, raised vesicles that itched. Within a few days, there was bleeding in the center and then it sank inwards. Now it looks black and leathery. Which question does the nurse ask in order to elicit **more** information about this patient's condition?
    a. "Do you remember being bitten by an insect?"
    b. "Do you work with or around animals?"
    c. "Have you noticed any mite or lice infestations?"
    d. "Have you had exposure to new soaps, lotions, or foods?"

64. A patient is diagnosed with chronic psoriasis and is prescribed a topical therapy of anthralin. What does the nurse teach the patient about proper use of this drug?
    a. Apply the paste every night before going to bed.
    b. Check for local tissue reaction and do not apply to surrounding skin.
    c. Apply the drug generously to the lesion and surrounding skin.
    d. Use two forms of contraception.

65. What does the nurse teach a patient about ultraviolet (UV) therapy for psoriasis?
    a. Use a commercial tanning bed service but limit exposure to 2-3 times per week.
    b. Use the sun as an inexpensive source of UV; inspect skin daily for overexposure.
    c. Wear dark glasses during and after treatment if psoralen is prescribed.
    d. Expect generalized redness with edema and tenderness after the treatment.

66. A patient is diagnosed with actinic keratoses. Which teaching point would the nurse emphasize?
    a. A follow-up appointment is needed for a premalignant condition.
    b. Clean the skin with a mild soap and lukewarm water.
    c. Keep fingernails short to prevent infection from scratching.
    d. Apply the topical ointment while skin is moist.

67. The nurse is examining the nevi on a patient's back and neck. Because most malignant melanomas arise from moles, which finding is a concern to warrant further investigation?
    a. Regular, well-defined borders
    b. Uniform dark-brown color
    c. Rough surface
    d. Sudden report of itching

68. Which occurrence is an example of conditions associated with Koebner's phenomenon?
    a. Chronic overexposure to sunlight
    b. Exposure to a dermatophyte infection
    c. Dormant herpes simplex virus infection
    d. Itching that worsens during the night

69. Which patient is the most likely candidate to be referred for Mohs' surgery?
    a. Has joint contractures from burn wounds
    b. Has squamous cell carcinoma
    c. Has pressure ulcer with infection in deep tissue layers
    d. Has excessive breast tissue

70. An older patient who is receiving chemotherapy is diagnosed with toxic epidermal necrolysis. In addition to identifying the causative agent, what does the nurse monitor for?
    a. Fluid and electrolyte imbalance, caloric intake, and hypothermia
    b. Shortness of breath, hypertension, and cardiac dysrhythmias
    c. Nausea, vomiting, diarrhea, and severe abdominal pain
    d. Severe itching with tenderness and edema of the skin

71. A patient with burns over a large amount of the body surface requires 2g/kg/day of protein for wound healing. The patient weighs 130 pounds. How many grams of protein does the patient need each day?
    a. 110 grams
    b. 112 grams
    c. 115 grams
    d. 118 grams

72. A patient had surgery 5 days ago. What is the **best** way for the nurse to determine the current state of healing or deterioration of the patient's surgical wound?
    a. Consult the wound specialist to examine the wound.
    b. Compare existing wound features to those previously documented.
    c. Ask the patient for subjective sensations of pain or discomfort.
    d. Review the objective criteria for the desired outcomes of healing.

73. Which data set is most likely to prompt the nurse to call the health care provider to obtain an order for a wound culture?
    a. Patient reports pain along the incision site.
    b. Wound is accidentally contaminated during a dressing change.
    c. Tissue surrounding surgical site is pink and swollen.
    d. Wound has moderate exudate that has a foul odor.

74. A patient with a clean laceration to the lower leg is seen in the emergency department (ED). The laceration is closed using sutures. The nurse recognizes this as which type of healing?
    a. Healing by first intention
    b. Healing by second intention
    c. Healing by third intention
    d. Healing by debridement

75. At the hospital, the patient was receiving whirlpool treatments to debride dead tissue. What could the home health nurse suggest as a substitute?
    a. Soaking in a hot tub until tissue softens
    b. Sitting in a warm sitz bath for 20 minutes
    c. Forceful irrigation of the wound with a 35-mL syringe
    d. Gently scrubbing the wound with a moist sponge

76. The nurse hears in report that an older patient has postherpetic neuralgia. Which sign/symptom is the patient **most** likely to report?
    a. Severe pain
    b. Severe itching
    c. Unsightly rash
    d. Dry skin

77. A 60-year-old patient requests a Zostavax vaccination. Which health history needs further investigation before Zostavax is administered?
    a. Being treated for an autoimmune disease
    b. Taking iron supplements for anemia
    c. History of deep vein thrombosis
    d. Allergy to iodine and shellfish

78. Which patient is at **highest** risk for development of skin cancer?
    a. Dark-skinned male who works as a lab technician
    b. Light-skinned female who works as a lifeguard every summer
    c. Older adult who enjoys gardening but wears a large hat
    d. Younger adult who works as a home health assistant

Care of Patients with Burns

26
CHAPTER

1. The nurse is caring for a patient with 45% total body surface area (TBSA) burns. Which are priority medical surgical concepts for this patient? **Select all that apply.**
   a. Tissue integrity
   b. Cellular regulation
   c. Perfusion
   d. Elimination
   e. Fluid and electrolyte balance
   f. Gas exchange

2. A patient was burned on the forearm after tripping and falling against a wood burning stove. There are currently several small blisters over the burn area. What does the nurse advise the patient to do about the blisters?
   a. Leave the blisters intact because they protect the wound from infection.
   b. Use a sterile needle to open a tiny hole in each blister to drain the fluid.
   c. Allow blisters to increase in size; then open them to release the fluid inside.
   d. Leave the blisters intact unless the pain and pressure increase.

3. The nurse is caring for a patient who has 30% total body surface area (TBSA) burn. During the first 12-36 hours, the nurse carefully monitors the patient for which status changes related to capillary leak syndrome?
   a. Bradycardia and pitting edema
   b. Hypertension and increased urine output
   c. Tachycardia and hypotension
   d. Respiratory depression and lung crackles

4. The home health nurse is visiting an older couple for the initial visit. In observing the household, the nurse identifies several behaviors and environmental factors to address. Which identified factors **increase** the risk for burns and/or household fires? **Select all that apply.**
   a. Several potholders hanging within easy reach of the stove
   b. Ashtray with old cigarette butts on the bedside table
   c. Space heater very close to the bed
   d. Single smoke detector in the kitchen
   e. Back exit hall of the house used as a storage space
   f. Small throw rug near the front door

5. The nurse is caring for several patients on the burn unit who have sustained extensive tissue damage. The nurse should monitor for which electrolyte imbalance that is typically associated with the **initial** third-spacing fluid shift?
   a. Hypercalcemia
   b. Hypernatremia
   c. Hypokalemia
   d. Hyperkalemia

6. The nurse is reviewing the hemoglobin and hematocrit results for a patient recently admitted for a severe burn. Which result is **most** likely related to vascular dehydration?
   a. Hematocrit of 58%
   b. Hemoglobin of 14 g/dL
   c. Hematocrit of 42%
   d. Hemoglobin of 10 g/dL

7. The nurse is performing a morning assessment on a patient admitted for serious burns to the extremities. For what reason does the nurse assess the patient's abdomen?
   a. To perform a daily full head-to-toe assessment
   b. To assess for nausea and vomiting related to pain medication
   c. To assess for a paralytic ileus secondary to reduced blood flow
   d. To monitor increased motility that may result in cramps and diarrhea

8. The nurse is interviewing and assessing an electrician who was brought to the emergency department (ED) after being "electrocuted." Bystanders report that he was holding onto the electrical source "for a long time." The patient is currently alert with no respiratory distress. During the interview, what does the nurse assess for?
   a. Knowledge of electrical safety
   b. Burn marks on the dominant hand
   c. Injuries based on reports of pain
   d. Entrance and exit wounds

9. A patient was involved in a house fire and suffered extensive full-thickness burns. In the long term, what issue may this patient have trouble with?
   a. Intolerance for vitamin C
   b. Metabolism of vitamin K
   c. Activation of vitamin D
   d. Absorption of vitamin A

10. During shift report, the nurse learns that a new patient was admitted for an inhalation injury. Auscultation of the lungs has revealed wheezing over the mainstem bronchi since admission. During the nurse's assessment of the patient, the wheezing sounds are absent. What does the nurse do **next**?
    a. Document these findings because they indicate that the patient is improving.
    b. Assess for respiratory distress because of potential airway obstruction.
    c. Obtain an order to discontinue oxygen therapy because it is no longer needed.
    d. Encourage use of incentive spirometry to prevent atelectasis.

11. The nurse is caring for several patients who have sustained burns. The patient with which **initial** injury is the least likely to experience severe pain when a sharp stimulus is applied?
    a. Severe sunburn after lying in the sun for several hours
    b. Deep full-thickness burn from an electrical accident
    c. Partial-thickness burn from picking up a hot pan
    d. Deep partial-thickness burn after a motorcycle accident

12. The nurse is reviewing arterial blood gas (ABG) results for a patient with 35% total body surface area (TBSA) burn in the resuscitation phase: pH is 7.26, Pco_2 is 36 mm Hg, and HCO_3^- is 19 mEq/L. What condition does the nurse suspect?
    a. Metabolic alkalosis
    b. Metabolic acidosis
    c. Respiratory acidosis
    d. Respiratory alkalosis

13. A patient comes to the clinic to be treated for burns from a barbecue fire. Although the patient does not appear to be in any respiratory distress, the nurse suspects an inhalation injury after observing which findings? **Select all that apply.**
    a. Burns to the face
    b. Bright cherry-red color to lips
    c. Singed nose hairs
    d. Edema of the nasal septum
    e. Black carbon particles around the mouth
    f. Sweet, sugary smell to the breath

14. The nurse is caring for a burn patient who received rigorous fluid resuscitation in the emergency department (ED) for hypotension and hypovolemic shock. In assessing renal function for the first 24 hours, what finding does the nurse anticipate?
    a. Output will be approximately equal to fluid intake.
    b. Output will be decreased compared to fluid intake.
    c. Urine will have a very low specific gravity and a pale-yellow color.
    d. Output will be managed with diuretics.

15. A patient sustained a superficial-thickness burn over a large area of the body. The patient is crying with discomfort and is very concerned about the long-term effects. What does the nurse tell the patient to expect?
    a. "Healing should occur in 3-6 days with no scarring or complications."
    b. "The pain should be less because more of the nerve endings were destroyed."
    c. "The wound will appear red and dry with some white areas."
    d. "The leathery eschar will have to be removed before healing can occur."

16. The nurse is caring for a patient brought to the emergency department (ED) with facial burns that occurred after the patient bent over the engine of his car. What is the **priority** for this patient?
    a. Initiate fluid resuscitation.
    b. Secure the airway.
    c. Manage pain and discomfort.
    d. Prevent infection.

17. The nurse is caring for a patient who sustained carbon monoxide poisoning. What assessment finding does the nurse anticipate?
    a. Patient will be cyanotic because of hypoxia.
    b. Blood gas value of Pao_2 will be very low.
    c. Patient will report a headache.
    d. Patient will report a dry and irritated throat.

18. For which patient would the rule of nines method of calculating burn size be most appropriate?
    a. Child who weighs at least 50 pounds
    b. Adult whose weight is proportionate to height
    c. Adult who weighs under 300 pounds
    d. Child whose weight is proportionate to height

19. Which criteria describes a full-thickness burn wound? **Select all that apply.**
    a. The wound is red, moist, and blanches easily.
    b. There is destruction to the epidermis and dermis.
    c. There are no skin cells for regrowth.
    d. The burned tissue is avascular.
    e. The burn wound will not be painful.
    f. The burn wound has a dry, hard, leathery eschar.

20. The nurse is assessing a patient with a burn wound to the back and chest area. Which assessment findings are consistent with a superficial-thickness burn wound? **Select all that apply.**
    a. Pink to red
    b. Pain
    c. Mild edema
    d. Moisture
    e. Eschar
    f. Blanch to pressure

21. The nurse observes peeling of dead skin on the legs of a patient with a superficial-thickness burn wound. What is the **most** accurate description of this assessment finding?
    a. Blanching
    b. Desquamation
    c. Slough
    d. Fluid shift

22. Which type of burn wound damages the epidermis, dermis, fascia, and tissues?
    a. Superficial
    b. Partial thickness
    c. Full thickness
    d. Deep full thickness

23. Which type of burn destroys the sweat glands, resulting in decreased excretory ability?
    a. Superficial
    b. Partial thickness
    c. Full thickness
    d. Deep full thickness

24. During the early phase of a burn injury, there is a drastic increase in capillary permeability. This physiologic change places the patient at risk for which problem?
    a. Acute kidney injury
    b. Fluid overload
    c. Increased cardiac output
    d. Hypovolemic shock

25. An adult patient is admitted to the burn unit after being burned in a house fire. Assessment reveals burns to the entire face, back of the head, and anterior torso and circumferential burns to both arms. Using the rule of nines, what is the extent of the burn injury?
    a. 18%
    b. 24%
    c. 45%
    d. 54%

26. What is the **most** effective intervention for preventing transmission of infection to a burn patient?
    a. Use of personal protective equipment (PPE) by anyone entering the patient's room
    b. Maintaining reverse isolation during the resuscitation phase
    c. Equipment designated for patient use
    d. Performing correct, proper, and consistent hand hygiene

27. Which vaccine is routinely administered when a burn patient is admitted to the hospital?
    a. Hepatitis B
    b. Tetanus
    c. Influenza
    d. Pneumonia

28. A patient has severe burns to the anterior surface of the body from a short exposure to high temperatures at a worksite furnace. Which area of the body is **most** vulnerable to a deep burn injury?
    a. Anterior chest
    b. Upper arms
    c. Palmar surface of hands
    d. Eyelids

29. A patient has sustained a burn that appears red and moist. The nurse gently applies pressure to the area to assess for what sign/symptom?
    a. Intensity of pain
    b. Blanching
    c. Pitting edema
    d. Fluid-filled blisters

30. What is the primary reason to prevent infection with burn injuries?
    a. Prevent extensive scar formation.
    b. Avoid sepsis.
    c. Avert worsening of pain.
    d. Avoid fever and inflammation.

31. The nurse is caring for several patients on the burn unit. Which patients have the **greatest** risk for developing respiratory problems? **Select all that apply.**
    a. Patient who was in a storage room where chemicals caught fire
    b. Patient who was working in an area where steam escaped from a pipe
    c. Patient who sustained a circumferential burn to the chest area
    d. Patient who was burned when a firecracker exploded prematurely
    e. Patient who was found unconscious in a slow-burning house fire
    f. Patient whose clothes caught fire while burning leaves

32. The nurse is caring for a firefighter who was trapped for a prolonged period of time by burning debris. During the shift, the nurse notes a progressive hoarseness, a brassy cough, and the patient reports increased difficulty with swallowing. How does the nurse interpret these changes?
    a. Temporary discomfort that can be treated with sips of cool fluids
    b. Signs and symptoms of probable carbon monoxide poisoning
    c. Signs indicating a pulmonary injury and possible airway obstruction
    d. Expected findings considering the mechanism of injury

33. The nurse has just received report on a patient admitted for steam inhalation burns. The patient is alert and conversant but reports that his throat feels raw. His wife says that he sounds hoarse compared to usual. Considering these findings, which order should the nurse **question**?
    a. Continuous pulse oximetry
    b. Vital signs and airway assessment twice a day
    c. Intubation equipment at the bedside
    d. Oxygen 2 L via nasal cannula to maintain saturation of greater than 90%

34. The nurse is caring for a burn patient who was stabilized by and transferred from a small rural hospital. The patient develops a new complaint of shortness of breath. On auscultation, the nurse hears crackles throughout the lung fields. What does the nurse suspect is causing this patient's symptoms?
    a. Pulmonary fluid overload due to fluid resuscitation
    b. Exposure to carbon monoxide that was undiagnosed
    c. Fat emboli secondary to extensive injury
    d. Excessive oxygen therapy at the first facility

35. The nurse is caring for several patients on the burn unit. Which of these patients has the **most** acute need for cardiac monitoring?
    a. Older adult woman who spilled hot water over her legs while boiling noodles
    b. Teenager with facial burns that occurred when he threw gasoline on a campfire
    c. Young woman who was struck by lightning while jogging on the beach
    d. Middle-aged man who fell asleep while smoking and sustained burns to the chest

36. A patient is transported to the emergency department (ED) for severe and extensive burns that occurred while he was trapped in a burning building. The patient is severely injured with respiratory distress, and the resuscitation team must immediately begin multiple interventions. Which task should be delegated to unlicensed assistive personnel (UAP)?
    a. Position the patient's head to open the airway and assist with intubation.
    b. Assist the respiratory therapist to maintain a seal during bag-valve-mask ventilation.
    c. Prepare the intubation equipment and set up the oxygen flowmeter.
    d. Elevate the head of the bed to achieve a high Fowler's position.

37. The nursing student notes on the care plan that the burn patient she is caring for is at risk for organ ischemia. Based on the student's knowledge of the pathophysiology of burns, which etiology does the nursing student select?
    a. Related to hypovolemia and hypotension
    b. Related to fluid overload and peripheral edema
    c. Related to prolonged resuscitation and hypoxia
    d. Related to direct blunt trauma to the kidneys

38. The student nurse is caring for a patient who has been in the burn unit for several weeks. The patient needs assistance with the bedpan to have a bowel movement, and the student nurse notes that the stool is black with a tarry appearance. What is the **most** important priority action at this time?
    a. Check the patient's CBC results including hematocrit and hemoglobin.
    b. Ask if the patient is currently taking an iron supplement.
    c. Test for the presence of occult blood with a Hemoccult card and reagent.
    d. Perform a dietary assessment to determine if the stool color is related to food.

39. A patient who lives in a rural community sustained severe burns during a house fire at 10 am. The rural emergency medical services (EMS) started a peripheral IV at 11:00 AM at a keep-vein-open (KVO) rate. The patient was admitted to the hospital at 1:00 PM. In calculating the fluid replacement, at what time is the fluid for the first 8-hour period completed?
    a. 6:00 PM
    b. 7:00 PM
    c. 8:00 PM
    d. 9:00 PM

40. A patient in the burn intensive care unit weighed 80 kg (preburn weight). The provider orders titration of IV fluid to achieve 0.5 mL/kg/hr urine output. What is the minimal hourly urine output for this patient?
    a. 30 mL/hr
    b. 35 mL/hr
    c. 40 mL/hr
    d. 45 mL/hr

41. A burn patient with which condition is most likely to have mannitol (Osmitrol) ordered as part of the drug therapy?
    a. Peripheral edema associated with burns on the lower extremities
    b. Inhalation burns around the mouth causing mucosal swelling
    c. Electrical burn with myoglobin in the urine
    d. Smoke inhalation and superficial burns to the forearms

42. A patient was admitted to the burn unit approximately 6 hours ago after being rescued from a burning building. In the emergency department (ED), he reported a dry, irritated throat "from breathing in the fumes" but otherwise had no airway complaints. During the shift, the nurse notes that the patient has suddenly developed marked stridor. The nurse anticipates preparing the patient for which emergency procedure?
    a. Bronchoscopy
    b. Intubation
    c. Needle thoracotomy
    d. Escharotomy

43. A patient was admitted for burns to the upper extremities after being trapped in a burning structure. The patient is also at risk for inadequate oxygenation related to inhalation of smoke and superheated fumes. Which diagnostic test **best** monitors this patient's gas exchange?
    a. Complete blood count
    b. Myoglobin level
    c. Carboxyhemoglobin level
    d. Chest x-ray

44. A patient in the burn intensive care unit is receiving vecuronium (Norcuron). What is the **priority** nursing intervention for this patient?
    a. Have emergency intubation equipment at the bedside.
    b. Ensure that all the equipment alarms are on and functional.
    c. Closely monitor the patient's urinary output every hour.
    d. Ensure that daily drug levels and electrolyte values are obtained.

45. The **priority** expected outcome during the resuscitation phase of a burn injury is to maintain which factor?
    a. The airway
    b. Cardiac output
    c. Fluid replacement
    d. Patient comfort

46. Which statement about the resuscitation phase of a burn injury is accurate?
    a. It occurs in the prehospital timeframe.
    b. It continues for about 8 hours after the burn.
    c. It continues for about 24-48 hours after the burn.
    d. It continues until the patient is stable.

47. The release of myoglobin from damaged muscle in patients with major burns can result in which potential complication?
    a. Paralytic ileus
    b. Acute kidney injury
    c. Limited mobility
    d. Hypovolemia

48. A burn patient in the fluid resuscitation phase is experiencing dyspnea. What are the **priority** interventions for this patient? **Select all that apply.**
    a. Elevate the head of bed to 45 degrees.
    b. Maintain patient in the supine position.
    c. Notify the Rapid Response Team.
    d. Administer an analgesic to calm the patient.
    e. Apply humidified oxygen.
    f. Attempt distraction using music therapy.

49. The vasodilating effects of carbon monoxide in patients with carbon monoxide poisoning cause what clinical manifestation?
    a. Cyanosis around the lips
    b. Generalized pallor
    c. Cherry-red skin color
    d. Mottled skin color

50. The nurse is caring for a burn patient about to undergo hydrotherapy. Which complementary therapies are appropriate for pain management in this patient? **Select all that apply.**
    a. Administering IV opioid analgesics
    b. Allowing the patient to make decisions regarding pain control
    c. Playing music in the background
    d. Using meditative breathing
    e. Using guided imagery
    f. Providing healing or therapeutic touch

51. A burn patient refuses to eat. The potential problem of weight loss related to increased metabolic rate and reduced calorie intake is identified for this patient. What method does the nurse use to weigh this patient correctly?
    a. Weigh once a week after morning hygiene and compare to previous weight.
    b. Weigh daily at the same time of day and compare to preburn weight.
    c. Use a bed scale and subtract the estimated weight of linens.
    d. Weigh daily without dressings or splints and compare to preburn weight.

52. The student nurse is preparing to assist with hydrotherapy for a burn patient. The supervising nurse instructs the student to obtain the necessary equipment before beginning the procedure. What equipment does the student nurse obtain? **Select all that apply.**
    a. Scissors and forceps
    b. Hydrogen peroxide
    c. Mild soap or detergent
    d. Pressure dressings
    e. Washcloths and gauze sponges
    f. Chlorhexidine sponges

53. The nurse is applying a dressing to cover a burn on a patient's left leg. What technique does the nurse use?
    a. Consider the depth of the injury and amount of drainage, and work distal to proximal.
    b. Change the dressing every 4 hours or when the drainage leaks through the dressing.
    c. Consider the patient's mobility and the area of injury, and work proximal to distal.
    d. Use multiple gauze layers and roller gauze to pad and protect the joint areas.

54. The nurse has just received phone report on a burn patient being transferred from the burn intensive care unit to the step-down burn unit. Which of these tasks is appropriate to delegate to unlicensed assistive personnel (UAP) in order to prepare the room?
    a. Place sterile sheets and a sterile pillowcase on the bed.
    b. Place a new disposable stethoscope in the room.
    c. Clear a space in the corner for the patient's flowers.
    d. Hang a sign on the door to prohibit entry of visitors.

55. The nurse is monitoring the nutritional status of a burn patient. Which indicators will the nurse use? **Select all that apply.**
    a. Amount of food the patient eats
    b. Weight to height ratio
    c. Serum albumin
    d. Amount of water the patient drinks
    e. Blood glucose
    f. Serum potassium

56. The nurse is educating a patient who has sustained burns to the dominant hand. What kind of active range-of-motion exercises does the nurse instruct the patient to perform?
    a. Exercise the hand, thumb, and fingers every hour while awake.
    b. Exercise the fingers and thumb at least three times a day.
    c. Use the hands to perform activities of daily living.
    d. Squeeze a soft rubber ball several times a day.

57. A burn patient must have pressure dressings applied to prevent contractures and reduce scarring. For **maximum** effectiveness, what procedure pertaining to the pressure garments is implemented?
    a. Changed every 24-48 hours to prevent infection
    b. Worn at least 23 hours a day until the scar tissue matures
    c. Removed for hygiene and during sleeping
    d. Applied with aseptic technique

58. The family reports that the burn patient is unable to perform self-care measures, so someone has been "doing everything for her." The nurse finds that the patient has the knowledge and the physical capacity to independently perform self-care. What is the nurse's **best** response?
    a. "What can your family do to help you feel better and stronger?"
    b. "You should be doing these things for yourself to increase your self-esteem."
    c. "Can you tell me about what's been happening since you were discharged from the hospital?"
    d. "Let's review the principles of self-care that you learned in the hospital."

59. A patient who sustained severe burns to the face with significant scarring and disfigurement will soon be discharged from the hospital. Which intervention is **best** to help the patient make the transition into the community?
    a. Discuss cosmetic surgery that could occur over the next several years.
    b. Focus on the positive aspects of going home and being with family.
    c. Teach the family to perform all aspects of care for the patient.
    d. Encourage visits from friends and short public appearances before discharge.

60. What does the process of full-thickness wound healing include? **Select all that apply.**
    a. Healing occurs by wound contraction.
    b. Eschar must be removed.
    c. Large blisters are protective and left undisturbed.
    d. Skin grafting may be necessary.
    e. Fasciotomy may be needed to relieve pressure and allow normal blood flow.
    f. Complete healing occurs within 3-6 weeks.

61. Which statement about the third-spacing or capillary leak syndrome in a patient with severe burns is accurate?
    a. It usually happens in the first 36-48 hours.
    b. It is a leak of plasma fluids into the interstitial space.
    c. It is present only in the burned tissues.
    d. It can usually be prevented with diuretics.

62. As a result of third-spacing, during the acute phase, which electrolyte imbalances may occur? **Select all that apply.**
    a. Hyperkalemia
    b. Hypokalemia
    c. Hypernatremia
    d. Hyponatremia
    e. Hypercalcemia
    f. Hypocalcemia

63. Because of the fluid shifts in burn patients, what effect on cardiac output does the nurse expect to see?
    a. An initial increase, then normalized in 24-48 hours
    b. Depressed up to 36 hours after the burn
    c. Improved with fluid restriction
    d. Responsive to diuretics as evidenced by urinary output

64. A patient with burn injuries is being discharged from the hospital. What important points does the nurse include in the discharge teaching? **Select all that apply.**
    a. Signs and symptoms of infection
    b. Drug regimens and potential medication side effects
    c. Definition of full-thickness burns
    d. Correct application and care of pressure garments
    e. Comfort measures to reduce scarring
    f. Dates for follow-up appointments

65. A patient has sustained significant burns that have created a hypermetabolic state. In planning care for this patient, what does the nurse consider?
    a. Increased retention of sodium
    b. Decreased secretion of catecholamines
    c. Increased caloric needs
    d. The decrease in core temperature

66. The nurse is reviewing the laboratory results for several burn patients who are approximately 24-36 hours postinjury. What laboratory results related to the fluid remobilization in these patients does the nurse expect to see?
    a. Anemia
    b. Metabolic alkalosis
    c. Hypernatremia
    d. Hyperkalemia

67. The nurse is changing a burn patient's dressing. Which factors would affect the number of gauze layers applied after a topical agent has been used to treat the wound? **Select all that apply.**
    a. Amount of drainage
    b. Patient mobility
    c. Amount of pain
    d. Depth of injury
    e. Positioning of patient
    f. Frequency of dressing changes

68. A patient was rescued from a burning house and treated with oxygen. Initially, the patient had audible wheezing and wheezing on auscultation, but after approximately 30 minutes the wheezing stopped. The patient now demonstrates substernal retractions and anxiety. What action does the nurse take at this time?
    a. Recognize an impending airway obstruction and prepare for immediate intubation.
    b. Continue to monitor the patient's respiratory status and initiate pulse oximetry.
    c. Document this finding as evidence of improvement and continue to observe.
    d. Stay with and encourage the patient to remain calm and breathe deeply.

69. The nurse is caring for a young woman who sustained burns on the upper extremities and anterior chest while attempting to put out a kitchen grease fire. Which laboratory results does the nurse expect to see during the resuscitation phase? **Select all that apply.**
    a. Potassium level of 3.2 mEq/L
    b. Glucose level of 180 mg/dL
    c. Hematocrit of 49%
    d. pH of 7.20
    e. Sodium level of 139 mEq/L
    f. Albumin level 2.9 g/dL

70. A patient has sustained a burn to the right ankle. The health care provider applied the initial dressing to the ankle, and the nurse assists the patient into bed and positions the ankle to prevent contracture. What is the correct position the nurse uses?
    a. Dorsiflexion
    b. Adduction
    c. External rotation
    d. Hyperextension

71. A patient has sustained a severe burn greater than 30% total body surface area (TBSA). What is the **best** way to assess renal function in this patient?
    a. Measure urine output and compare this value with fluid intake.
    b. Weigh the patient every day and compare that to the dry weight.
    c. Note the amount of edema and measure abdominal girth.
    d. Assist the patient with a urinal or bedpan every 2 hours.

72. The nurse is caring for an African-American patient with a burn injury. The patient is experiencing severe pain and discomfort that are unrelated to the burned areas. The nurse advocates that the provider order which additional test?
    a. Sickle cell for trait
    b. Drug screen for opiate abuse
    c. X-rays to identify bone injuries
    d. ECG to identify cardiac dysrhythmias

73. The health care provider has ordered an escharotomy for a patient because of constriction around the patient's chest. The nurse is teaching the patient and family about the procedure. Which statement by the family indicates a need for **additional** teaching?
    a. "He will have to receive general anesthesia."
    b. "He'll be awake for the procedure."
    c. "He will receive medication for sedation and pain."
    d. "We could stay with him at the bedside during the procedure."

74. The nurse is caring for a firefighter who was brought in for burns around the face and upper chest. Airway maintenance for this patient with respiratory involvement includes what action?
    a. Monitoring for signs and symptoms of upper airway edema during fluid resuscitation
    b. Inserting a nasopharyngeal airway when the patient's airway is completely obstructed
    c. Obtaining an order for as-needed (PRN) oxygen per nasal cannula
    d. Frequently suctioning the mouth with Yankauer suction

75. At what point does fluid mobilization occur in patients with burns?
    a. After the scar tissue is formed and fluids are no longer being lost
    b. Within the first 4 hours after the burns were sustained
    c. About 24 hours after the burn injury when the fluid is reabsorbed from the interstitial tissue
    d. Immediately after the burns occur

76. The nurse is caring for a patient with chronic pain associated with an old burn injury. Which nonpharmacologic intervention does the nurse use to help relieve the patient's pain?
    a. Cooling blanket to decrease edema
    b. Lower room temperature to reduce discomfort
    c. Massaging nonburned areas
    d. Range-of-motion exercises

77. A patient with a burn injury had an autograft. The nurse learns in report that the donor site is on the upper thigh. What type of wound does the nurse expect to find at the donor site?
    a. Stage 1
    b. Partial thickness
    c. Full thickness
    d. Stage 4

78. To prevent the complication of Curling's ulcer, what does the nurse anticipate the health care provider will order?
    a. Nasogastric tube insertion
    b. Histamine-2 blockers
    c. Abdominal assessment every 4 hours
    d. Systemic antibiotic

79. Several patients are transported from an industrial fire to a local emergency department (ED). Which factors increase the risk of death for these patients? **Select all that apply.**
    a. Male gender
    b. Age greater than 60 years
    c. Burn greater than 40% TBSA
    d. Presence of an inhalation injury
    e. Presence of contact burns
    f. History of kidney disease

80. What is the **most** essential patient data needed for calculating the fluid rates, energy requirements, and drug doses for the burn patient?
    a. Age
    b. Health history
    c. Preburn weight
    d. Current weight

81. Which drug therapy reduces the risk of wound infection for burn patients?
    a. Large doses of oral antifungal medications every 4 hours
    b. Silver nitrate solution covered by dry dressings applied every 4 hours
    c. Silver sulfadiazine on full-thickness injuries every 4 hours
    d. Broad-spectrum antibiotics given intravenously

82. A patient has sustained a relatively large burn. The nurse anticipates that the patient's nutritional requirements may **exceed** how many kcal/day?
    a. 1500
    b. 2000
    c. 3000
    d. 5000

83. Which feelings are **most** typically expressed by the burn patient? **Select all that apply.**
    a. Suspicion
    b. Regression
    c. Apathy
    d. Denial
    e. Suicidal ideations
    f. Anger

84. A patient has been depressed and withdrawn since her injury and has expressed that "life will never be the same." Which nursing intervention **best** promotes a positive image for this burn patient?
    a. Discussing the possibility of reconstructive surgery with the patient
    b. Allowing the patient to choose a colorful scarf to cover the burned area
    c. Playing cards or board games with the patient
    d. Encouraging the patient to consider how fortunate she is to be alive

85. A 28-year-old male patient sustained second- and third-degree burns on his legs (30%) when his clothing caught fire while he was burning leaves. He was hosed down by his neighbor and arrived at the emergency department (ED) in severe discomfort. What is the **priority** problem for the patient at this time?
    a. Acute pain related to damaged or exposed nerve endings
    b. Decreased fluid volume related to electrolyte imbalance
    c. Potential for inadequate oxygenation
    d. Diminished self-image related to the appearance of legs

86. Which patient has the **highest** risk for a fatal burn injury?
    a. 4-year-old child
    b. 32-year-old man
    c. 45-year-old woman
    d. 77-year-old man

87. The nurse is providing care for a burn patient who recently received a graft. On assessment of the patient's wound, redness and swelling as well as some foul-smelling drainage is noted. What does the nurse suspect?
    a. Partial thickness burn
    b. Local infection of burn wound
    c. Failure of the graft
    d. Systemic sepsis

88. Which factors in the older adult increase the risk of complications from a burn injury?
Select all that apply.
   a. Slower healing time
   b. Thinner skin
   c. Increased inflammatory response
   d. Increased pulmonary compliance
   e. Altered glucose metabolism
   f. History of heart failure

89. Over a period of 4 days the patient developed an elevated temperature associated with disorientation and lethargy. Lab values include a normal platelet level. Which type of infection does the nurse suspect?
   a. Viral
   b. Fungal
   c. Gram-positive bacterial
   d. Gram-negative bacterial

90. Which are expected outcomes when evaluating the care of a patient with burn injuries?
Select all that apply.
   a. Patient's infection was treated rapidly.
   b. Patient's airway remained patent.
   c. Patient's pain was decreased or relieved.
   d. Patient's perception of self is positive.
   e. Patient's weight loss was only 10%.
   f. Patient's wounds are all in the process of healing.

Assessment of the Respiratory System

1. What is the **priority** medical-surgical concept for the nurse when performing an assessment of a patient's respiratory system?
   a. Perfusion
   b. Gas exchange
   c. Acid-base balance
   d. Cellular regulation

2. Which factor is the **most** common cause of chronic respiratory problems and physical limitations?
   a. Exposure to coal dust
   b. Decreased strength of respiratory muscles
   c. Use of smokeless products such as chewing tobacco
   d. Smoking cigarettes or exposure to cigarette smoke

3. A patient comes to the health care provider's office for an annual physical. The patient reports a persistent, nagging cough. Which question does the nurse ask first about this symptom?
   a. "How long has your cough been present?"
   b. "Do you have a family history of lung cancer?"
   c. "Have you been running a fever?"
   d. "Do you have sneezing and congestion?"

4. When blood passes through the lungs, what happens to oxygen?
   a. It diffuses from the alveoli into the red blood cells.
   b. It diffuses from the red blood cells into the alveoli.
   c. It decreases concentration in the blood.
   d. It increases concentration in the alveoli.

5. Which substances from cigarette smoke have been implicated in the development of serious lung diseases? **Select all that apply.**
   a. Carbon dioxide
   b. Nicotine
   c. Tar
   d. Carbon monoxide
   e. Dust particles
   f. Nitrogen

6. A patient reports smoking a pack of cigarettes a day for 9 years. He quit for 2 years and then smoked 2 packs a day for the last 30 years. What are the pack-years for this patient?
   a. 39 years
   b. 69 years
   c. 19.5 years
   d. 41 years

7. The nurse is explaining third-hand passive smoking to a patient. Which explanation is **most** accurate?
   a. Sitting in a car with a person who is smoking
   b. Exposure to smoke on the clothes of a smoker
   c. Walking through a group of people smoking outside
   d. Entering a room where several people have been smoking

8. Which statement made by a patient who is a smoker indicates the need for additional teaching?
   a. "I don't worry about lung problems because I don't smoke, but my husband smokes."
   b. "I worry about lung diseases because I borrow cigarettes when I'm out with friends."
   c. "I use a hookah when I smoke but I'm trying to quit because I know it's not good for me."
   d. "I'm using e-cigarettes to try to stop smoking but I worry because I don't know the long-term effects."

9. Pulmonary function tests are scheduled for a patient with a history of smoking who reports dyspnea and chronic cough. What will patient teaching information about this procedure include?
   a. Do not smoke for at least 2 weeks before the test.
   b. Bronchodilator drugs may be withheld 2 days before the test.
   c. The patient will breathe through the mouth and wear a nose clip during the test.
   d. The patient will be expected to walk on a treadmill during the test.

10. Which groups of people are at high risk for nicotine addiction from smoking? **Select all that apply.**
    a. White collar workers
    b. Native Americans and African Americans
    c. College graduates
    d. Women who work full time
    e. Gay and lesbian people
    f. High school dropouts

11. The nurse is providing care for a patient who would like to quit smoking. Which important teaching points must be included when teaching this patient? **Select all that apply.**
    a. Talk with your health care provider about nicotine replacement therapies.
    b. Ask for help from family and friends who have quit smoking.
    c. Smoking while using a nicotine patch is acceptable as long as you are gradually decreasing how much you smoke.
    d. Remove all ashtrays, cigarettes, pipes, cigars, and lighters from your home to decrease the temptation to smoke.
    e. If you are used to having a cigarette after eating, get up from the table as soon as you are finished eating.
    f. Avoid starting an exercise program at the same time you quit smoking because making two big changes at the same time is setting yourself up for failure.

12. The health care provider has prescribed varenicline for the patient who wishes to quit smoking. What **specific** priority teaching must the nurse provide for the patient and his family?
    a. Avoid spending time in enclosed spaces with active smokers.
    b. Make a list of all the reasons that you wish to quit smoking cigarettes.
    c. Plan to reward yourself with the money you save from not smoking cigarettes.
    d. Be sure to report any changes in behavior or thought processes to your health care provider.

13. In which situation would the oxygen-hemoglobin dissociation curve shift to the left?
    a. Decreased pH (acidosis)
    b. Increased pH (alkalosis)
    c. Increased body temperature
    d. Increased body carbon dioxide concentration

14. Which respiratory changes occur as a result of aging? **Select all that apply.**
    a. Increased elastic recoil
    b. Dilation of alveolar ducts
    c. Decreased ability to cough
    d. Alveolar surface tension increases
    e. Diffusion capacity decreases
    f. Diaphragm muscle strength decreases

15. A patient is scheduled to have a pulmonary function test (PFT). Which type of information does the nurse include in the nursing history so that PFT results can be appropriately determined?
    a. Age, gender, race, height, weight, and smoking status
    b. Occupational status, activity tolerance for activities of daily living
    c. Medication history and history of allergies to contrast media
    d. History of chronic medical conditions and surgical procedures

16. Which description best explains residual volume (RV)?
    a. Amount of air in the lungs at the end of maximal inhalation
    b. Amount of air remaining in the lungs at the end of full forced exhalation
    c. Amount of air remaining in the lungs after normal exhalation
    d. Maximal amount of forced air that can be exhaled after maximal inspiration

17. Which airway structure is part of the immune system?
    a. Eustachian tubes
    b. Turbinates
    c. Paranasal sinuses
    d. Palatine tonsils

18. Which structure protects the patient from the risk of aspiration?
    a. Larynx
    b. Glottis
    c. Epiglottis
    d. Cricoid cartilage

19. The nurse is caring for a patient with dyspnea described as fair to moderate with activity. The patient has no dyspnea at rest. He sometimes experiences dyspnea while showering or dressing and has to stop to catch his breath when going up a flight of stairs. The nurse recognizes that the patient has which class of dyspnea?
    a. Class II
    b. Class III
    c. Class IV
    d. Class V

20. The nurse is assessing a patient's respiratory system. On auscultation the nurse hears squeaky, musical continuous sounds when the patient inhales and exhales. The nurse recognizes that these sounds are which abnormal finding?
    a. Fine crackles
    b. Coarse crackles
    c. Wheezes
    d. Rhonchi

21. Which assessment finding reflects an immediate gas exchange and perfusion problem?
    a. Clubbed fingers
    b. Barrel chest
    c. Weight loss
    d. Cyanosis

22. The nurse is caring for an older adult who uses a wheelchair and spends over half of each day in bed. Which intervention is important in promoting pulmonary hygiene **related to** age and decreased mobility?
    a. Obtain an order for as-needed (prn) oxygen via nasal cannula.
    b. Encourage the patient to turn, cough, and deep-breathe.
    c. Reassure the patient that immobility is temporary.
    d. Monitor the respiratory rate and check pulse oximetry readings.

23. The nurse is assessing a middle-aged patient who reports a decreased tolerance for exercise and that she must work harder to breathe. Which questions assist the nurse in determining what these changes are related to? **Select all that apply.**
    a. "Do you have anemia?"
    b. "When did you first notice these symptoms?"
    c. "Do you or have you ever smoked cigarettes?"
    d. "How often do you exercise?"
    e. "Are you coughing up any colored sputum?"
    f. "Does your sputum clear with coughing?"

24. A patient who received a bronchoscopy was nothing by mouth (NPO) for several hours before the test. A few hours after the test, the patient is hungry and would like to eat a meal. What does the nurse do before allowing the patient to eat?
    a. Order a meal because the patient is now alert and oriented.
    b. Check pulse oximetry to be sure oxygen saturation has returned to normal.
    c. Check for a gag reflex before allowing the patient to eat.
    d. Assess for nausea from the medications given for the test.

25. After a bronchoscopy procedure, the patient coughs up sputum that contains blood. What is the **best** nursing action at this time?
    a. Assess vital signs and respiratory status and notify the provider of the findings.
    b. Monitor the patient for 24 hours to see if blood continues in the sputum.
    c. Send the sputum to the lab for cytology for possible lung cancer.
    d. Reassure the patient that this is a normal response after a bronchoscopy.

26. Before a bronchoscopy procedure, the patient received benzocaine spray as a topical anesthetic to numb the oropharynx. The nurse is assessing the patient after the procedure. Which finding suggests that the patient is developing methemoglobinemia?
    a. The patient has a decreased hematocrit level.
    b. The patient has cyanosis that does not respond to supplemental oxygen.
    c. The blood sample is a bright cherry-red color.
    d. The patient experiences sedation and amnesia.

27. The nurse is caring for several patients who had diagnostic testing for respiratory disorders. Which diagnostic test has the **highest** risk for the postprocedure complication of pneumothorax?
    a. Bronchoscopy
    b. Laryngoscopy
    c. Computed tomography of lungs
    d. Thoracentesis

28. A patient's pulse oximetry reading is 89%. What is the nurse's **first** priority action?
    a. Recheck the reading with a different oximeter.
    b. Apply supplemental oxygen and recheck the oximeter reading in 45 minutes.
    c. Assess the patient for respiratory distress and recheck the oximeter reading.
    d. Place the patient in the recovery position and monitor frequently.

29. A patient demonstrates labored, shallow respirations and a respiratory rate of 32/min with a pulse oximetry reading of 85%. What is the **priority** nursing intervention?
    a. Notify respiratory therapy to give the patient a breathing treatment.
    b. Start oxygen via nasal cannula at 2 L/min.
    c. Obtain an order for a stat arterial blood gas (ABG).
    d. Encourage coughing and deep-breathing exercises.

30. The patient is scheduled for a computed tomography (CT) scan. Which **priority** question must the nurse be sure to ask before the procedure?
    a. "Do you have a history of any form of cancer?"
    b. "Have you ever had a CT scan before?"
    c. "Are you allergic to iodine or shellfish?"
    d. "Can you lie very still for at least an hour or more?"

31. Which factors or conditions cause a decreased (below normal) partial pressure of end-tidal carbon dioxide ($PEtCO_2$) level due to poor pulmonary ventilation? **Select all that apply.**
    a. Hyperthermia
    b. Malpositioned endotracheal tube
    c. Apnea
    d. Hypoventilation
    e. Airway obstruction
    f. Pulmonary embolism

32. The nurse is reviewing arterial blood gas (ABG) results from an 86-year-old patient. Which results would be considered normal findings for a patient of this age?
    a. Normal pH, normal Pao_2, normal $Paco_2$
    b. Normal or acidotic pH, decreased Pao_2, normal $Paco_2$
    c. Normal or alkalotic pH, decreased Pao_2, normal $Paco_2$
    d. Decreased pH, decreased Pao_2, decreased $Paco_2$

33. While auscultating lung sounds in the anterior chest, the nurse hears moderately loud sounds on inspiration that are equal in length with expiration. In what area is this lung sound considered normal?
    a. Trachea
    b. Major bronchi
    c. Lung fields
    d. Larynx

34. Which sounds in the smaller bronchioles and the alveoli indicate normal lung sounds?
    a. Harsh, hollow, and tubular blowing
    b. Nothing; normally no sounds are heard
    c. Soft, low rustling; like wind in the trees
    d. Flat, dull tones with a moderate pitch

35. Upon assessing the lungs, the nurse hears short, discrete popping sounds "like hair being rolled between fingers near the ear" in the bilateral lower lobes. How is this assessment documented?
    a. Rhonchi
    b. Wheezes
    c. Fine crackles
    d. Coarse crackles

36. The nurse is taking a history on a patient who reports sleeping in a recliner chair at night because lying on the bed causes shortness of breath. How is this documented?
    a. Orthopnea
    b. Paroxysmal nocturnal dyspnea
    c. Orthostatic nocturnal dyspnea
    d. Tachypnea

37. What conditions shift the oxyhemoglobin dissociation curve to the right? **Select all that apply.**
    a. Increased carbon dioxide concentration
    b. Chronic hypoxia
    c. Increased tissue pH (alkalosis)
    d. Decreased tissue temperature
    e. Decreased tissue pH (acidosis)
    f. Increased body temperature

38. What observations does the nurse make when performing a general assessment of a patient's lungs and thorax? **Select all that apply.**
    a. Symmetry of chest movement
    b. Rate, rhythm, and depth of respirations
    c. Use of accessory muscles for breathing
    d. Comparison of the anteroposterior diameter with the lateral diameter
    e. Measurement of the length of the chest cavity
    f. Assessment of chest expansion and respiratory excursion

39. Which assessment finding is an objective sign of chronic oxygen deprivation?
    a. Continuous cough productive of clear sputum
    b. Audible inspiratory and expiratory wheeze
    c. Chest pain that increases with deep inspiration
    d. Clubbing of fingernails and a barrel-shaped chest

40. The nurse is palpating a patient's chest and identifies an increased tactile fremitus or vibration of the chest wall produced when the patient speaks. What does the nurse do **next**?
    a. Observe for other findings associated with subcutaneous emphysema.
    b. Document the observation as an expected normal finding.
    c. Observe the patient for other findings associated with a pneumothorax.
    d. Document the observation as a pleural friction rub.

41. The nurse reviews the complete blood count results for the patient who has chronic obstructive pulmonary disease (COPD) and lives in a high mountain area. What lab results does the nurse expect to see for this patient?
    a. Increased red blood cells
    b. Decreased neutrophils
    c. Decreased eosinophils
    d. Increased lymphocytes

42. The nurse is inspecting a patient's chest and observes an increase in anteroposterior diameter of the chest. When is this an expected finding?
    a. With a pulmonary mass
    b. Upon deep inhalation
    c. In older adult patients
    d. With chest trauma

43. What is the best position for a patient to assume for a thoracentesis?
    a. Side-lying, affected side exposed, head slightly raised
    b. Lying flat with arm on affected side across the chest
    c. Sitting up, leaning forward on the over-bed table
    d. Prone position with arms above the head

44. Which procedure has a risk for the complication of pneumothorax?
    a. Thoracentesis
    b. Use of incentive spirometry
    c. Pulmonary function test (PFT)
    d. Ventilation-perfusion scan

45. A patient has undergone a percutaneous lung biopsy. After the procedure, what tests may be ordered to confirm that there is no pneumothorax? **Select all that apply.**
    a. Computed tomography
    b. Pulmonary function test
    c. Magnetic resonance imaging
    d. Digital chest radiography
    e. Chest x-ray
    f. Fluoroscopy

46. The respiratory therapist consults with and reports to the nurse that a patient is producing frothy pink sputum. What does the nurse suspect is occurring with this patient?
    a. Pneumothorax
    b. Pulmonary edema
    c. Pulmonary infection
    d. Pulmonary infarction

47. A patient who had a thoracentesis is now experiencing rapid shallow respirations, rapid heart rate, and pain on the affected side that is worse at the end of inhalation. What complication does the nurse suspect this patient has developed?
    a. Hemoptysis
    b. Lung abscess
    c. Pneumothorax
    d. Lung cancer

48. For what reasons would a patient have a bronchoscopy? **Select all that apply.**
    a. Obtain samples for cultures
    b. Diagnose pulmonary disease
    c. View upper airway structures
    d. Administer medications
    e. Obtain samples for biopsy
    f. Lung cancer staging

49. The nurse has received a patient from the recovery room who is somewhat drowsy but is capable of following instructions. Pulse oximetry has dropped from 95% to 90%. What is the **priority** nursing intervention?
    a. Administer oxygen at 2 L/min by nasal cannula, then reassess.
    b. Have the patient perform coughing and deep-breathing exercises, then reassess.
    c. Administer naloxone to reverse narcotic sedation effect.
    d. Withhold narcotic pain medication to reduce sedation effect.

50. What is a pulse oximeter used to measure?
    a. Oxygen perfusion in the extremities
    b. Pulse and perfusion in the extremities
    c. Generalized tissue perfusion
    d. Hemoglobin saturation with oxygen

51. Which aspect of pulmonary function testing (PFT) would be considered a normal result in the older adult?
    a. Increased forced vital capacity
    b. Decline in forced expiratory volume in 1 second
    c. Decrease in diffusion capacity of carbon monoxide
    d. Increased functional residual capacity

52. In the older adult with chronic pulmonary disease, there is a loss of elastic recoiling of the lung and decreased chest wall compliance. What is the result of this occurrence?
    a. The thoracic area becomes shorter.
    b. The patient has an increased activity tolerance.
    c. There is an increase in anteroposterior ratio.
    d. The patient has severe shortness of breath.

53. In the older adult, there is a decreased number of functional alveoli. To assist the patient to compensate for this change related to aging, what does the nurse do?
    a. Encourage the patient to ambulate and change positions.
    b. Allow the patient to rest and sleep frequently.
    c. Have face-to-face conversations when possible.
    d. Obtain an order for supplemental oxygen.

54. The nurse teaches a patient who wants to quit smoking about the impact of cigarette smoking on the lower respiratory tract. Which statement by the patient indicates an understanding of the information?
    a. "Using nicotine replacement therapy will increase my chances of success."
    b. "If I stop smoking, the damage to my lungs will be reversed."
    c. "Cigarette smoke affects my ability to cough out secretions from the lungs."
    d. "Smoking makes the large and small airways get bigger."

55. A patient reports fatigue and shortness of breath when getting up to walk to the bathroom; however, the pulse oximetry reading is 99%. Which laboratory value is consistent with the patient's subjective symptoms?
    a. Blood urea nitrogen (BUN) of 15 mg/dL
    b. White blood cell count (WBC) of 8000/mm^3
    c. Hemoglobin of 9 g/dL
    d. Blood glucose 160 mg/dL

56. The nurse is performing a respiratory assessment including pulse oximetry on several patients. Which conditions or situations may cause an artificially low reading? **Select all that apply.**
    a. Fever
    b. Anemia
    c. Receiving narcotic pain medications
    d. Peripheral artery disease
    e. History of respiratory disease such as cystic fibrosis or tuberculosis
    f. Edema

57. A patient who had neck surgery for removal of a tumor reports "not being able to breathe very well." The nurse observes that the patient has decreased chest movement and an elevated pulse. A bronchoscopy is ordered. For what reason did the provider order a bronchoscopy for this patient?
    a. Reverse and relieve any obstruction caused during the neck surgery.
    b. Assess the function of vocal cords or remove foreign bodies from the larynx.
    c. Aspirate pleural fluid or air from the pleural space.
    d. Visualize the larynx (airway structures) to use as a guide for intubation.

58. A patient returns to the unit after bronchoscopy. In addition to respiratory status assessment, which assessment does the nurse make in order to prevent aspiration?
    a. Presence of pain or soreness in throat
    b. Time and amount of last oral fluid intake
    c. Type and location of chest pain
    d. Presence or absence of gag reflex

59. The nurse hears fine crackles during a lung assessment of the patient who is in the initial postoperative period. Which nursing intervention helps relieve this respiratory problem?
    a. Monitor the patient with a pulse oximeter.
    b. Encourage coughing and deep-breathing.
    c. Obtain an order for a chest x-ray.
    d. Obtain an order for high-flow oxygen.

60. A patient having respiratory difficulty has a pH of 7.48. What is the nurse's **best** interpretation of this value?
    a. Acidosis
    b. Alkalosis
    c. Hypoxia
    d. Hypercarbia

61. The nurse is performing a respiratory assessment on an older adult patient. Which questions would the nurse be sure to ask? **Select all that apply.**
    a. "When was your last chest x-ray?"
    b. "Do you now or have you ever smoked?"
    c. "Have you had influenza or pneumonia vaccinations?"
    d. "Do you have enough energy to do what you like to do?"
    e. "When was the last time you had a tetanus shot?"
    f. "Does anyone in your family have a history of chronic illnesses?"

62. Tissue oxygen delivery through dissociation from hemoglobin is based on which factor?
    a. Saturation
    b. Oxygen tension
    c. Unloading from hemoglobin
    d. Tissues' need for oxygen

63. The nurse makes observations about several respiratory patients' abilities to perform activities of daily living in order to quantify the level of dyspnea. Which patient is considered to have class V dyspnea?
    a. Experiences subjective shortness of breath when walking up a flight of stairs
    b. Limited to bed or chair and experiences shortness of breath at rest
    c. Can independently shower and dress but cannot keep pace with similarly aged people
    d. Experiences shortness of breath during aerobic exercise such as jogging

64. The nurse is reviewing the arterial blood gas results for a 25-year-old trauma patient who has new-onset shortness of breath and demonstrates shallow and irregular respirations. The arterial blood gas results are pH 7.26, Pco_2 47%, Po_2 89%, HCO_3^- 24. What imbalance does the nurse suspect this patient has?
    a. Respiratory acidosis
    b. Respiratory alkalosis
    c. Metabolic acidosis
    d. Metabolic alkalosis

65. While assessing a patient's chest and lung fields, the nurse notes rapid heart rate, rapid shallow respirations, tracheal deviation toward the right side, and new-onset nagging cough. What is the nurse's **priority** action?
    a. Document this expected finding and apply oxygen after checking pulse oximetry.
    b. Notify the health care provider because the patient has an airway obstruction.
    c. Assess the patient for air hunger or pain at the end of inhalation and exhalation.
    d. Palpate for crackling sensation underneath the skin or for localized tenderness.

66. The nurse is assisting the health care provider to perform a thoracentesis. What does the nurse do prior to the beginning of the procedure?
    a. Position the patient in semi-Fowler's position.
    b. Apply goggles and mask to prevent oral or eye splashes.
    c. Provide a bottle without a vacuum for specimen collection.
    d. Shave the patient's entire back.

28 CHAPTER

Care of Patients Requiring Oxygen Therapy or Tracheostomy

1. What is the most important interrelated medical-surgical concept for nursing care of patients requiring oxygen therapy?
   a. Gas exchange
   b. Perfusion
   c. Tissue integrity
   d. Cellular regulation

2. In what situations is oxygen therapy needed for a patient? **Select all that apply.**
   a. To treat hypoxia
   b. To treat hypothermia
   c. To treat hypoxemia
   d. When the normal 35% oxygen level in the air is inadequate
   e. When the normal 21% oxygen level in the air is inadequate
   f. To treat acute and chronic respiratory illnesses

3. Which conditions will increase the body's need for more oxygen? **Select all that apply.**
   a. Hypothyroid state
   b. Infection in the blood
   c. Diabetes mellitus
   d. Body temperature of 101°F
   e. Hemoglobin level of 8.7 g/dL
   f. Heart failure

4. To improve a patient's oxygenation to a normal level, the amount of oxygen administered is based on which factors? **Select all that apply.**
   a. Symptom management only
   b. Pulse oximetry reading
   c. Respiratory assessment
   d. The patient's subjective complaints
   e. Arterial blood gas results
   f. Presence of chronic hypercarbia

5. What are the hazards of administering oxygen therapy? **Select all that apply.**
   a. Oxygen supports and enhances combustion.
   b. Oxygen itself can burn.
   c. Each electrical outlet in the room must be covered if not in use.
   d. All electrical equipment in the room must be grounded to prevent fires.
   e. Solutions with high concentrations of alcohol or oil cannot be used in the room.
   f. Alcohol-based hand rubs should be removed from rooms with oxygen therapy.

6. Which parameters does the nurse monitor to ensure that a patient's response to oxygen therapy gas exchange is adequate? **Select all that apply.**
   a. Level of consciousness
   b. Respiratory pattern
   c. Oxygen flow rate
   d. Pulse oximetry
   e. Respiratory rate
   f. Blood pressure

7. The patient has been on oxygen therapy at 70% for over 48 hours. For which complication must the nurse monitor?
   a. Oxygen-induced hypoventilation
   b. Hypercarbia
   c. Oxygen toxicity
   d. Absorptive atelectasis

8. The nurse is monitoring a patient receiving oxygen therapy. On auscultation the nurse notes that the patient developed new onset of crackles and decreased breath sounds. Which condition does the nurse recognize?
   a. Oxygen toxicity
   b. Hypoxemia
   c. Hypercarbia
   d. Absorptive atelectasis

9. A patient requires home oxygen therapy. When the home health nurse enters the patient's home for the initial visit, the nurse observes several issues that are safety hazards related to the patient's oxygen therapy. What hazards do these include? **Select all that apply.**
   a. Bottle of wine in the kitchen area
   b. Package of cigarettes on the coffee table
   c. Several decorative candles on the mantelpiece
   d. Grounded outlet with a green dot on the plate
   e. Electric fan with a frayed cord in the bathroom
   f. Computer with a three-pronged plug

10. The patient is receiving oxygen at 5 L/min by nasal cannula. What **priority** intervention must the nurse use at this time?
    a. Switch to a mask delivery system.
    b. Humidify the oxygen with sterile water.
    c. Monitor for manifestations of oxygen toxicity.
    d. Add extension tubing for patient mobility.

11. The home health nurse has been caring for a patient with a chronic respiratory disorder. Today the patient seems confused when she is normally alert and oriented × 3. What is the **priority** nursing action?
    a. Notify the provider about the mental status change.
    b. Check the pulse oximeter reading.
    c. Ask the patient's family when this behavior started.
    d. Perform a mental status examination.

12. The nurse is caring for several patients on a general medical-surgical unit. The nurse would question the need for oxygen therapy for a patient with which condition?
    a. Pulmonary edema with decreased arterial Po_2 levels
    b. Valve replacement with increased cardiac output
    c. Anemia with a decreased hemoglobin and hematocrit
    d. Sustained fever with an increased metabolic demand

13. When a patient is requiring oxygen therapy, what is important for the nurse to know?
    a. Patients require 1-10 L/min by nasal cannula in order for oxygen to be effective.
    b. Oxygen-induced hypoventilation is the priority when $Paco_2$ levels are unknown.
    c. Why the patient is receiving oxygen, expected outcomes, and complications.
    d. The goal is the highest Fio_2 possible for the particular device being used.

14. The nurse is caring for a patient receiving humidified oxygen. Which precaution does the nurse take to prevent bacterial contamination and infection?
    a. Never drain fluid from the water trap back into the nebulizer.
    b. Always wear gloves when cleaning the patient's nasal cannula.
    c. Do not allow live or cut flowers into the patient's room.
    d. Administer ordered antibiotic therapy.

15. The nurse is administering oxygen to a patient who is hypoxic and has chronic high levels of carbon dioxide. Which oxygen therapy prevents a respiratory complication for this patient?
    a. Fio_2 higher than the usual 2-4 L/min per nasal cannula
    b. Venturi mask of 40% for the delivery of oxygen
    c. Lower concentration of oxygen (1-2 L/min) per nasal cannula
    d. Variable Fio_2 via partial rebreather mask

16. The patient is prescribed home oxygen. Which criteria are important when choosing the oxygen delivery system? **Select all that apply.**
    a. Oxygen concentration required by the patient
    b. Importance of accuracy and control of the oxygen concentration
    c. Importance of humidity
    d. Need to teach patient to suction self
    e. Patient pain medication administration
    f. Patient mobility

17. A patient is receiving a high concentration of oxygen as a temporary emergency measure. Which nursing action is the **most** appropriate to prevent complications associated with high-flow oxygen?
    a. Auscultate the lungs every 4 hours for oxygen toxicity.
    b. Increase the oxygen if the PaO_2 level is less than 93 mm Hg.
    c. Monitor the prescribed oxygen level and length of therapy.
    d. Decrease the oxygen if the patient's condition does not improve.

18. Increased risk for oxygen toxicity is related to which factors? **Select all that apply.**
    a. Continuous delivery of oxygen at greater than 50% concentration
    b. Family members smoking while patient is receiving oxygen therapy
    c. The severity and extent of lung disease
    d. Neglecting to monitor the patient's status and reducing oxygen concentration as soon as possible
    e. Adding continuous positive airway pressure (CPAP) or positive end-expiratory pressure (PEEP)
    f. Delivery of a high concentration of oxygen over 24-48 hours

19. A patient is receiving warmed and humidified oxygen. The respiratory therapist informs the nurse that several other patients on other units have developed hospital-acquired infections and *Pseudomonas aeruginosa* has been identified as the organism. What does the nurse do?
    a. Place the patient in respiratory isolation.
    b. Obtain an order for a sputum culture.
    c. Change the humidifier every 24 hours.
    d. Obtain an order to discontinue the humidifier.

20. A patient is receiving warmed and humidified oxygen. In discarding the moisture formed by condensation, why does the nurse minimize the time that the tubing is disconnected?
    a. To prevent the patient from desaturating
    b. To reduce the patient's risk of infection
    c. To minimize the disturbance to the patient
    d. To facilitate overall time management

21. What is the best description of the nurse's role in the delivery of oxygen therapy?
    a. Receiving the therapy report from the respiratory therapist
    b. Evaluating the patient's response to oxygen therapy
    c. Contacting respiratory therapy for the devices
    d. Being familiar with the devices and techniques used in order to provide proper care

22. Which complication is the result of constant pressure exerted by a tracheostomy cuff causing tracheal dilation and erosion of cartilage?
    a. Tracheomalacia
    b. Tracheal stenosis
    c. Tracheoesophageal fistula
    d. Trachea–innominate artery fistula

23. A patient requires oxygen therapy with a nasal cannula. Which interventions will the nurse teach the student nurse providing care for this patient? **Select all that apply.**
    a. "Make sure that the prongs on the nasal cannula are properly positioned in the nares."
    b. "Apply a water-soluble gel to the nares as needed."
    c. "Adjust the flow rate between 1 and 8 liters/minute based on how the patient is feeling."
    d. "Be sure to assess the patency of both nares."
    e. "Assess the patient for any changes in respiratory rate and pattern."
    f. "Nasal cannula can provide a patient with between 24% and 50% oxygen flow."

24. A patient is receiving oxygen therapy through a nonrebreather mask. What is the correct nursing intervention?
    a. Maintain oxygen liter flow so that the reservoir bag is up to one-half full.
    b. Maintain 60%-75% FiO_2 at 6-11 L/min.
    c. Ensure that valves and rubber flaps are patent, functional, and not stuck.
    d. Assess for effectiveness and switch to partial rebreather mask for more precise FiO_2.

25. A patient receiving oxygen via a face mask at 5 L/min is able to eat. Which nursing intervention is performed at mealtimes?
    a. Change the mask to a nasal cannula of 6 L/min or more.
    b. Have the patient work around the face mask as best as possible.
    c. Obtain a provider order for a nasal cannula at 5 L/min.
    d. Obtain a provider order to remove the mask at meals.

26. The provider orders transtracheal oxygen therapy for a patient with respiratory difficulty. What does the nurse tell the patient's family about the purpose of this type of oxygen delivery system?
    a. Delivers oxygen directly into the lungs
    b. Keeps the small air sacs open to improve gas exchange
    c. Prevents the need for an endotracheal tube
    d. Provides high humidity with oxygen delivery

27. A patient is at risk for aspiration. Which instructions must the nurse provide to the unlicensed assistive personnel (UAP) prior to feeding the patient? **Select all that apply.**
    a. Position the patient in the most upright position possible.
    b. Provide adequate time; do not "hurry" the patient.
    c. Provide sips of water or milk between bites of food to help with swallowing.
    d. Encourage the patient to "tuck" his or her chin down and move the forehead forward while swallowing.
    e. If the patient coughs, stop the feeding until he or she indicates that the airway has been cleared.
    f. Allow the patient to indicate when he or she is ready for the next bite.

28. Which high flow oxygen delivery system delivers the **most** accurate concentration of oxygen without intubation?
    a. Partial rebreather mask
    b. Nonrebreather mask
    c. High flow nasal cannula
    d. Venturi mask

29. A patient requires long-term airway maintenance following surgery for cancer of the neck. The nurse is using a piece of equipment to explain the procedure and mechanism that are associated with this long-term therapy. Which piece of equipment is the nurse **most** likely use for this patient teaching session?
    a. Tracheostomy tube
    b. Nasal trumpet
    c. Endotracheal tube
    d. Nasal cannula

30. Which patients could benefit from the use of noninvasive positive-pressure ventilation (NPPV)? **Select all that apply.**
    a. Patient with acute exacerbation of COPD
    b. Patient with acute pneumothorax
    c. Patient with cardiogenic pulmonary edema
    d. Patient with cardiopulmonary arrest
    e. Patient with an acute asthma attack
    f. Patient with sleep apnea

31. A patient is receiving preoperative teaching for a partial laryngectomy and will have a tracheostomy postoperatively. How does the nurse define a tracheostomy to the patient?
    a. Opening in the trachea that enables breathing
    b. Temporary procedure that will be reversed at a later date
    c. Technique using positive pressure to improve gas exchange
    d. Procedure that holds open the upper airways

32. A patient returns from the operating room and the nurse assesses for subcutaneous emphysema, a potential complication associated with tracheostomy. How does the nurse assess for this complication?
    a. Checking the volume of the pilot balloon
    b. Listening for airflow through the tube
    c. Inspecting and palpating for air under the skin
    d. Assessing the tube for patency

33. A patient with a tracheostomy stoma in place develops increased coughing, inability to expectorate secretions, and difficulty breathing. What are these assessment findings related to?
    a. Overinflation of the pilot balloon
    b. Tracheoesophageal fistula
    c. Cuff leak and rupture
    d. Tracheal stenosis

34. A patient returns from the operating room after having a tracheostomy. While assessing the patient, which observation made by the nurse warrants **immediate** notification of the health care provider?
    a. Patient is alert but unable to speak and has difficulty communicating his needs.
    b. There is a small amount of bleeding present at the incision.
    c. Skin is puffy at the neck area with a crackling sensation.
    d. Respirations are audible and noisy with an increased respiratory rate.

35. A patient was intubated for acute respiratory failure, and there is an endotracheal tube in place. Which nursing interventions are appropriate for this patient? **Select all that apply.**
    a. Ensure that the oxygen is warmed and humidified.
    b. Suction the airway and then the mouth, and give oral care.
    c. Suction the airway with the oral suction equipment.
    d. Position the tubing so it does not pull on the airway.
    e. Apply suction only when withdrawing the suction catheter.
    f. Keep a resuscitation bag at the bedside at all times.

36. To prevent accidental decannulation of a tracheostomy tube, what does the nurse do?
    a. Obtain an order for continuous upper extremity restraints.
    b. Secure the tube in place using ties or fabric fasteners.
    c. Allow some flexibility in motion of the tube while coughing.
    d. Instruct the patient to hold the tube with a tissue while coughing.

37. A patient has a recent tracheostomy. What necessary equipment does the nurse ensure is kept at the bedside? **Select all that apply.**
    a. Resuscitation bag
    b. Pair of wire cutters
    c. Oxygen tubing
    d. Suction equipment
    e. Tracheostomy tube with obturator
    f. Endotracheal (ET) tube

38. The nurse is assessing a patient after surgery for placement of a tracheostomy tube and notes these findings: difficulty breathing; noisy respirations; difficulty inserting a suction catheter; and thick, dry secretions. Which complication of a tracheostomy does the nurse suspect?
    a. Tube obstruction
    b. Tube dislodgement
    c. Accidental decannulation
    d. Pneumothorax

39. Which statement by the nursing student indicates an understanding of the purpose of administering oxygen by nasal cannula?
    a. "With a nasal cannula, a wide range of oxygen flow rates and concentrations can be delivered."
    b. "A minimum flow rate of 5 L/min is needed to prevent the rebreathing of exhaled air."
    c. "It works by pulling in a proportional amount of room air for each liter flow of oxygen."
    d. "It is often used for chronic lung disease and for any patient needing long-term oxygen therapy."

40. A patient has a temporary tracheostomy following surgery to the neck area to remove a benign tumor. Which nursing intervention is performed to prevent obstruction of the tracheostomy tube?
    a. Provide tracheal suctioning when there are noisy respirations.
    b. Provide oxygenation to maintain pulse oximeter readings.
    c. Inflate the cuff to maximum pressure and check it once per shift.
    d. Suction regularly and as needed (PRN) with an oral suction device.

41. A patient sustained a serious crush injury to the neck and had a tracheostomy tube placed 3 days ago. As the nurse is performing tracheostomy care, the patient suddenly sneezes very forcefully and the tracheostomy tube falls out onto the bed linens. What does the nurse do?
    a. Ventilate the patient with 100% oxygen and notify the provider.
    b. Quickly and gently replace the tube with a clean cannula kept at the bedside.
    c. Quickly rinse the tube with sterile solution and gently replace it.
    d. Give the patient oxygen; call for assistance and a new tracheostomy kit.

42. Patients with a tracheostomy or endotracheal tube need suctioning. Which nursing interventions apply to proper suctioning technique? **Select all that apply.**
    a. Preoxygenate the patient for at least 30 seconds before suctioning.
    b. Instruct the patient that he or she is going to be suctioned.
    c. Quickly insert the suction catheter until resistance is met.
    d. Suction the patient for at least 30 seconds to remove secretions.
    e. Repeat suctioning as needed for four to five total suction passes.
    f. Apply suction only when withdrawing the suction catheter.

43. What are possible complications that can occur with suctioning from an artificial airway? **Select all that apply.**
    a. Infection
    b. Coughing
    c. Hypoxia
    d. Tissue (mucosa) trauma
    e. Vagal stimulation
    f. Bronchospasm

44. A patient required emergency intubation and currently has an artificial airway in place. Oxygen is being administered directly from the wall source. Why would warmed and humidified oxygen be a **more** appropriate choice for this patient?
    a. Helps prevent drying damage to mucous membranes
    b. Promotes thick secretions, which are easier to suction
    c. Is more comfortable for the patient
    d. Is less likely to cause oxygen toxicity

45. A patient has an endotracheal tube and requires frequent suctioning for copious secretions. Which is a **major** complication of tracheal suctioning?
    a. Atelectasis
    b. Hypoxia
    c. Hypercarbia
    d. Bronchodilation

46. While the nursing student changes a patient's tracheostomy dressing, the nurse observes the student using a pair of scissors to cut a 4×4 gauze pad to make a split dressing that will fit around the tracheostomy tube. What is the nurse's **best** action?
    a. Give the student positive reinforcement for use of materials and technique.
    b. Report the student to the instructor for remediation of the skill.
    c. Change the dressing immediately after the student has left the room.
    d. Direct the student in the correct use of materials and explain the rationale.

47. The nurse is caring for a patient with a tracheostomy who has recently been transferred from the intensive care unit (ICU), where he has had no unusual occurrences related to the tracheostomy or his oxygenation status. What does the routine care for this patient include?
    a. Thorough respiratory assessment at least every 2 hours
    b. Maintaining the cuff pressure between 50 and 100 mm Hg
    c. Suctioning as needed; maximum suction time of 20 seconds
    d. Changing the tracheostomy dressing four times a day

48. A patient with a tracheostomy is being discharged to home. In patient teaching, what does the nurse instruct the patient to do?
    a. Use sterile technique when suctioning.
    b. Instill tap water into the artificial airway.
    c. Clean the tracheostomy tube with soap and water.
    d. Increase the humidity in the home.

49. A patient with a permanent tracheostomy is interested in developing an exercise regimen. Which activity does the nurse advise the patient to **avoid?**
    a. Aerobics
    b. Tennis
    c. Golf
    d. Swimming

50. A patient with an endotracheal tube in place has dry mucous membranes of the mouth and lips related to the tube and the partial open mouth position. What technique does the nurse use to provide this patient with frequent oral care?
    a. Cleanses the mouth with glycerin swabs
    b. Provides alcohol-based mouth rinse and oral suction
    c. Cleanses with a mixture of hydrogen peroxide and water
    d. Uses oral swabs or a soft-bristled brush moistened in water

51. A patient with a tracheostomy who receives unnecessary suctioning can experience which complications? **Select all that apply.**
    a. Bronchospasm
    b. Mucosal damage
    c. Impaired gag reflex
    d. Bronchodilation
    e. Bleeding
    f. Tracheostomy obstruction

52. A patient who is breathing on his own has a fenestrated tracheostomy tube with a cuff. Which precaution must the nurse instruct the student about when caring for this patient?
    a. Always keep the cuff inflated to prevent secretions from entering the lungs.
    b. Suction the patient every 30-60 minutes.
    c. Always deflate the cuff before capping the tube with the decannulation cap.
    d. To reduce the risk for tracheal damage, keep the cuff pressure between 22 and 30 mm Hg.

53. A patient has a cuffed tracheostomy tube without a pressure relief valve. To prevent tissue damage of the tracheal mucosa, what does the nurse do?
    a. Deflate the cuff every 2-4 hours and maintain as needed.
    b. Change the tracheostomy tube every 3 days or per hospital policy.
    c. Assess and record cuff pressures each shift using the occlusive technique.
    d. Assess and record cuff pressures each shift using minimal leak technique.

54. An older adult patient is at risk for aspirating food or fluids. Which are the most appropriate nursing actions to prevent this problem? **Select all that apply.**
    a. Provide close supervision when the patient is self-feeding.
    b. Instruct the patient to tilt the head back when swallowing.
    c. Obtain an order for a clear liquid diet and offer small, frequent amounts.
    d. Instruct the patient to tuck the chin down when swallowing.
    e. Place the patient in an upright position.
    f. Keep emergency suctioning equipment at hand and turned on.

55. An older adult patient sustained a stroke several weeks ago and is having difficulty swallowing. To prevent aspiration during mealtimes, what does the nurse do?
    a. Hyperextend the head to allow food to enter the stomach and not the lungs.
    b. Give thin liquids after each bite of food to help "wash the food down."
    c. Encourage "dry swallowing" after each bite to clear residue from the throat.
    d. Maintain a low Fowler's position during eating and for 2 hours afterwards.

56. A patient with a tracheostomy tube is currently alert and cooperative but is coughing more frequently and producing more secretions than usual. The nurse determines that there is a need for suctioning. Which nursing intervention does the nurse use to prevent hypoxia for this patient?
    a. Allow the patient to breathe room air prior to suctioning.
    b. Avoid prolonged suctioning time.
    c. Suction frequently when the patient is coughing.
    d. Use the largest available catheter.

57. The nurse is suctioning the secretions from a patient's endotracheal tube. The patient demonstrates a vagal response by a drop in heart rate to 54/min and a drop in blood pressure to 90/50 mm Hg. After stopping suctioning, what is the nurse's **priority** action?
    a. Allow the patient to rest for at least 10 minutes.
    b. Monitor the patient and call the Rapid Response Team.
    c. Oxygenate with 100% oxygen and monitor the patient.
    d. Administer atropine according to standing orders.

58. A patient with a tracheostomy is unable to speak. He is not in acute distress but is gesturing and trying to communicate with the nurse. Which nursing intervention is the **best** approach in this situation?
    a. Rely on the family to interpret for the patient.
    b. Ask questions that can be answered with a "yes" or "no" response.
    c. Obtain an immediate consult with the speech therapist.
    d. Encourage the patient to rest rather than struggle with communication.

59. Which clinical finding in a patient with a recent tracheostomy is the **most** serious and requires immediate intervention?
    a. Increased cough and difficulty expectorating secretions
    b. Food particles in the tracheal secretions
    c. Pulsating tracheostomy tube in synchrony with the heartbeat
    d. Set tidal volume on the ventilator not being received by the patient

60. The nurse is caring for a patient with a tracheostomy. Which interventions for bronchial and oral hygiene should the nurse delegate to the unlicensed assistive personnel (UAP)? **Select all that apply.**
    a. Turn and reposition the patient every 2 hours.
    b. Teach the patient to cough and deep-breathe.
    c. Elevate the head of the bed for mouth care.
    d. Assist the patient to the bathroom as needed.
    e. Help the patient rise mouth with saline every 4 hours while awake.
    f. Keep glycerin swabs at the bedside for oral care as needed.

29 CHAPTER

Care of Patients with Noninfectious Upper Respiratory Problems

1. Which medical-surgical concepts take priority when the nurse is caring for a patient with a noninfectious upper respiratory problem? **Select all that apply.**
   a. Gas exchange
   b. Acid-base balance
   c. Fluid and electrolyte balance
   d. Cellular regulation
   e. Tissue integrity
   f. Elimination

2. Following radiation therapy for head and neck cancer, the nurse instructs the patient about which potential side effects? **Select all that apply.**
   a. Skin redness and tenderness
   b. Numbness of the mouth, lips, or face
   c. Difficulty swallowing
   d. Hoarseness
   e. Dry mouth
   f. Impaired taste

3. What type of treatment has the **highest** cure rate for small cancers of the head and neck?
   a. Surgery
   b. Chemotherapy
   c. Laser surgery
   d. Radiation therapy

4. The nursing student is preparing patient teaching materials about head and neck cancer. Which statement is accurate and included in the patient teaching information?
   a. It metastasizes often to the brain.
   b. It usually develops over a short time.
   c. It is often seen as red edematous areas.
   d. It is often seen as white patchy mucosal lesions.

5. The nurse is interviewing a patient to assess for risk factors related to head and neck cancer. Which questions are appropriate to include? **Select all that apply.**
   a. "How many servings per day of alcohol do you typically drink?"
   b. "Have you had frequent episodes of acute or chronic visual problems?"
   c. "Have you had a problem with sores in your mouth?"
   d. "When was the last time you saw your dentist?"
   e. "Do you have recurrent laryngitis or frequent episodes of sore throat?"
   f. "How many packs per day do you smoke and for how many years?"

6. Which patient with the highest risk for developing cancer of the larynx should be alerted about relevant lifestyle modifications to decrease this risk?
   a. 57-year-old male with alcoholism
   b. 18-year-old marijuana smoker
   c. 28-year-old female with diabetes
   d. 34-year-old male who snorts cocaine

7. In order to facilitate comfort and breathing for the patient with a laryngeal tumor, the nurse should use which position?
   a. Sims'
   b. Supine
   c. Fowler's
   d. Prone

8. Which intervention does the nurse use to assist the patient who suffers from chronic xerostomia secondary to past radiation treatments?
    a. Offer small frequent meals.
    b. Suggest a moisturizing spray.
    c. Explain fluid restrictions.
    d. Teach to wash with mild soap and water.

9. The patient with laryngeal cancer that is being treated with radiation therapy is experiencing hoarseness. What teaching points must the nurse stress with this patient? **Select all that apply.**
    a. "Your voice should improve within 4-6 weeks after the radiation therapy is completed."
    b. "Typically the hoarseness becomes worse during the radiation therapy."
    c. "Gargle 4-6 times a day with an alcohol-based mouthwash."
    d. "Rest your voice and use alternative communication methods during radiation therapy."
    e. "Wash your neck 3 times daily with a strong antiseptic soap."
    f. "The speech therapist can offer options for alternative communication methods."

10. The nurse is assessing a patient's skin at the site of radiation therapy to the neck. Which skin condition is expected in relation to the radiation treatments?
    a. Red, tender, and peeling
    b. Shiny, pale, and tight
    c. Puffy and edematous
    d. Pale, dry, and cool

11. Which surgical procedure of the neck area poses no risk postoperatively for aspiration?
    a. Total laryngectomy
    b. Transoral cordectomy
    c. Hemilaryngectomy
    d. Partial laryngectomy

12. The patient with a total laryngectomy has a laryngectomy button in place. What important teaching points must the nurse include when teaching the patient about a laryngectomy button? **Select all that apply.**
    a. A laryngectomy button is shorter and softer than a laryngectomy tube.
    b. A laryngectomy button comes in only one size.
    c. A laryngectomy button is more comfortable than a laryngectomy tube.
    d. A laryngectomy button requires use of an alternative form of communication.
    e. A laryngectomy button requires use of sterile procedure when it is changed.
    f. A laryngectomy button is longer and narrow like an endotracheal tube.

13. The nurse is caring for a postoperative patient who had a neck dissection. Which assessment finding is expected?
    a. Bulky gauze dressing is present that is dry and intact over the site.
    b. The patient can speak normally but reports a sore throat.
    c. Permanent gastrostomy tube is present with continuous tube feedings.
    d. The patient has shoulder drop and limited range of motion.

14. The nursing student is caring for an older adult patient who sustained a stroke, is confused, and is having trouble swallowing. Which statement by the nursing student indicates an understanding of aspiration precautions for this patient?
    a. "I will administer pills as whole tablets; they are easier to swallow."
    b. "If the patient coughs, I will discontinue feeding and contact the physician."
    c. "I will keep the head of the bed elevated during and after feeding."
    d. "I will encourage small amounts of fluids such as water, tea, or juices."

15. The nurse observes that a patient is having difficulty swallowing and has initiated aspiration precautions. Which procedure does the nurse expect the health care provider to order for this patient?
    a. Chest x-ray of the neck and chest
    b. CT scan of the head and neck
    c. Dynamic swallow study under fluoroscopy
    d. Direct and indirect laryngoscopy

16. A patient has had neck dissection surgery with a reconstructive flap over the carotid artery. Which intervention is appropriate for the flap care?
    a. Evaluate the flap every hour for the first 72 hours.
    b. Monitor the flap by gently placing a Doppler on the flap.
    c. Position the patient so that the flap is in the dependent position.
    d. Apply a wet-to-dry dressing to the flap.

17. The nurse is caring for several patients who require treatment for laryngeal cancer. Which treatment/procedure requires patient education about aspiration precautions?
    a. Total laryngectomy
    b. Laser surgery
    c. Radiation therapy
    d. Supraglottic laryngectomy

18. Which statement by the patient indicates understanding about radiation therapy for neck cancer?
    a. "My voice will initially be hoarse but should improve over time."
    b. "There are no side effects other than a hoarse voice."
    c. "Dry mouth after radiation therapy is temporary and short-term."
    d. "My throat is not directly affected by radiation."

19. What does the nurse include in the teaching session for a patient who is scheduled to have a partial laryngectomy?
    a. Supraglottic method of swallowing
    b. Presence of a tracheostomy tube and nasogastric tube for feeding due to postoperative swelling
    c. Not being able to eat solid foods
    d. Permanence of the tracheostomy, referred to as a laryngectomy stoma

20. A patient has been transferred from the intensive care unit to the medical-surgical unit after a laryngectomy. What does the nurse suggest to encourage the patient to participate in self-care?
    a. Changing the tracheostomy collar
    b. Suctioning the mouth with an oral suction device
    c. Checking the stoma with a flashlight
    d. Observing the color of the reconstructive flap

21. The nurse is caring for a patient who had reconstructive neck surgery and observes bright red blood spurting from the tissue flap that is covering the carotid artery. Which action must the nurse take **first**?
    a. Call the surgeon and alert the operating room.
    b. Call the Rapid Response Team.
    c. Apply immediate, direct pressure to the site.
    d. Apply a bulky sterile dressing and secure the airway.

22. A patient is experiencing acute anxiety related to hospitalization stress and an inability to accept changes related to laryngeal cancer. The patient wants to leave the hospital but agrees to try a medication to "help me calm down." For which medication does the nurse obtain a prn order?
    a. Amitriptyline
    b. Modafinil
    c. Morphine sulfate
    d. Lorazepam

23. A patient with a recent diagnosis of sinus cancer states that he wants another course of antibiotics because he believes he simply has another sinus infection. What is the nurse's **best** response?
    a. "I'll call the physician for the antibiotic prescription."
    b. "Why are you doubting your doctor's diagnosis?"
    c. "Let me bring you some information about sinus cancer."
    d. "What did the doctor say to you about your condition?"

24. A patient is unable to speak following a cordectomy. Which action is delegated to the unlicensed assistive personnel (UAP) to assist the patient in dealing with communication issues?
    a. Politely tell the patient not to communicate.
    b. Teach the patient how to use hand signals.
    c. Allow extra time to accomplish ADLs because of communication limitations.
    d. Give step-by-step instructions during the ADLs and discourage two-way communication.

25. The nurse is assessing a patient who has had a neck dissection with removal of muscle tissue, lymph nodes, and the 11th cranial nerve. Which assessment finding is anticipated because of the surgical procedure?
    a. Shoulder drop with an increased limitation of movement
    b. Asymmetrical eye movements and a change of visual acuity
    c. Weak, hoarse voice
    d. Facial swelling with discoloration and bruising around the eyes

26. A patient is having radiation therapy to the neck and reports a sore throat and difficulty swallowing. Which statement by the nursing student indicates a correct understanding of symptom relief for this patient?
    a. "The patient should not swallow anything too cold or too hot."
    b. "I will give the patient a mouthwash with an alcohol base."
    c. "I will help the patient with a saline gargle."
    d. "The patient should be reassured that the sore throat is temporary."

27. The health care provider orders the discontinuation of the nasogastric tube for a patient with a total laryngectomy. Before discontinuing the tube, which action must be performed?
    a. The health care provider and the nurse will assess the patient's ability to swallow.
    b. Reassure the patient that eating and swallowing will be painless and natural.
    c. The nutritionist will evaluate the patient's nutritional status.
    d. The patient will be offered a prn analgesic or an anxiolytic medication.

28. A patient has had surgery for cancer of the neck. Which behavior indicates that the patient understands how to perform self-care to prevent aspiration?
    a. Chooses thin liquids that cause coughing but knows to take small sips
    b. Eats small frequent meals that include a variety of textures and nutrients
    c. Asks for small frequent sips of nutrition supplement as a bedtime snack
    d. Positions self upright before eating or drinking anything

29. A patient is receiving enteral feedings and a nasogastric tube is in place. In order to prevent aspiration, which precautions are used? **Select all that apply.**
    a. No bolus feedings are given at night.
    b. Hold the feeding if the residual volume exceeds 20 mL.
    c. Vary the time of feedings according to the patient's preference.
    d. Elevate the head of the bed during and after feedings.
    e. Evaluate the patient's tolerance of the feedings.
    f. Allow the patient to indicate when he or she is ready for the next bite.

30. A patient has demonstrated anxiety since a diagnosis of neck cancer. The surgery and radiation therapy are completed. Which behavior indicates that the patient's fears are decreasing?
    a. Repeatedly asks the same questions and seeks to revalidate all information
    b. States that he is less anxious but is irritable and tense whenever questioned
    c. Makes a plan to contact the American Cancer Society Visitor Program
    d. Makes a plan to share personal belongings with friends and family

31. Which are warning signs of head and neck cancer? **Select all that apply.**
    a. Difficulty swallowing
    b. Change in fit of dentures
    c. Intermittent bilateral ear pain
    d. Weight gain
    e. Numbness in the mouth, lips, or face
    f. Lump in mouth, neck, or throat

32. Which symptom suggests the possibility of sinus cancer?
    a. Intermittent nasal obstruction
    b. Little to no nasal drainage
    c. Bloody nasal discharge
    d. Lymph node enlargement on opposite side from tumor

33. The nurse is providing preoperative teaching for a patient who will have a malignant sinus tumor surgically removed. Which **key** teaching point would the nurse be sure to include?
    a. Patients often have changes in the sensations of taste and smell.
    b. Problems with speech rarely occur with this type of surgery.
    c. Often patients gain weight and need dietary consults for weight loss.
    d. After the surgery, you will need to have irrigations with an alcohol-based solution.

34. The nurse is caring for a patient with a nasal fracture. The patient has clear secretions that react positively when tested for glucose. Which complication does the nurse suspect?
    a. Jaw fracture
    b. Facial fracture
    c. Vertebral fracture
    d. Skull fracture

35. The patient with a nasal fracture has clear fluid draining from the nose that dries on a piece of filter paper and leaves a yellow "halo" ring at the dried edge of the fluid. What is the nurse's **first** action?
    a. Document the finding.
    b. Notify the health care provider.
    c. Send a sample to the lab.
    d. Place the patient in a supine position.

36. The nurse is caring for several patients who are at risk because of problems related to the upper airway. Which are the **priority** assessments and actions for these patients?
    a. Thickness of oral secretions; encourage ingestion of oral fluids
    b. Anxiety and pain; provide reassurance and NSAIDs
    c. Adequacy of oxygenation; ensure an unobstructed airway
    d. Evidence of spinal cord injuries; obtain order for x-rays

37. On postoperative assessment, the nurse notes that the patient with a rhinoplasty repeatedly swallows. What is the nurse's **first** action?
    a. Examine the throat for bleeding.
    b. Provide ice chips to ease swallowing.
    c. Notify the health care provider.
    d. Ask if the patient is hungry.

38. Which instructions must the nurse give to a patient after rhinoplasty to prevent bleeding? **Select all that apply.**
    a. Limit or avoid straining during bowel movements (e.g., Valsalva maneuver).
    b. Do not sniff upwards or blow your nose.
    c. Sneeze with your mouth closed for a few days after packing is removed.
    d. Forceful coughing should be done to keep the airways clear.
    e. Avoid aspirin-containing products or NSAIDs.
    f. Use a humidifier to prevent mucosal drying.

39. Which factors contribute to sleep apnea? **Select all that apply.**
    a. Smoking
    b. A short neck
    c. Athletic lifestyle
    d. Small uvula
    e. Enlarged tonsils or adenoids
    f. Underweight for height and gender

40. Which side effects would a patient with obstructive sleep apnea report? **Select all that apply.**
    a. Excessive daytime sleepiness
    b. Excessive daytime hyperactivity
    c. Inability to concentrate
    d. Excessive production of sputum
    e. Irritability
    f. Heavy snoring

41. A patient has been diagnosed with sleep apnea. Which assessment findings indicate that the patient is having complications associated with sleep apnea?
    a. Side effects of hypoxemia, hypercapnia, and sleep deprivation
    b. Decrease in arterial carbon dioxide levels and sleep deprivation
    c. Respiratory alkalosis with retention of carbon dioxide
    d. Irritability, obesity, and enlarged tonsils or adenoids

42. A patient has been diagnosed with airway obstruction during sleep. The nurse will likely include patient education about which device for home use?
    a. Continuous positive airway pressure (CPAP) to deliver a positive airway pressure
    b. Oxygen via face mask to prevent hypoxia
    c. Neck brace to support the head and facilitate breathing
    d. Nebulizer treatments with bronchodilators

43. The patient has a diagnosis of mild sleep apnea. Which interventions will the nurse teach the patient that may correct this condition? **Select all that apply.**
    a. Change sleeping positions.
    b. Use continuous positive airway pressure (CPAP) every night.
    c. Look into a weight loss program.
    d. A position fixing device can prevent tongue subluxation.
    e. You may need surgery to remodel your posterior oropharynx.
    f. A prescription for modafinil may help promote wakefulness during the day.

44. The nurse is assessing a patient who reports being struck in the face and head several times. During the assessment, pink-tinged drainage from the nares is observed. Which nursing action provides relevant assessment data?
    a. Have the patient gently blow the nose and observe for bloody mucus.
    b. Test the drainage with a reagent to check the pH.
    c. Ask the patient to describe the appearance of the face before the incident.
    d. Place a drop of the drainage on a filter paper and look for a yellow ring.

45. While playing football at school, a patient injured his nose, resulting in a possible simple fracture. The patient's parents call the nurse seeking advice. What does the nurse tell the parents to do?
    a. Ask the school nurse to insert a nasal airway to ensure patency.
    b. Apply an ice pack and allow the patient to rest in a supine position.
    c. Seek medical attention within 24 hours to minimize further complications.
    d. Monitor the symptoms for 24 hours and contact the physician if there is bleeding.

46. A patient had a rhinoplasty and is preparing for discharge home. A family member is instructed by the nurse to monitor the patient for postnasal drip by using a flashlight to look in the back of the throat. If bleeding is noted, what does the nurse tell the family member to do?
    a. Place ice packs on the back of the neck and apply pressure to the nose.
    b. Hyperextend the neck and apply pressure and ice packs as needed.
    c. Seek immediate medical attention for the bleeding.
    d. Monitor for 24 hours if the bleeding appears to be a small amount.

47. The nurse is teaching a patient about post-rhinoplasty care. Which patient statement indicates an understanding of the instruction?
    a. "I will have a very large dressing on my nose."
    b. "I will have bruising around my eyes, nose, and face."
    c. "There will be swelling that will cause a loss of sense of smell."
    d. "My nose will be three times its normal size for 3 weeks."

48. An older adult with dehydration has altered mental status and inspissated (thickly crusted) oral and nasopharyngeal secretions. What **priority** instruction would the nurse give to the unlicensed assistive personnel (UAP) when providing care for this patient?
    a. Bathe the patient twice a day.
    b. Provide comprehensive oral care every 2 hours.
    c. Ambulate the patient in the hall every 4 hours.
    d. Check vital signs including temperature every 6 hours.

49. A patient with an active nosebleed (epistaxis) is admitted to the emergency department. Which intervention does the nurse use **first**?
    a. Have the patient sit upright with the head forward.
    b. Insert nasal packing.
    c. Apply direct lateral pressure to the nose.
    d. Place a nasal catheter.

50. After being treated in the emergency department for posterior nosebleed, the patient is admitted to the hospital. The nasal packing is in place and vital signs are stable. The patient has an IV of normal saline at 125 mL/hr. What is the **priority** for nursing care?
    a. Airway management
    b. Managing potential dehydration
    c. Managing potential decreased cardiac output
    d. Monitoring for potential infection

51. A patient is admitted for a posterior nosebleed. Posterior packing is in place and the patient is on oxygen therapy, antibiotics, and opioid analgesics. What is the **priority** assessment?
    a. Tolerance of packing or tubes
    b. Gag and cough reflexes
    c. Mouth breathing
    d. Skin breakdown around the nares

52. Packing has been removed from a patient with epistaxis. Which discharge instructions would the nurse be sure to teach the patient and his family? **Select all that apply.**
    a. Use saline spray to add moisture and prevent rebleeding.
    b. Use lots of petrolatum jelly to coat the inside and outside of the nasal passages for comfort.
    c. Avoid vigorous nose blowing.
    d. Do not take aspirin-containing products or NSAIDs.
    e. No strenuous lifting for at least a month.
    f. Consume only small meals for 2 weeks.

53. A patient returns from surgery following a rhinoplasty. The unlicensed assistive personnel (UAP) places the patient in a supine position to encourage rest and sleep. Which action should the nurse take **first**?
    a. Teach the patient how to use the bed controls to position herself.
    b. Explain the purpose of the semi-Fowler's position to the nursing assistant.
    c. Place the patient in a semi-Fowler's position and assess for aspiration.
    d. Post a notice at the head of the bed to remind personnel about positioning.

54. The nurse is caring for a patient who had a nasoseptoplasty. Which action is the **best** to assign to the licensed practical nurse?
    a. Administer a stool softener to ease bowel movements.
    b. Assess the patient's airway and breathing after general anesthesia.
    c. Evaluate the patient's emotional reaction to the facial edema and bruising.
    d. Take vital signs every 4 hours as ordered by the physician.

55. The nurse is providing postoperative nursing care for a patient with surgical correction of a deviated septum. Which intervention is part of the standard care for this patient?
    a. Apply ice to the nasal area and eyes to decrease swelling and pain.
    b. Encourage deep coughing to prevent atelectasis and clear secretions.
    c. Administer NSAIDs or Tylenol every 4-6 hours for pain relief.
    d. Apply moist heat and humidity to the nasal area for comfort and circulation.

56. A patient arrives in the emergency department with a severe crush injury to the face with blood gurgling from the mouth and nose and obvious respiratory distress. The nurse prepares to assist the physician with which procedure to manage the airway?
    a. Performing a needle thoracotomy
    b. Inserting an endotracheal tube
    c. Performing a tracheotomy
    d. Inserting a nasal airway and giving oxygen

57. A patient with facial trauma has undergone surgical intervention to wire the jaw shut. In performing discharge teaching with this patient, which topics does the nurse cover? **Select all that apply.**
    a. Oral care
    b. Activity
    c. Use of wire cutters
    d. Communication
    e. Aspiration prevention
    f. Dental liquid diet

58. The nurse is assessing a patient with significant and obvious facial trauma after being struck repeatedly in the face. Which finding is the **priority** and requires immediate intervention?
    a. Asymmetry of the mandible
    b. Restlessness with high-pitched respirations
    c. Nonparallel extraocular movements
    d. Pain upon palpation over the nasal bridge

59. A patient has an inner maxillary fixation. The nurse encourages the patient to eat which kind of food?
    a. Milkshakes
    b. Cottage cheese
    c. Tea and toast
    d. Tuna and noodle casserole

60. A patient enters the emergency department after being punched in the throat. What does the nurse monitor for?
    a. Aphonia
    b. Dry cough
    c. Crepitus
    d. Loss of gag reflex

61. A patient has sustained a mandible fracture and the surgeon has explained that the repair will be made using a resorbable plate. The patient discloses to the nurse that he has not told the surgeon about his substance abuse and illicit drug dependence. What is the nurse's **best** response?
    a. "Why didn't you talk to your surgeon about this issue?"
    b. "You should tell the surgeon, but it is your choice."
    c. "It is important for your surgeon to know about this information."
    d. "You shouldn't be ashamed; your surgeon will still repair your fracture."

62. A patient has had an inner maxillary fixation for a mandibular fracture. Which piece of equipment should be kept at the bedside at **all** times?
    a. Waterpik
    b. Wire cutters
    c. Pair of hemostats
    d. Emesis basin

63. A patient who was in a motor vehicle accident and sustained laryngeal trauma is being treated in the emergency department with humidified oxygen and is being monitored every 15-30 minutes for respiratory distress. Which assessment finding indicates the **urgent** need for further intervention?
    a. Respiratory rate 24, Pao_2 80-100, no difficulty with communication
    b. Pulse oximetry 96%, anxious, fatigued, blood in sputum, abdominal breathing
    c. Confused and disoriented, difficulty producing sounds, pulse oximetry 80%
    d. Anxious, respiratory rate 30, talking rapidly about the accident, warm to touch

64. A patient in the emergency department with laryngeal trauma has developed shortness of breath with stridor and decreased oxygen saturation. What is the **priority** action?
    a. Insert an oral or nasal airway.
    b. Assess for tachypnea, anxiety, and nasal flaring.
    c. Obtain the equipment for a tracheostomy.
    d. Apply oxygen and stay with the patient.

65. An older adult patient who is talking and laughing while eating begins to choke on a piece of meat. What is the **initial** emergency management for this patient?
    a. Several sharp blows between the scapulae
    b. Call the Rapid Response Team
    c. Nasotracheal suctioning
    d. Abdominal thrusts (Heimlich maneuver)

66. The patient with laryngeal trauma develops stridor. What is the nurse's **highest** priority intervention?
    a. Apply oxygen by nasal cannula.
    b. Obtain an arterial blood gas sample.
    c. Call the Rapid Response Team (RRT).
    d. Perform a maneuver to open the airway.

30

CHAPTER

Care of Patients with Noninfectious Lower Respiratory Problems

1. What is the **priority** medical-surgical concept for patients with noninfectious lower respiratory problems such as emphysema?
   a. Perfusion
   b. Gas exchange
   c. Cellular regulation
   d. Tissue integrity

2. Which of the following are characteristics of chronic pulmonary emphysema? **Select all that apply.**
   a. Decreased surface area of alveoli
   b. Chronic thickening of bronchial walls
   c. High arterial oxygen level
   d. Hypercapnia
   e. Arterial blood gases (ABGs) show chronic respiratory acidosis
   f. Increased eosinophils

3. Which are characteristics of asthma? **Select all that apply.**
   a. Narrowed airway lumen due to inflammation
   b. Increased eosinophils
   c. Increased secretions
   d. Intermittent bronchospasm
   e. Loss of elastic recoil
   f. Stimulation of disease process by allergies

4. The nurse is caring for an older adult patient with a chronic respiratory disorder. Which interventions are **best** to use in caring for this patient? **Select all that apply.**
   a. Provide rest periods between activities such as bathing, meals, and ambulation.
   b. Place the patient in a supine position after meals to allow for rest.
   c. Schedule drug administration around routine activities to increase adherence to drug therapy.
   d. Arrange chairs in strategic locations to allow the patient to walk and rest.
   e. Teach the patient to avoid getting the pneumococcal vaccine.
   f. Encourage the patient to have an annual flu vaccination.

5. The nurse is caring for an older adult patient with a history of chronic asthma. Which problem related to aging can influence the care and treatment of this patient?
   a. Asthma usually resolves with age, so the condition is less severe in older adult patients.
   b. It is more difficult to teach older adult patients about asthma than to teach younger patients.
   c. With aging, the beta-adrenergic drugs do not work as effectively.
   d. Older adult patients have difficulty manipulating handheld inhalers.

6. A patient with chronic obstructive pulmonary disease (COPD) is likely to have which findings on assessment? **Select all that apply.**
   a. Body odor and unkempt hair
   b. Sitting in a chair leaning forward with elbows on knees
   c. Unintentional weight gain
   d. Decreased appetite
   e. Unexplained weight loss
   f. Crooked fingers

7. The nurse is helping a patient learn about managing her asthma. What does the nurse instruct the patient to do?
   a. Keep a symptom diary to identify what triggers the asthma attacks.
   b. Make an appointment with an allergist for allergy therapy.
   c. Take a low dose of aspirin every day for the anti-inflammatory action.
   d. Drink large amounts of clear fluid to keep mucus thin and watery.

8. The nurse is taking a medical history on a new patient who has come to the office for a checkup. The patient states that he was supposed to take a medication called montelukast, but that he never got the prescription filled. What is the best response by the nurse?
   a. "When were you first diagnosed with a respiratory disorder?"
   b. "Why didn't you get the prescription filled?"
   c. "Tell me how you feel about your decision to not fill the prescription."
   d. "Are you having any problems with your asthma?"

9. The nurse teaches a patient with asthma to perform which intervention before exercising?
   a. Rest for at least an hour.
   b. Use the short-acting beta-adrenergic (SABA) medication.
   c. Dress in extra clothing during cold weather.
   d. Practice pursed-lip breathing.

10. A patient with asthma is repeatedly noncompliant with the medication regimen, which has resulted in the patient being hospitalized for a severe asthma attack. Which interventions does the nurse suggest to help the patient manage asthma on a daily basis? **Select all that apply.**
    a. Encourage active participation in the plan of care.
    b. Help the patient develop a flexible plan of care.
    c. Have the pharmacist establish a plan of care.
    d. Teach the patient about asthma and the treatment plan.
    e. Assess symptom severity using a peak flowmeter 1-2 times per week.
    f. Educate the patient about implementation of his or her personal asthma action plan.

11. A child attending day camp has asthma, and her parent sent with her all of her medicine in a small carry bag. The child has an asthma attack that is severe enough to warrant a rescue drug. Which medication from the child's bag is **best** to use for the acute symptoms?
    a. Omalizumab
    b. Fluticasone
    c. Salmeterol
    d. Albuterol

12. Which are main purposes of asthma treatment? **Select all that apply.**
    a. Prevent asthma episodes.
    b. Avoid secondhand smoke.
    c. Improve airflow.
    d. Relieve symptoms.
    e. Improve exercise tolerance.
    f. Control asthma episodes.

13. A patient admitted for a respiratory workup has baseline pulmonary function tests (PFTs). After treatment with a bronchodilator the forced expiratory volume (FEV_1) increases by 14%. How does the nurse **best** interpret this value?
    a. The patient has emphysema.
    b. The patient has asthma.
    c. The patient has chronic bronchitis.
    d. The patient has acute bronchitis.

14. A patient who is allergic to dogs experiences a sudden "asthma attack." Which assessment finding does the nurse expect for this patient?
    a. Slow, deep, pursed-lip respirations
    b. Breathlessness and difficulty completing sentences
    c. Clubbing of the fingers and cyanosis of the nail beds
    d. Bradycardia and irregular pulse

15. A patient is experiencing an asthma attack and shows an increased respiratory effort. Which arterial blood gas (ABG) value is more associated with the **early** phase of the attack?
    a. $Paco_2$ of 60 mm Hg
    b. $Paco_2$ of 30 mm Hg
    c. pH of 7.40
    d. Pao_2 of 98 mm Hg

16. A patient who has well-controlled asthma has what kind of airway changes?
    a. Chronic, leading to hyperplasia
    b. Temporary and reversible
    c. Acute loss of smooth muscle mass
    d. Permanent and irreversible

17. Which are key elements for a personal asthma action plan? **Select all that apply.**
    a. A schedule for prescribed daily controller drug(s) and directions for prescribed reliever drug
    b. A list of possible triggers for each asthma attack
    c. Patient-specific daily asthma control assessment questions
    d. Directions for adjusting the daily controller drug schedule
    e. Emergency actions to take when asthma is not responding to controller and reliever drugs
    f. When to contact the health care provider (in addition to regularly scheduled visits)

18. What are the goals for drug therapy in the treatment of asthma? **Select all that apply.**
    a. Drugs are used to stop an attack once it has started.
    b. Weekly drugs are used to reduce the asthma response.
    c. Combination drugs are avoided in the treatment of asthma.
    d. Some patients only require drug therapy during an asthma episode.
    e. Drugs are used to change airway responsiveness.
    f. Some drugs are used to decrease inflammation.

19. The nurse is teaching a patient how to interpret peak expiratory flow (PEF) readings and to use this information to manage drug therapy at home. Which statement by the patient indicates a need for additional teaching?
    a. "If the reading is in the green zone, there is no need to increase the drug therapy."
    b. "Red is 50% below my 'personal best.' I should try a rescue drug and seek help."
    c. "If the reading is in the yellow zone, I should increase my use of my inhalers."
    d. "If frequent yellow readings occur, I should see my doctor for a change in medications."

20. A neighbor with asthma is experiencing a severe and prolonged asthma attack that is unresponsive to treatment with a short-acting beta-adrenergic (SAB_2A) drug. What is the nurse's **best** action?
    a. Continue to administer the patient's SAB_2A drug at 5-minute intervals.
    b. Call the patient's health care provider.
    c. Apply the supplemental oxygen that is in the patient's home.
    d. Call 911 and get the patient to emergency care as soon as possible.

21. A patient with a history of asthma enters the emergency department with severe dyspnea, accessory muscle involvement, neck vein distention, and severe inspiratory/expiratory wheezing. The nurse is prepared to assist the physician with which procedure if the patient does not respond to initial interventions?
    a. Emergency intubation
    b. Emergency needle thoracentesis
    c. Emergency chest tube insertion
    d. Emergency pleurodesis

22. A patient presents to the walk-in clinic with extremely labored breathing and a history of asthma that is unresponsive to prescribed inhalers or medications. What is the **first priority** nursing action?
    a. Establish IV access to give emergency medications.
    b. Obtain the equipment and prepare the patient for intubation.
    c. Place the patient in a high Fowler's position, and start oxygen.
    d. Call 911 and report that the patient has probable status asthmaticus.

23. A patient with chronic bronchitis often shows signs of hypoxia. Which clinical manifestation is the **priority** to monitor for in this patient?
    a. Chronic, nonproductive, dry cough
    b. Clubbing of fingers
    c. Large amounts of thick mucus
    d. Barrel chest

24. For a patient who is a nonsmoker, which classic assessment finding is particularly **important** in diagnosing asthma?
    a. Cough
    b. Dyspnea
    c. Audible wheezing
    d. Tachypnea

25. The nurse is taking a history for a patient with chronic pulmonary disease. The patient reports often sleeping in a chair that allows his head to be elevated rather than going to bed. The patient's behavior is a strategy to deal with which condition?
    a. Paroxysmal nocturnal dyspnea
    b. Orthopnea
    c. Tachypnea
    d. Cheyne-Stokes

26. The patient has one gene allele for alpha-1 antitrypsin (AAT) that is faulty and one that is normal. Which statement is true about this patient?
    a. The patient will have an alpha-1 antitrypsin deficiency and is at risk for COPD.
    b. The patient will not be at risk for development of COPD.
    c. The patient will be a carrier for alpha-1 antitrypsin deficiency.
    d. The patient will make enough alpha-1 antitrypsin to avoid COPD even if exposed to smoking.

27. A patient has chronic bronchitis. The nurse plans interventions for inadequate oxygenation based on which set of clinical manifestations?
    a. Chronic cough, thin secretions, and chronic infection
    b. Respiratory alkalosis, decreased $Paco_2$, and increased Pao_2
    c. Areas of chest tenderness and sputum production (often with hemoptysis)
    d. Large amounts of thick secretions and repeated infections

28. A patient has COPD with chronic difficulty breathing. In planning this patient's care, what condition must the nurse acknowledge is present in this patient?
    a. Decreased need for calories and protein requirements since dyspnea causes activity intolerance
    b. COPD has no effect on calorie and protein needs, meal tolerance, satiety, appetite, and weight
    c. Increased metabolism and the need for additional calories and protein supplements
    d. Anabolic state, which creates conditions for building body strength and muscle mass

29. In obtaining a history for a patient with chronic obstructive pulmonary disease, which risk factors are related to potentially causing or triggering the disease process? **Select all that apply.**
    a. Cigarette smoking
    b. Occupational and air pollution
    c. Genetic tendencies
    d. Smokeless tobacco
    e. Occupation
    f. Food or drug allergies

30. Which statement is true about the relationship of smoking cessation to the pathophysiology of chronic obstructive pulmonary disease (COPD)?
    a. Smoking cessation completely reverses the damage to the lungs.
    b. Smoking cessation slows the rate of disease progression.
    c. Smoking cessation is an important therapy for asthma but not for COPD.
    d. Smoking cessation reverses the effects on the airways but not the lungs.

31. A patient has a history of chronic obstructive pulmonary disease (COPD) but is admitted for a surgical procedure that is unrelated to the respiratory system. To prevent any complications related to the patient's COPD, what action does the nurse take?
    a. Assess the patient's respiratory system every 8 hours.
    b. Monitor for signs and symptoms of pneumonia.
    c. Give high-flow oxygen to maintain pulse oximetry readings.
    d. Instruct the patient to use a tissue if coughing or sneezing.

32. The nurse is instructing a patient regarding complications of chronic obstructive pulmonary disease (COPD). Which statement by the patient indicates the need for additional teaching?
    a. "I have to be careful because I am susceptible to respiratory infections."
    b. "I could develop heart failure, which could be fatal if untreated."
    c. "My COPD is serious, but it can be reversed if I follow my doctor's orders."
    d. "The lack of oxygen could cause my heart to beat in an irregular pattern."

33. What is the purpose of pulmonary function testing, especially airflow rates and lung volume measurements, when classifying chronic obstructive pulmonary disease (COPD)?
    a. Determines the oxygen liter flow rates required by the patient
    b. Measures blood gas levels before bronchodilators are administered
    c. Evaluates the movement of oxygenated blood from the lung to the heart
    d. Distinguishes airway disease (obstructive) from interstitial lung disease (restrictive)

34. A patient with respiratory difficulty has completed a pulmonary function test before starting any treatment. The peak expiratory flow (PEF) is 15%-20% below what is expected for this adult patient's age, gender, and size. The nurse anticipates this patient will need additional information about which topic?
    a. Further diagnostic tests to confirm pulmonary hypertension
    b. How to manage asthma medications and identify triggers
    c. Smoking cessation and its relationship to COPD
    d. How to manage the acute episode of respiratory infection

35. Patients with asthma are taught self-care activities and treatment modalities according to the "step method." Which symptoms and medication routines relate to step 3?
    a. Symptoms occur daily; daily use of inhaled corticosteroid and a long-acting beta agonist
    b. Symptoms occur more than once per week; daily use of anti-inflammatory inhaler
    c. Symptoms occur less than once per week; use of rescue inhalers once per week
    d. Frequent exacerbations with limited physical activity; increased use of rescue inhalers

36. What principle guides the nurse when providing oxygen therapy for a patient with chronic obstructive pulmonary disease (COPD)?
    a. The patient depends on a high serum carbon dioxide level to stimulate the drive to breathe.
    b. The patient requires a low serum oxygen level for the stimulus to breathe to work.
    c. The patient who receives oxygen therapy at a high flow rate is at risk for a respiratory arrest.
    d. The patient should receive oxygen therapy at rates to reduce hypoxia and bring SpO2 levels up between 88% and 92%.

37. In assisting a patient with chronic obstructive pulmonary disease (COPD) to relieve dyspnea, which sitting positions are beneficial to the patient for breathing? **Select all that apply.**
    a. On edge of chair, leaning forward with arms folded and resting on a small table
    b. In a low semireclining position with the shoulders back and knees apart
    c. Forward in a chair with feet spread apart and elbows placed on the knees
    d. Head slightly flexed, with feet spread apart and shoulders relaxed
    e. Low semi-Fowler's with knees elevated
    f. Side lying to facilitate diaphragm movement

38. The nurse is developing a teaching plan for a patient with chronic airflow limitation using the priority patient problem of insufficient knowledge related to energy conservation. What does the nurse advise the patient to **avoid**?
    a. Performing activities at a relaxed pace throughout the day with rest periods
    b. Working on activities that require using arms at chest level or lower
    c. Eating three large meals per day
    d. Talking and performing activities separately

39. A patient with chronic obstructive pulmonary disease (COPD) has meal-related dyspnea. To address this issue, which drug does the nurse offer the patient 30 minutes **before** the meal?
    a. Albuterol
    b. Guaifenesin
    c. Fluticasone
    d. Pantoprazole sodium

40. Drugs for the treatment of chronic obstructive pulmonary disease (COPD) are the same as those used for management of asthma. Which additional class of drugs would the nurse expect to administer for a patient with COPD?
    a. Beta-blocker drugs
    b. Corticosteroids
    c. Xanthines
    d. Mucolytics

41. A patient is receiving ipratropium and reports nausea, blurred vision, headache, and inability to sleep. What action does the nurse take?
    a. Administer a prn medication for nausea and a mild prn sedative.
    b. Report these symptoms to the physician as signs of overdose.
    c. Obtain a physician's request for an ipratropium level.
    d. Tell the patient that these side effects are normal and not to worry.

42. A patient with asthma has been prescribed a fluticasone inhaler. What is the purpose of this drug for the patient?
    a. Relaxes the smooth muscles of the airway.
    b. Acts as a bronchodilator in severe episodes.
    c. Reduces obstruction of airways by decreasing inflammation.
    d. Reduces the histamine effect of the triggering agent.

43. What is the advantage of using the aerosol route for administering short-acting beta$_2$ agonists?
   a. Achieves a rapid and effective anti-inflammatory action
   b. Reduces the risk for fungal infections
   c. Increases patient compliance because it is easy to use
   d. Provides rapid therapy with fewer systemic side effects

44. The nurse is teaching a patient with chronic obstructive pulmonary disease (COPD) about his medications. Which statement by the patient indicates the need for additional teaching?
   a. "I will carry my albuterol (Proventil) with me at all times."
   b. "I will use my salmeterol (Serevent) whenever I start to feel short of breath."
   c. "I will check my heart rate before and after my exercise period."
   d. "I will use my ipratropium (Atrovent) 4 times a day."

45. A patient has been prescribed cromolyn sodium for the treatment of asthma. Which statement by the patient indicates a correct understanding of this drug?
   a. "It opens my airways and provides short-term relief."
   b. "It is the medication that should be used 30 minutes before exercise."
   c. "It is not intended for use during acute episodes of asthma attacks."
   d. "It is a steroid medication, so there are severe side effects."

46. After the nurse has instructed a patient with chronic obstructive pulmonary disease (COPD) in the proper coughing technique, which action the next day by the patient indicates the need for additional teaching or intervention?
   a. Coughing upon rising in the morning
   b. Coughing before meals
   c. Coughing after meals
   d. Coughing at bedtime

47. A family member of a patient with chronic obstructive pulmonary disease (COPD) asks the nurse, "What is the purpose of making him cough on a routine basis?" What is the nurse's **best** response?
   a. "We have to check the color and consistency of his sputum."
   b. "We don't want him to feel embarrassed when coughing in public, so we actively encourage it."
   c. "It improves air exchange by increasing airflow in the larger airways."
   d. "If he cannot cough, the physician may elect to do a tracheostomy."

48. A patient with a history of bronchitis for greater than 20 years is hospitalized. With this patient's history, what is a potential complication?
   a. Right-sided heart failure
   b. Left-sided heart failure
   c. Renal disease
   d. Stroke

49. The nurse is caring for a patient with chronic bronchitis and notes the following clinical findings: fatigue, dependent edema, distended neck veins, and cyanotic lips. These assessment findings are consistent with which disease process?
   a. COPD
   b. Cor pulmonale
   c. Asthma
   d. Lung cancer

50. A patient is admitted with asthma. Which assessment findings are **most** likely to indicate that the patient's asthma condition is deteriorating and progressing toward respiratory failure?
   a. Crackles, rhonchi, and productive cough with yellow sputum
   b. Tachypnea, thick and tenacious sputum, and hemoptysis
   c. Audible breath sounds, wheezing, and use of accessory muscles
   d. Respiratory alkalosis; slow, shallow respiratory rate

51. A patient has returned several times to the clinic for treatment of respiratory problems. Which action does the nurse perform **first**?
    a. Obtain a history of the patient's previous respiratory problems and response to therapy.
    b. Ask the patient to describe his compliance to the prescribed therapies.
    c. Obtain a request for diagnostic testing, including a tuberculosis and human immunodeficiency virus (HIV) evaluation.
    d. Listen to the patient's lungs, obtain a pulse oximetry reading, and count the respiratory rate.

52. The nurse assesses a patient and finds a dusky appearance with bluish mucous membranes and production of lots of mucous secretions. What illness does the nurse suspect?
    a. Asthma
    b. Emphysema
    c. Chronic bronchitis
    d. Acute bronchitis

53. The patient with chronic obstructive pulmonary disease (COPD) is undergoing pulmonary rehabilitation by walking. What does the nurse teach this patient about when to **increase** his or her walking time?
    a. "You should increase your walking time when your rest periods decrease."
    b. "You should increase your walking time when your heart rate remains less than 80/minute."
    c. "You should increase your walking time when you are no longer short of breath."
    d. "You should increase your walking time when you do not need to use an inhaler."

54. What is the most serious complication of cystic fibrosis (CF)?
    a. Pancreatic insufficiency
    b. Constant presence of thick, sticky mucus
    c. Intestinal obstruction
    d. Cirrhosis of the liver

55. A patient is undergoing diagnostic testing for possible cystic fibrosis (CF). Which nonpulmonary assessment findings does the nurse expect to observe in a patient with CF? **Select all that apply.**
    a. Peripheral edema
    b. Abdominal distention
    c. Steatorrhea
    d. Constipation
    e. Gastroesophageal reflux
    f. Malnourished appearance

56. The nurse is caring for a patient who has cystic fibrosis (CF). Which assessment findings indicate the need for exacerbation therapy? **Select all that apply.**
    a. New-onset crackles
    b. Increased activity tolerance
    c. Increased frequency of coughing
    d. Increased chest congestion
    e. Increased SaO_2
    f. At least a 10% decrease in FEV_1

57. The patient is receiving high-frequency chest wall oscillation (HFCWO). What are the actions of this therapy? **Select all that apply.**
    a. It dislodges mucus from the bronchial walls.
    b. It increases mobilization of mucus.
    c. It causes bronchodilation of the airways.
    d. It moves mucus upward toward the central airways.
    e. It decreases inflammation within the lung tissues.
    f. It thins secretions, making them easier to clear from the lungs.

58. A patient with cystic fibrosis (CF) is admitted to the medical-surgical unit for an elective surgery. Which infection control measure is **best** for this patient?
    a. It is best to put two patients with CF in the same room.
    b. Standard Precautions including hand-washing are sufficient.
    c. The patient is to be placed on contact isolation.
    d. Measures that limit close contact between people with CF are needed.

59. The nurse is taking a history from a patient with chronic cystic fibrosis (CF). Which symptoms would the nurse expect? **Select all that apply.**
    a. Frequent respiratory infections
    b. Occasional respiratory congestion
    c. Decreased exercise tolerance
    d. Arterial blood gases that show respiratory alkalosis
    e. Increased sputum production
    f. Decreased carbon dioxide levels on ABGs

60. A patient is diagnosed with cor pulmonale secondary to pulmonary hypertension and is receiving an infusion of epoprostenol through a small portable IV pump. What is the **critical priority** for this patient?
    a. Strict aseptic technique must be used to prevent sepsis.
    b. Infusion must not be interrupted, even for a few minutes.
    c. The patient must have a daily dose of warfarin.
    d. The patient must be assessed for angina-like chest pain and fatigue.

61. A patient has developed pulmonary arterial hypertension (PAH). What is the goal of drug therapy for this patient?
    a. Dilate pulmonary vessels and prevent clot formation.
    b. Decrease pain and make the patient comfortable.
    c. Improve or maintain gas exchange.
    d. Maintain and manage pulmonary exacerbation.

62. Which are the most common early symptoms of pulmonary arterial hypertension (PAH)?
    a. Shortness of breath and dizziness
    b. Hypotension and headache
    c. Dyspnea and fatigue
    d. Chest pain and orthopnea

63. A patient with pulmonary arterial hypertension (PAH) is prescribed bosentan. For which side effect must the nurse monitor?
    a. Bradycardia
    b. Increased risk for blood clotting
    c. Decreased urine output
    d. Hypotension

64. Which drugs are essential for slowing the progression of the disease in a patient with pulmonary fibrosis?
    a. Immunosuppressants
    b. Opioids
    c. Antibiotics
    d. Bronchodilators

65. The patient is diagnosed with early pulmonary fibrosis. Which finding indicates that the patient's disease is progressing?
    a. The patient is short of breath with exertion.
    b. The patient is becoming increasingly more short of breath.
    c. The patient is experiencing respiratory infections.
    d. The patient is experiencing side effects from his or her drugs.

66. The nurse is providing discharge instructions to a patient with pulmonary fibrosis and the patient's family. What instructions are appropriate for this patient? **Select all that apply.**
    a. Using home oxygen
    b. Maintaining activity level as before
    c. Preventing respiratory infections
    d. Limiting fluid intake
    e. Energy conservation measures
    f. Encouraging patient to complete all ADLs

67. A patient had prolonged occupational exposure to petroleum distillates and subsequently developed a chronic lung disease. This patient is advised to seek frequent health examinations because there is a **high** risk for developing which respiratory disease condition?
    a. Tuberculosis
    b. Cystic fibrosis
    c. Lung cancer
    d. Pulmonary hypertension

68. The nurse has completed a community presentation about lung cancer. Which statement from a participant demonstrates an understanding of the information presented?
    a. "The primary prevention for reducing the risk of lung cancer is to stop smoking and avoid secondhand smoke."
    b. "The overall 5-year survival rate for all patients with lung cancer is 85%."
    c. "The death rate for lung cancer is less than prostate, breast, and colon cancer combined."
    d. "Cures are most likely for patients who undergo treatment for stage III disease."

69. Which sites are commonly affected by lung cancer metastasis? **Select all that apply.**
    a. Heart
    b. Bone
    c. Liver
    d. Colon
    e. Brain
    f. Adrenal glands

70. Which of the following may be warning signs of lung cancer? **Select all that apply.**
    a. Dyspnea
    b. Dark yellow-colored sputum
    c. Persistent cough or change in cough
    d. Abdominal pain and frequent stools
    e. Use of accessory muscles for breathing
    f. Labored or painful breathing

71. Which statement is true about radiation therapy for lung cancer patients?
    a. It is given daily in "cycles" over the course of several months.
    b. It causes hair loss, nausea, and vomiting for the duration of treatment.
    c. It causes dry skin at the radiation site, fatigue, and changes in appetite with nausea.
    d. It is the best method of treatment for systemic metastatic disease.

72. The nurse is taking a report on a patient who had a pneumonectomy 4 days ago. Which question is the **best** to ask during the shift report?
    a. "Does the physician want us to continue encouraging use of the spirometer?"
    b. "How much drainage did you see in the Pleur-evac during your shift?"
    c. "Do we have a request to 'milk' the patient's chest tube?"
    d. "Does the surgeon want the patient placed on the operative or nonoperative side?"

73. A patient is fearful that she might develop lung cancer because her father and grandfather died of cancer. She seeks advice about how to modify lifestyle factors that contribute to cancer. How does the nurse advise this patient?
    a. Not to worry about air pollution unless there is hydrocarbon exposure
    b. Quit her job if she has continuous exposure to lead or other heavy metals
    c. Avoid situations where she would be exposed to "secondhand" smoke
    d. Not to be concerned because there are no genetic factors associated with lung cancer

74. A patient is receiving a chemotherapy agent for lung cancer. The nurse anticipates that the patient is likely to have which common side effect?
    a. Diarrhea
    b. Nausea
    c. Flatulence
    d. Constipation

75. A patient is having pain resulting from bone metastases caused by lung cancer. What is the **most** effective intervention for relieving the patient's pain?
    a. Support the patient through chemotherapy.
    b. Handle and move the patient very gently.
    c. Administer analgesics around the clock.
    d. Reposition the patient, and use distraction.

76. Which intervention promotes comfort in dyspnea management for a patient with lung cancer?
   a. Administer morphine only when the patient requests it.
   b. Place the patient in a supine position with a pillow under the knees and legs.
   c. Encourage coughing and deep-breathing and independent ambulation.
   d. Provide supplemental oxygen via cannula or mask.

77. The nurse is caring for a patient with a chest tube. What is the correct nursing intervention for this patient?
   a. The patient is encouraged to cough and do deep-breathing exercises frequently.
   b. "Stripping" of the chest tubes is done routinely to prevent obstruction by blood clots.
   c. Water level in the suction chamber need not be monitored, just the collection chamber.
   d. Drainage containers are positioned upright or on the bed next to the patient.

78. Upon observation of a chest tube setup, the nurse reports to the physician that there is a leak in the chest tube and system. How has the nurse identified this problem?
   a. Drainage in the collection chamber has decreased.
   b. The bubbling in the suction chamber has suddenly increased.
   c. Fluctuation in the water seal chamber has stopped.
   d. There was onset of continuous vigorous bubbling in the water seal chamber.

79. The physician's prescriptions indicate an increase in the suction to –20 cm for a patient with a chest tube. To implement this, the nurse performs which intervention?
   a. Increases the wall suction to the medium setting and observes gentle bubbling in the suction chamber
   b. Adds water to the suction and drainage chambers to the level of –20 cm
   c. Stops the suction, adds sterile water to the level of –20 cm in the water seal chamber, and resumes the wall suction
   d. Has the patient cough and deep-breathe and monitors the level of fluctuation to achieve –20 cm

80. A patient has a chest tube in place. What does the water in the water seal chamber do when the system is functioning correctly?
   a. Bubbles vigorously and continuously
   b. Bubbles gently and continuously
   c. Fluctuates with the patient's respirations
   d. Stops fluctuation, and bubbling is not observed

81. The nurse is caring for a patient with a chest tube in place. Over the past hour the drainage from the tube was 110 mL. What is the nurse's **best** action?
   a. Gently "milk" the tubing to remove clots.
   b. Check the chest tube system for leaks.
   c. Instruct the patient to cough and deep-breathe.
   d. Notify the surgeon immediately.

82. The nurse is working for a manufacturing company and is responsible for routine employee health issues. Which primary prevention is most important for those employees at **high** risk for occupational pulmonary disease?
   a. Screen all employees by use of chest x-ray films twice a year.
   b. Advise employees not to smoke and to use masks and ventilation equipment.
   c. Perform pulmonary function tests once a year on all employees.
   d. Refer at-risk employees to a social worker for information about pensions.

31 CHAPTER

Care of Patients with Infectious Respiratory Problems

1. Which patient is at most risk for development of rhinosinusitis?
   a. Patient with a deviated nasal septum
   b. Patient with an ear infection
   c. Patient with an infected heart valve
   d. Patient with a cellulitis

2. Which prescribed drug order for an older adult diagnosed with rhinosinusitis would the nurse clarify with the health care provider?
   a. Acetaminophen
   b. Diphenhydramine
   c. Montelukast
   d. Cromolyn sodium

3. Which signs and symptoms suggest that a patient's rhinosinusitis is bacterial? **Select all that apply.**
   a. Facial trauma
   b. Purulent drainage
   c. Headache
   d. Fever
   e. Drop in blood pressure
   f. No response to decongestants

4. Which statement by a patient indicates correct understanding of drug therapy for rhinosinusitis?
   a. "A side effect of my antihistamine drug can be increased itching."
   b. "When I am feeling better I can stop taking my antibiotics."
   c. "I will take two acetaminophen tablets every 4 hours to prevent fever."
   d. "My decongestant will decrease the swelling so I can breathe better."

5. An adult patient is diagnosed with rhinosinusitis. What does the nurse instruct the patient to do? **Select all that apply.**
   a. Get plenty of rest, at least 8-10 hours per day.
   b. Keep fluid intake between 1000 and 1200 mL per day.
   c. Use a humidifier to help relieve congestion.
   d. Use nasal saline irrigation to safely relieve symptoms.
   e. Try sleeping with the head of your bed flat for better drainage.
   f. Limit exposure to any allergic causes.

6. Drug therapy with **first-generation** antihistamines to treat sinusitis is used with caution in the older adult because of which possible side effects? **Select all that apply.**
   a. Reduced clearance
   b. Hypotension
   c. Confusion
   d. Dry mouth
   e. Constipation
   f. Decreased risk of confusion

7. A patient comes to the walk-in clinic reporting seasonal nasal congestion, sneezing, rhinorrhea, and itchy, watery eyes. The nurse identifies that the patient most likely has rhinosinusitis and should also be assessed for sinusitis. Which manifestations does the nurse assess in a patient with rhinosinusitis? **Select all that apply.**
   a. Pain over the cheek radiating to the teeth
   b. Tenderness to percussion over the sinuses
   c. Generalized musculoskeletal achiness
   d. General facial pain when bending forward
   e. Referred pain to the temple or back of the head
   f. Generalized swelling of the face and neck

8. To reduce the spread of colds, which points must the nurse include when teaching patients? **Select all that apply.**
   a. Stay home from work, school, or other places where people gather.
   b. Seek medical attention at the first sign of an oncoming cold.
   c. Cover both mouth and nose when coughing or sneezing.
   d. Dispose of used tissues properly.
   e. Thorough handwashing is essential.
   f. Avoid crowds of people.

9. A patient reports throat soreness and swelling, purulent nasal drainage, postnasal drip, fever, dental pain, and ear pressure. Which disorder does the nurse suspect?
   a. Bacterial rhinosinusitis
   b. Tonsillitis
   c. Viral rhinosinusitis
   d. Pneumonia

10. For which complications does the nurse monitor when a patient is diagnosed with rhinosinusitis? **Select all that apply.**
    a. Pneumonia
    b. Meningitis
    c. Abscess
    d. Tuberculosis
    e. Cellulitis
    f. Tonsillitis

11. Which factors can contribute to acute rhinosinusitis? **Select all that apply.**
    a. Viruses
    b. Coughing
    c. Irritants
    d. Bacteria
    e. Facial trauma
    f. Antibiotic therapy

12. A patient reporting a "sore throat" also has a temperature of 101.4°F (38.5°C), pus behind the tonsils, and swollen lymph nodes. This patient will **most** likely be treated for which type of bacterial infection?
    a. Staphylococcus
    b. Pneumococcus
    c. Streptococcus
    d. Epstein-Barr virus

13. Which patients are at risk for developing health care–acquired pneumonia? **Select all that apply.**
    a. Confused patient
    b. Patient with atrial fibrillation who is alert and oriented
    c. Patient with Gram-negative colonization of the mouth
    d. Patient with hyperthyroid disease
    e. Malnourished patient
    f. Patient with influenza

14. The nurse is teaching the patient and family about care of a peritonsillar abscess at home. For what symptoms does the nurse indicate the need for the patient to go to the emergency department (ED) **immediately**? **Select all that apply.**
    a. Persistent cough
    b. Hoarseness
    c. Stridor
    d. Drooling
    e. Nausea and vomiting
    f. Fever

15. A 35-year-old male patient with no health problems states that he had a flu shot last year and asks if it is necessary to have it again this year. What is the **best** response by the nurse?
    a. "No, because once you get a flu shot, it lasts for several years and is effective against many different viruses."
    b. "Yes, because the immunity against the virus wears off, increasing your chances of getting the flu."
    c. "Yes, because the vaccine guards against a specific virus and reduces your chances of acquiring flu and is only effective for one year."
    d. "No, flu shots are only for high-risk patients and you are not considered to be high risk."

16. An active 55-year-old schoolteacher with chronic obstructive pulmonary disease (COPD) taking prednisone asks if it is necessary to get a flu shot. What is the **best** response by the nurse?
    a. "Yes, flu shots are highly recommended for patients with chronic illness and/or patients who are receiving immunotherapy."
    b. "No, flu shots are only recommended for patients 60 years old and older."
    c. "Yes, it will help minimize the risk of triggering an exacerbation of COPD."
    d. "No, patients who are active, not living in a nursing home, and not health care providers do not need a flu shot."

17. A patient with rapid onset of severe headache, muscle aches, fever, chills, fatigue, and weakness comes to the emergent care unit. On further assessment, he tells the nurse that additional symptoms include sore throat and sneezing cough. What instructions should be given to the patient for his cough? **Select all that apply.**
    a. "Be sure to wash your hands carefully whenever you cough or sneeze."
    b. "Don't try to stop your sneezing because it will get worse."
    c. "Cover your mouth with a tissue whenever you cough or sneeze."
    d. "Be sure to perform oral hygiene at least four times every day."
    e. "If you don't have a tissue, cough into your upper sleeve, not your hand."
    f. "Be sure to dispose of used tissues immediately."

18. The nurse is giving discharge instructions to a patient diagnosed with a viral influenza. Which statement by the patient indicates the need for further teaching?
    a. "I should try to rest, increase my fluid intake, and get a humidifier for the house."
    b. "I will wait for my test results; then I can get a prescription for antibiotics."
    c. "Over-the-counter analgesics, like Tylenol or ibuprofen, can be used for pain."
    d. "I should gargle several times a day with warm salt water and use throat lozenges."

19. A patient with COPD needs instruction in measures to prevent pneumonia. What information does the nurse include? **Select all that apply.**
    a. Avoid going outside.
    b. Clean all respiratory equipment you have at home.
    c. Avoid indoor pollutants such as dust and aerosols.
    d. Get plenty of rest and sleep daily.
    e. Limit alcoholic beverages to 4-5 per week.
    f. Be sure to get the pneumonia vaccinations.

20. A patient who presents with symptoms of influenza that started 24 hours ago is seen by the health care provider. Which intervention does the nurse expect for this patient?
    a. Prescription for antibiotics
    b. Admission to an acute care facility
    c. An order for an antiviral agent such as oseltamivir
    d. Instructions to rest and decrease fluid intake

21. A patient with a history of frequent and recurrent episodes of tonsillitis now reports a severe sore throat with pain that radiates behind the ear and difficulty swallowing. The nurse suspects the patient may have a peritonsillar abscess. On physical assessment, which deviated structure supports the nurse's supposition?
    a. Uvula
    b. Trachea
    c. Tongue
    d. Mucous membranes

22. A parent calls the emergency department (ED) about her child who reports a severe sore throat and refuses to drink fluids or to take liquid pain medication. What is the **most** important question for the nurse to ask in order to determine the urgency of seeking immediate medical attention?
    a. "Does the child seem to be refusing fluids and medications because of the sore throat?"
    b. "Is the child drooling or do you hear stridor, a raspy rough sound when the child breathes?"
    c. "When did the symptoms start and how long have you been encouraging fluids?"
    d. "Is the throat red or do you see any white patches in the back of the throat?"

23. In a long-term care facility caring for older adults and those who are immunocompromised, one employee and several patients have been diagnosed with influenza (flu). What does the supervising nurse do to decrease risk of infection to other patients?
    a. Ask employees who have flu to stay at home for at least 24 hours.
    b. Place any patient with a sore throat, cough, or rhinorrhea into isolation for 1-2 weeks.
    c. Ask employees with flu symptoms to stay at home for up to 5 days after onset of symptoms.
    d. Recommend that all patients and employees be immediately vaccinated for flu.

24. Which are examples of a pandemic influenza? **Select all that apply.**
    a. H1N1 "swine flu"
    b. Seasonal flu
    c. Spanish influenza
    d. H5N1 "bird flu"
    e. Viral influenza
    f. H7N9 "avian flu"

25. A cluster of H5N1 bird influenza cases occurs. Which intervention is **most** appropriate for this outbreak of flu?
    a. Administer two Vepacel injections 28 days apart.
    b. Avoid the use of antiviral drugs such as zanamivir.
    c. Give oral antibiotics as directed by the health care provider.
    d. Restrict fluids for all infected individuals.

26. Which statements about Middle East respiratory syndrome (MERS) are accurate? **Select all that apply.**
    a. MERS is caused by a virus that causes many respiratory illnesses including the common cold.
    b. The patient with MERS displays only respiratory symptoms such as cough and shortness of breath.
    c. Diagnostic tests for MERS include blood, urine, and sputum for culture and sensitivity.
    d. Interventions for MERS can include IV fluids, mechanical ventilation, and dialysis.
    e. A patient being treated for MERS should be maintained on airborne, contact, and reverse isolation.
    f. "Convalescent serum" may be given if the patient and convalescent person are the same blood type.

27. Which patient is at **highest** risk for developing health care–acquired (HCA) pneumonia?
    a. Any hospitalized patient between the ages 18 and 65 years
    b. 32-year-old trauma patient on a mechanical ventilator
    c. Disabled 54-year-old with osteoporosis, discharged to home
    d. Any patient who has not received the vaccine for pneumonia

28. Which statement **best** describes pneumonia?
    a. An infection of just the "windpipe" because the lungs are "clear" of any problems
    b. A serious inflammation of the bronchioles, alveoli, and interstitial spaces from various causes
    c. Only an infection of the lungs with mild to severe effects on breathing
    d. An inflammation resulting from lung damage caused by long-term smoking

29. A patient is seen in the health care provider's office and is diagnosed with community-acquired pneumonia (CAP). What are the **most** common symptoms associated with CAP? **Select all that apply.**
    a. Dyspnea
    b. Abdominal pain
    c. Back pain
    d. Chest discomfort
    e. Increased sputum production
    f. Fever

30. Which diagnostic tests are most likely to be done for an older patient suspected of having pneumonia? **Select all that apply.**
    a. Sputum Gram stain
    b. Pulmonary function test
    c. Fluorescein bronchoscopy
    d. Peak flowmeter measurement
    e. Chest x-ray
    f. Complete blood count (CBC)

31. The nurse is reviewing laboratory results for a patient who has pneumonia. Which laboratory value does the nurse expect to see for this patient?
    a. Decreased hemoglobin
    b. Increased red blood cells (RBCs)
    c. Decreased neutrophils
    d. Increased white blood cells (WBCs)

32. A patient is diagnosed with pneumonia. During auscultation of the lower lung fields, the nurse hears coarse crackles and identifies the patient problem of impaired oxygenation. What is the underlying physiologic condition associated with the patient's condition?
    a. Hypoxemia
    b. Hyperemia
    c. Hypocapnia
    d. Hypercapnia

33. Which patient is the **least** likely to be at risk for developing pneumonia?
    a. Patient with a 5-year history of smoking
    b. Renal transplant patient
    c. Postoperative patient with a bedside commode
    d. Postoperative patient with a hip replacement

34. A patient is admitted to the hospital with pneumonia. What does the nurse expect the chest x-ray results to reveal?
    a. Patchy areas of increased density
    b. Tension pneumothorax
    c. Thick secretions causing airway obstruction
    d. Large hyperinflated airways

35. What nursing intervention may help to prevent the complication of pneumonia for a surgical patient?
    a. Monitoring chest x-rays and WBC counts for early signs of infection
    b. Monitoring lung sounds every shift and encouraging fluids
    c. Teaching coughing, deep-breathing exercises, and use of incentive spirometry
    d. Encouraging hand hygiene among all caregivers, patients, and visitors

36. The nurse is conducting an in-service for the hospital staff about practices that help prevent pneumonia among at-risk patients. Which nursing intervention is encouraged as standard practice?
    a. Administering vaccines to patients at risk
    b. Implementing isolation for debilitated patients
    c. Restricting foods from home in immuno-suppressed patients
    d. Decontaminating respiratory therapy equipment weekly

37. A patient hospitalized for pneumonia has ineffective airway clearance related to fatigue, chest pain, excessive secretions, and muscle weakness. What nursing intervention helps to correct this problem?
    a. Administer oxygen to prevent hypoxemia and atelectasis.
    b. Push fluids to greater than 3000 mL/day to ensure adequate hydration.
    c. Administer bronchodilator therapy in a timely manner to decrease broncho-spasms.
    d. Maintain semi-Fowler's position to facilitate breathing and prevent further fatigue.

38. A patient is admitted to the hospital for treatment of pneumonia. Which nursing assessment finding **best** indicates that the patient is responding to antibiotics?
    a. Wheezing, oxygen at 2 L/min, respiratory rate 26, no shortness of breath or chills
    b. Temperature 99°F, lung sounds clear, pulse oximetry on 2 L/min at 98%, cough with yellow sputum
    c. Cough, clear sputum, temperature 99°F, pulse oximetry at 96% on room air
    d. Feeling tired, respiratory rate 28 on 2 L/min of oxygen, audible breath sounds

39. The nurse is reviewing the laboratory results for an older adult patient with pneumonia. Which laboratory value frequently seen in patients with pneumonia may **not** be seen in this patient?
    a. RBC 4.0-5.0
    b. Hgb 12-16 gm/dL
    c. Hct 36%-48%
    d. WBC 12,000-18,000 cells/µL

40. Which condition **increases** the risk for a patient to develop community-acquired pneumonia (CAP)?
    a. Patient has received the pneumococcal vaccination.
    b. Patient uses tobacco and alcohol often and regularly.
    c. Patient lives alone and eats alone.
    d. Patient received influenza shot in November rather than September.

41. A critical concern for a patient returning to the unit after a surgical procedure is related to impaired oxygenation caused by inadequate ventilation. Which arterial blood gas value and assessment finding indicates to the nurse that oxygen and incentive spirometry must be administered?
    a. Pao_2 is 89 mm Hg with crackles.
    b. Pao_2 is 90 mm Hg with wheezing.
    c. Pco_2 is 38 mm Hg with clear lung sounds.
    d. Pco_2 is 45 mm Hg with atelectasis.

42. The nurse has identified the problem of ineffective airway clearance with bronchospasms for a patient with pneumonia. The patient has no previous history of chronic respiratory disorders. The nurse obtains an order for which nursing intervention?
    a. Increased liters of humidified oxygen via face mask
    b. Scheduled and prn (as needed) aerosol nebulizer bronchodilator treatments
    c. Handheld bronchodilator inhaler as needed
    d. Corticosteroid via inhaler or IV to reduce the inflammation

43. An older adult patient asks the nurse how often one should receive the pneumococcal vaccine for pneumonia prevention. What is the nurse's **best** response?
    a. Every year, when the patient is receiving the "flu shot."
    b. The standard is vaccination every 3 years.
    c. It is usually given once 6-12 months after the Prevnar 13 vaccine.
    d. There is no set schedule; it depends on the patient's history and risk factors.

44. The nurse is providing discharge instructions about pneumonia to a patient and family. Which discharge information must the nurse be sure to include?
    a. Complete antibiotics as prescribed, rest, drink fluids, and minimize contact with crowds.
    b. Take all antibiotics as ordered, resume diet and all activities as before hospitalization.
    c. No restrictions regarding activities, diet, and rest because the patient is fully recovered when discharged.
    d. Continue antibiotics only until no further signs of pneumonia are present; avoid exposing immunosuppressed individuals.

45. A patient is admitted to the hospital with cough, purulent sputum production, temperature of 37.9°C (100.3°F), and reports of shortness of breath. Which intervention does the nurse provide **first**?
    a. Set up oxygen equipment and administer oxygen.
    b. Instruct the patient about the importance of keeping the oxygen delivery device on.
    c. Monitor the effectiveness of oxygen therapy (pulse oximetry, ABGs) as appropriate.
    d. Monitor the patient's anxiety related to the need for oxygen delivery.

46. A patient treated for pneumonia is being prepared for discharge by the nurse. The patient is capable of performing self-care and is anxious to return to his job at the construction site. Which discharge instructions does the nurse give to this patient?
    a. "You are not contagious to others, so you can return to work as soon as you like."
    b. "You will continue to feel tired and will fatigue easily for the next several weeks."
    c. "Try to drink 4 quarts of water per day, especially if you are very physically active."
    d. "You should be able to return to work full-time in 2 weeks when your energy returns."

47. A patient being treated for pneumonia reports pain that increases on inspiration. The nurse suspects which complication has occurred?
    a. Pleuritic chest pain
    b. Pulmonary emboli
    c. Pleural effusion
    d. Meningitis

48. Which conditions may cause patients to be at risk for aspiration pneumonia? **Select all that apply.**
    a. Continuous tube feedings
    b. Bronchoscopy procedure
    c. Magnetic resonance imaging (MRI) procedure
    d. Decreased level of consciousness
    e. Stroke
    f. Chest tube

49. An older adult patient often coughs and chokes while eating or trying to take medication. The patient insists that he is okay, but the nurse identifies the priority patient problem of risk for aspiration. Which nursing interventions are used to prevent aspiration pneumonia? **Select all that apply.**
    a. Head of bed should always be elevated during feeding.
    b. Monitor the patient's ability to swallow small bites.
    c. Give thin liquids to drink in small, frequent amounts.
    d. Consult a nutritionist and obtain swallowing studies.
    e. Monitor the patient's ability to swallow saliva.
    f. Place the patient on NPO (nothing by mouth) status until swallowing is normal.

50. Which condition causes a patient to have the **greatest** risk for ventilator-associated pneumonia?
    a. History of alcohol use
    b. Presence of feeding tube
    c. Weight loss
    d. IV therapy with normal saline

51. In the event of a new severe acute respiratory syndrome (SARS) outbreak, what is the nurse's **primary** role?
    a. Immediately report new cases of SARS to the Centers for Disease Control and Prevention (CDC).
    b. Administer oxygen, standard antibiotics, and supportive therapies to patients.
    c. Prevent the spread of infection to other employees and patients.
    d. Initiate and strictly enforce contact isolation procedures.

52. The nurse is preparing a community information packet about "bird flu." What information does the nurse include in the packet? **Select all that apply.**
    a. In the event of an outbreak, do not eat any cooked or uncooked poultry products.
    b. Prepare a minimum of 2 weeks' supply of food, water, and routine prescription drugs.
    c. Listen to public health announcements and early warning signs for disease outbreaks.
    d. Avoid traveling to areas where there has been a suspected outbreak of disease.
    e. Obtain a supply of antiviral drugs such as oseltamivir.
    f. In the event of an outbreak, avoid going to public areas such as churches or schools.

53. A patient reports experiencing mild fatigue and a dry, harsh cough. There is a possibility of exposure to inhalation anthrax 3-4 days ago, but the patient currently reports feeling much better. What does the nurse advise the patient to do?
    a. Have a complete blood count to rule out the disease.
    b. Monitor for and immediately seek attention for respiratory symptoms.
    c. Consult a health care provider for diagnostic testing and antibiotic therapy.
    d. Stay at home, rest, increase fluid intake, and avoid public places.

54. A patient with human immunodeficiency virus (HIV) is admitted to the hospital with a temperature of 99.6°F (37.5°C) and reports of bloody sputum, night sweats, feeling of tiredness, and shortness of breath. What are these assessment findings consistent with?
    a. *Pneumocystis jiroveci* pneumonia (PJP)
    b. Tuberculosis
    c. Superinfection as a result of a low CD4 count
    d. Severe bronchitis

55. Which statements about the precautions of caring for a hospitalized patient with tuberculosis (TB) are true? **Select all that apply.**
    a. Health care workers must wear a mask that covers the face and mouth.
    b. Negative airflow rooms are required for these patients.
    c. Health care workers must wear an N95 or high-efficiency particulate air (HEPA) mask.
    d. Gown and gloves are included in appropriate barrier protection.
    e. Strict contact precautions must be maintained.
    f. Careful handwashing is required before and after providing patient care.

56. Which people are at **greatest** risk for developing tuberculosis (TB) in the United States? **Select all that apply.**
    a. An alcoholic homeless man who occasionally stays in a shelter
    b. A college student sharing a room in a dormitory
    c. A person with immune dysfunction or HIV
    d. A homemaker who does volunteer work at a homeless shelter
    e. Immigrants (especially those from the Philippines and Mexico)
    f. An adult living in a crowded area such as a long-term-care facility

57. After several weeks of "not feeling well," a patient is seen in the health care provider's office for possible tuberculosis (TB). If TB is present, which assessment findings does the nurse expect to observe? **Select all that apply.**
    a. Fatigue
    b. Weight gain
    c. Night sweats
    d. Chest soreness
    e. Low-grade fever
    f. Shortness of breath

58. Which test is the **most** accurate and rapid test for tuberculosis (TB)?
    a. Chest x-ray
    b. Nucleic acid amplification test (NAAT)
    c. Tuberculin test (Mantoux test)
    d. Sputum cultures

59. After receiving the subcutaneous Mantoux skin test, a patient with no risk factors returns to the clinic in the required 48-72 hours for the test results. Which assessment finding indicates a positive result?
    a. Test area is red, warm, and tender to touch.
    b. There is induration or a hard nodule of any size at the site.
    c. Induration/hardened area measures 5 mm or greater.
    d. Induration/hardened area measures 10 mm or greater.

60. A patient has a positive skin test result for tuberculosis (TB). What explanation does the nurse give to the patient?
    a. "There is active disease, but you are not yet infectious to others."
    b. "There is active disease, and you need immediate treatment."
    c. "You have been infected, but this does not mean active disease is present."
    d. "A repeat skin test is necessary because the test could give a false-positive result."

61. A patient has been compliant with drug therapy for tuberculosis (TB) and has returned as instructed for follow-up. Which result indicates that the patient is **no longer** infectious/communicable?
    a. Negative chest x-ray
    b. No clinical symptoms
    c. Negative skin test
    d. Three negative sputum cultures

62. A patient diagnosed with tuberculosis (TB) agrees to take the medication as instructed and to complete the therapy. When does the nurse tell the patient is the **best** time to take the medication?
    a. Before breakfast
    b. After breakfast
    c. Midday
    d. Bedtime

63. A patient has active tuberculosis (TB). Which drugs will the health care provider order during the **initial** phase of treatment? **Select all that apply.**
    a. Bedaquiline fumarate
    b. Isoniazid
    c. Rifampin
    d. Bacille Calmette-Guérin
    e. Ethambutol
    f. Pyrazinamide

64. A patient diagnosed with tuberculosis (TB) has been receiving treatment for 3 months and has clinically shown improvement. The family asks the nurse if the patient is still infectious. What is the nurse's **best** reply?
    a. "The patient is still infectious until the entire treatment is completed."
    b. "The patient is likely not infectious but needs to continue treatment for at least 6 months."
    c. "The patient is infectious until there is a negative chest x-ray."
    d. "The patient may or may not be infectious; a purified protein derivative test (PPD) must be done."

65. The female patient is receiving isoniazid (INH) to treat tuberculosis (TB). Which teaching points are essential for the nurse to review with the patient? **Select all that apply.**
    a. Do not take medications such as Maalox with this medication.
    b. Avoid drinking alcoholic beverages.
    c. The urine will be orange in color.
    d. Take a multivitamin with B complex.
    e. If going out in the sun, be sure to wear protective clothing and sunscreen.
    f. This drug reduces the effectiveness of oral contraceptives.

66. A patient with suspected tuberculosis (TB) is admitted to the hospital. Along with a private room, which nursing intervention is appropriate **related to** isolation procedures?
    a. Airborne and contact isolation for sputum only
    b. Strict airborne precautions and use of specially fitted respirator face masks
    c. Airborne isolation with surgical masks until diagnosis is confirmed
    d. Only standard precautions are necessary until the diagnosis is confirmed

67. A patient is admitted to the hospital with a diagnosis of tuberculosis (TB). While providing medication teaching, the patient asks the nurse why she must give the drugs by directly observed therapy (DOT). What is the nurse's **best** response?
    a. "DOT can be done by having any person other than the patient observe that the drugs are swallowed."
    b. "DOT is to assure that the drug regimen is followed and drug-resistant TB organisms do not occur."
    c. "DOT was developed because too many patients do not take their drug as prescribed."
    d. "DOT is used only with homeless people who cannot be trusted to take the drugs as prescribed."

68. After being discharged from the hospital, a patient is diagnosed with tuberculosis (TB) at the outpatient clinic. What is the correct procedure regarding public health policy in this case?
    a. Contact the infection control nurse at the hospital because the hospital is responsible for follow-up of this case.
    b. There are no regulations because the patient was diagnosed at the clinic and not during hospitalization.
    c. Contact the public health nurse so that all individuals who have come in contact with the patient can be screened.
    d. Have the patient sign a waiver regarding the hospital and clinic's liability for treatment.

69. Patients who are at high risk for tuberculosis (TB) would be asked which questions upon assessment? **Select all that apply.**
    a. "What does your diet normally consist of?"
    b. "Do you have an immune dysfunction or HIV?"
    c. "Do you use alcohol or inject recreational drugs?"
    d. "Where do you live in the United States?"
    e. "Do you work in a crowded area such as a prison or mental health facility?"
    f. "Have you ever had a bacille Calmette-Guérin (BCG) vaccine?"

70. The nurse is making home visits to an older adult recovering from a hip fracture and identifies the problem of risk for respiratory infection. Which condition represents a factor of normal aging that would contribute to this **increased** risk?
    a. Inability to force a cough
    b. Decreased strength of respiratory muscles
    c. Increased elastic recoil of alveoli
    d. Increased macrophages in alveoli

71. A 30-year-old is admitted with severe coughing "fits" lasting several minutes. He tells you that he developed cold symptoms a little over a week ago. Which **priority** question would the nurse ask him?
    a. "Has your health care provider prescribed antibiotics for your symptoms?"
    b. "On average, how often do you experience cold symptoms each winter?"
    c. "Did you receive the usual childhood immunization when you were a child?"
    d. "Do you smoke or did you ever smoke or use any tobacco products?"

72. A 42-year-old patient is admitted with a diagnosis of coccidioidomycosis. Which statements about this diagnosis are accurate? **Select all that apply.**
    a. Symptoms of coccidioidomycosis resemble those of other respiratory infections.
    b. Coccidioidomycosis is a viral infection caused by the *coccidioides* organism.
    c. The *coccidioides* organism is present in the soil but is inactive.
    d. Coccidioidomycosis is sometimes misdiagnosed as flu or pneumonia.
    e. Most younger healthy adults recover from the infection without treatment.
    f. Severe coccidioidomycosis is treated with drugs such as fluconazole (Diflucan).

Care of Critically Ill Patients with Respiratory Problems

1. Which are **major** risk factors for venous thromboembolism (VTE) leading to pulmonary embolism (PE)? **Select all that apply.**
   a. Malnutrition
   b. Central venous catheters
   c. Chronic obstructive pulmonary disease (COPD)
   d. Obesity
   e. Prolonged immobility
   f. Conditions that decrease blood clotting

2. What is the **most** common site of origin for a clot to occur, causing a pulmonary embolism (PE)?
   a. Right side of the heart
   b. Deep veins of the legs and pelvis
   c. Antecubital vein in upper extremities
   d. Subclavian veins

3. What is the **most** common cause of an embolism?
   a. Amniotic fluid
   b. Bolus of air
   c. Blood clot
   d. Arterial plaque

4. Which conditions define respiratory failure? **Select all that apply.**
   a. Ventilatory failure
   b. Circulatory failure
   c. Oxygenation failure
   d. Severe anemia
   e. Combination of ventilatory and oxygenation failure
   f. Chronic emphysema

5. A patient in the hospital is receiving a continuous infusion of heparin for a pulmonary embolism (PE). When the nurse enters the room, the patient has blood on the front of his chest and is holding a tissue saturated with blood to his nose. What is the **first** priority action the nurse must take?
   a. Have the patient sit up and lean forward, pinching the nostrils.
   b. Have a UAP set up oral suctioning to suction excess blood from the patient's mouth.
   c. Stop the heparin IV infusion.
   d. Obtain laboratory results for prothrombin time and complete blood count.

6. The nurse's young neighbor who smokes is going on an overseas flight. The neighbor knows he is at risk for deep vein thrombosis (DVT) and pulmonary embolism (PE) and asks the nurse for advice. What does the nurse suggest?
   a. Exercise regularly and walk around before boarding the flight.
   b. Get a prescription for heparin therapy and take it before the flight.
   c. Drink water and get up every hour for at least 5 minutes during the flight.
   d. Elevate the legs as much as possible during and after the flight.

7. The nurse is caring for several postoperative patients at risk for developing pulmonary embolism (PE). Which interventions does the nurse use to help prevent the development of PE in these patients? **Select all that apply.**
   a. Start passive and active range-of-motion exercises for the extremities.
   b. Ambulate postoperative patients soon after surgery.
   c. Use antiembolism devices postoperatively.
   d. Elevate legs in an extended position.
   e. Change patient position every 4-6 hours.
   f. Administer stool softeners to prevent constipation.

8. The nurse suspects a patient has a pulmonary embolism (PE) and notifies the provider, who orders an arterial blood gas. The health care provider is on the way to the facility. The nurse anticipates and prepares the patient for which additional diagnostic test?
   a. Ultrasound
   b. Pulmonary angiography
   c. 12-lead ECG
   d. Venous Dopplers

9. The health care provider orders heparin therapy for a patient with a relatively small pulmonary embolism (PE). The patient states, "I didn't tell the doctor my complete medical history." Which condition may affect the health care provider's decision to **immediately** start heparin therapy?
   a. Type 2 diabetes mellitus
   b. Recent cerebral hemorrhage
   c. Newly diagnosed osteoarthritis
   d. Asthma since childhood

10. A patient with a pulmonary embolism (PE) asks for an explanation of heparin therapy. What is the nurse's **best** response?
    a. "It keeps the clot from getting larger by preventing platelets from sticking together to improve blood flow."
    b. "It will improve your breathing and decrease chest pain by dissolving the clot in your lung."
    c. "It promotes the absorption of the clot in your leg that originally caused the PE."
    d. "It increases the time it takes for blood to clot, therefore preventing further clotting and improving blood flow."

11. A patient is being treated with heparin therapy for a pulmonary embolism (PE). What does the nurse monitor in relation to the heparin therapy and potential for bleeding?
    a. Lab values for any elevation of prothrombin time (PT) or partial thromboplastin time (PTT) value
    b. PTT values for greater than 2.5 times the control and/or the patient for bleeding
    c. Occurrence of a pulmonary infarction by blood in sputum
    d. PT values for International Normalized Ratio (INR) for a therapeutic range of 2 to 3 and/or the patient for bleeding

12. Acute respiratory failure is classified by which critical arterial blood gas (ABG) values? **Select all that apply.**
    a. $PaCO_2$ 39 mm Hg
    b. $PaCO_2$ 52 mm Hg
    c. PaO_2 78 mm Hg
    d. PaO_2 55 mm Hg
    e. pH value of < 7.3
    f. SaO_2 90%

13. Upon diagnosis of a submassive pulmonary embolism (PE), the nurse expects to perform which therapeutic intervention for the patient?
    a. Provide oral anticoagulant therapy.
    b. Maintain bedrest in the supine position.
    c. Give oxygen therapy via mechanical ventilator.
    d. Administer parenteral low molecular weight heparin (LMWH).

14. The nurse is caring for a patient with a postoperative complication of pulmonary embolism (PE). The nurse determines the patient has adequate perfusion by which data? **Select all that apply.**
    a. Pulse oximetry of 95%
    b. Arterial blood gas, pH of 7.28
    c. Patient's subjective desire to go home
    d. Absence of pallor or cyanosis
    e. Mental status at patient's baseline
    f. Palpable peripheral pulses

15. Which are extrapulmonary causes of ventilatory failure? **Select all that apply.**
    a. Stroke
    b. Use of opioid analgesics
    c. Pulmonary edema
    d. Chronic obstructive pulmonary disease
    e. Massive obesity
    f. Increased intracranial pressure

16. The nurse is caring for several postoperative patients with high risk for a pulmonary embolism (PE). All of these patients have preexisting chronic respiratory problems. Which assessment finding suggests that a patient has developed a PE with pulmonary infarction?
    a. Dyspnea
    b. Sudden dry cough
    c. Hemoptysis
    d. Audible wheezing

17. The nurse is caring for several patients at risk for deep vein thrombosis (DVT) and pulmonary embolism (PE). Which condition causes the patient to be a candidate for placement of a vena cava filter?
    a. Presence of symptoms of shock
    b. Signs of deteriorating cardiopulmonary status
    c. Recurrent bleeding while receiving anticoagulants
    d. No response to oxygen therapy

18. A patient with a massive pulmonary embolism (PE) has hypotension and shock and is receiving IV crystalloids. The patient's cardiac output does not improve. The nurse anticipates an order for which drug?
    a. Hydromorphone
    b. Alteplase
    c. Diltiazem
    d. Dobutamine

19. An older adult patient on anticoagulation therapy for a pulmonary embolism (PE) is somewhat confused and requires assistance with activities of daily living (ADLs). Which instruction **specific** to this therapy does the nurse give to the unlicensed assistive personnel (UAP)?
    a. Count and report episodes of urinary incontinence.
    b. Use a lift sheet when moving or turning the patient in bed.
    c. Assist with ambulation because the patient is likely to have dizziness.
    d. Give the patient an extra blanket, because the patient is likely to feel cold.

20. A patient with a pulmonary embolism (PE) is receiving anticoagulant therapy. Which assessment **related to** the therapy does the nurse perform?
    a. Measure abdominal girth because the medication causes fluid retention.
    b. Check skin turgor because dehydration contributes to anticoagulation.
    c. Monitor for nausea, vomiting, and diarrhea.
    d. Examine skin every 2 hours for evidence of bleeding.

21. What does the nurse monitor for in a patient with a pulmonary embolism (PE)? **Select all that apply.**
    a. Vomiting
    b. Cyanosis
    c. Rapid heart rate
    d. Dyspnea
    e. Paradoxical chest movement
    f. Crackles in the lung fields

22. After receiving parenteral heparin anticoagulant therapy, patients are often discharged from the hospital with a prescription and instructions for which drug?
    a. Protamine sulfate
    b. Prednisone
    c. Warfarin
    d. Oral heparin

23. A patient is following up on a postoperative complication of pulmonary embolism (PE). The patient must have blood drawn to determine the therapeutic range for warfarin (Coumadin). Which lab test determines this therapeutic range?
    a. Partial thromboplastin time (PTT) level
    b. Platelets
    c. International Normalized Ratio (INR)
    d. Coumadin peak and trough

24. The nurse is reviewing lab results for a patient with a new-onset pulmonary embolism (PE). What is the INR therapeutic range?
    a. 1.0-1.5
    b. 2.5-3.0
    c. 3.1-4.5
    d. 4.6-5.0

25. A patient demonstrates chest pain, dyspnea, dry cough, and change in level of consciousness. The nurse suspects pulmonary embolism (PE) and notifies the health care provider, who orders an arterial blood gas (ABG). In the early stage of a PE, what would ABG results probably indicate?
    a. Respiratory alkalosis
    b. Respiratory acidosis
    c. Metabolic acidosis
    d. Metabolic alkalosis

26. A patient recently received anticoagulant therapy for complications of pulmonary embolism (PE) after knee surgery. The patient is now in a rehabilitation facility and is receiving warfarin (Coumadin). What is the nursing responsibility **related to** warfarin (Coumadin)?
    a. Have protamine sulfate available as an antidote.
    b. Administer NSAIDs or aspirin for pain related to the knee.
    c. Teach the patient about foods high in vitamin K.
    d. Monitor platelets for thrombocytopenia.

27. Ventilatory failure is the result of what processes? **Select all that apply.**
    a. Hematologic disease
    b. Defect in the respiratory control center of the brain
    c. Physical problem of the lungs
    d. Poor function of the diaphragm
    e. Physical problem of the chest wall
    f. Infectious diseases such as pneumonia

28. Which conditions are related to acute respiratory distress syndrome (ARDS)? **Select all that apply.**
    a. Lung fluid increases.
    b. A systemic inflammatory response occurs.
    c. The lungs dry out and become stiff.
    d. Lung volume is decreased.
    e. Hypoxemia results.
    f. Surfactant production is increased.

29. The nurse is reviewing the arterial blood gas (ABG) results for a patient. The latest ABGs show pH 7.48, HCO_3^- 23 mEq/L, $Paco_2$ 25 mm Hg, and Pao_2 98 mm Hg. What is the correct interpretation of these lab findings?
    a. Chronic respiratory alkalosis with compensation
    b. Acute respiratory alkalosis and hyperventilation
    c. Acute respiratory acidosis and hypoventilation
    d. Chronic respiratory acidosis and hypoventilation

30. The nurse is caring for a patient with acute hypoxemia. Which nursing interventions are **best** for the care of this patient? **Select all that apply.**
    a. Minimal self-care
    b. Sedatives prn
    c. Upright position
    d. Oxygen therapy
    e. Remain NPO while dyspneic
    f. Prescribed metered-dose inhalers

31. A patient reports pain with inspiration after falling off a skateboard. The provider makes the diagnosis of rib fracture. The nurse prepares to do patient teaching for which treatment?
    a. Mechanical ventilation
    b. Tight bandage around chest
    c. Pain control for adequate breathing
    d. Opioid analgesics for pain

32. The nurse is assessing a patient who sustained significant chest trauma during a motor vehicle accident. What significant assessment finding suggests tension pneumothorax?
    a. Tracheal deviation to the unaffected side
    b. Inspiratory stridor and respiratory distress
    c. Diminished breath sounds over the affected hemothorax
    d. Hyperresonant percussion note over the affected side

33. The nurse is assessing a patient with a hemothorax. When the nurse performs percussion of the chest on the affected side, what type of sound is expected?
    a. Hypertympanic
    b. Dull
    c. Hyperresonant
    d. Crackles

34. On arrival to the emergency department (ED), the patient develops extreme respiratory distress and the provider identifies a tension pneumothorax. The nurse prepares to assist with which **initial** urgent procedure?
    a. Endotracheal intubation with mechanical ventilation
    b. Placement of a chest tube to reduce pneumothorax on the affected side
    c. Insertion of an 8-inch (20.3-cm), 16- or 18-gauge pericardial needle
    d. Insertion of a large-bore needle into the second intercostal space on the affected side

35. The nurse is performing patient teaching for a patient who will be taking anticoagulants at home. What does the nurse include in the instructions? **Select all that apply.**
    a. Use a soft-bristled toothbrush and floss frequently.
    b. Do not take aspirin or any aspirin-containing products.
    c. Do not participate in activities that will cause bumps, scratches, or scrapes.
    d. If you are bumped, apply ice to the site for at least 24 hours.
    e. Eat warm, cool, or cold foods to avoid burning your mouth.
    f. If you must blow your nose, do so gently without blocking either nasal passage.

36. Which patient has the **greatest** risk for developing adult respiratory distress syndrome (ARDS)?
    a. 74-year-old who aspirates a tube feeding
    b. 34-year-old with chronic renal failure
    c. 56-year-old with uncontrolled diabetes mellitus
    d. 18-year-old with a fractured femur

37. Which assessment finding is considered an **early** sign of adult respiratory distress syndrome (ARDS)?
    a. Adventitious lung sounds
    b. Hyperthermia and hot, dry skin
    c. Intercostal and suprasternal retractions
    d. Heightened mental acuity and surveillance

38. A patient with which condition is a potential candidate for autotransfusion, should the need arise?
    a. Tension pneumothorax
    b. Hemothorax
    c. Abdominal bleeding
    d. Esophageal bleeding

39. A patient sustained a chest injury resulting from a motor vehicle accident. The patient is asymptomatic at first but slowly develops decreased breath sounds, crackles, wheezing, and tachypnea. The mechanism of injury and physical findings are consistent with which condition?
    a. Flail chest
    b. Rib fractures
    c. Pneumothorax
    d. Pulmonary contusion

40. A patient is admitted after a near-drowning and develops adult respiratory distress syndrome (ARDS), which is confirmed by the health care provider. The nurse prepares equipment for which treatment?
    a. Oxygen therapy via continuous positive airway pressure (CPAP)
    b. Mechanical ventilation and endotracheal tube
    c. High-flow oxygen via face mask
    d. Tracheostomy tube

41. A 19-year-old patient was seen in the emergency department after a motorcycle accident for multiple rib fractures that resulted in free-floating ribs, paradoxical breathing, and inadequate oxygenation. What is this condition called?
    a. Tension pneumothorax
    b. Flail chest
    c. Pulmonary contusion
    d. Subcutaneous emphysema

42. The high-pressure alarm of a patient's mechanical ventilator goes off. What are the potential causes for this? **Select all that apply.**
    a. Mucus plug
    b. Air leak in endotracheal tube cuff
    c. Patient fighting the ventilator
    d. Bronchospasm
    e. Patient coughing
    f. Ventilator tubing disconnected

43. The low-pressure alarm of a patient's mechanical ventilator goes off. What are potential causes for this? **Select all that apply.**
    a. Blockage in the circuit
    b. Cuff leak in the endotracheal or tracheostomy tube
    c. Patient stopping breathing
    d. Cuff of the endotracheal or tracheostomy tube overinflated
    e. Leak in the circuit
    f. Patient biting on oral endotracheal tube

44. A patient with adult respiratory distress syndrome (ARDS) is currently in the exudative management stage. What is the focus of the nursing assessment?
    a. Monitor closely for progressive hypoxemia.
    b. Note early changes in dyspnea and tachypnea.
    c. Review the x-ray reports for evidence of patchy infiltrates.
    d. Monitor for multiple organ dysfunction syndrome.

45. The nurse is caring for a patient at risk for pulmonary contusion. Why is this a potentially lethal chest injury?
    a. The patient could have broken ribs.
    b. The patient could develop laryngospasm.
    c. Respiratory failure develops over time.
    d. There is a risk of infection from chest tubes.

46. A patient has been successfully intubated by the health care provider, and the nurse and respiratory therapist are securing the tube in place. What does the nurse include in the documentation regarding the intubation procedure? **Select all that apply.**
    a. Presence of bilateral and equal breath sounds
    b. Level of the tube
    c. Changes in vital signs during the procedure
    d. Rate of the IV fluids
    e. Presence (or absence) of dysrhythmias
    f. Placement verification by end-tidal carbon dioxide levels

47. The nurse is assisting with an emergency intubation for a patient in severe respiratory distress. Although the health care provider is experienced, the procedure is difficult because the patient has severe kyphosis. At what point does the nurse intervene?
    a. First intubation attempt lasts longer than 15 seconds.
    b. First intubation attempt lasts longer than 30 seconds.
    c. Second intubation attempt is unsuccessful.
    d. Second intubation attempt causes the patient to struggle.

48. A patient in the emergency department required emergency intubation for status asthmaticus. **Immediately** after the insertion of an endotracheal (ET) tube, what is the most accurate method for the nurse and/or health care provider to use to verify correct placement?
    a. Observe for chest excursion.
    b. Listen for expired air from the ET tube.
    c. Check end-tidal CO_2 level.
    d. Wait for the results of the chest x-ray.

49. The nurse is caring for several patients on the medical-surgical unit who are experiencing acute respiratory problems. Which conditions may eventually require a patient to be intubated? **Select all that apply.**
    a. Trouble maintaining a patent airway because of mucosal swelling
    b. History of congestive heart failure and demonstrating orthopnea
    c. Copious secretions and lacking muscular strength to cough
    d. Pulse oximetry of 93% with a high-flow oxygen face mask
    e. Increasing fatigue because of the work of breathing
    f. COPD patient with SaO_2 of 90% able to cough up secretions

50. The nurse receives report on a patient with adult respiratory distress syndrome (ARDS) who has been intubated for 6 days and has progressive hypoxemia that responds poorly to high levels of oxygen. This patient is in which phase of ARDS case management?
    a. Exudative phase
    b. Fibroproliferative phase
    c. Resolution phase
    d. Recovery phase

51. A postoperative patient reports sudden onset of shortness of breath and pleuritic chest pain. Assessment findings include diaphoresis, hypotension, crackles in the left lower lobe, and pulse oximetry of 85%. What does the nurse suspect has occurred with this patient?
    a. Atelectasis
    b. Pneumothorax
    c. Pulmonary embolism
    d. Flail chest

52. The nurse hears in shift report that a patient has been agitated and pulling at the endotracheal tube (ET). Soft restraints have recently been ordered and placed, but the patient continues to move his head and chew at the tube. What does the nurse do to ensure proper placement of the ET tube?
    a. Suction the patient frequently through the oral airway.
    b. Talk to the patient and tell him to calm down.
    c. Mark the tube where it touches the patient's teeth.
    d. Auscultate for breath sounds every 4 hours.

53. The nurse is caring for a patient on a mechanical ventilator. What does the nurse monitor to assess for the **most** likely cardiac problem associated with this therapy?
    a. Check blood pressure.
    b. Check for ventricular dysrhythmias.
    c. Take an apical pulse before giving medications.
    d. Ask the patient about chest pain.

54. A patient in the critical care unit requires an emergency ET intubation. The nurse immediately obtains and prepares which supplies to assist with performing this procedure? **Select all that apply.**
    a. Tracheostomy tube or kit
    b. Resuscitation bag-valve-mask device
    c. Source for 100% oxygen
    d. Suction equipment
    e. Airway equipment box (e.g., laryngoscope)
    f. Oral airway

55. A patient on a ventilator is biting and chewing at the endotracheal tube (ET). Which nursing intervention is used for ET management?
    a. Reassure the patient that everything is okay.
    b. Administer a paralyzing agent.
    c. Insert an oral airway.
    d. Frequently suction the mouth.

56. The nurse is performing a check of the ventilator equipment. What is included during the equipment check?
    a. Drain the condensed moisture back into the humidifier.
    b. Empty the humidifier and the drainage tubing.
    c. Note the prescribed and actual settings.
    d. Turn off the alarms during the system check.

57. The nursing student is assisting in the care of a critically ill patient on a ventilator. Which action by the student nurse requires intervention by the supervising nurse?
    a. Deflates the cuff on the ET tube to check placement.
    b. Applies soft wrist restraints as ordered.
    c. Suctions the patient for 10 seconds at a time.
    d. Maintains the correct placement of the ET tube.

58. A patient has a history of COPD on a mechanical ventilator. The nurse obtains an order for which type of dietary therapy for this patient?
    a. High-fat nutritional supplement
    b. High-protein nutritional supplement
    c. High-carbohydrate nutritional supplement
    d. High-calorie nutritional supplement

59. The nursing student is assisting in the care of a patient on a mechanical ventilator. Which action by the student contributes to the prevention of ventilator-acquired pneumonia (VAP)?
    a. Suctions the patient frequently
    b. Performs oral care every 2 hours
    c. Encourages visitors to wear masks
    d. Obtains a sputum specimen for culture

60. The nurse is caring for a patient on a mechanical ventilator. During the shift, the nurse hears the patient talking to himself. What does the nurse do **next**?
    a. See if the patient has a change of mental status.
    b. Check the inflation of the pilot balloon.
    c. Assess the pulse oximetry for saturation level.
    d. Evaluate the patient's readiness to be weaned.

61. The nurse notices that a patient has a gradual increase in peak inspiratory pressure over the last several days. What is the **best** nursing intervention for this patient?
    a. Assess for a reason such as adult respiratory distress syndrome (ARDS) or pneumonia.
    b. Continue to increase peak airway pressure as needed.
    c. Change to another mode such as intermittent mandatory ventilation (IMV).
    d. Make arrangements for permanent ventilatory support.

62. A patient is intubated and has mechanical ventilation with positive end-expiratory pressure (PEEP). Because this patient is at risk for a tension pneumothorax, what is the nurse's **priority** action?
    a. Assess lung sounds every 30-60 minutes.
    b. Obtain an order for an arterial blood gas.
    c. Have chest tube equipment on standby.
    d. Direct the unlicensed assistive personnel to turn the patient every 2 hours.

63. The nurse is caring for a patient on a mechanical ventilator. Which assessments does the nurse perform for this patient? **Select all that apply.**
    a. Observe the patient's mouth around the tube for pressure ulcers.
    b. Auscultate the lungs for crackles, wheezes, equal breath sounds, and decreased or absent breath sounds.
    c. Assess the placement of the ET.
    d. Check at least every 24 hours to be sure the ventilator settings are as prescribed.
    e. Check to be sure alarms are set.
    f. Observe the patient's need for tracheal, oral, or nasal suctioning every 2 hours.

64. What are the characteristics of a mechanical ventilator that is pressure-cycled? **Select all that apply.**
    a. Preset inspiration and expiration rate is programmed with possible variation of tidal volume and pressure.
    b. It is a positive-pressure ventilator.
    c. It pushes air into the lungs until a preset airway pressure is reached.
    d. There is no need for an artificial airway such as a tracheostomy or endotracheal tube.
    e. Tidal volumes and inspiratory times are varied.
    f. The ventilator is used for a short period of time.

65. What are the characteristics of a mechanical ventilator that is time-cycled? **Select all that apply.**
    a. It needs an artificial airway such as a tracheostomy or endotracheal tube.
    b. It is a positive-pressure ventilator.
    c. Its tidal volumes are variable.
    d. Preset inspiration and expiration rate can be set with possible variation of tidal volume.
    e. Inspiratory time is variable.
    f. A preset volume of air is delivered with each breath.

66. What are the characteristics of a noninvasive pressure support such as Bi-PAP? **Select all that apply.**
    a. It provides noninvasive pressure support ventilation by nasal mask or face mask.
    b. It takes over most of the work of breathing for the patient.
    c. It is most often used for patients with sleep apnea.
    d. It delivers a breath when a patient does not breathe.
    e. It may be used for patients with respiratory muscle fatigue.
    f. It can be used for impending respiratory failure to avoid more invasive ventilation methods.

67. Which statement about a microprocessor ventilator is true?
    a. Positive pressure is maintained throughout the entire respiratory cycle to prevent alveolar collapse.
    b. Positive pressure is exerted during expiration to keep lungs partially inflated.
    c. Noninvasive pressure support ventilation is provided by nasal mask or face mask.
    d. A computer monitors ventilatory functions, alarms, and patient condition.

68. What are the characteristics of a mechanical ventilator that is volume-cycled? **Select all that apply.**
    a. It pushes air into the lungs until a preset volume is delivered.
    b. A constant volume of air is delivered regardless of the pressure needed to deliver it.
    c. Pressure limits vary to prevent damage to the structures of the lungs.
    d. Tidal volume delivered varies based on chest wall compliance.
    e. It is a positive-pressure ventilator.
    f. This ventilator is primarily used during surgery and postoperatively.

69. The nurse hears an alarm go off on a mechanical ventilator that signals the ventilator is not able to give the patient a breath. What are the possible reasons that would make this alarm go off? **Select all that apply.**
    a. The tubing has become disconnected.
    b. The patient is not breathing on his or her own.
    c. The pulse oximetry reading is below 90%.
    d. The patient has become disconnected from the ventilator.
    e. The patient needs to be suctioned.
    f. The patient has a mucous plug blocking the airway.

70. A patient with a tracheostomy who is on a mechanical ventilator is beginning to take spontaneous breaths at his own rate and tidal volume between set ventilator breaths. Which mode is the ventilator on?
    a. Assist-control (AC) ventilation
    b. Bi-level positive airway pressure (Bi-PAP)
    c. Synchronized intermittent ventilation (SIMV)
    d. Continuous flow (flow-by)

71. A patient who is on a mechanical ventilator needs a set volume and set rate delivered because the patient is not able to do the work of breathing. To what mode must the ventilator be set?
    a. Positive end-expiratory pressure (PEEP)
    b. Continuous positive airway pressure (CPAP)
    c. Bi-level positive airway pressure (Bi-PAP)
    d. Assist control

72. The provider instructs the nurse to watch for and report signs and symptoms of improvement so the patient can be weaned from the ventilator. Which assessment finding indicates the patient is ready to be weaned?
    a. Indications that respiratory infection is resolving
    b. Showing signs of becoming ventilator-dependent
    c. Maintaining blood gases within normal limits
    d. Patient receiving only 1-2 mechanical ventilator breaths per minute

73. An older adult patient arrives in the emergency department after falling off a roof. The nurse observes "sucking inward" of the loose chest area during inspiration and a "puffing out" of the same area during expiration. Arterial blood gas (ABG) results show severe hypoxemia and hypercarbia. Which procedure does the nurse prepare for?
    a. Chest tube insertion
    b. Endotracheal intubation
    c. Needle thoracotomy
    d. Tracheostomy

74. The charge nurse in the intensive care unit is reviewing the patient census and caseload to identify staffing needs and potential transfers. Which patient might take the **longest** time to wean from a ventilator?
    a. 54-year-old man with metastatic colon cancer who has been intubated for 6 days
    b. 32-year-old woman recovering from a general anesthetic following a tubal ligation
    c. 25-year-old man intubated for 28 hours after an anaphylactic reaction
    d. 49-year-old man with a gunshot wound to the chest who was intubated for 8 hours

75. A patient is being extubated and the nurse has emergency equipment at the bedside. Which intervention is implemented during extubation?
    a. Ensure that the cuff is inflated at all times.
    b. Remove the tube during expiration.
    c. Instruct the patient to pant while the tube is removed.
    d. Instruct the patient to cough after the tube is removed.

76. The nurse is caring for a patient who was recently extubated. What is an expected assessment finding for this patient?
    a. Stridor
    b. Dyspnea
    c. Restlessness
    d. Hoarseness

77. The patient is to be extubated. What action does the nurse perform **first**?
    a. Hyperoxygenate the patient.
    b. Rapidly deflate the cuff of the ET tube.
    c. Thoroughly suction both the ET tube and the oral cavity.
    d. Explain the procedure.

78. Which patients on mechanical ventilators are at high risk for barotraumas? **Select all that apply.**
    a. Patient with adult respiratory distress syndrome (ARDS)
    b. Patient with underlying chronic airflow limitation
    c. Patient on bi-level positive airway pressure (Bi-PAP)
    d. Patient on positive end-expiratory pressure (PEEP)
    e. Patient on synchronized intermittent mechanical ventilation (SIMV)
    f. Patient receiving low level of pressure support

79. The nurse is caring for a patient who has just been extubated. What interventions will the nurse use in caring for this patient? **Select all that apply.**
    a. Monitor vital signs every 30 minutes at first.
    b. Assess the ventilatory pattern for manifestations of respiratory distress.
    c. Place the patient in a recumbent position.
    d. Instruct the patient to take deep breaths every half hour.
    e. Encourage use of an incentive spirometer every 2 hours.
    f. Advise the patient to limit speaking right after extubation.

80. The nurse is assessing a patient who was extubated several hours ago. Which patient finding warrants notification of the Rapid Response Team?
    a. Hoarseness
    b. Report of sore throat
    c. Inability to expectorate secretions
    d. 90% saturation on room air

81. A patient is admitted to the trauma unit following a front-end motor vehicle collision. The patient is currently asymptomatic, but the health care provider advises the nurse that the patient has a **high** risk for pulmonary contusion. What does the nurse carefully monitor for?
    a. Tracheal deviation
    b. Paradoxical chest movements
    c. Progressive chest pain
    d. Decreased breath sounds

82. Which finding might delay weaning a patient from mechanical ventilation support?
    a. Hematocrit = 42%
    b. Arterial Po_2 = 70 mm Hg on a 40% Fio_2
    c. Apical heart rate = 72 beats per minute
    d. Oral temperature = 101°F

83. A patient in respiratory failure is diagnosed with a flail chest. After the patient is intubated, which treatment does the nurse expect to be implemented?
    a. Positive end-expiratory pressure (PEEP)
    b. Synchronized intermittent mechanical ventilator (SIMV)
    c. Bi-level positive airway pressure (Bi-PAP)
    d. Peak inspiratory pressure (PIP)

84. A patient in a motor vehicle accident was unrestrained and appears to have hit the front dashboard. The patient has severe respiratory distress, inspiratory stridor, and extensive subcutaneous emphysema. The ED physician identifies tracheobronchial trauma. Which procedure does the nurse **immediately** prepare for?
    a. Cricothyroidotomy
    b. Chest tube insertion
    c. Cardiopulmonary resuscitation
    d. Pericardiocentesis

85. What causes the potential cardiac problems that can result from mechanical ventilation?
    a. Negative pressure increases in the chest.
    b. Positive pressure increases in the chest.
    c. Positive pressure decreases in the heart.
    d. Negative pressure decreases in the lungs.

86. What is the cardiac problem that can occur from mechanical ventilation?
    a. Hypotension
    b. Dehydration
    c. Bradycardia
    d. Hypertension

87. Which clinical manifestations can occur from cardiac problems due to mechanical ventilation? **Select all that apply.**
    a. Decreased cardiac output
    b. Diuresis
    c. Bradycardia
    d. Fluid retention
    e. Atrial fibrillation
    f. Increased urine output

88. Which conditions indicate the need to suction a mechanically ventilated patient? **Select all that apply.**
    a. Presence of ronchi when listening to breath sounds
    b. Presence of moisture in the ventilator tubing
    c. Audible secretions in the endotracheal tube
    d. Low pressure alarm sounds off
    e. Increased peak inspiratory pressure (PIP)
    f. Tubing becomes disconnected from the ventilator

89. Which actions are essential for the nurse caring for a mechanically ventilated patient to prevent ventilator-acquired pneumonia (VAP)? **Select all that apply.**
    a. Keep the HOB elevated at least 30 degrees.
    b. Perform oral care every 12 hours.
    c. Prevent aspiration.
    d. Suction every 1-2 hours around the clock.
    e. Turn and reposition patient every 2 hours.
    f. Prevent pressure ulcers around the mouth.

90. The patient is to be weaned from the mechanical ventilator by taking him off the ventilator for short periods of time and then assessing how well he tolerates being off the machine for progressively longer periods of time. The nurse recognizes this as which method of weaning from the ventilator?
    a. Synchronous intermittent mandatory ventilation method
    b. T-piece method
    c. Pressure support ventilation method
    d. Continuous positive airway pressure method

Assessment of the Cardiovascular System

33 CHAPTER

1. Which description **best** defines the cardiovascular concept of afterload?
   a. Degree of myocardial fiber stretch at end of diastole and just before heart contracts
   b. Amount of resistance the ventricles must overcome to eject blood through the semilunar valves and into the peripheral blood vessels
   c. Pressure that the ventricle must overcome to open the tricuspid valve
   d. Force of contraction independent of preload

2. Which are risk factors for cardiovascular disease (CVD) in women? **Select all that apply.**
   a. Waist and abdominal obesity
   b. Excess fat in the buttocks, hips, and thighs
   c. Postmenopausal
   d. Diabetes mellitus
   e. Asian ethnicity
   f. Elevated homocysteine level

3. The nurse is assessing a patient's nicotine dependence. Which questions does the nurse ask for an accurate assessment? **Select all that apply.**
   a. "How soon after you wake up in the morning do you smoke?"
   b. "What kind of cigarettes do you smoke?"
   c. "Do you wake up in the middle of the night to smoke?"
   d. "Do you find it difficult not to smoke in places where smoking is prohibited?"
   e. "Do you smoke when you are ill?"
   f. "What happened the last time you tried to quit smoking?"

4. The nurse is talking to a patient who has been trying to quit smoking. Which statement by the patient indicates an understanding of cigarette usage as it relates to reducing cardiovascular risks?
   a. "I need to be completely cigarette-free for at least 3 years."
   b. "I don't smoke as much as I used to; I'm down to one pack a day."
   c. "I started smoking a while ago, but I'll quit in a couple of years."
   d. "I only smoke to relax, when I drink, or when I go out with friends."

5. The nurse is providing health teaching for a patient at risk for heart disease. Which factor is the **most** modifiable, controllable risk factor?
   a. Obesity
   b. Diabetes mellitus
   c. Ethnic background
   d. Family history of cardiovascular disease

6. The nurse is giving a community presentation about heart disease in women. What information does the nurse include in the presentation? **Select all that apply.**
   a. Dyspnea on exertion may be the first and only symptom of heart failure.
   b. Symptoms are subtle or atypical.
   c. Pain is often relieved by rest.
   d. Having waist and abdominal obesity is a higher risk factor than having fat in buttocks and thighs.
   e. Pain always responds to nitroglycerin.
   f. Common symptoms include back pain, indigestion, nausea, vomiting, and anorexia.

7. Which blood pressure readings require further assessment? **Select all that apply.**
   a. 90 mm Hg systolic
   b. 139 mm Hg systolic
   c. 115 mm Hg systolic
   d. 66 mm Hg diastolic
   e. 100 mm Hg diastolic
   f. 96 mm Hg diastolic

8. The nurse is assessing a patient with cardiovascular disease (CVD). What is the **priority** medical-surgical concept for this patient?
   a. Fluid and electrolyte balance
   b. Perfusion
   c. Gas exchange
   d. Acid-base balance

9. Which category of cardiovascular drugs increases heart rate and contractility?
   a. Diuretics
   b. Beta blockers
   c. Catecholamines
   d. Benzodiazepines

10. Which category of cardiovascular drugs blocks sympathetic stimulation to the heart and **decreases** the heart rate?
    a. Beta blockers
    b. Catecholamines
    c. Steroids
    d. Benzodiazepines

11. What different pathophysiologic conditions can the healthy heart adapt to? **Select all that apply.**
    a. Menses
    b. Stress
    c. Gastroesophageal reflux disease
    d. Infection
    e. Hemorrhage
    f. Kidney stones

12. Which statements about blood pressure are accurate? **Select all that apply.**
    a. Pulse pressure is the difference between the systolic and diastolic pressures.
    b. The right ventricle of the heart generates the greatest amount of blood pressure.
    c. Diastolic blood pressure is primarily determined by the amount of peripheral vasoconstriction.
    d. To maintain adequate blood flow through the coronary arteries, mean arterial pressure (MAP) must be at least 60 mm Hg.
    e. Diastolic blood pressure is the highest pressure during contraction of the ventricles.
    f. Systolic blood pressure is the amount of pressure/force generated by the left ventricle to distribute blood into the aorta with each contraction of the heart.

13. The nurse is assessing a 62-year-old native Hawaiian woman. She is postmenopausal, has had diabetes for 10 years, has smoked one pack a day of cigarettes for 20 years, walks twice a week for 30 minutes, is an administrator, and describes her lifestyle as sedentary. For her weight and height she has a body mass index of 32. Which risk factors for this patient are controllable for cardiovascular disease (CVD)? **Select all that apply.**
    a. Ethnic background
    b. Smoking
    c. Age
    d. Obesity
    e. Postmenopausal
    f. Sedentary lifestyle

14. The health care provider orders orthostatic vital signs on a patient who experienced dizziness and feeling lightheaded. What is the nurse's **first** action?
    a. Instruct the patient to change position to sitting or standing.
    b. Measure the blood pressure when the patient is supine.
    c. Place the patient in supine position for at least 3 minutes.
    d. Wait for at least 1 minute before auscultating blood pressure and counting the radial pulse.

15. In a hypovolemic patient, stretch receptors in the blood vessels sense a reduced volume or pressure and send fewer impulses to the central nervous system. As a result, which signs/symptoms does the nurse expect to observe in the patient?
    a. Reddish mottling to skin and a blood pressure elevation
    b. Cool, pale skin and tachycardia
    c. Warm, flushed skin with low blood pressure
    d. Pale pink skin with bradycardia

16. Which term describing the difference between systolic and diastolic values is an **indirect** measure of cardiac output?
    a. Paradoxical blood pressure
    b. Pulse pressure
    c. Ankle-brachial index
    d. Normal blood pressure

17. The nurse is performing a dietary assessment on a 45-year-old business executive at risk for cardiovascular disease (CVD). Which assessment method used by the nurse is the **most** reliable and accurate?
    a. Ask the patient to identify foods he or she eats that contain sodium, sugar, cholesterol, fiber, and fat.
    b. Ask the patient's spouse, who does the cooking and shopping, to identify the types of foods that are consumed.
    c. Ask the patient how cultural beliefs and economic status influence the choice of food items.
    d. Ask the patient to recall the intake of food, fluids, and alcohol during a typical 24-hour period.

18. Based on the physiologic force that propels blood forward in the veins, which patient has the **greatest** risk for venous stasis?
    a. Older adult patient with hypertension who rides a bicycle daily
    b. Middle-aged construction worker taking warfarin (Coumadin)
    c. Bedridden patient in the end stage of Alzheimer's disease
    d. Teenage patient with a broken leg who sits and plays video games

19. Which statement about the peripheral vascular system is true?
    a. Veins are equipped with valves that direct blood flow to the heart and prevent backflow.
    b. The velocity of blood flow depends on the diameter of the vessel lumen.
    c. Blood flow decreases and blood tends to clot as the viscosity decreases.
    d. The parasympathetic nervous system has the largest effect on blood flow to organs.

20. A patient comes to the clinic stating, "My right foot turns a darkish red color when I sit too long, and when I put my foot up, it turns pale." Which condition does the nurse suspect?
    a. Central cyanosis
    b. Peripheral cyanosis
    c. Arterial insufficiency
    d. Venous insufficiency

21. Which exercise regimen for an older adult meets the recommended guidelines for physical fitness to promote heart health?
    a. 6-hour bike ride every Saturday
    b. Golfing for 4 hours two times a week
    c. Running for 15 minutes three times a week
    d. Brisk walk 30 minutes every day

22. The patient has smoked half a pack of cigarettes per day for 2 years. How many pack-years has this patient smoked?
    a. 1/2 pack-year
    b. 1 pack-year
    c. 1 1/5 pack-years
    d. 2 pack-years

23. In assessing a patient who has come to the clinic for a physical exam, the nurse notes that the patient has decreased skin temperature. What is this finding **most** indicative of?
    a. Anemia
    b. Heart failure
    c. Arterial insufficiency
    d. Stroke

24. Emergency personnel discovered a patient lying outside in the cool evening air for an unknown length of time. The patient is in a hypothermic state. What other assessment finding does the nurse expect to see?
    a. Blood pressure and heart rate lower than normal
    b. Heart rate and respiratory rate higher than normal
    c. Normal vital signs as a result of compensatory mechanisms
    d. Gradually improved vital signs with enteral nutrition

25. The advanced practice nurse is assessing the vascular status of a patient's lower extremities using the ankle-brachial index. What is the correct technique for this assessment method?
    a. A blood pressure cuff is applied to the lower extremities and the systolic pressure is measured by Doppler ultrasound at both the dorsalis pedis and posterior tibial pulses.
    b. The dorsalis pedis and posterior tibial pulses are manually palpated and compared bilaterally for strength and equality and compared to the standard index.
    c. A blood pressure cuff is applied to the lower extremities to observe for an exaggerated decrease in systolic pressure by more than 10 mm Hg during inspiration.
    d. Blood pressure on the legs is measured with the patient supine; then the patient stands for several minutes and blood pressure is measured in the arms.

26. What is the correct technique for assessing a patient with arterial insufficiency in the right lower leg?
    a. Use the Doppler to find the dorsalis pedis and posterior tibial pulses on the right leg.
    b. Palpate the peripheral arteries in a head-to-toe approach with a side-to-side comparison.
    c. Check all the pulse points in the right leg in dependent and supine positions.
    d. Palpate the major arteries, such as the radial and femoral, and observe for pallor.

27. The nurse is performing a cardiac assessment on an older adult. What is a common assessment finding for this patient?
    a. S_4 heart sound
    b. Leg edema
    c. Pericardial friction rubs
    d. Change in point of maximum impulse (PMI) location

28. A patient's chart notes that the examiner has heard S_1 and S_2 on auscultation of the heart. What does this documentation refer to?
    a. First and second heart sounds
    b. Pericardial friction rub
    c. Murmur
    d. Gallop

29. The nurse is taking report on a patient who will be transferred from the cardiac intensive care unit to the general medical-surgical unit. The reporting nurse states that S_4 is heard on auscultation of the heart. This is **most** closely associated with which situation?
    a. Heart murmur
    b. Pericardial friction rub
    c. Ventricular hypertrophy
    d. Normal heart sounds

30. Which patient has an abnormal heart sound?
    a. S_1 in a 45-year-old patient
    b. S_2 in a 30-year-old patient
    c. S_3 in a 15-year-old patient
    d. S_3 in a 54-year-old patient

31. The nurse is caring for a patient at risk for heart problems. What are normal findings for the cardiovascular assessment of this patient? **Select all that apply.**
    a. Presence of a thrill
    b. Splitting of S_2; decreases with expiration
    c. Jugular venous distention to level of the mandible
    d. Point of maximal impulse (PMI) in fifth intercostal space at midclavicular line
    e. Paradoxical chest movement with inspiration and expiration
    f. Accentuated or intensified S_1 after exercise

32. The nurse practitioner reads in a patient's chart that a carotid bruit was heard during the last two annual checkups. Today on auscultation, the bruit is absent. How does the nurse practitioner evaluate this data?
    a. The problem has resolved spontaneously.
    b. There may have been an anomaly in previous findings.
    c. The occlusion of the vessel may have progressed past 90%.
    d. The antiplatelet therapy is working.

33. The nurse is assessing a patient with suspected cardiovascular disease (CVD). When assessing the precordium, which assessment technique does the nurse begin with?
    a. Percussion
    b. Palpation
    c. Auscultation
    d. Inspection

34. In assessing a patient, the nurse finds that the point of maximal impulse (PMI) appears in more than one intercostal space and has shifted lateral to the midclavicular line. How does the nurse interpret this data?
    a. Left ventricular hypertrophy
    b. Superior vena cava obstruction
    c. Pulmonary hypertension
    d. Constrictive pericarditis

35. When the nurse assesses a patient with cardiovascular disease (CVD), there is difficulty auscultating the first heart sound (S_1). What is the nurse's **best** action?
    a. Ask the patient to lean forward or roll to his or her left side.
    b. Instruct the patient to take a deep breath and hold it.
    c. Auscultate with the bell instead of the diaphragm.
    d. Ask the unlicensed assistive personnel (UAP) to complete a 12-lead electrocardiogram (ECG) immediately.

36. While listening to a patient's heart sounds, the nurse detects a murmur. What does the nurse understand about the cause of murmurs?
    a. A murmur is caused by the closing of the aortic and pulmonic valves.
    b. A murmur is caused when blood flows from the atrium to a noncompliant ventricle.
    c. A murmur is caused by anemia, hypertension, or ventricular hypertrophy.
    d. A murmur is caused when there is turbulent blood flow through normal or abnormal valves.

37. The patient has a diagnosis of angina. Which assessment data would the nurse expect to find? **Select all that apply.**
    a. Sudden onset of pain
    b. Intermittent pain relieved with sitting upright
    c. Substernal pain that may spread across chest, back, and arms
    d. Pain usually lasts less than 15 minutes
    e. Sharp, stabbing pain that is moderate to severe
    f. Pain relieved with rest

38. The nurse working in a women's health clinic is reviewing the risk factors for several patients for stroke and myocardial infarction (MI). Which patient has the **highest** risk for MI?
    a. 49-year-old on estrogen replacement therapy
    b. 55-year-old with unstable angina
    c. 23-year-old with diabetes that is currently not well controlled
    d. 60-year-old with well-controlled hypertension

39. A patient comes to the emergency department (ED) reporting chest pain. In evaluating the patient's pain, which questions does the nurse ask the patient? **Select all that apply.**
    a. "How long does the pain last and how often does it occur?"
    b. "How do you feel about the pain?"
    c. "Is the pain different from any other episodes of pain you've had?"
    d. "What activities were you doing when the pain first occurred?"
    e. "Where is the chest pain? What does it feel like?"
    f. "Have you had other signs and symptoms that occur at the same time?"

40. The nurse is instructing a patient with congestive heart failure (CHF) on what signs to look for when experiencing an exacerbation of CHF. Which are appropriate teaching points for this patient? **Select all that apply.**
    a. "It is possible to gain 10-15 lbs before edema develops."
    b. "Notify the provider of a weight loss of 3-5 lbs within 2 weeks."
    c. "Notify the provider of a weight gain of 2 lbs within 1-2 days."
    d. "Notify the provider if you notice that your shoes or rings feel tight."
    e. "Notify the provider if your skin becomes dry and scaly."
    f. "Sitting up or standing will relieve orthopnea."

41. A 65-year-old patient comes to the clinic reporting fatigue. The patient would like to start an exercise program but thinks "anemia might be causing the fatigue." What is the nurse's **first** action?
    a. Advise the patient to start out slowly and gradually build strength and endurance.
    b. Obtain an order for a complete blood count and nutritional profile.
    c. Assess the onset, duration, and circumstances associated with the fatigue.
    d. Perform a physical assessment to include testing of muscle strength and tone.

42. A young patient reports having frequent episodes of palpitations but denies having chest pain. Which follow-up question does the nurse ask to assess the patient's symptom of palpitations?
    a. "Have you noticed a worsening of shortness of breath when you are lying flat?"
    b. "Do your shoes feel unusually tight, or are your rings tighter than usual?"
    c. "Do you feel dizzy or have you lost consciousness with the palpitations?"
    d. "Does anyone in your family have a history of palpitations?"

43. Syncope in the aging person can likely occur with which actions by the patient? **Select all that apply.**
    a. Laughing
    b. Turning the head
    c. Performing a Valsalva maneuver
    d. Walking briskly for 20-30 minutes
    e. Shrugging the shoulders
    f. Swallowing fluids

44. The nurse performing a physical assessment on a patient with a history of cardiovascular disease (CVD) observes that the patient has ascites, jaundice, and anasarca. How does the nurse interpret these findings?
    a. Late signs of severe right-sided heart failure
    b. Early signs of mild right-sided heart failure
    c. Late signs of mild left-sided heart failure
    d. Early signs of left- and right-sided heart failure

45. The nurse is performing an assessment on a patient brought in by emergency personnel. The nurse immediately observes that the patient has spontaneous respirations and the skin is cool, pale, and moist. What is the **priority** patient problem?
    a. Abnormal body temperature
    b. Decreased perfusion
    c. Altered skin integrity
    d. Potential for peripheral neurovascular dysfunction

46. The nurse is caring for a patient at risk for a myocardial infarction (MI). For what **primary** reason does the nurse plan interventions to prevent anxiety or overexertion?
    a. An increase in heart rate increases myocardial oxygen demand.
    b. A release of epinephrine and norepinephrine causes MI.
    c. An increase in activity or emotion affects preload and afterload.
    d. Cardiac output is decreased by anxiety or physical stress.

47. Which nonspecific signs and symptoms are frequently seen in women who present with coronary artery disease (CAD)? **Select all that apply.**
    a. Malaise
    b. Hypoventilation
    c. Shortness of breath
    d. Anxiety
    e. Fatigue
    f. Diaphoresis

48. A patient reports severe cramping in the legs while attempting to walk for exercise. The health care provider diagnoses the patient with intermittent claudication. What does the nurse advise the patient to do?
    a. Elevate the legs on a pillow.
    b. Buy and wear supportive shoes.
    c. Massage the legs before walking.
    d. Rest the legs in a dependent position.

49. A patient entering the cardiac rehabilitation unit seems optimistic and at times unexpectedly cheerful and upbeat. Which statement by the patient causes the nurse to suspect a maladaptive use of denial in the patient?
    a. "I am sick and tired of talking about these dietary restrictions. Could we talk about it tomorrow?"
    b. "Oh, I don't really need that medication information. I'm sure that I'll soon be able to get by without it."
    c. "This whole episode of heart problems has been an eye-opener for me, but I really can't wait to get out of here."
    d. "That doctor is driving me crazy with all his instructions. Could you put all that information away in my suitcase?"

50. The nurse taking a medical history of a patient makes a special notation to follow up on valvular abnormalities of the heart. Which recurrent condition in the patient's history causes the nurse to make this notation?
    a. Streptococcal infections of the throat
    b. Staphylococcal infections of the skin
    c. Vaginal yeast infections
    d. Fungal infections of the feet or inner thighs

51. The nurse interprets a patient's serum lipid tests. Which results suggest an **increased** risk for cardiovascular disease (CVD)? **Select all that apply.**
    a. LDL 160 mg/dL
    b. HDL 60 mg/dL
    c. Total cholesterol 180 mg/dL
    d. Triglycerides 175 mg/dL
    e. Lp(a) 45 mg/dL
    f. Total cholesterol 250 mg/dL

52. What is the **most** significant laboratory cardiac marker in a patient who has had a myocardial infarction (MI)?
    a. Presence of troponin T and I
    b. Elevation of myoglobin levels
    c. Decreased creatine kinase levels
    d. Elevation of the white blood cell count

53. A patient in the emergency department (ED) with chest pain has a possible myocardial infarction (MI). Which laboratory test is done to determine this diagnosis?
    a. Troponin T and I
    b. Serum potassium
    c. Homocysteine
    d. Highly sensitive C-reactive protein

54. Which laboratory tests are used to predict a patient's risk for coronary artery disease (CAD)? **Select all that apply.**
    a. Cholesterol level
    b. Triglyceride level
    c. Prothrombin time
    d. Low-density lipoprotein level
    e. Albumin level
    f. Protein level

55. The patient with a history of allergy to iodine-based contrast dyes is scheduled for a cardiac catheterization. What action does the nurse expect with regard to the scheduled test?
    a. Delay the test for a week or more.
    b. Administer an antihistamine and/or steroid before the test.
    c. The test will be performed without administration of contrast dye.
    d. The patient will receive anticoagulation therapy before the test.

56. A patient is undergoing diagnostic testing for reports of chest pain. Which test is done to determine the location and extent of coronary artery disease (CAD)?
    a. Electrocardiogram (ECG)
    b. Echocardiogram
    c. Cardiac catheterization
    d. Chest x-ray

57. Which medications will the nurse hold until **after** a patient's cardiac catheterization?
    a. Daily vitamin and enteric-coated aspirin
    b. Atenolol and IV antibiotic
    c. Potassium and folic acid
    d. Warfarin and furosemide

58. Which interventions and actions does the nurse perform to detect and prevent kidney toxicity when caring for a patient after cardiac catheterization? **Select all that apply.**
    a. Provide IV and oral fluids for 12-24 hours.
    b. Assess pedal pulses every 15 minutes.
    c. Check the catheterization site every hour.
    d. Monitor intake and output.
    e. Keep the catheterized extremity straight for 6 hours.
    f. Restrict oral fluids for 3-6 hours before the procedure.

59. Microalbuminuria has been shown to be a clear marker of widespread endothelial dysfunction in cardiovascular disease (CVD). Which conditions should prompt patients to be tested annually for microalbuminuria? **Select all that apply.**
    a. Hypertension
    b. Metabolic syndrome
    c. Smoking cigarettes
    d. Use of anticoagulant therapy
    e. Sedentary lifestyle
    f. Diabetes mellitus

60. A patient is being discharged with a prescription for warfarin. Which tests will the nurse instruct the patient to routinely have done for follow-up monitoring?
    a. Prothrombin time (PT) and International Normalized Ratio (INR)
    b. Partial thromboplastin time (PTT) and serum potassium
    c. Complete blood count and platelet count
    d. Sodium and potassium levels

61. What is the significance of a sodium level of 130 mEq/L for a patient with heart failure?
    a. Increased risk for ventricular dysrhythmias
    b. Dilutional hyponatremia and fluid retention
    c. Potential for electrical instability of the heart
    d. Slowed conduction of impulse through the heart

62. Which test is performed to determine valve disease of the mitral valve, left atrium, or aortic arch?
    a. Transesophageal echocardiogram (TEE)
    b. Electrocardiogram (ECG)
    c. Myocardial nuclear perfusion imaging (MNPI)
    d. Phonocardiography

63. A patient is scheduled to have an exercise electrocardiography test. What instruction does the nurse provide to the patient before the procedure takes place?
    a. "Have nothing to eat or drink after midnight."
    b. "Avoid smoking or drinking alcohol for at least 2 weeks before the test."
    c. "Wear comfortable, loose clothing and rubber-soled, supportive shoes."
    d. "Someone must drive you home because of possible sedative effects of the medications."

64. A nurse is monitoring the patient's blood pressure and electrocardiogram (ECG) during a stress test. Which parameter indicates the patient should **stop** exercising?
    a. Increase in heart rate
    b. Increase in blood pressure
    c. ECG showing the P wave and QRS complex
    d. ECG showing ST-segment depression

65. What measures are taken to prepare a patient for a pharmacologic stress echocardiogram? **Select all that apply.**
    a. Patient can eat his/her diet as ordered.
    b. IV access needs to be present.
    c. Oxygen at 2 L per nasal cannula is placed on patient 3 hours prior to test.
    d. An oral laxative is given the day before the test.
    e. Patient is to be NPO for 3-6 hours before the test.
    f. Teach the patient that blood pressure and heart rate will be continuously monitored.

66. The nurse is explaining the purposes of angiography to a patient. Which material will the nurse explain to the patient? **Select all that apply.**
    a. Determine an abnormal structure of the heart.
    b. Identify an arterial obstruction.
    c. Assess the cardiovascular response to increased workload.
    d. Identify an arterial narrowing.
    e. Identify an aneurysm.
    f. Determine if cardiac enlargement is present.

67. What is included in postprocedural care of a patient after a cardiac catheterization? **Select all that apply.**
    a. Patient remains on bedrest for 12-24 hours.
    b. Patient is placed in a high Fowler's position.
    c. Dressing is assessed for bloody drainage or hematoma.
    d. Peripheral pulses in the affected extremity, as well as skin temperature and color, are monitored with every vital sign check.
    e. Adequate oral and IV fluids are provided for hydration.
    f. Vital signs are monitored every hour for 24 hours.

68. Which assessment finding in a patient who has had a cardiac catheterization does the nurse report **immediately** to the health care provider?
    a. Pain at the catheter insertion site
    b. Catheterized extremity dusky with decreased peripheral pulses
    c. Small hematoma at the catheter insertion site
    d. Pulse pressure of 40 mm Hg with a slow, bounding pulse

69. The nurse is providing discharge instructions for a patient who had a cardiac catheterization. Which instructions must the nurse include? **Select all that apply.**
    a. Notify the health care provider for increased swelling, redness, warmth, or pain.
    b. Leave the dressing in place for the first day.
    c. Limit activity for at least 2-3 weeks.
    d. Avoid lifting and exercise for a few days.
    e. Report any bruise or hematoma to the health care provider.
    f. Bruising or a small hematoma is expected.

70. The patient is scheduled for an exercise stress test. Which medications does the nurse expect the cardiologist will want held **before** the procedure?
    a. Atenolol and Cardizem
    b. Vitamins and potassium
    c. Colace and enteric-coated aspirin
    d. Acetaminophen and metered-dose bronchodilator

71. Which statement about veterans and risk for heart disease is **most** accurate?
    a. Veterans are not at increased risk for heart disease because most are relatively young.
    b. Veterans' increased risk for heart disease may be independent of health behaviors and chronic medical conditions.
    c. Veterans are at increased risk for heart disease because many are homeless and without proper health care.
    d. Veterans are at increased risk for heart disease because of increased incidence of poor physical and mental health.

72. The patient is a 48-year-old female who came to the emergency department (ED) with symptoms of indigestion with abdominal fullness, chronic fatigue even with rest, and feeling of an "inability to catch my breath." What is the nurse's **best** interpretation of these symptoms?
    a. These symptoms are not indicative of the presence of heart disease.
    b. The patient may need a workup for fibromyalgia.
    c. Women with heart disease present with atypical symptoms.
    d. This patient may be experiencing signs of painful gastric ulcers.

73. Which measure is **most** accurate when assessing a patient for fluid retention?
    a. Documenting edema as mild, moderate, or severe
    b. Measuring and monitoring daily patient weight
    c. Assessing peripheral swelling as 1+ to 4+
    d. Auscultating lungs for abnormal sounds such as crackles

74. The patient with constrictive pericarditis has a paradoxical blood pressure. How does the nurse measure this for a patient?
    a. Assess for a decrease in systolic pressure by more than 10 mm Hg during the inspiratory phase of the respiratory cycle.
    b. Assess for an increase in systolic pressure by more than 10 mm Hg during the inspiratory phase of the respiratory cycle.
    c. Measure the difference between systolic blood pressure and diastolic blood pressure.
    d. Check the blood pressure by Doppler ultrasound at both the dorsalis pedis and posterior tibial pulses.

75. Which statement about a hypokinetic pulse is accurate?
    a. It is a large, "bounding" pulse caused by an increased ejection of blood.
    b. It is caused by high cardiac output as with exercise, sepsis, or thyrotoxicosis.
    c. It may occur with increased sympathetic system activity caused by pain, fever, or anxiety.
    d. It is a weak pulse with a narrow pulse pressure seen with decreased cardiac output.

76. The nurse assesses a pericardial friction rub in a cardiac patient. What is the nurse's **best** interpretation of this finding? **Select all that apply.**
    a. It occurs with movements of the heart during the cardiac cycle.
    b. It originates in the septum between the ventricles.
    c. It is a transient sign of inflammation.
    d. It is often heard with cardiac valve insufficiency.
    e. It can occur after myocardial infarction.
    f. It is very loud and can be heard without a stethoscope.

77. The patient is admitted to the emergency department (ED) with sudden onset of chest pain that is intense, is substernal radiating to the left arm, and has lasted over an hour. What is the **most** likely cause of this chest pain?
    a. Angina
    b. Myocardial infarction
    c. Pericarditis
    d. Pleuropulmonary

78. The health care provider's note describes the patient's New York Heart Association Functional Classification of Cardiovascular Disability as Class III. Which statement **best** describes this patient's functional ability?
    a. Ordinary physical activity results in fatigue, palpitation, dyspnea, or anginal pain.
    b. Less than ordinary physical activity causes fatigue, palpitation, dyspnea, or anginal pain.
    c. Ordinary physical activity does not cause undue fatigue, palpitation, dyspnea, or anginal pain.
    d. If any physical activity is undertaken, discomfort is increased.

34 CHAPTER

Care of Patients with Dysrhythmias

1. What does stimulation of the sympathetic nervous system produce?
   a. Delayed electrical impulse causing hypotension
   b. Increased the heart rate
   c. Virtually no effect on the ventricles of the heart
   d. Slowed atrioventricular (AV) conduction time that results in a slow heart rate

2. The primary pacemaker of the heart, the sino-atrial (SA) node, is functional if a patient's pulse is at what regular rate?
   a. Fewer than 60 beats/min
   b. 60-100 beats/min
   c. 80-100 beats/min
   d. Greater than 100 beats/min

3. The nurse is taking vital signs and reviewing the electrocardiogram (ECG) of a patient who is training for a marathon. The heart rate is 45 beats/min and the ECG shows sinus brady-cardia. How does the nurse interpret this data?
   a. A rapid filling rate that lengthens diastolic filling time and leads to decreased cardiac output
   b. The body's attempt to compensate for a decreased stroke volume by decreasing the heart rate
   c. An adequate stroke volume that is associated with cardiac conditioning
   d. A common finding in the healthy adult that would be considered normal

4. The nurse is performing an assessment on a cardiac patient. In order to determine if the patient has a pulse deficit, what does the nurse do?
   a. Take the patient's blood pressure and subtract the diastolic from the systolic pressure.
   b. Take the patient's pulse in a supine position and then in a standing position.
   c. Assess the apical and radial pulses for a full minute and calculate differences in rate.
   d. Take the radial pulse, have the patient rest for 15 minutes, and then retake the pulse.

5. What does the P wave in an electrocardiogram (ECG) represent?
   a. Atrial depolarization
   b. Atrial repolarization
   c. Ventricular depolarization
   d. Ventricular repolarization

6. What is the normal measurement of the PR interval in an electrocardiogram (ECG)?
   a. Less than 0.11 second
   b. 0.06-0.10 second
   c. 0.12-0.20 second
   d. 0.16-0.26 second

7. What is the normal measurement of QRS complex in an electrocardiogram (ECG) normally?
   a. Less than 0.12 second
   b. 0.10-0.16 second
   c. 0.12-0.20 second
   d. 0.16-0.24 second

8. What is the normal position of the ST segment in an electrocardiogram (ECG)?
   a. Isoelectric
   b. Elevated
   c. Depressed
   d. Biphasic

9. What is the total time required for ventricular depolarization and repolarization as represented on the electrocardiogram (ECG)?
   a. PR interval
   b. QRS complex
   c. ST segment
   d. QT interval

10. The nurse is performing a 12-lead electrocardiogram (ECG) on a patient with chest pain. Because the positioning of the electrodes is crucial, how does the nurse place the ECG electrodes?
   a. Four leads are placed on the limbs and six are placed on the chest.
   b. The negative electrode is placed on the left arm and the positive electrode is placed on the right leg.
   c. Four leads are placed on the limbs and four are placed on the chest.
   d. The negative electrode is placed on the right arm and the positive electrode is placed on the left leg.

11. Because cardiac dysrhythmias are abnormal rhythms of the heart's electrical system, the heart is unable to perform what function?
   a. It cannot oxygenate the blood throughout the body.
   b. It cannot remove carbon dioxide from the body.
   c. It cannot effectively pump oxygenated blood throughout the body.
   d. It cannot effectively conduct impulses with increased activity.

12. The nurse is caring for several patients in the telemetry unit who are being remotely watched by a monitor technician. What is the nurse's **primary** responsibility in the monitoring process of these patients?
   a. Watching the bank of monitors on the unit
   b. Printing ECG rhythm strips routinely and as needed
   c. Interpreting rhythms
   d. Assessment and management of patients

13. A patient in the telemetry unit who has continuous electrocardiogram (ECG) monitoring is scheduled for a test in the radiology department. Who is responsible for determining when monitoring can be suspended?
   a. Telemetry technician
   b. Charge nurse
   c. Health care provider
   d. Primary nurse

14. The nurse is reviewing preliminary electrocardiogram (ECG) results of a patient admitted for mental status changes. The nurse alerts the health care provider about ST elevation or depression in the patient because it is an indication of which condition?
   a. Myocardial injury or ischemia
   b. Ventricular irritability
   c. Subarachnoid hemorrhage
   d. Prinzmetal's angina

15. The nurse is reviewing electrocardiogram (ECG) results of a patient admitted for fluid and electrolyte imbalances. The T waves are tall and peaked. The nurse reports this finding to the health care provider and obtains an order for which serum level test?
   a. Sodium
   b. Glucose
   c. Potassium
   d. Phosphorus

16. Which actions are the responsibilities of the monitor technician? **Select all that apply.**
   a. Watch the bank of monitors on a unit.
   b. Notify the health care provider of any changes.
   c. Print routine ECG strips.
   d. Apply battery-operated transmitter leads to patients.
   e. Interpret the rhythms.
   f. Report patient rhythm and significant changes to the nurse.

17. The nurse is notified by the telemetry monitor technician about a patient's heart rate. Which method does the nurse use to confirm the technician's report?
    a. Count QRS complexes in a 6-second strip and multiply by 10.
    b. Analyze an ECG rhythm strip by using an ECG caliper.
    c. Run an ECG rhythm strip and use the memory method.
    d. Assess the patient's heart rate directly by taking an apical pulse.

18. The nurse is analyzing the electrocardiogram (ECG) rhythm strips for assigned patients. What is the nurse's **first** action?
    a. Analyze the P waves.
    b. Determine the heart rate.
    c. Measure the QRS duration.
    d. Measure the PR interval.

19. A patient's electrocardiogram (ECG) rhythm strip is irregular. Which method does the nurse use for an accurate assessment?
    a. 6-second strip method
    b. Memory method
    c. Big block method
    d. Commercial ECG rate ruler

20. The nurse is assessing a patient's electrocardiogram (ECG) rhythm strip and checking the regularity of the atrial rhythm. What is the correct technique?
    a. Place one caliper point on a QRS complex; place the other point on the precise spot on the next QRS complex.
    b. Place one caliper point on a P wave; place the other point on the precise spot on the next P wave.
    c. Place one caliper point at the beginning of the P wave; place the other point at the end of the P-R segment.
    d. Place one caliper point at the beginning of the QRS complex; place the other point where the S-T segment begins.

21. The nurse is assessing a patient's electrocardiogram (ECG) rhythm strip and analyzing the P waves. Which questions does the nurse use to evaluate the P waves? **Select all that apply.**
    a. Are P waves present?
    b. Are the P waves occurring regularly?
    c. Does one P wave follow each QRS complex?
    d. Are the P waves greater than 0.20 second?
    e. Do all the P waves look similar?
    f. Are the P waves smooth, rounded, and upright in appearance?

22. The nurse is assessing a patient's electrocardiogram (ECG) rhythm strip and notes that occasionally the QRS complex is missing. How does the nurse interpret this finding?
    a. A junctional impulse
    b. A supraventricular impulse
    c. Ventricular tachycardia
    d. A dysrhythmia

23. The student nurse is looking at a patient's electrocardiogram (ECG) rhythm strip and suspects a normal sinus rhythm (NSR). Which ECG criteria are included for NSR? **Select all that apply.**
    a. Rate: Atrial and ventricular rates of 40-120 beats/min
    b. Rhythm: Atrial and ventricular rhythms regular
    c. P waves: Present, consistent configuration
    d. One P wave before each QRS complex
    e. P-R interval: 0.24 second
    f. QRS duration: 0.04-0.10 second and constant

24. The heart monitor of a patient shows a rhythm that appears as a wandering or fuzzy baseline. What is the **priority** action for the nurse?
    a. Immediately obtain a 12-lead ECG to assess the actual rhythm.
    b. Assess the patient to differentiate artifact from actual lethal rhythms.
    c. Check to see if the patient has a do-not-resuscitate order.
    d. Ask the patient care technician to take vital signs on the patient.

25. What does the T wave on an electrocardiogram (ECG) represent?
    a. Ventricular depolarization
    b. Atrial repolarization
    c. Atrial depolarization
    d. Ventricular repolarization

26. The remote telemetry technician calls the nurse to report that a patient's electrocardiogram (ECG) signal transmission is not very clear. What does the nurse do to enhance the transmission?
    a. Clean the skin with povidone-iodine solution before applying the electrodes.
    b. Ensure that the area for electrode placement is dry and nonhairy.
    c. Apply tincture of benzoin to the electrode sites and allow it to dry.
    d. Abrade the skin by rubbing briskly with a rough washcloth.

27. With the speed set for 25 mm/second, the segment between the dark lines on a monitor ECG strip represents how many seconds?
    a. 3
    b. 6
    c. 10
    d. 20

28. Which components measure electrocardiogram (ECG) waveforms?
    a. Blood pressure (BP) and cardiac output (CO)
    b. Seconds (sec) and minutes (min)
    c. Heart rate per minute (HR/min)
    d. Amplitude (voltage) and duration (time)

29. The nurse is evaluating a patient's electrocardiogram (ECG) strip. ST segment elevation of 1.5 mm (1.5 small blocks) is noted. Which conditions may be indicated by this ST elevation? **Select all that apply.**
    a. Myocardial infarction
    b. Hyperkalemia
    c. Hypokalemia
    d. Ventricular hypertrophy
    e. Pericarditis
    f. Endocarditis

30. What is the heart rate shown on a 6-second electrocardiogram (ECG) strip when the number of R-R intervals is 5? What is this rhythm?
    a. 30/minute bradycardia
    b. 40/minute bradycardia
    c. 50/minute bradycardia
    d. 60/minute normal

31. How does the nurse interpret the measurement of the P-R interval when the interval is six small boxes on the ECG strip?
    a. Atrium is taking longer to repolarize.
    b. Longer-than-normal impulse time from the SA node to the ventricles is shown.
    c. There is a problem with the length of time the ventricles are depolarizing.
    d. This is the normal length of time for the P-R interval.

32. The nurse hears in report that a patient has sinus arrhythmia. In order to validate that this is associated with changes in intrathoracic pressure, what does the nurse do **next**?
    a. Count the respiratory and pulse rate at rest and then count both rates after moderate exertion.
    b. Observe that the heart rate increases slightly during inspiration and decreases slightly during exhalation.
    c. Ask the patient to hold the breath and take an apical pulse; then have the patient resume normal breathing.
    d. Have the patient take a deep breath; then count the patient's apical pulse rate while the patient slowly exhales.

33. The nurse is reviewing a patient's electrocardiogram (ECG) and notes a wide distorted QRS complex of 0.14 second followed by a P wave. What does this finding indicate?
    a. Wide but normal complex, and no cause for concern
    b. Premature ventricular contraction
    c. Problem with the speed set on the ECG machine
    d. Delayed time of the electrical impulse through the ventricles

34. Which clinical manifestations are reflections of sustained tachydysrhythmias? **Select all that apply.**
    a. Chest discomfort
    b. Moist cyanotic skin
    c. Palpitations
    d. Hypertension
    e. Syncope
    f. Restlessness

35. The nurse is monitoring a patient who is sleeping. The monitor shows that the patient's heart rate increases slightly during inspiration and decreases slightly during exhalation. Which cardiac rhythm does the nurse document?
    a. Normal sinus rhythm
    b. Sinus arrhythmia
    c. Sinus bradycardia
    d. Sinus tachycardia

36. Which definition **best** describes the synchronous (demand) pacing mode?
    a. The pacemaker continues to fire at a fixed rate as set on the generator.
    b. The pacemaker's sensitivity is set to sense the patient's own beats.
    c. Electrical pulses are transmitted through two large external electrodes and then transcutaneously to stimulate ventricular depolarization.
    d. External battery-operated pulse generator on one end and wires in contact with the heart on the other end.

37. The nurse is assisting the health care provider to perform temporary pacing for a patient who has atropine-refractory symptomatic bradycardia. What is the desired outcome for this patient as evidenced by the cardiac monitor?
    a. No spike, but a complete QRS complex indicating atrial depolarization
    b. A spike followed by a QRS complex indicating ventricular depolarization
    c. Two spikes, followed by a QRS complex indicating ventricular depolarization
    d. A spike before and after a QRS complex indicating atrial depolarization

38. The health care provider has completed the placement of lead wires for the invasive temporary pacemaker in a patient who is asystolic. In turning on the pacing unit, which setting does the nurse use?
    a. Synchronous pacing mode
    b. Demand pacing mode
    c. Asynchronous pacing mode
    d. Temporary pacing mode

39. The nurse in the telemetry unit must perform transcutaneous pacing. When should transcutaneous pacing be used?
    a. When a patient's rhythm strip shows atrial fibrillation.
    b. Only when a patient's ECG demonstrates a bradydysrhythmia.
    c. When a patient is experiencing syncope and dizziness.
    d. Only as a temporary emergency measure until a more permanent pacing method can be started.

40. A patient has an invasive temporary pacemaker. In what ways does the nurse ensure the patient's safety related to electrical issues with the pacemaker? **Select all that apply.**
    a. Ensure that external ends of the lead wires are insulated with rubber gloves.
    b. Loop the wire ends and cover with nonconductive tape.
    c. Ensure that no electrical equipment is used in the patient's room.
    d. Report frayed wire to the biomedical engineering department.
    e. Wash hands before touching any of the wires.
    f. Notify the health care provider if the pacemaker fails to capture and pace the heart.

41. Which statements about permanent pacemakers are accurate? **Select all that apply.**
    a. Permanent pacemakers treat conduction disorders such as complete heart block.
    b. Permanent pacemakers are powered by lithium batteries that can last for 20 years or more.
    c. Permanent pacemakers are available as pacemaker/defibrillator devices.
    d. Biventricular permanent pacemakers allow synchronized depolarization of the ventricles.
    e. The pulse generator of a permanent pacemaker is usually implanted in the subclavian area.
    f. The patient with a permanent pacemaker should be taught to avoid lifting his or her arm over the head for at least 6 months.

42. A patient has had a permanent pacemaker surgically implanted. What are the nursing responsibilities for the care of this patient following surgical implantation? **Select all that apply.**
    a. Administer short-acting sedatives.
    b. Assess the implantation site for bleeding, swelling, redness, tenderness, or infection.
    c. Teach about and monitor for the initial activity restrictions.
    d. Observe for overstimulation of the chest wall, which could lead to pneumothorax.
    e. Monitor the ECG rhythm to check that the pacemaker is working correctly.
    f. Assess that the implantation site dressing is clean and dry.

43. The nurse is teaching a patient with a permanent pacemaker. What information about the pacemaker does the nurse tell the patient? **Select all that apply.**
    a. Report any pulse rate lower than what is set on the pacemaker.
    b. If the surgical incision is near the shoulder, avoid overextending the joint.
    c. Keep handheld cellular phones at least 6 inches away from the generator.
    d. Avoid sources of strong electromagnetic fields, such as magnets.
    e. Avoid strenuous activities that may cause the device to discharge inappropriately.
    f. Carry a pacemaker identification card and wear a medical alert bracelet.

44. Which dysrhythmia results in asynchrony of atrial contraction and decreased cardiac output?
    a. Sinus tachycardia
    b. Atrial flutter
    c. Atrial fibrillation
    d. First-degree atrioventricular block

45. Which dysrhythmia causes the ventricles to quiver, resulting in absence of cardiac output?
    a. Ventricular tachycardia
    b. Ventricular fibrillation
    c. Asystole
    d. Third-degree heart block

46. Which are causes of atrial irritability and premature atrial contractions (PACs)? **Select all that apply.**
    a. Stress
    b. Caffeine
    c. Syncope
    d. Anxiety
    e. Infection
    f. Pulmonary hypotension

47. A patient is diagnosed with recurrent supraventricular tachycardia (SVT). What does the nurse do in order to accomplish the preferred treatment?
    a. Place the patient on the cardiac monitor and perform carotid massage.
    b. Give oxygen and establish IV access for antidysrhythmic drugs.
    c. Assist the provider in attempting atrial overdrive pacing.
    d. Provide information about radiofrequency catheter ablation therapy.

48. The patient has sustained supraventricular tachycardia (SVT), and the health care provider orders IV adenosine. Which important actions must the nurse perform when administering this drug? **Select all that apply.**
    a. Inject the drug slowly over 1 minute.
    b. Have emergency equipment at the bedside.
    c. Follow the drug injection with a normal saline bolus.
    d. Have injectable beta-blocker drugs at the bedside.
    e. Monitor the patient for bradycardia, nausea, and vomiting.
    f. Prepare for synchronized cardioversion immediately after giving adenosine.

49. Based on the prevalence and risk factors for atrial fibrillation (AF), which patient group is at highest risk for AF?
    a. Older adults
    b. Diabetics
    c. Substance abusers
    d. Pediatric cardiology patients

50. What are the risk factors for atrial fibrillation (AF)? **Select all that apply.**
    a. Chronic obstructive pulmonary disease (COPD)
    b. Hypertension
    c. Peripheral vascular disease
    d. Diabetes mellitus
    e. Valvular disease
    f. Excessive alcohol use

51. A patient with atrial fibrillation (AF) suddenly develops shortness of breath, chest pain, hemoptysis, and a feeling of impending doom. The nurse recognizes these symptoms as which complication?
    a. Pulmonary embolism
    b. Embolic stroke
    c. Absence of atrial kick
    d. Increased cardiac output

52. A patient scheduled to have elective cardioversion for atrial fibrillation (AF) will receive drug therapy for about 6 weeks **before** the procedure. What information about the drug therapy does the nurse teach the patient?
    a. Manage orthostatic hypotension
    b. Watch for bleeding signs
    c. Eat potassium-rich food sources
    d. Report muscle weakness or tremors

53. The patient has a diagnosis of paroxysmal atrial fibrillation (AF). Which statement is **most** accurate about this diagnosis?
    a. The patient experiences an episode within 7 days that converts back to sinus rhythm.
    b. The patient experiences episodes of AF that occur for longer than 7 days.
    c. The patient remains in AF and a decision is made not to restore or maintain sinus rhythm.
    d. The patient experiences AF in the absence of mitral valve disease or repair.

54. Traditionally, what medications will **most** likely be ordered for a patient with atrial fibrillation (AF)? **Select all that apply.**
    a. Diltiazem hydrochloride
    b. Furosemide
    c. Heparin
    d. Enoxaparin
    e. Sodium warfarin
    f. Metoprolol

55. A patient is about to undergo elective cardioversion. The nurse sets the defibrillator for synchronized mode so that the electrical shock is not delivered on the T wave. This is done to **avoid** which complication?
    a. Electrical burns to the skin
    b. Ventricular standstill
    c. Arcing from the electrodes
    d. Ventricular fibrillation (VF)

56. A patient has an implantable cardioverter defibrillator (ICD). In cardioversion shock, why is the defibrillator set in the synchronized mode?
    a. Avoid discharging the shock during the T wave
    b. Discharging the shock during the R wave
    c. Discharging the shock during the T wave
    d. Avoid discharging the shock during the Q wave

57. A patient with atrial fibrillation (AF) is scheduled to have an elective cardioversion. The nurse ensures that the patient has a prescription for a 4- to 6-week supply of which type of medication?
    a. Anticoagulants
    b. Digitalis
    c. Diuretics
    d. Potassium supplements

58. Which are nursing responsibilities after a patient receives an elective cardioversion to establish a normal heart rhythm? **Select all that apply.**
    a. Maintain an open airway.
    b. Remove oxygen devices.
    c. Assess vital signs and level of consciousness.
    d. Document results of the cardioversion.
    e. Provide sips of water or ice chips.
    f. Monitor for dysrhythmias.

59. The patient with atrial fibrillation (AF) is not a candidate for long-term anticoagulation therapy. Which procedure is **contraindicated** for this patient?
    a. Biventricular pacing
    b. Elective cardioversion
    c. Transthoracic pacing
    d. Radiofrequency catheter ablation

60. The nurse is caring for a patient with coronary artery disease (CAD). The patient reports palpitations and chest discomfort, and the nurse notes a tachydysrhythmia on the electrocardiogram (ECG) monitor. What does the nurse do next?
    a. Analyze the ECG strip.
    b. Notify the health care provider.
    c. Give supplemental oxygen.
    d. Administer a narcotic analgesic.

61. The nurse is taking the initial history and vital signs on a patient with fatigue. The nurse notes a regular apical pulse of 130 beats/min. The nurse assesses the patient for what contributing factors? **Select all that apply.**
    a. Anxiety or stress
    b. Fever
    c. Hypovolemia
    d. Anemia or hypoxemia
    e. Hypothyroidism
    f. Constipation

62. The nurse is taking a history and vital signs on a patient who has come to the clinic for a routine checkup. The patient has a pulse rate of 50 beats/min but denies any distress. What does the nurse do **next**?
    a. Give supplemental oxygen.
    b. Establish IV access.
    c. Complete the health history.
    d. Check the blood pressure.

63. The nurse is reviewing the monitored rhythms of several patients in the cardiac stepdown unit. The patient with which cardiac dysrhythmia has the greatest need of **immediate** attention?
    a. Chronic atrial fibrillation
    b. Paroxysmal supraventricular tachycardia (PSVT) that is suddenly terminated
    c. Sustained rapid ventricular response
    d. Sinus tachycardia with premature atrial complexes

64. The cardiac monitor of a postoperative patient shows four successive premature ventricular complexes (PVCs). How does the nurse interpret this finding?
    a. The ECG monitor is showing artifact.
    b. The patient had an episode of nonsustained ventricular tachycardia (NSVT).
    c. The monitor is showing two PVC couplets in a row.
    d. This rhythm may lead to idioventricular rhythm as seen in the dying heart.

65. The remote telemetry monitor technician alerts the nurse to the presence of premature ventricular contractions (PVCs) in a newly admitted patient. The patient's room has a bedside monitor. How does the nurse assess whether the premature complexes are providing perfusion to the extremities?
    a. Palpate peripheral arteries while observing the monitor for widened complexes.
    b. Auscultate for the apical heart sounds and listen for irregularities or pauses.
    c. Check the color and temperature of extremities and capillary refill of fingers and toes.
    d. Assess the ECG strip for regularity and width of QRS complexes.

66. What is the **primary** significance of ventricular tachycardia (VT) in a cardiac patient?
    a. It increases the ventricular filling time, therefore increasing cardiac output.
    b. It signals that the patient needs potassium supplement for replacement.
    c. It warrants immediate initiation of cardiopulmonary resuscitation.
    d. It is commonly the initial rhythm before deterioration into ventricular fibrillation (VF).

67. The nurse is interviewing a patient who suddenly becomes faint, immediately loses consciousness, and becomes pulseless and apneic. There is no blood pressure, and heart sounds are absent. The nurse has called for help. What does the nurse do **next**?
    a. Begin compressions.
    b. Defibrillate the patient.
    c. Establish IV access.
    d. Give supplemental oxygen.

68. A patient is in full cardiac arrest, and CPR is in progress. The electrocardiogram (ECG) monitor shows ventricular fibrillation. What does the nurse expect will be the **next** intervention?
    a. The patient will have an endotracheal tube placed.
    b. The patient will be defibrillated using the asynchronous mode.
    c. The health care provider will insert a central line for emergency drugs.
    d. Family members will be escorted to a waiting area and updated as needed.

69. A patient is diagnosed with torsades de pointes. The nurse prepares to administer which emergency medication?
    a. Magnesium sulfate
    b. Epinephrine
    c. Adenosine
    d. Calcium chloride

70. In a patient's record, the nurse notes frequent episodes of bradycardia and hypotension related to unintended vagal stimulation. Which instruction for this patient's care does the nurse relay to the unlicensed assistive personnel (UAP)?
    a. Avoid raising the patient's arms above the head during hygiene.
    b. Ambulate the patient slowly and stop frequently for brief rests.
    c. Generously lubricate rectal thermometer probes and insert very cautiously.
    d. Monitor the heart rate and rhythm if the patient is vomiting.

71. Excessive vagal stimulation can result from which activities? **Select all that apply.**
    a. Jogging outside
    b. Carotid sinus massage
    c. Suctioning a patient
    d. Voiding in a urinal
    e. Valsalva maneuver
    f. Bearing down as if having a bowel movement

72. The nurse is caring for several patients who have a dysrhythmia. What does the nurse teach each of the patients to do?
    a. Stay at least 4 feet away from a microwave oven that is operating.
    b. Avoid electronic metal detectors, such as those at airports.
    c. Learn the procedure for assessing the pulse.
    d. Purchase an automatic external defibrillator (AED) for home use.

73. A patient reports chest pain and dizziness after exertion, and the family reports a concurrent new onset of mild confusion in the patient, as well as difficulty concentrating. What is the **priority** problem for this patient?
    a. Activity intolerance
    b. Decreased cardiac output
    c. Acute confusion
    d. Inadequate oxygenation

74. According to the Vaughn-Williams classification of antidysrhythmics, which Class II drug controls dysrhythmias associated with excessive beta-adrenergic stimulation?
    a. Amiodarone hydrochloride
    b. Propranolol hydrochloride
    c. Diltiazem
    d. Verapamil hydrochloride

75. Which drug for symptomatic bradycardia does the nurse prepare to administer to a patient with a bradydysrhythmia?
    a. Epinephrine
    b. Atropine
    c. Calcium
    d. Lidocaine

76. Which safety precaution must be taken before defibrillating a patient with ventricular fibrillation (VF) or pulseless ventricular tachycardia (VT)?
    a. Make sure that the defibrillator is set on the synchronous mode.
    b. Disconnect the monitor leads to prevent electrical shorts.
    c. Be sure to hyperventilate the patient before the defibrillation.
    d. Command all health care team members to stand clear of the patient's bed.

77. The respiratory therapist (RT) and the medical student are ventilating a patient in cardiac arrest, while the nurse and health care provider are preparing the patient and equipment for intubation. At which point does the nurse intervene?
    a. The RT inserts an oropharyngeal airway.
    b. The medical student sets the oxygen flowmeter at 2 L/min.
    c. The RT ventilates with a manual resuscitation bag and mask.
    d. The medical student uses the chin-lift position on the patient.

78. The patient with episodes of stable ventricular tachycardia (VT) is scheduled to have an elective cardioversion. Which patient information will the nurse report **immediately** to the health care provider?
    a. The patient is prescribed digoxin 0.125 mg daily.
    b. The patient's urine output for the past 24 hours was 2100 mL.
    c. The patient's monitor shows runs of 12-20 PVCs.
    d. The patient takes a multivitamin every day.

79. A patient has had synchronized cardioversion for unstable ventricular tachycardia (VT). Which interventions does the nurse include in this patient's care **after** the procedure? **Select all that apply.**
    a. Administer therapeutic hypothermia.
    b. Assess vital signs and the level of consciousness.
    c. Administer antidysrhythmic drug therapy.
    d. Monitor for dysrhythmias.
    e. Monitor for loss of capture.
    f. Assess for chest burns from electrodes.

80. The nurse discovers a patient is unconscious and without palpable pulses and immediately initiates CPR. For what reason is CPR started on this patient?
    a. To identify the underlying heart rhythm
    b. For the rapid return of a pulse, blood pressure, and consciousness
    c. To prevent rib fractures or lacerations of the liver and spleen
    d. To mimic cardiac function until the defibrillator arrives

81. Automatic external defibrillator (AED) electrodes are placed on a patient who is unconscious and has no pulse. The nurse prepares to **immediately** defibrillate if the monitor analyzes which cardiac dysrhythmia?
    a. Third-degree heart block
    b. Pulseless electrical activity
    c. Ventricular fibrillation
    d. Idioventricular rhythm

82. A patient is found pulseless, and the cardiac monitor shows a rhythm that has no recognizable deflections, but instead has coarse "waves" of varying amplitudes. What is the **priority** Advanced Cardiac Life Support (ACLS) intervention for this rhythm?
    a. Immediate defibrillation
    b. Administration of epinephrine IV push
    c. Endotracheal intubation
    d. Noninvasive temporary pacing

83. For the patient who has been defibrillated due to ventricular fibrillation, what other essential interventions are needed as soon as possible **after** defibrillation? **Select all that apply.**
    a. High-quality CPR
    b. Placement of an invasive temporary pacemaker
    c. Administration of epinephrine, vasopressin, and atropine, as appropriate
    d. Identification and correction of the cause of the pulseless rhythm
    e. Continuous ECG monitoring
    f. Initiation of ACLS protocols as soon as possible

84. A patient has no pulse, and the cardiac monitor shows ventricular fibrillation (VF). Which drugs does the nurse prepare to administer during ACLS resuscitation? **Select all that apply.**
    a. Lidocaine
    b. Epinephrine
    c. Calcium chloride
    d. Amiodarone hydrochloride
    e. Dopamine hydrochloride
    f. Magnesium sulfate

85. Once ACLS resuscitation is begun after a patient's cardiac arrest, what is the medical-surgical nurse's role?
    a. To provide information about the patient including a brief summary of the patient's medical condition and the events that occurred up until the time of cardiac arrest
    b. To take the role of medication nurse and administer drugs as ordered by the team leader
    c. To remove all unnecessary equipment and people from the room so that the ACLS interventions can be performed more effectively
    d. To take any family members or friends to a quiet area and remain with them, offering emotional support

86. A patient's monitor shows new-onset atrial fibrillation, and the patient is scheduled for an elective cardioversion. The nurse sets the biphasic defibrillator on synchronous mode to deliver how many joules?
    a. 40-80 joules
    b. 80-120 joules
    c. 120-200 joules
    d. 200-360 joules

87. The nurse is performing defibrillation with an automated external defibrillator (AED). Which step is **most** vital this procedure?
    a. Placing the gel pads anterior over the apex and posterior for better conduction
    b. Allowing 1 minute for recharging before delivering another shock
    c. Ensuring that no personnel touch the patient at the time a shock is delivered
    d. Continuously ventilating the patient via a mouth-to-mask device during the defibrillation

88. What effect does Class IV drugs have on the cardiac conduction system?
    a. Stabilize membranes to decrease myocardial contractility
    b. Decrease heart rate and conduction velocity
    c. Lengthen the absolute refractory period and prolong repolarization
    d. Slow the flow of calcium into the cell during depolarization to depress automaticity

89. Which descriptions are characteristic of a Class III antidysrhythmic medication? **Select all that apply.**
    a. Lengthen the absolute refractory period
    b. Increase the force of the contraction
    c. Include hypertension as a side effect
    d. Prolong repolarization
    e. Include bradycardia as a side effect
    f. Prolong the QT interval

90. The nurse is teaching a patient with an implanted cardioverter defibrillator (ICD). What instruction does the nurse emphasize to the patient?
    a. Rest for several hours after an internal defibrillator shock before resuming activities.
    b. Have family members step away during the internal defibrillator shock for safety.
    c. Expect to cope with the discomfort and fear associated with having an ICD shock the heart.
    d. Report any pulse rate higher than what is set on the pacemaker.

91. The nurse is teaching a community group how to use an automatic external defibrillator (AED). What is the **first** step for using the AED that the nurse teaches?
    a. Rescuer presses the "analyze" button on the machine.
    b. Place the patient on a firm, dry surface.
    c. Rescuer stops CPR and directs anyone present to move away.
    d. Place two large adhesive-patch electrodes on the patient's chest.

92. The nurse is interviewing a patient with spontaneous ventricular tachycardia (VT) who may be a possible candidate for an implanted cardioverter defibrillator (ICD). The nurse senses that the patient is anxious. What is the nurse's **most** therapeutic response?
    a. "Your feelings are natural; patients report psychological distress related to ICD."
    b. "ICD is similar to defibrillation, which saved your life during the last episode."
    c. "You seem anxious. What are your concerns about having this treatment?"
    d. "Would you like to talk to the doctor about the details of the procedure?"

93. Which beta-blocker drug approved for use in treating dysrhythmias is also a Class III antidysrhythmic drug?
    a. Sotalol
    b. Esmolol
    c. Acebutolol
    d. Propanolol

*Interpret each ECG strip below. **Write your answers in the blanks provided.***

94.

RATE _____ RHYTHM _____ P WAVES _____

PR INTERVAL _____ QRS DURATION _____

INTERPRETATION _____

95.

RATE _____ RHYTHM _____ P WAVES _____

PR INTERVAL _____ QRS DURATION _____

INTERPRETATION _____

96.

RATE _____ RHYTHM _____ P WAVES _____

PR INTERVAL _____ QRS DURATION _____

INTERPRETATION _____

97.

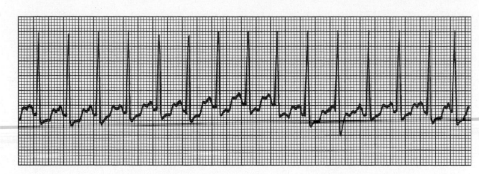

RATE _____   RHYTHM _____   P WAVES _____

PR INTERVAL _____   QRS DURATION _____

INTERPRETATION _____

98.

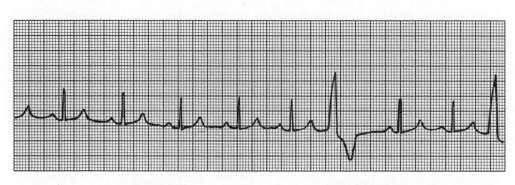

RATE _____   RHYTHM _____   P WAVES _____

PR INTERVAL _____   QRS DURATION _____

INTERPRETATION _____

99.

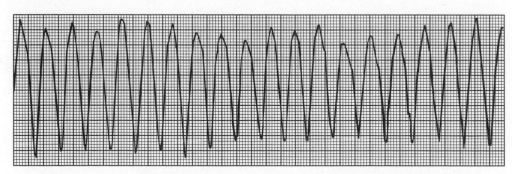

RATE _____   RHYTHM _____   P WAVES _____

PR INTERVAL _____   QRS DURATION _____

INTERPRETATION _____

100.

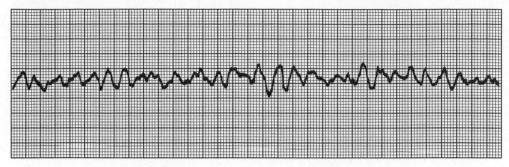

RATE _____   RHYTHM _____   P WAVES _____

PR INTERVAL _____   QRS DURATION _____

INTERPRETATION _____

101.

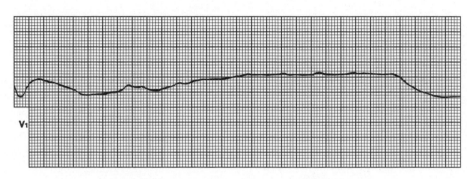

RATE _____   RHYTHM _____   P WAVES _____

PR INTERVAL _____   QRS DURATION _____

INTERPRETATION _____

102.

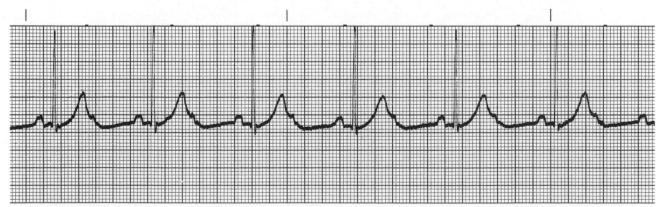

RATE _____   RHYTHM _____   P WAVES _____

PR INTERVAL _____   QRS DURATION _____

INTERPRETATION _____

35

CHAPTER

Care of Patients with Cardiac Problems

1. Which definition **best** describes left-sided heart failure?
   a. Increased volume and pressure develop and result in peripheral edema.
   b. It can occur when cardiac output remains normal or above normal.
   c. There is decreased tissue perfusion from poor cardiac output and pulmonary congestion from increased pressure in the pulmonary vessels.
   d. It is the percentage of blood ejected from the heart during systole.

2. During assessment of a patient with heart failure, the nurse notes that the patient's pulses alternate in strength. What does this assessment indicate to the nurse?
   a. Pulsus paradoxus
   b. Orthostatic hypotension
   c. Hypotension
   d. Pulsus alternans

3. When heart failure develops, what is the **initial** compensatory mechanism of the heart that maintains cardiac output?
   a. Sympathetic stimulation
   b. Parasympathetic stimulation
   c. Renin-angiotensin activation system (RAAS)
   d. Myocardial hypertrophy

4. When is B-type natriuretic peptide (BNP) produced and released for a patient with heart failure?
   a. When a patient has an enlarged liver
   b. When a patient has fluid overload
   c. When a patient's ejection fraction is lower than normal
   d. When a patient has ventricular hypertrophy

5. The nurse is taking a history on a patient recently diagnosed with heart failure. The patient admits to "sometimes having trouble catching my breath" but is unable to provide more specific details. What question does the nurse ask to gather more data about the patient's symptoms?
   a. "Do you have any medical problems, such as high blood pressure?"
   b. "What did your doctor tell you about your diagnosis?"
   c. "What was your most strenuous activity in the past week?"
   d. "How do you feel about being told that you have heart failure?"

6. The night shift nurse is listening to report and hears that a patient has paroxysmal nocturnal dyspnea. What does the nurse plan to do **next**?
   a. Instruct the patient to sleep in a side-lying position and then check on the patient every 2 hours to help with switching sides.
   b. Make the patient comfortable in a bedside recliner with several pillows to keep the patient more upright throughout the night.
   c. Check on the patient several hours after bedtime and assist the patient to sit upright and dangle the feet when dyspnea occurs.
   d. Check the patient frequently because the patient has insomnia due to a fear of suffocation.

7. The nurse is assessing a patient with right-sided heart failure. Which assessment findings does the nurse expect to see in this patient? **Select all that apply.**
   a. Dependent edema
   b. Weight loss
   c. Jugular venous distention
   d. Hypotension
   e. Hepatomegaly
   f. Angina

8. The nurse is assessing a patient with left-sided heart failure. Which assessment findings does the nurse expect to see in this patient? **Select all that apply.**
   a. Ascites
   b. S_3 heart sound
   c. Paroxysmal nocturnal dyspnea
   d. Jugular venous distention
   e. Oliguria during the day
   f. Wheezes or crackles

9. Based on the etiology and the **main** cause of heart failure, which patient has the greatest need for health promotion measures to prevent heart failure?
   a. Patient with Alzheimer's
   b. Patient with cystitis
   c. Patient with asthma
   d. Patient with hypertension

10. What is an **early** sign of left ventricular failure that a patient is most likely to report?
    a. Nocturia
    b. Weight gain
    c. Swollen legs
    d. Nocturnal coughing

11. The nurse is reviewing diagnostic test results for a patient who is hypertensive. Which laboratory result is an early warning sign of decreased heart compliance and prompts the nurse to **immediately** notify the health care provider?
    a. Normal B-type natriuretic peptide
    b. Decreased hemoglobin
    c. Elevated thyroxine (T_4)
    d. Presence of microalbuminuria

12. The nurse is interviewing a patient with a history of high blood pressure and heart problems. Which statement by the patient causes the nurse to suspect the patient may have heart failure?
    a. "I noticed a very fine red rash on my chest."
    b. "I had to take off my wedding ring last week."
    c. "I've had fever quite frequently."
    d. "I have pain in my shoulder when I cough."

13. A patient who was admitted for newly diagnosed heart failure is now being discharged. The nurse instructs the patient and family on how to manage heart failure at home. What **major** self-management categories should the nurse include? **Select all that apply.**
    a. Medications
    b. Weight
    c. Heart transplants
    d. Activity
    e. Diet
    f. What to do when symptoms get worse

14. A patient's bilateral radial pulses are occasionally weak and irregular. Which assessment technique does the nurse use **first** to investigate this finding?
    a. Check the color and the capillary refill in the upper extremities.
    b. Check the peripheral pulses in the lower extremities.
    c. Take the apical pulse for 1 minute, noting any irregularity in heart rhythm.
    d. Check the cardiac monitor for irregularities in rhythm.

15. A patient is at risk for heart failure but currently has no official medical diagnosis. While assessing the patient's lungs, the nurse hears profuse fine crackles. What does the nurse do **next**?
    a. Report the finding to the health care provider.
    b. Document the finding as a baseline for later comparison.
    c. Give the patient low-flow supplemental oxygen.
    d. Ask the patient to cough and reauscultate the lungs.

16. A patient is admitted for heart failure and has edema, neck vein distention, and ascites. What is the **most** reliable way to monitor fluid gain or loss in this patient?
    a. Check for pitting edema in the dependent body parts.
    b. Auscultate the lungs for crackles or wheezing.
    c. Assess skin turgor and the condition of mucous membranes.
    d. Weigh the patient daily at the same time with the same scale.

17. The home health nurse is evaluating a patient being treated for heart failure. Which statement by the patient is the **best** indicator of hope and well-being as a desired psychological outcome?
    a. "I'm taking the medication and following the doctor's orders."
    b. "I'm looking forward to dancing with my wife on our wedding anniversary."
    c. "I'm planning to go on a long trip; I'll never go back to the hospital again."
    d. "I want to thank you for all that you have done. I know you did your best."

18. The nurse is reviewing the laboratory results for a patient who was admitted with dyspnea. Which diagnostic test **best** differentiates between heart failure and lung dysfunction?
    a. Arterial blood gas
    b. B-type natriuretic peptide
    c. Hemoglobin
    d. Serum electrolytes

19. The nursing student is assisting in the care of a patient with advanced right-sided heart failure. In addition to bringing a stethoscope, what additional piece of equipment does the student bring in order to assess this patient?
    a. Tape measure
    b. Glasgow Coma Scale
    c. Portable Doppler
    d. Bladder ultrasound scanner

20. Which test is the **best** tool for diagnosing heart failure?
    a. Echocardiography
    b. Pulmonary artery catheter
    c. Radionuclide studies
    d. Multigated angiographic (MUGA) scan

21. A patient with heart failure has inadequate tissue perfusion. Which nursing interventions are included in the plan of care for this patient? **Select all that apply.**
    a. Monitor respiratory rate, rhythm, and quality every 1-4 hours.
    b. Auscultate breath sounds every 4-8 hours.
    c. Provide supplemental oxygen to maintain oxygen saturation at 90% or greater.
    d. Place the patient in a supine position with pillows under each leg.
    e. Assist the patient in performing coughing and deep-breathing exercises every 2 hours.
    f. Encourage the patient to perform all ADLs even when tired.

22. Which interventions are effective for a patient with a potential for pulmonary edema caused by heart failure? **Select all that apply.**
    a. Sodium and fluid restriction
    b. Slow infusion of hypotonic saline
    c. Administration of potassium
    d. Administration of loop diuretics
    e. Position in semi-Fowler's to high Fowler's position
    f. Weekly weight monitoring

23. An older adult patient with heart failure is volume depleted and has a low sodium level. The health care provider has ordered valsartan, an angiotensin receptor blocker (ARB). After the initial dose, for what complication does the nurse carefully monitor in this patient?
    a. Hypotension
    b. Cough
    c. Fluid retention
    d. Chest pain

24. The health care provider has ordered an angiotensin receptor blocker (ARB) for a patient with heart failure. The parameters are to maintain a systolic blood pressure ranging from 90 to 110 mm Hg. Today the patient has a blood pressure of 110/80 mm Hg but feels dizzy and lightheaded. What is the nurse's **first** priority action?
    a. Give the medication because blood pressure is within the parameters.
    b. Call the health care provider about the new onset of confusion.
    c. Hold the medication and document the new findings.
    d. Assess the patient for other symptoms of decreased tissue perfusion.

25. A patient with heart failure has excessive aldosterone secretion and is experiencing thirst and continuously asking for water. What instruction does the nurse give the unlicensed assistive personnel (UAP)?
    a. Severely restrict fluid to 500 mL plus output from the previous 24 hours.
    b. Give the patient as much water as desired to prevent dehydration.
    c. Restrict fluid to 2 L daily, with accurate intake and output.
    d. Frequently offer the patient ice chips and moistened toothettes.

26. A patient is prescribed diuretics for treatment of heart failure. Because of this therapy, the nurse pays particular attention to which laboratory test level?
    a. Peak and trough levels of the drugs
    b. Serum potassium
    c. Serum sodium
    d. Prothrombin time (PT)

27. An older adult patient is taking digoxin for treatment of heart failure. What is the **priority** nursing action for this patient related to the medication therapy?
    a. Give the medication in conjunction with an antacid.
    b. Keep the patient on the cardiac monitor and observe for ventricular dysrhythmias.
    c. Monitor for early signs of toxicity such as bradycardia on the ECG tracing.
    d. Advise the patient that there is increased mortality related to toxicity.

28. A patient is receiving digoxin therapy for heart failure. What assessment does the nurse perform **before** administering the medication?
    a. Auscultate the apical pulse rate and heart rhythm.
    b. Assess for nausea and abdominal distention.
    c. Auscultate the lungs for crackles.
    d. Check for increased urine output.

29. The nurse is reviewing the ECG of a patient on digoxin therapy. What **early** sign of digitalis toxicity does the nurse look for?
    a. Tachycardia
    b. Peaked T wave
    c. Atrial fibrillation
    d. Loss of P wave

30. Which laboratory test does the nurse monitor for potential cardiac problems and digoxin toxicity?
    a. Complete blood count
    b. Blood urea nitrogen (BUN)
    c. Serum potassium
    d. International Normalized Ratio (INR)

31. A patient is receiving an infusion of nesiritide for treatment of heart failure. What is the **priority** nursing assessment while administering this medication?
    a. Monitor for hypotension.
    b. Assess for cardiac dysrhythmias.
    c. Observe for respiratory depression.
    d. Monitor for peripheral vasoconstriction.

32. A patient has recently been diagnosed with acute heart failure. Which medication order does the nurse question?
    a. Dobutamine, a beta-adrenergic agonist
    b. Milrinone, a phosphodiesterase inhibitor
    c. Levosimendan, a positive inotropic
    d. Carvedilol, a beta blocker

33. A patient has an ejection fraction of less than 30%. The nurse prepares to provide patient education about which potential treatment?
    a. Automatic implantable cardioverter/defibrillator
    b. Heart transplant
    c. Mechanical implanted pump
    d. Ventricular reconstructive procedures

34. The nurse identifies a priority problem of fatigue and weakness for the patient with heart failure. After the patient ambulates 200 feet down the hall, the patient's blood pressure change is decreased by more than 20 mm Hg. How does the nurse interpret this data?
    a. The patient is building endurance.
    b. The activity is too stressful.
    c. The patient could walk farther.
    d. The activity is appropriate.

35. A patient with heart failure is anxious to recover quickly. After the patient ambulates with the UAP, the nurse observes that the patient has dyspnea. The nurse asks the patient to rate her exertion on a scale of 1 to 20, and the patient says, "I can keep going. It's only about a 15." What is the nurse's **best** response?
    a. "Slow down a bit; ideally you should be less than 12."
    b. "As long as you are less than 18, you can keep going."
    c. "Stop right now; you should not tax your heart beyond 5."
    d. "You should go slower; you cannot reach level 0 in one day."

36. Why does the nurse document the precise location of crackles auscultated in the lungs of a patient with heart failure?
    a. Crackles will eventually change to wheezes as the pulmonary edema worsens.
    b. The level of the fluid spreads laterally as the pulmonary edema worsens.
    c. The level of the fluid ascends as the pulmonary edema worsens.
    d. Crackles will eventually diminish as the pulmonary edema worsens.

37. A patient comes to the emergency department (ED) extremely anxious, tachycardic, struggling for air, and with a moist cough productive of frothy, blood-tinged sputum. What is the **priority** nursing intervention?
    a. Apply a pulse oximeter and cardiac monitor.
    b. Administer high-flow oxygen therapy via face mask.
    c. Prepare for continuous positive airway pressure ventilation.
    d. Prepare for intubation and mechanical ventilation.

38. A patient is treated for acute pulmonary edema. Which medications does the nurse prepare to administer to this patient? **Select all that apply.**
    a. Nitroglycerin SL
    b. Furosemide IV
    c. Morphine sulfate IV
    d. Metoprolol IV
    e. Nitroglycerin IV
    f. Oxygen by nasal cannula at 1 L/minute

39. What is the expected outcome for a patient with the collaborative problem of preventing and managing pulmonary edema?
    a. No dysrhythmias
    b. Clear lung sounds
    c. Less fatigue
    d. No disorientation

40. The nurse is teaching a patient with heart failure about signs and symptoms that suggest a return or worsening of heart failure. What does the nurse include in the teaching? **Select all that apply.**
    a. Rapid weight loss of 3 lbs in a week
    b. Increase in exercise tolerance lasting 2-3 days
    c. Cold symptoms (cough) lasting more than 3-5 days
    d. Excessive awakening at night to urinate
    e. Development of dyspnea or angina at rest or worsening angina
    f. Increased swelling in the feet, ankles, or hands

41. A patient is prescribed bumetanide. What is an important teaching point for the nurse to include about this medication?
    a. Caution to move slowly when changing positions, especially from lying to sitting
    b. Information about potassium-rich foods to include in the diet
    c. Written instructions on how to count the radial pulse rate
    d. Information about low-sodium diets and reading food labels for sodium content

42. The nurse is teaching a patient about the treatment regimen for heart failure. Which statement by the patient indicates a need for further instruction?
    a. "I must weigh myself once a month and watch for fluid retention."
    b. "If my heart feels like it is racing, I should call the doctor."
    c. "I'll need to consider my activities for the day and rest as needed."
    d. "I'll need periods of rest and activity, and I should avoid activity after meals."

43. Which characteristics describe mitral valve stenosis? **Select all that apply.**
    a. Classic signs of dyspnea, angina, and syncope.
    b. Rumbling apical diastolic murmur.
    c. S₃ often present due to severe regurgitation.
    d. Right-sided failure results in neck vein distention.
    e. The patient may experience palpitations while lying on the left side.
    f. Mild mitral stenosis is usually asymptomatic.

44. Which characteristics describe mitral valve prolapse? **Select all that apply.**
    a. Hepatomegaly is a late sign.
    b. Leaflets enlarge and fall back into left atrium during systole.
    c. Most patients are asymptomatic.
    d. Patients have normal heart rate and blood pressure.
    e. Mitral valve prolapse is becoming a disorder of aging populations.
    f. A midsystolic click and late systolic murmur can be heard at the apex of the heart.

45. A patient is diagnosed with moderate mitral valve stenosis. Which findings is the nurse most likely to encounter during the physical assessment of this patient? **Select all that apply.**
    a. Dyspnea on exertion
    b. Orthopnea
    c. Palpitations
    d. Asymptomatic
    e. Neck vein distention
    f. Early wet productive cough

46. The nurse hears in report that a patient has been diagnosed with mitral regurgitation (insufficiency). Which **early** symptom is most likely to be first reported by the patient?
    a. Atypical chest pain
    b. Chronic weakness
    c. Anxiety
    d. Dyspnea

47. A patient is diagnosed with mitral valve stenosis. Which finding warrants immediate notification of the health care provider because of the potential for decompensation?
    a. Irregular heart rhythm signifying atrial fibrillation
    b. Slow, bounding peripheral pulses associated with bradycardia
    c. An increase and decrease in pulse rate that follows inspiration and expiration
    d. An increase in pulse rate and blood pressure after exertion

48. The nurse is assessing the pulses of a patient with valvular disease and finds "bounding" arterial pulses. What is this finding **most** characteristic of?
    a. Aortic regurgitation
    b. Aortic stenosis
    c. Mitral valve prolapse
    d. Mitral insufficiency

49. A patient with a history of valvular heart disease requires an invasive dental procedure. The nurse notifies the health care provider to obtain a patient prescription for which type of medication?
    a. Anticoagulants
    b. Antihypertensives
    c. Antibiotics
    d. Antianginals

50. The patient is admitted with aortic stenosis. Diagnostic testing reveals that the surface area of the valve is less than 1 cm. Which **urgent** intervention is required at this time?
    a. Therapy with drugs that increase myocardial contractility
    b. Physical therapy consult to create an individualized exercise program
    c. Surgical heart valve replacement
    d. Aortic valvuloplasty in the cardiac catheterization lab

51. The nurse is assessing a patient at risk for valvular disease and finds pitting edema. This finding is a sign for which type of valvular disease?
    a. Mitral valve stenosis and insufficiency
    b. Aortic valve stenosis and insufficiency
    c. Tricuspid valve prolapse
    d. Mitral valve prolapse

52. The health care provider recommends to a patient that diagnostic testing be performed to assess for valvular heart disease. The nurse teaches the patient about which test that is commonly used for this purpose?
    a. Echocardiography
    b. Electrocardiography
    c. Exercise testing
    d. Thallium scanning

53. Long-term anticoagulant therapy for a patient with valvular heart disease and chronic atrial fibrillation includes which drug?
    a. Heparin sodium
    b. Warfarin sodium
    c. Diltiazem
    d. Enoxaparin

54. The surgical noninvasive intervention of a balloon valvuloplasty is often used for which type of patient?
    a. Young adults with a genetic valve defect
    b. Older adults who are nonsurgical candidates
    c. Adults whose open heart surgery failed
    d. Older adults who need replacement valves

55. The nurse is caring for a patient who had a valvuloplasty. The nurse monitors for which common complication in the **postprocedural** period?
    a. Myocardial infarction
    b. Angina
    c. Bleeding and emboli
    d. Infection

56. A patient with a prosthetic valve replacement must understand that postoperative care will include lifelong therapy with which type of medication?
    a. Antibiotics
    b. Anticoagulants
    c. Immunosuppressants
    d. Pain medication

57. A patient is a candidate for a xenograft valve. The nurse emphasizes that this type of valve does not require anticoagulant therapy but will require which intervention?
    a. Replacement in about 7-10 years
    b. An exercise program to develop collateral circulation
    c. Daily temperature checks to watch for signs of rejection
    d. Frequent monitoring for pulmonary edema

58. A patient is scheduled for valve surgery. Which medication does the nurse instruct the patient to discontinue at least 72 hours before the procedure?
    a. Antihypertensives
    b. Diuretics
    c. Anticoagulants
    d. Antibiotics

59. What is the **most** common problem for the patient with valvular heart disease?
    a. Reduced cardiac output
    b. Difficulty coping
    c. Shortness of breath
    d. Altered body image

60. The nurse is giving discharge instructions to a patient who had valve surgery. Which home care instructions does the nurse include in the teaching plan? **Select all that apply.**
    a. Increase consumption of foods high in vitamin K.
    b. Use an electric razor to avoid skin cuts.
    c. Report any bleeding or excessive bruising.
    d. Watch for and report any fever, drainage, or redness at the site.
    e. Avoid heavy lifting for 3-6 weeks.
    f. Report dyspnea, syncope, dizziness, edema, and palpitations.

61. The nurse assesses a patient and notes red, flat, pinpoint spots on the mucous membranes. Which finding has the nurse assessed?
    a. Pericardial friction rub
    b. Splinter hemorrhages
    c. Petechiae
    d. Systemic emboli

62. The patient has excess fluid in the pericardial cavity seen on echocardiogram. For which complication is the patient at increased risk?
    a. Pericardial friction rub
    b. Pulsus paradoxus
    c. Cardiac tamponade
    d. Systemic emboli

63. The patient has infective endocarditis. Which findings does the nurse expect when assessing this patient? **Select all that apply.**
    a. Pericardial friction rub
    b. Osler's nodes
    c. Petechiae
    d. A new regurgitant murmur
    e. Grating pain that is aggravated by breathing
    f. Fever associated with chills and night sweats

64. Which patients are at greatest risk of developing infective endocarditis? **Select all that apply.**
    a. IV drug user
    b. Patient with a myocardial infarction
    c. Patient with a prosthetic mitral valve replacement, postoperative
    d. Patient with mitral stenosis who recently had an abscessed tooth removed
    e. Older adult patient with urinary tract infection and valve damage
    f. Patient with cardiac dysrhythmias

65. A patient with aortic valve endocarditis reports fatigue and shortness of breath. Crackles are heard on lung auscultation. What do these assessment findings **most** likely indicate?
    a. Emboli to the lung
    b. Valve incompetence resulting in heart failure
    c. Valve stenosis resulting in increased chamber size
    d. Coronary artery disease

66. A patient is admitted for possible infective endocarditis. Which test does the nurse anticipate will be performed to confirm a positive diagnosis?
    a. CT scan
    b. MRI
    c. Blood cultures
    d. Echocardiogram

67. A patient is diagnosed with new-onset infective endocarditis. Which recent procedure is the patient **most** likely to report?
    a. Teeth cleaning
    b. Urinary bladder catheterization
    c. Chest radiography
    d. ECG

68. In what way does arterial embolization to the brain manifest itself in a patient with infective endocarditis?
    a. Dysarthria
    b. Dysphagia
    c. Atelectasis
    d. Electrolyte imbalances

69. Which treatment intervention applies to a patient with infective endocarditis?
    a. Administration of oral penicillin for 6 weeks or more
    b. Hospitalization for initial IV antibiotics; then home to continue IV therapy
    c. Complete bedrest for the duration of treatment
    d. Long-term anticoagulation therapy with heparin followed by oral warfarin

70. What is the definitive treatment for a patient with chronic constrictive pericarditis?
    a. Antibiotic therapy
    b. Surgical excision of the pericardium
    c. Administration of beta blockers and corticosteroids
    d. Pericardiocentesis

71. A patient is admitted to the unit with assessment findings that include substernal pain that radiates to the left shoulder. The pain is described by the patient as grating, and is worse with inspiration and coughing. What likely is the cause of this patient's symptoms?
    a. Chronic constrictive pericarditis
    b. Cardiac tamponade
    c. Hypertrophic cardiomyopathy
    d. Acute pericarditis

72. Which signs/symptoms occur with chronic constrictive pericarditis? **Select all that apply.**
    a. Thick, rigid pericardium
    b. Stiff heart valves
    c. Jugular venous distention
    d. Crackles and wheezes
    e. Exertional fatigue and dyspnea
    f. Dependent edema

73. The nurse is assessing a patient with pericarditis. In order to hear a pericardial friction rub, which stethoscope technique does the nurse use?
    a. Place the diaphragm at the apex of the heart.
    b. Place the diaphragm at the left lower sternal border.
    c. Place the bell just below the left clavicle.
    d. Place the bell at several points while the patient holds his or her breath.

74. A patient is admitted for pericarditis. In order to assist the patient to feel more comfortable, what does the nurse instruct the patient to do?
    a. Sit in a semi-Fowler's position with pillows under the arms.
    b. Lie on the side in a fetal position.
    c. Sit up and lean forward.
    d. Lie down and bend the legs at the knees.

75. The nurse is reviewing the ECG of a patient admitted for acute pericarditis. Which ECG change does the nurse anticipate?
    a. Normal ECG
    b. ST-T spiking
    c. Peaked T waves
    d. Wide QRS complexes

76. A patient is admitted for pericarditis. How will the patient likely describe his pain?
    a. Grating substernal pain that is aggravated by inspiration
    b. Sharp pain that radiates down the left arm
    c. Dull ache that feels vaguely like indigestion
    d. Continuous boring pain that is relieved with rest

77. Which are proposed criteria for diagnosis of acute pericarditis? **Select all that apply.**
    a. Pericardial chest pain
    b. Chest pain lasts longer than 3 months
    c. Presence of pericardial friction rub
    d. New ST elevation on all ECG leads
    e. Hepatic engorgement
    f. New or worsening pericardial effusion

78. What is the common treatment for rheumatic carditis?
    a. Pericardiocentesis
    b. Antibiotics for 10 days
    c. Pain medication for substernal pain control
    d. Rest with observation for further necessary treatment

79. Which are signs and symptoms of rheumatic carditis? **Select all that apply.**
    a. Cardiomegaly (enlarged heart)
    b. Bradycardia
    c. New murmur development
    d. Existing streptococcal infection
    e. Metabolic acidosis
    f. Pericardial friction rub

80. Assessment findings for a patient with acute pericarditis include neck vein distention, clear lungs, muffled heart sounds, tachycardia, tachypnea, and a greater than 10 mm Hg difference in systolic pressure on inspiration than on expiration. What is the nurse's first response to these assessment findings?
    a. Continue to monitor the patient; these are normal signs of pericarditis.
    b. Administer oxygen and immediately report the findings to the health care provider.
    c. Monitor oxygen saturation and seek order for pain medication to control symptoms.
    d. Check ECG, administer morphine for pain, and administer diuretics.

81. A patient had an emergency pericardiocentesis for cardiac tamponade. Which nursing interventions are included in the postprocedural care of this patient? **Select all that apply.**
    a. Closely monitor for the recurrence of tamponade.
    b. Be prepared to provide adequate fluid volumes to increase cardiac output.
    c. Prepare the patient for emergency sternotomy if tamponade recurs.
    d. Administer diuretics to decrease fluid volumes around the heart.
    e. Send the pericardial effusion specimen to the laboratory for culture.
    f. Keep the patient on bedrest and supine for at least 24 hours.

82. Which is a characteristic of dilated cardiomyopathy?
    a. Results from replacement of myocardial tissue with fibrous tissue
    b. Causes stiff ventricles that restrict filling during diastole
    c. Causes symptoms of left ventricular failure
    d. Causes right ventricular failure early in the disease

83. Which type of cardiomyopathy results from replacement of myocardial tissue with fibrous and fatty tissue?
    a. Hypertrophic cardiomyopathy
    b. Arrhythmogenic right ventricular cardiomyopathy
    c. Dilated cardiomyopathy
    d. Restrictive cardiomyopathy

84. A patient may die without any symptoms from which type of cardiomyopathy?
    a. Dilated cardiomyopathy
    b. Arrhythmogenic right ventricular cardiomyopathy
    c. Restrictive cardiomyopathy
    d. Hypertrophic cardiomyopathy

85. The cause of dilated cardiomyopathy may include which factors? **Select all that apply.**
    a. Alcohol abuse
    b. Sedentary lifestyle
    c. Infection
    d. Chemotherapy
    e. Poor nutrition
    f. Cigarette smoking

86. Which descriptions accurately characterize restrictive cardiomyopathy? **Select all that apply.**
    a. Prognosis is poor.
    b. Symptoms are similar to left- or right-sided heart failure.
    c. Some patients die without any symptoms.
    d. It is the most common type of cardiomyopathy.
    e. It is the rarest of cardiomyopathies.
    f. Filling is restricted during diastole.

87. A patient who reports having a sore throat 2 weeks ago now reports chest pain. On physical assessment, the nurse hears a new murmur, pericardial friction rub, and tachycardia. The electrocardiogram (ECG) shows a prolonged P-R interval. What condition does the nurse suspect in this patient?
    a. Rheumatic carditis
    b. Heart failure
    c. Cardiomyopathy
    d. Aortic stenosis

88. A patient has received a heart transplant for dilated cardiomyopathy. Because the patient has a high risk for cardiac tamponade, for which signs/symptoms does the nurse **immediately** notify the health care provider?
    a. Crackles and wheezes of the lungs
    b. Pulsus paradoxus and muffled heart sounds
    c. Hepatomegaly and ascites
    d. Dependent edema and fluid retention

89. The nurse is assessing a patient who has received a heart transplant. Which clinical manifestations suggest transplant rejection? **Select all that apply.**
    a. Shortness of breath
    b. Depression
    c. Severe abdominal pain
    d. New bradycardia
    e. Hypotension
    f. Decreased activity tolerance

90. Which patient meets the criteria for selection as a candidate for heart transplant surgery?
    a. Patient with life expectancy of 3-5 years
    b. Patient who is over 75 years of age
    c. Patient who is New York Heart Association (NYHA) class III
    d. Patient who drinks 5-6 beers every day

91. Which priority medical surgical concept applies to a patient with heart failure?
    a. Gas exchange
    b. Infection
    c. Perfusion
    d. Comfort

36 CHAPTER

Care of Patients with Vascular Problems

1. Atherosclerosis affects which larger arteries? **Select all that apply.**
   a. Renal
   b. Femoral
   c. Coronary
   d. Brachial cephalic
   e. Aorta
   f. Carotid

2. An African-American male is being seen for a blister on the right toe. What factors **increase** this patient's risk for developing atherosclerosis? **Select all that apply.**
   a. 20-year history of type 1 diabetes
   b. Sedentary lifestyle
   c. Father with history of colon cancer
   d. 35 lbs overweight
   e. Grandmother who died after myocardial infarction
   f. Drinking 2-3 diet sodas per day

3. Which factors can increase systemic arterial pressure? **Select all that apply.**
   a. Decreased cardiac output
   b. Increased heart rate
   c. Increased peripheral vascular resistance
   d. Increased stroke volume
   e. Decreased blood pressure
   f. Decreased stroke volume

4. Which blood pressure is considered normal for an adult patient over 60 years of age?
   a. 162/92 mm Hg
   b. 150/94 mm Hg
   c. 156/90 mm Hg
   d. 144/88 mm Hg

5. A patient is admitted with a vascular problem. Based on the pathophysiology of systemic arterial pressure, the systemic arterial pressure is a product of what factors? **Select all that apply.**
   a. Cardiac output
   b. Norepinephrine
   c. Preload
   d. Total peripheral vascular resistance
   e. Diastolic blood pressure
   f. Afterload

6. A patient's cholesterol screening shows a low-density lipoprotein cholesterol (LDL-C) value greater than 190 mg/dL. What is the nurse's **best** interpretation of these results?
   a. All patients with LDL-C equal to or greater than 190 mg/dL should be evaluated for secondary causes of hyperlipidemia and treated with statin therapy.
   b. Any patient with a low LDL-C value should be routinely followed with every 6 month lipid profile values monitoring to see trends in this value.
   c. This patient should be taught to exercise 6-7 days a week to help bring the LDL-C value down over time.
   d. Repeat total cholesterol and LDL-C cholesterol testing during the next routine exam.

7. The nurse is counseling a group of women about cholesterol-lowering drugs. Which drug will decrease blood pressure while decreasing triglycerides (TGs), increasing high-density lipoprotein (HDL), and lowering low-density lipoprotein (LDL)?
   a. Ezetimibe
   b. Caduet
   c. Vytorin
   d. Advicor

8. The nurse is conducting dietary teaching with a patient. Which statement by the patient indicates an understanding of fat sources and the need to limit saturated fats?
   a. "Coconut oil has a rich flavor and is a good cooking oil."
   b. "Sunflower oil is high in saturated fats, so I should avoid it."
   c. "Meat and eggs mostly contain unsaturated fats."
   d. "Canola oil has monounsaturated fat and is recommended."

9. The nurse educates and advises a patient to follow the Dietary Approaches to Stop Hypertension (DASH) diet. Which instructions does the nurse give to the patient? **Select all that apply.**
   a. Consume a dietary pattern that emphasizes intake of lean protein.
   b. Consume low-fat dairy products, poultry, and fish.
   c. Lower sodium intake to no more than 2400 mg per day.
   d. Engage in aerobic physical activity 6-7 times a week.
   e. Limit intake of sweets and red meats.
   f. Eat legumes, nontropical vegetable oils (e.g., canola), and nuts.

10. A patient is prescribed atorvastatin. The nurse instructs the patient to watch for and report which side effect?
    a. Nausea and vomiting
    b. Cough
    c. Headaches
    d. Muscle cramps

11. A patient gets a new prescription for Pravigard for treatment of high cholesterol. Because this is a combination drug, the nurse alerts the physician when the patient discloses an allergy to which drug?
    a. Sulfa
    b. Aspirin
    c. Some calcium channel blockers
    d. Some diuretics

12. A patient is prescribed niacin (Niaspan) to lower low-density lipoprotein cholesterol (LDL-C) and very-low-density lipoprotein (VLDL). Why are lower doses prescribed to the patient?
    a. To reduce side effects of flushing and feeling warm
    b. To prevent muscle myopathies
    c. To prevent elevation of blood pressure
    d. To prevent undesirable hypokalemia

13. The nurse is conducting an initial cardiovascular assessment on a middle-aged patient. What techniques does the nurse employ in the assessment? **Select all that apply.**
    a. Take blood pressure on the dominant arm.
    b. Palpate pulses at all of the major sites.
    c. Palpate for temperature differences in the lower extremities.
    d. Perform bilateral but separate palpation on the carotid arteries.
    e. Auscultate for bruits in the radial and brachial arteries.
    f. Check for orthostatic hypotension.

14. The nurse is performing blood pressure screening at a community center. Which patients are referred for evaluation of their blood pressure? **Select all that apply.**
    a. Diabetic patient with a blood pressure of 118/78 mm Hg
    b. Patient with heart disease with a blood pressure of 134/90 mm Hg
    c. Patient with no known health problems who has a blood pressure of 125/86 mm Hg
    d. Diabetic patient with a blood pressure of 180/80 mm Hg
    e. Patient with no known health problems who has a blood pressure of 106/70 mm Hg
    f. Patient with muscle cramping who is prescribed a statin drug

15. The home health nurse is making the initial visit to an older adult patient with hypertension. The nurse recommends that the patient obtain which item for home use?
    a. Ambulatory blood pressure monitoring device
    b. Exercise bicycle
    c. Blood glucose monitor scale
    d. Food scale

16. The nurse is evaluating the blood pressure of a 75-year-old woman. Based on current research, which finding is the **better** indicator of heart disease risk for this patient?
    a. Diastolic of 86 mm Hg
    b. Systolic of 160 mm Hg
    c. Blood pressure of 138/68 mm Hg
    d. Blood pressure of 110/90 mm Hg

17. A 32-year-old patient with diabetes reports sudden onset of headaches, blurred vision, and dyspnea. The patient's blood pressure is normally 120/80 mm Hg but today is 200/130 mm Hg. What condition does the nurse suspect?
    a. Sustained hypertension
    b. Malignant hypertension
    c. Primary hypertension
    d. Secondary hypertension

18. Which are risk factors for hypertension? **Select all that apply.**
    a. Age greater than 40 years
    b. Family history of hypertension
    c. Excessive calorie consumption
    d. Physical inactivity
    e. Excessive alcohol intake
    f. Hypolipidemia

19. The nurse is reviewing the results of urine tests for a patient with a medical diagnosis of essential hypertension. The presence of catecholamines in the urine is evidence of which disorder?
    a. Renal failure
    b. Primary aldosteronism
    c. Cushing's syndrome
    d. Pheochromocytoma

20. The nurse is reviewing the electrocardiogram (ECG) for a patient with a medical diagnosis of essential hypertension. What is the first ECG sign of heart disease resulting from hypertension?
    a. Left atrial and ventricular hypertrophy
    b. Right atrial and ventricular atrophy
    c. Malfunction of the sinoatrial (SA) node
    d. Malfunction of the atrioventricular (AV) node

21. Which blood pressure finding for a 55-year-old adult patient with no other medical problems would warrant **further** evaluation for hypertension?
    a. 128/78 mm Hg
    b. 134/80 mm Hg
    c. 146/88 mm Hg
    d. 152/94 mm Hg

22. A middle-aged patient with no health insurance has tried lifestyle modifications to control uncomplicated hypertension but continues to struggle. What is considered a **first** drug of choice for this patient?
    a. Calcium channel blocker
    b. Alpha blocker
    c. Thiazide-type diuretic
    d. Angiotensin-converting enzyme inhibitor

23. The nurse is reviewing the medication schedule for an older adult patient who needs medication for hypertension. The patient lives alone but is able to manage self-care. What frequency of drug therapy does the nurse advocate for this patient?
    a. Once a day
    b. Two times a day
    c. Three times a day
    d. Four times a day

24. The nurse is reviewing prescriptions for a patient recently diagnosed with hypertension. The nurse **questions** a prescription for which type of drug?
    a. Angiotensin II receptor blockers
    b. Alpha blocker
    c. Thiazide diuretic
    d. ACE inhibitor

25. For which patient does the nurse question the use of hydrochlorothiazide?
    a. Asthmatic patient
    b. Patient with chronic airway limitation
    c. Patient with hyperkalemia
    d. Patient with hypokalemia

26. The nurse is teaching a patient about taking hydrochlorothiazide. Which foods does the nurse instruct the patient to eat in conjunction with the use of this drug?
    a. Bananas and oranges
    b. Milk and cheese
    c. Cranberries and prunes
    d. Cabbage and cauliflower

27. A patient reports dizziness when changing positions from sitting to standing and a sudden dry cough after starting a prescription for captopril. Which nursing intervention is **most** useful for this patient?
    a. Instruct the patient to change positions slowly and take an over-the-counter cough syrup.
    b. Tell the patient to take the medication at bedtime and use over-the-counter throat lozenges.
    c. Notify the health care provider because the medication should be discontinued.
    d. Teach the patient to increase her fluid intake.

28. Which intervention renders angiotensin II receptor blockers (ARBs) and ACE inhibitors effective in African Americans?
    a. Drug is taken with a diuretic, a beta blocker, or a calcium channel blocker.
    b. Give at a much higher dosage than for other ethnic groups.
    c. Combine with rigorous lifestyle modification.
    d. Take around the clock on a very individualized schedule.

29. The nurse is reviewing antihypertensive medication orders for a patient with asthma. The nurse **questions** the use of which type of medication?
    a. Cardioselective beta blockers because they reduce cardiac output
    b. Noncardioselective beta blockers because they may cause bronchoconstriction
    c. ACE inhibitors because they cause a nagging cough
    d. Thiazide diuretics because they promote potassium excretion

30. The nurse prepares to teach a patient recovering from a myocardial infarction (MI) about combination drug therapy based on "best practices" for controlling hypertension. Which drugs does the nurse include in the teaching plan? **Select all that apply.**
    a. Beta blockers
    b. ACE inhibitors
    c. Acetaminophen
    d. Angiotensin II receptor blockers
    e. Central alpha-agonists
    f. NSAIDs

31. The student nurse is giving a patient with benign prostatic hyperplasia a morning dose of furosemide. The student says, "This is your blood pressure medicine," but the patient responds, "I don't have high blood pressure." What does the student nurse do next?
    a. Explain to the patient that his blood pressure is not high because the drug is controlling it.
    b. Stop and recheck the medication administration record and then do additional drug research.
    c. Recheck the blood pressure and then hold the drug if the blood pressure is not elevated.
    d. Contact the charge nurse for advice about how to handle the patient's refusal.

32. A patient admits difficulty with long-term adherence to antihypertensive therapy. Which nursing interventions promote compliance for this patient? **Select all that apply.**
    a. Carefully review all medication instructions with the patient.
    b. Give the patient a list of resources for finding information on the medications.
    c. Reinforce the fact that damage to organs occurs even if there are no symptoms.
    d. Teach the patient about the continuous ambulatory blood pressure monitoring device.
    e. Assess the patient's resources to obtain medications.
    f. Advocate for medications that are taken three times a day for better BP control.

33. The nurse is reviewing medical records for several patients with kidney problems and hypertension or the potential for hypertension. Which patient does the nurse expect to be screened for renal artery stenosis?
    a. Patient with a history of kidney stones
    b. Patient taking multiple antihypertensive drugs at high doses
    c. Patient with newly diagnosed hypertension
    d. Patient with a history of frequent urinary tract infections

34. The nurse assesses a patient and documents the following findings: "edema 2+ bilateral ankles, brown pigmentation of lower extremities skin, aching pain of lower extremities when standing that is relieved with elevation." What condition does the patient likely have?
    a. Deep vein thrombosis
    b. Venous insufficiency
    c. Peripheral arterial disease
    d. Raynaud's syndrome

35. The nurse assesses a patient and documents the following findings: "decreased pedal and posterior tibial pulses bilateral (1+), skin is cool-to-cold to touch, loss of hair on lower extremities, patient reports that lower extremity pain is reproducible when walking and relieved by rest, and also noted are thickened toenails." What condition does the patient likely have?
    a. Peripheral venous disease
    b. Deep vein thrombosis
    c. Raynaud's syndrome
    d. Peripheral arterial disease

36. Which patients are at risk for peripheral arterial disease (PAD)? **Select all that apply.**
    a. Patient with hypertension
    b. Patient with diabetes mellitus
    c. Patient who is a cigarette smoker
    d. Patient with anemia
    e. Patient who is very thin
    f. African-American patient

37. For which symptom do most patients seek medical attention when they have peripheral arterial disease?
    a. Intermittent claudication
    b. Pain at rest
    c. Redness in the extremity
    d. Muscle atrophy

38. The nurse is caring for a patient with a medical diagnosis of inflow peripheral arterial disease. Which symptom does the nurse expect the patient to report?
    a. Very frequent episodes of rest pain
    b. Discomfort in the lower back, buttocks, or thighs after walking
    c. Burning or cramping in the calves, ankles, feet, or toes after walking
    d. Waking frequently at night to hang the feet off the bed

39. The nurse is assessing the lower extremity of a patient with peripheral arterial disease. What pulse(s) does the nurse palpate?
    a. Posterior tibial pulse of the affected leg
    b. Pedal pulse in both feet
    c. All pulses in both legs
    d. Strength of the pulses in the affected leg

40. While assessing a patient, the nurse sees a small, round ulcer with a "punched out" appearance and well-defined borders on the great toe. The patient reports the ulcer is painful. How does the nurse interpret this finding?
    a. Venous stasis ulcer
    b. Diabetic ulcer
    c. Gangrenous ulcer
    d. Arterial ulcer

41. A patient is undergoing diagnostic testing for pain and burning sensation in the legs. What does an ankle-brachial index (ABI) of less than 0.9 in either leg indicate?
    a. Normal arterial circulation to the lower extremities
    b. Presence of peripheral arterial disease
    c. Severe venous disease of the lower extremities
    d. Need for immediate surgical intervention

42. The nurse is consulting with the physical therapist to design an exercise program for patients with peripheral vascular disease. Which patient is a candidate for an exercise program?
    a. Patient with severe rest pain
    b. Patient with intermittent claudication
    c. Patient with gangrene
    d. Patient with venous ulcers

43. A patient with peripheral arterial disease asks, "Why should I exercise when walking several blocks seems to make my leg cramp up?" What is the nurse's **best** response?
    a. "Exercise may improve blood flow to your leg because small vessels will compensate for blood vessels that are blocked off."
    b. "This type of therapy is free and you can do it by yourself to improve the muscles in your legs."
    c. "The cramping will eventually stop if you continue the exercise routine. If you have too much pain, just rest for a while."
    d. "Exercise is a noninvasive nonsurgical technique that is used to increase arterial flow to the affected limb."

44. The nurse is teaching a patient with peripheral arterial disease about positioning and position changes. What suggestion does the nurse give to the patient?
    a. Sit upright in a chair if legs are not swollen.
    b. Sleep with legs above the heart level if legs are swollen.
    c. Avoid crossing the legs at all times.
    d. Change positions slowly when getting out of bed.

45. The nurse is instructing a patient with peripheral arterial disease (PAD) about ways to promote vasodilation. What information does the nurse include? **Select all that apply.**
    a. Maintain a warm environment at home.
    b. Wear socks or insulated shoes at all times.
    c. Apply direct heat to the limb by using a heating pad.
    d. Prevent cold exposure of the affected limb.
    e. Limit fluids to prevent increased blood viscosity.
    f. Completely abstain from smoking or chewing tobacco.

46. The nurse is assessing a patient at risk for peripheral vascular disease. Which assessment finding indicates arterial ulcers rather than diabetic or venous ulcers?
    a. Ulcer located over the pressure points of the feet
    b. Ulcer located on plantar surface of foot
    c. Severe pain or discomfort occurring at the ulcer site
    d. Associated ankle discoloration and edema

47. Which are complications that can result from severe peripheral arterial disease? **Select all that apply.**
    a. Gangrene
    b. Varicose veins
    c. Aneurysm
    d. Amputation
    e. Ulcer formation
    f. Valve damage

48. Which drugs are used to promote circulation in a patient with chronic peripheral arterial disease? **Select all that apply.**
    a. Pentoxifylline
    b. Propranolol hydrochloride
    c. Aspirin
    d. Clopidogrel
    e. Ezetimibe
    f. Cilostazol

49. Which statements pertaining to a percutaneous transluminal balloon angioplasty are correct? **Select all that apply.**
    a. One or more arteries are dilated with a balloon catheter to open the vessel.
    b. It is a minor surgical procedure.
    c. Stents may be placed to ensure adequate blood flow.
    d. Placement of stents results in a longer hospital stay.
    e. Some patients are occlusion-free for 3-5 years.
    f. Patients must have occlusions or stenoses that are accessible to the catheter.

50. A patient with peripheral arterial disease is scheduled to have percutaneous transluminal intervention. What information does the nurse give the patient about this procedure?
    a. It is usually used when amputation is inevitable.
    b. Reocclusion may occur afterwards and the procedure may be repeated.
    c. Most patients are occlusion-free afterwards, particularly if stents are placed.
    d. It is painless and there are very few risks or dangers.

51. A patient has returned to the unit after having percutaneous transluminal intervention. What nursing actions are included in the routine **postprocedural** care of this patient? **Select all that apply.**
    a. Observe for bleeding at the puncture site.
    b. Observe vital signs frequently.
    c. Perform frequent checks of the distal pulses in both limbs.
    d. Encourage bedrest with the limb straight for about 1 to 2 hours.
    e. Administer antiplatelet therapy as ordered.
    f. Provide supplemental oxygen via nasal cannula.

52. A patient has returned to the unit after surgery for arterial revascularization with graft placement. The nurse monitors for graft occlusion, which is **most** likely to occur within which time frame?
    a. First 2 hours
    b. First 24 hours
    c. Next 2 days
    d. First week

53. A patient is in the postanesthesia care unit (PACU) after surgery for arterial revascularization with graft placement. Which procedure does the nurse use to check the patency of the graft?
    a. Check the extremity every 15 minutes for the first hour, then hourly, for changes in color, temperature, and pulse intensity.
    b. Check the dorsalis pedis pulse every 15 minutes for the first hour, then hourly.
    c. Ask the patient if there is any pain or loss of sensation anywhere in the extremity, and withhold patient-controlled analgesia.
    d. Gently palpate the site every 15 minutes for the first hour and assess for warmth, redness, and edema.

54. A patient has returned to the unit after a percutaneous transluminal intervention. What is the postprocedural nursing priority?
    a. Pain management
    b. Checking the distal pulses
    c. Early ambulation to prevent complications
    d. Monitoring for bleeding at the puncture site

55. The student nurse is assisting in the care of a patient returning from the PACU after aortofemoral bypass. The nurse intervenes when the student performs which action?
    a. Offers to obtain a meal tray for the patient
    b. Demonstrates to the patient how to use the incentive spirometer
    c. Encourages the patient to deep-breathe every 1-2 hours
    d. Explains to the patient the purpose of 24-hour bedrest

56. A patient has had surgery for arterial revascularization with graft placement. The nurse notes swelling and tenseness of the skin tissue, and the patient reports an increasing pain with numbness and tingling, as well as a decrease in the ability to wiggle toes and ankles. What does the nurse suspect is occurring with this patient?
    a. Graft infection
    b. Compartment syndrome
    c. Graft occlusion
    d. Reaction to thrombolytic therapy

57. A patient has had aortoiliac bypass surgery with graft placement. The nurse notes induration, erythema, tenderness, warmth, edema, and drainage at the site. Before calling the physician, what **additional** assessment does the nurse perform?
    a. Palpates the patient's abdomen and checks for the last bowel movement
    b. Auscultates the patient's lung sounds and checks the pulse oximeter reading
    c. Assesses the patient for signs of occult bleeding and looks at the prothrombin time results
    d. Checks the patient's temperature and looks at the white blood cell results

58. A patient is admitted with a medical diagnosis of acute arterial occlusion. What documentation does the nurse expect to see in this patient's medical record?
    a. Acute MI and/or atrial fibrillation within the previous weeks
    b. History of chronic venous stasis disease treated with debridement and wound care
    c. History of Marfan syndrome or Ehlers-Danlos syndrome
    d. Episode of blunt trauma that occurred several months ago

59. A patient with an acute arterial occlusion requires abciximab. What nursing responsibilities are associated with the administration of this medication?
    a. Platelet counts must be monitored at 3, 6, and 12 hours after the start of the infusion.
    b. For platelet counts over 100,000/mm^3, infusion must be readjusted or discontinued.
    c. Monitor for manifestations of rash, itching, or swelling.
    d. Monitor for edema, pain on passive movement, or poor capillary refill.

60. Which is a postoperative nursing intervention for a patient with arterial revascularization?
    a. Promote graft patency by limiting IV fluid infusion.
    b. Instruct the patient to avoid bending at the hips or knees.
    c. Resume regular diet immediately after surgery.
    d. Avoid coughing and deep-breathing exercises.

61. Which statements are accurate about true aneurysms? **Select all that apply.**
    a. Permanent dilatation of an artery
    b. Enlarged artery to at least 2 times the normal diameter
    c. Formed when blood accumulates in the wall of the artery
    d. Are a result of arterial injury or trauma
    e. Arterial wall is congenitally weakened
    f. Aneurysms can be described as false aneurysms or true aneurysms.

62. The nurse is reviewing a patient's abdominal CT scan and notes that the patient has an out-pouched segment coming off of the abdominal aorta. What is the nurse's **best** interpretation of these results?
    a. Dissecting aneurysm
    b. Saccular aneurysm
    c. Fusiform aneurysm
    d. False aneurysm

63. What is the most common location for an aneurysm?
    a. Abdominal aorta
    b. Thoracic aorta
    c. Femoral arteries
    d. Popliteal arteries

64. What is the most common cause of an aneurysm?
    a. Emboli
    b. Trauma
    c. Atherosclerosis
    d. Thrombus formation

65. A patient is suspected to have an abdominal aortic aneurysm (AAA). What does the nurse assess for?
    a. Abdominal, flank, or back pain
    b. Chest pain and shortness of breath
    c. Hoarseness and difficulty swallowing
    d. Disruption of bowel and bladder patterns

66. A 75-year-old man with a history of atherosclerosis comes to the emergency department (ED) with abdominal pain. What findings indicate a possible abdominal aortic aneurysm? **Select all that apply.**
    a. Left-sided chest pain
    b. Abdominal, flank, or back pain
    c. Visible pulsation on the upper abdominal wall
    d. Hoarseness
    e. Difficulty swallowing
    f. An abdominal bruit on auscultation

67. A patient with an abdominal aortic aneurysm (AAA) is admitted to the hospital. Which tests does the health care provider order to confirm an accurate diagnosis as well as to determine the size and location of the AAA? **Select all that apply.**
    a. Chest x-ray
    b. Ultrasound
    c. Electrocardiogram
    d. Magnetic resonance imaging
    e. Computed tomography
    f. Cardiac catheterization

68. A patient is diagnosed with a 3-cm abdominal aortic aneurysm. What is the **best** nonsurgical intervention to decrease the risk of rupture of an aneurysm and to slow the rate of enlargement?
    a. Maintenance of normal blood pressure and avoidance of hypertension
    b. Bedrest until there is shrinkage of the aneurysm
    c. Heparin and Coumadin therapy to decrease clotting
    d. Intraarterial thrombolytic therapy

69. A patient with a ruptured aneurysm may exhibit which symptoms? **Select all that apply.**
    a. Bradypnea
    b. Tachycardia
    c. Increased systolic pressure
    d. Decreased blood pressure
    e. Severe pain
    f. Decreased level of consciousness

70. Which are complications of endovascular stent grafts when an emergent repair of an abdominal aortic aneurysm (AAA) is needed? **Select all that apply.**
    a. Aneurysm rupture
    b. Peripheral embolization
    c. Septic shock
    d. Misplacement of stent graft
    e. Aneurysm dissection
    f. Bleeding

71. A patient has an abdominal aortic aneurysm that is small and asymptomatic. What priority teaching must the nurse complete with this patient?
    a. "You will need an elective AAA repair as soon as possible."
    b. "Your aneurysm could rupture at any time, causing you to go into shock."
    c. "You will have frequent CT scans or ultrasounds to monitor the growth of the aneurysm."
    d. "The preferred surgical repair for your aneurysm is an open abdominal procedure."

72. A patient has had an aneurysm repair. Which activity does the nurse suggest as an example of appropriate exercise during the **recovery** period?
    a. Playing golf
    b. Washing dishes
    c. Climbing stairs
    d. Driving a car

73. A patient is admitted for a medical diagnosis of detectable abdominal aortic aneurysm. What does the nurse expect to find documented in the patient's description of symptoms?
    a. Hematuria and painful urination that started very suddenly
    b. Steady and gnawing abdominal pain unaffected by movement, lasting for days
    c. No subjective complaints of pain, but episodes of dizziness
    d. Pain in the lower extremities exacerbated by walking and relieved by rest

74. While assessing a patient with abdominal aortic aneurysm, the nurse notes a pulsation in the upper abdomen slightly to the left of the midline between the xiphoid process and the umbilicus. What does the nurse do next?
    a. Measure the mass with a ruler.
    b. Palpate the mass for tenderness.
    c. Percuss the mass to determine the borders.
    d. Auscultate for a bruit over the mass.

75. A patient was admitted for abdominal aortic aneurysm with a pulsating abdominal mass. The nurse notes a sudden onset of diaphoresis, decreased level of consciousness, a blood pressure of 88/60 mm Hg, and an irregular apical pulse. Oxygen is in place via mask. What is the **priority** nursing action at this time?
    a. Establish IV access.
    b. Alert the Rapid Response Team.
    c. Auscultate for a bruit and assess the mass.
    d. Place the patient on the cardiac monitor.

76. The nurse is reviewing the radiologist's report of the abdominal x-ray of a patient suspected of having an abdominal aortic aneurysm (AAA). The report notes an "eggshell" appearance. How does the nurse interpret this data?
    a. Validates the presence of a fusiform aneurysm
    b. Suggests an artifact, so the x-ray should be repeated
    c. Indicates a congenital anomaly that will obscure the aneurysm
    d. Indicates the aneurysm is the size of an egg

77. The nurse is designing a teaching plan for a patient with a 4-cm abdominal aortic aneurysm (AAA). The patient is currently asymptomatic. What is the nurse's goal for nonsurgical management of this patient?
    a. Teach lifestyle modifications that will minimize the growth of the aneurysm.
    b. Monitor the growth of the aneurysm and follow the antihypertensive medication regimen.
    c. Encourage compliance with anticoagulant drugs and laboratory follow-up appointments.
    d. Stabilize the patient's condition and improve overall health so surgery can be safely performed.

78. The nurse is performing preoperative teaching for a patient who is having an elective endovascular stent graft repair for an abdominal aortic aneurysm (AAA). What key points are included in teaching for this patient? **Select all that apply.**
    a. "This type of repair has decreased hospital stays."
    b. "The stents are inserted through the skin into the femoral artery."
    c. "You will be receiving general anesthesia."
    d. "In the OR you will receive a large volume of IV fluids."
    e. "This procedure has resulted in improved mortality for AAA repairs."
    f. "After the procedure you will be in the surgical ICU for at least 1-2 days."

79. Which are signs of a thoracic aortic aneurysm (TAA)? **Select all that apply.**
    a. Tachycardia
    b. Shortness of breath
    c. Hoarseness
    d. Paralytic ileus
    e. Difficulty swallowing
    f. Visible mass above the suprasternal notch

80. The nurse notes a change in pulses, a cool extremity below the graft, bluish discoloration to the flanks, and abdominal distention in a patient who has had an endoscopic stent graft repair of an abdominal aortic aneurysm. These symptoms are consistent with which postoperative complication?
    a. Ischemic colitis
    b. Spinal cord ischemia
    c. Graft occlusion or rupture
    d. Thoracic outlet syndrome

81. A patient is admitted through the emergency department (ED) for emergency surgery of a ruptured aneurysm. Why does the nurse monitor the patient for renal failure?
    a. A urinary catheter was inserted under potentially nonsterile conditions.
    b. Aggressive fluid management in the ED could overload the kidneys.
    c. Hypovolemia associated with rupture can result in decreased urinary output.
    d. Medications used in the emergency procedure are nephrotoxic.

82. A patient who had an endoscopic stent graft repair for an abdominal aortic aneurysm (AAA) was transferred to the unit from the PACU. Which action does the nurse take when caring for this patient over the next 24 hours?
    a. Assess the patient's ability to climb stairs.
    b. Teach the patient that he or she may drive 1-2 days after discharge.
    c. Discourage coughing and deep-breathing.
    d. Assist the patient to a bedside chair.

83. The nurse is assessing a patient with a suspected ruptured thoracic aortic aneurysm. Which assessment finding is **most likely** to be present?
    a. Loss of pulses distal to the aneurysm
    b. Decreased level of consciousness
    c. Sudden and excruciating back or chest pain
    d. Disruption of bowel and bladder patterns

84. A patient who had a thoracic aortic aneurysm repair has been progressing well for several days after the surgery but today tells the nurse, "My toes and lower legs feel a little numb and tingly." What is the nurse's **best** first action?
    a. Encourage the patient to do active range-of-motion exercises in bed.
    b. Help the patient get up, dangle the legs, and then ambulate.
    c. Assess extremities for sensation, movement, or pulse changes.
    d. Instruct unlicensed assistive personnel (UAP) to assist the patient in elevating the legs.

85. Which actions does the nurse instruct the patient to avoid after discharge with an abdominal aortic aneurysm repair? **Select all that apply.**
    a. Lifting heavy objects
    b. Going up stairs
    c. Using the bathroom
    d. Sitting in a chair for meals
    e. Pushing, pulling, or straining
    f. Vacuuming the carpets

86. A patient is considering endovascular stent grafts. What is one of the advantages of this procedure?
    a. Decreased length of hospital stay
    b. Less risk for hemorrhage
    c. Decreased incidence of postprocedural rupture
    d. Use of local, rather than general, anesthesia

87. The home health nurse is making the first visit to a patient who had an abdominal aortic aneurysm repair. In evaluating the home situation, what does the nurse observe that is cause for concern?
    a. The patient has been having groceries delivered for several weeks.
    b. There is a calendar hanging on the refrigerator with medication times.
    c. The patient's bedroom and bathroom access are on the ground floor.
    d. The patient decides to mow the lawn and clean out the garage.

88. A patient comes to the emergency department (ED) with anterior chest pain described as a "tearing" sensation. The patient is diaphoretic, nauseated, faint, and apprehensive, and blood pressure is 200/130 mm Hg. Which medication is **most likely** to be ordered for this patient?
    a. Antianginal such as nitroglycerin
    b. IV beta blocker such as esmolol
    c. Calcium channel antagonist such as amlodipine
    d. Beta blocker such as propranolol

89. The patient has a pulsating mass that is visible over the femoral artery. What action must the nurse **avoid**?
    a. Auscultation of the mass
    b. Turning the patient on his or her side
    c. Palpating the pulsatile mass
    d. Assessing distal pulses

90. Which are characteristics of Raynaud's disease? **Select all that apply**.
    a. Occurs in smokers, often in young men
    b. Claudication in feet and lower extremities is present
    c. Occurs mostly in young women
    d. Is episodic, causing white, then blue, fingers
    e. Cold intolerance is present
    f. Occurs only in upper extremities

91. A young male patient is diagnosed with early stage Buerger's disease. What assessment finding does the nurse expect to find in the patient's record?
    a. Claudication in feet that is worse at night
    b. Intolerance of warm environments
    c. Dizziness and lightheadedness
    d. Pain in the lower back with ambulation

92. The nurse is teaching a patient with Buerger's disease about self-care. What is the **most important** point that the nurse emphasizes?
    a. Lower intake of fat and reduce cholesterol to reverse the disease process.
    b. Perform daily exercise of fingers or toes to slow the progress of the disease.
    c. Limit exposure to extreme or prolonged cold temperatures because of vasoconstriction.
    d. Cease cigarette smoking and tobacco use to arrest the disease process.

93. A patient reports tiredness in the arm with exertion, paresthesia, dizziness, and exercise-induced pain in the forearm when the arms are elevated. The nurse suspects subclavian steal. What physical assessment does the nurse perform?
    a. Check blood pressure in both arms.
    b. Auscultate for a carotid bruit.
    c. Check for orthostatic hypotension.
    d. Observe the arm for redness or edema.

94. A patient who is an avid golfer is diagnosed with thoracic outlet syndrome. What does the nurse advise the patient that is specific to this syndrome?
    a. Rest if shortness of breath occurs.
    b. Avoid walking long distances.
    c. Avoid elevating the arms above the head.
    d. Perform deep-breathing exercises.

95. A 25-year-old woman reports bilateral blanching of both upper extremities that occurs in cold temperatures. She reports numbness and cold sensation, and afterwards the arms become very red. Which condition are these symptoms most consistent with?
    a. Raynaud's disease
    b. Buerger's disease
    c. Subclavian steal
    d. Thoracic outlet syndrome

96. Which medication is a patient with Raynaud's disease **most likely** to be prescribed?
    a. Lovastatin
    b. Coumadin
    c. Nifedipine
    d. Captopril

97. A patient has been on bedrest following a motor vehicle accident. While assessing the patient, the nurse notes that the patient's left lower extremity has edema and is warm to the touch. The patient reports the calf of the left leg is slightly painful. The nurse suspects that this assessment may indicate which disorder?
    a. Raynaud's syndrome
    b. Cellulitis
    c. Aneurysm
    d. Venous thromboembolism

98. A patient is admitted to the hospital with deep vein thrombosis (DVT). Which drugs are preferred for treatment and prevention of DVT?
    a. Subcutaneous low–molecular-weight heparins (LMWHs)
    b. IV unfractionated heparin
    c. Novel oral anticoagulants (NOACs)
    d. Thrombolytic therapy

99. The patients with which conditions are candidates for an inferior vena cava filter placement? **Select all that apply.**
    a. Abdominal aortic aneurysm
    b. Chronic obstructive pulmonary disease
    c. Recurrent deep vein thrombosis
    d. No response to medical treatment
    e. Intolerance to anticoagulation drug therapy
    f. Recurrent pulmonary emboli

100. What is the recommended therapeutic range for the International Normalized Ratio (INR) for a patient receiving warfarin sodium?
    a. 0.5-1.0
    b. 1.0-1.5
    c. 1.5-2.0
    d. 2.0-2.5

101. A patient prescribed warfarin sodium is instructed that certain foods decrease the effect of the drug. Which foods, if eaten, must be consumed in consistent and small amounts each day?
    a. Fresh fruits
    b. Chicken and beef
    c. Spinach and asparagus
    d. Milk and cheese

102. The nurse is teaching a patient who is at risk for venous thromboembolism (VTE). The patient is currently asymptomatic and is living in the community. What interventions does the nurse instruct the patient to do to minimize the risk of VTE? **Select all that apply.**
    a. Avoid oral contraceptives.
    b. Drink adequate fluids to avoid dehydration.
    c. Exercise the legs during long periods of bedrest or sitting.
    d. Arise early in the morning for ambulation.
    e. Use a venous plexus foot pump.
    f. Avoid potential trauma such as contact sports.

103. The nurse is reviewing the diagnostic test results for a patient suspected of having a deep vein thrombosis (DVT). The results show a negative D-dimer test. How does the nurse interpret this data?
    a. The test can exclude DVT without an ultrasound.
    b. Venous duplex ultrasonography is needed.
    c. The patient has arterial disease.
    d. Impedance plethysmography is needed.

104. The health care provider has ordered unfractionated heparin (UFH) for a patient with a deep vein thrombosis (DVT). Before administering the drug, the nurse ensures that which laboratory tests were obtained for baseline measurement? **Select all that apply.**
    a. Prothrombin time (PT)
    b. Activated partial thromboplastin time (APTT or aPTT)
    c. International Normalized Ratio (INR)
    d. Complete blood count (CBC) with platelet count
    e. Arterial blood gas
    f. Urinalysis

105. The nurse notes that the platelet count for a patient who is to receive unfractionated heparin (UFH) is 100,000/mm³. How does the nurse interpret this result?
    a. It is slightly lowered and worth monitoring for trends.
    b. It is significantly low, so the health care provider should be notified.
    c. It is insignificant unless other values such as PT or APTT are abnormal.
    d. It is higher than expected but within normal limits for therapy.

106. The medication order for unfractionated heparin (UFH) is for 80 units/kg of body weight. How does the nurse interpret this order?
    a. Appropriate dose for the continuous IV infusion
    b. Higher than expected dose for the initial IV bolus
    c. Appropriate dose for the initial IV bolus
    d. Appropriate dose for maintenance therapy

107. A patient is receiving anticoagulant therapy. The nurse instructs the unlicensed assistive personnel (UAP) in which task related to the anticoagulant therapy?
    a. Observe the skin for ecchymosis, bruising, and petechiae during morning hygiene.
    b. Replace the antiembolism devices after bathing or ambulating.
    c. Check on the patient every 2 hours and report changes in mental status.
    d. Watch for and report blood in the stool when assisting the patient with toileting.

108. A patient receiving unfractionated heparin (UFH) therapy is ordered to discontinue the therapy and begin low–molecular-weight heparin (LMWH) with enoxaparin. What is the **priority** nursing intervention?
    a. Discontinue the UFH at least 30 minutes before the first LMWH injection.
    b. Check the APTT results after giving the first LMWH injection.
    c. Assess the patient's IV site before starting the LMWH.
    d. Check the PT and INR results before giving the first LMWH injection.

109. For which side effects does the nurse monitor when a patient is prescribed idarucizumab? **Select all that apply.**
    a. Hypokalemia
    b. Confusion
    c. Diarrhea
    d. Hypernatremia
    e. Fever
    f. Pneumonia

110. Which novel oral anticoagulant (NOAC) drug currently has an antidote?
    a. Dabigatran
    b. Rivaroxaban
    c. Apixaban
    d. Idarucizumab

111. The nurse is teaching a patient about the side effects and potential problems associated with taking warfarin sodium. Which statement by the patient indicates a correct understanding of the nurse's instruction?
    a. "If I notice bleeding of the gums, I should skip one or two doses of the medication."
    b. "I should eat a lot of cabbage, cauliflower, and broccoli to prevent bleeding."
    c. "For injury and bleeding, I should apply direct pressure and seek medical assistance."
    d. "I should avoid going to the dentist while I am taking this medication."

112. A patient with a venous stasis ulcer is prescribed the topical agent Accuzyme. What are the purposes of this drug? **Select all that apply.**
    a. Eliminate infection
    b. Promote healing
    c. Chemically debride the ulcer
    d. Improve circulation
    e. Eliminate necrotic tissue
    f. Prevent stasis

113. The nurse is instructing a patient and caregiver on warfarin (Coumadin) therapy at home. Which items does the nurse include in the teaching plan? **Select all that apply.**
    a. "Eat small amounts of broccoli and spinach."
    b. "Avoid beta blockers and ACE inhibitors."
    c. "Inform your dentist of taking warfarin prior to treatment."
    d. "Eat small amounts of oranges and bananas."
    e. "Avoid NSAIDs and birth control pills."
    f. "Be sure to have your INR lab checked as ordered."

114. Which statements pertaining to the use of the Unna boot are correct? **Select all that apply.**
    a. It is used to heal peripheral arterial disease ulcers.
    b. It is applied from the toes to the knee.
    c. It promotes venous return and prevents stasis.
    d. It is changed by a health care provider every 3-4 days.
    e. It forms a sterile environment for the ulcer.
    f. The patient is instructed to report any increase in pain.

115. The nurse is assessing an obese patient's lower leg and notes a small irregularly shaped ulcer over the medial malleolus with brownish discoloration. The patient reports that the "leg has been that way for a long time." What do these findings suggest to the nurse?
    a. Varicose vein
    b. Venous stasis ulcer
    c. Phlebitis
    d. Raynaud's phenomenon

116. The nurse is consulting with the registered dietitian about diet therapy for a patient with chronic venous stasis ulcers. What are the dietary recommendations to help this patient promote wound healing?
    a. High-protein foods
    b. Vitamin D and B supplements
    c. Low-fat foods
    d. High-calcium foods

117. A patient has a venous stasis ulcer that requires a dressing. Which dressing materials are selected for this type of wound? **Select all that apply.**
    a. Oxygen-permeable polyethylene film
    b. Oxygen-impermeable hydrocolloid dressing
    c. Dry gauze dressings
    d. Artificial skin products
    e. Unna boot
    f. Vacuum-assisted wound closure

118. The nurse is assessing a patient with distended, protruding veins. In order to assess for varicose veins, what technique does the nurse use?
    a. Place the patient in a supine position with elevated legs; as the patient sits up, observe the veins filling from the proximal end.
    b. Place the patient in the Trendelenburg position and observe the distention and protruding of the veins.
    c. Ask the patient to stand and observe the leg veins; then ask the patient to sit or lie down and observe the veins.
    d. Ask the patient to walk around the room and observe the veins; then have the patient rest for several minutes and reassess the veins.

119. A patient with varicose veins asks the nurse to provide a list of all available treatment options. Which options does the nurse include on the list for the patient? **Select all that apply.**
    a. Elastic stockings and elevation of the extremities
    b. Thrombolytic therapy
    c. Application of radiofrequency (RF) energy
    d. Endovenous ablation
    e. Anticoagulant therapy
    f. Sclerotherapy

120. The nurse is assessing the IV site of a patient who has been receiving a normal saline infusion. There is redness and warmth radiating up the arm with pain, soreness, and swelling. What does the nurse do next?
    a. Discontinue the IV and apply warm, moist soaks.
    b. Slow the infusion rate and reassess within 1 hour.
    c. Discontinue the IV and apply a cold pack.
    d. Contact the health care provider for an order for an antidote.

121. Which patient has the **greatest** risk for a pulmonary embolus related to a venous disorder?
    a. Patient with bilateral varicose veins
    b. Patient with phlebitis of superficial veins
    c. Patient with thrombophlebitis in a deep vein of the lower extremity
    d. Patient with venous insufficiency throughout the leg

122. What information does the nurse include when teaching a patient with chronic venous stasis? **Select all that apply.**
    a. Elevate the legs when sitting.
    b. Avoid crossing the legs.
    c. Wear antiembolic stockings at night during sleep.
    d. Avoid standing still for any length of time.
    e. Avoid wearing tight girdles, tight pants, and narrow-banded knee-high socks.
    f. Keep legs positioned below the heart at night for better perfusion.

123. Which patient is at greatest risk for developing varicose veins?
    a. 37-year-old mail carrier
    b. 39-year-old retail store clerk
    c. 40-year-old operating room scrub technician
    d. 25-year-old pregnant woman in the first trimester

124. Which intervention is used for conservative treatment of varicose veins?
    a. Dry heat
    b. Ice packs
    c. Elevation
    d. Massage

125. Which type of exercise should the nurse teach a patient with varicose veins is best for improving venous return?
    a. Jogging
    b. Walking
    c. Strength training
    d. Horseback riding

126. The nurse observes diminished pulses, cold skin, and a pulsatile mass over the femoral artery in a patient reporting pain in the right leg. What condition does the nurse suspect in this patient?
    a. Venous thromboembolism
    b. Buerger's disease
    c. Femoral aneurysm
    d. Popliteal entrapment

127. The nurse is providing care for a patient with venous insufficiency. Which medical-surgical concepts have priority with this patient? **Select all that apply.**
    a. Perfusion
    b. Fluid and electrolyte balance
    c. Immunity
    d. Clotting
    e. Tissue integrity
    f. Cellular regulation

37
CHAPTER

Care of Patients with Shock

1. Which medical-surgical concept has the **high-est** priority when a patient develops shock?
   a. Perfusion
   b. Fluid and electrolyte balance
   c. Tissue integrity
   d. Cellular regulation

2. Which statements about shock are true? **Select all that apply.**
   a. Shock is a whole-body response to tissues not receiving enough oxygen.
   b. Shock is widespread abnormal cellular metabolism.
   c. Shock occurs only in the acute care setting.
   d. Shock may occur in older adults in response to urinary tract infections.
   e. Shock is mostly classified as a disease.
   f. Shock affects all body organs.

3. Which hormones are released in response to **decreased** mean arterial pressure (MAP)? **Select all that apply.**
   a. Insulin
   b. Renin
   c. Antidiuretic hormone (ADH)
   d. Epinephrine
   e. Aldosterone
   f. Serotonin

4. Which condition results in blood vessels that are normally partially constricted?
   a. Hypoxia
   b. Vasodilation
   c. Sympathetic tone
   d. Decreased mean arterial pressure

5. The patient has decreased oxygenation and impaired tissue perfusion. Which clinical manifestations are evidence of onset of the nonprogressive or compensatory stages of shock? **Select all that apply.**
   a. Decreased urine output
   b. Low-grade fever
   c. Narrowing pulse pressure
   d. Decreased heart rate
   e. Increased heart rate
   f. Increased sodium reabsorption

6. Which statement about the systemic effects of shock is correct?
   a. The liver is essentially unaffected, but liver enzymes may be lower than normal.
   b. The current heart rate and blood pressure indicate the cardiac system is at baseline.
   c. The brain and neurologic system can withstand 10-15 minutes of severe hypoperfusion.
   d. The kidneys can tolerate hypoxia and anoxia up to 1 hour without permanent damage.

7. Which patients are at risk for shock related to fluid shifts? **Select all that apply.**
   a. Hypoglycemic patient
   b. Severely malnourished patient
   c. Patient with ascites
   d. Patient with kidney disease
   e. Patient with minor burns
   f. Patient with a large wound

8. A young woman comes to the emergency department (ED) with lightheadedness and "a feeling of impending doom." Pulse is 110 beats/min; respirations are 30/min; and blood pressure is 140/90 mm Hg. Which factors does the nurse ask about that could contribute to shock? **Select all that apply.**
   a. Recent accident or trauma
   b. Prolonged diarrhea or vomiting
   c. History of depression or anxiety
   d. Possibility of pregnancy
   e. Use of over-the-counter medications
   f. Recent hospitalization

9. Which are specific causes or risk factors for cardiogenic shock? **Select all that apply.**
   a. Anesthesia
   b. Myocardial infarction
   c. Cardiac tamponade
   d. Ventricular dysrhythmias
   e. Constrictive pericarditis
   f. Cardiomyopathy

10. Which patient is at risk for obstructive shock?
    a. Patient with a history of angina
    b. Patient with chronic atrial fibrillation
    c. Patient with a pulmonary embolus
    d. Patient with a history of heart failure

11. A patient has cardiac dysrhythmias and pulmonary problems as a result of receiving the first dose of a new IV antibiotic. The nurse recognizes that this represents what type of shock?
    a. Hypovolemic
    b. Cardiogenic
    c. Anaphylactic
    d. Septic

12. A patient with head trauma was treated for a cerebral hematoma. **After** surgery, this patient is at risk for what type of shock?
    a. Obstructive
    b. Cardiogenic
    c. Chemical-induced distributive
    d. Neural-induced distributive

13. The nurse is performing a morning shift assessment on several patients. For which patient is the nurse **immediately** concerned about decreased tissue perfusion if the capillary refill time was delayed?
    a. Patient with diabetes mellitus
    b. Anemic patient
    c. Patient with peripheral vascular disease
    d. Patient with severe dehydration

14. The nursing student takes the morning blood pressure of a postoperative patient, and the reading is 90/50 mm Hg. What does the student do next? **Select all that apply.**
    a. Report the reading to the primary nurse as a possible sign of hypovolemia.
    b. Assess the patient for subjective feelings of dizziness or shortness of breath.
    c. Check the patient's chart for trends in morning vital sign readings.
    d. Notify the instructor to verify the significance of the finding.
    e. Call a "code blue."
    f. Place the patient in reverse Trendelenburg position.

15. A patient at risk for shock has had some small, subtle changes in behavior within the past hour. How does the nurse evaluate the patient's mental status throughout the night?
    a. Assess the patient while he or she is awake and then allow him or her to sleep until morning.
    b. Ask the patient and family to describe the patient's normal sleep and behavior patterns.
    c. Periodically attempt to awaken the patient and document how easily he or she is aroused.
    d. Allow the patient to sleep but assess respiratory effort and skin temperature.

16. For which indications would the nurse be prepared to administer a colloid product? **Select all that apply.**
    a. Hemorrhagic shock
    b. Dehydration
    c. Peripheral tissue hypoxia
    d. Fluid replacement
    e. Restore osmotic pressure
    f. Increase hematocrit and hemoglobin levels

17. The patient at risk for hypovolemic shock tells the nurse that he is very thirsty. Which action should the nurse delegate to the unlicensed assistive personnel (UAP) **first**?
    a. Give the patient a cup of ice water.
    b. Assist the patient to the bathroom.
    c. Check the patient's vital signs.
    d. Ask the patient if he would like some juice.

18. Which questions can help guide the nurse when evaluating the mental status of a patient at risk for shock? **Select all that apply.**
    a. Is it necessary to repeat questions to obtain a response?
    b. Can the patient answer "yes" or "no" questions?
    c. Does the response answer the question asked?
    d. Does the patient have difficulty making word choices?
    e. Is the patient irritated or upset by the questions?
    f. How long is the patient's attention span?

19. The nurse is caring for a patient at risk for hypovolemic shock. What is the **first** sign of hypovolemic shock the nurse should monitor?
    a. Elevated body temperature
    b. Decreasing urine output
    c. Vasodilation
    d. Increasing heart rate

20. Assessment findings of a patient with trauma injuries reveal cool and pale skin, reported thirst, urine output 100 mL/8 hr, blood pressure 122/78 mm Hg, pulse 102 beats/min, and respirations 24/min with decreased breath sounds. The nurse recognizes that the patient is in which phase of shock?
    a. Nonprogressive
    b. Progressive
    c. Refractory
    d. Multiple organ dysfunction

21. A patient with blunt trauma to the abdomen has been NPO for several hours in preparation for a procedure and now reports thirst. What is the nurse's **priority** action?
    a. Get the patient a few ice chips or a moistened swab.
    b. Obtain an order for a stat hematocrit and hemoglobin.
    c. Take the patient's vital signs and compare to baseline.
    d. Obtain an order to increase the IV rate.

22. A patient is brought to the emergency department (ED) with a gunshot wound. What are the **early** signs of hypovolemic shock the nurse should monitor? **Select all that apply.**
    a. Elevated serum potassium level
    b. Increase in heart rate
    c. Decrease in oxygen saturation
    d. Marked decrease in blood pressure
    e. Increase in respiratory rate
    f. Decreased MAP of 10-15 mm Hg

23. The unlicensed assistive personnel (UAP) reports repeatedly and unsuccessfully trying to take a patient's blood pressure with the electronic and manual devices. The nurse notes that the patient's apical pulse is elevated and the patient is at risk for hypovolemic shock. What is the **best** method for the nurse to determine the systolic blood pressure?
    a. Apply the electronic device to a lower extremity.
    b. Instruct the UAP to immediately get the Doppler.
    c. Apply the manual cuff and palpate for the systolic.
    d. Tell the UAP to try the electronic device on the other arm.

24. The nurse identifies signs and symptoms of internal hemorrhage in a postoperative patient. What is included in the care of this patient for hypovolemic shock? **Select all that apply.**
    a. Elevate the feet with the head flat or elevated 30 degrees.
    b. Monitor vital signs every 5 minutes until they are stable.
    c. Administer clotting factors or plasma.
    d. Provide oxygen therapy.
    e. Ensure IV access.
    f. Leave the patient and notify the Rapid Response Team.

25. A young trauma patient is at risk for hypovolemic shock related to occult hemorrhage. What baseline indicator allows the nurse to recognize the **early** signs of shock?
    a. Urine output
    b. Pulse rate
    c. Fluid intake
    d. Skin color

26. Which statement about assessment of skin during shock is accurate?
    a. For a patient with dark skin, pallor or cyanosis is best assessed in the oral mucous membranes.
    b. For all patients in shock, the skin is expected to feel warm and dry to the touch.
    c. For a lighter skinned patient, skin is usually a whitish blue color.
    d. For a patient with dark skin, color will be bluish gray.

27. A patient in hypovolemic shock is receiving sodium nitroprusside to enhance myocardial perfusion. What is an important nursing assessment when administering this drug?
    a. Assess the patient for headache because it is an early symptom of drug excess.
    b. Assess blood pressure at least every 15 minutes because hypertension is a symptom of overdose.
    c. Assess blood pressure at least every 15 minutes because systemic vasodilation can cause hypotension.
    d. Assess the patient every 30 minutes for extravasation because nitroprusside can cause severe vasoconstriction and tissue ischemia.

28. A patient with hypovolemic shock is receiving an infusion of dopamine. Which nursing interventions are essential when a patient is receiving this drug? **Select all that apply.**
    a. Take the blood pressure at least every 15 minutes.
    b. Monitor urine output every hour.
    c. Cover the infusion bag to protect it from light.
    d. Assess the patient for chest pain.
    e. Check the infusion site every 30 minutes for extravasation.
    f. Ask a patient receiving this drug about headaches.

29. A patient with hypovolemia is restless and anxious. The skin is cool and pale, pulse is thready at a rate of 135 beats/min, blood pressure is 92/50 mm Hg, and respirations are 32/min. What actions must the nurse take? **Select all that apply.**
    a. Obtain a stat order for an IV normal saline bolus.
    b. Check vital signs at least every 15 minutes.
    c. Notify the Rapid Response Team.
    d. Place the patient in a semi-Fowler's position.
    e. Call a "code blue."
    f. Administer supplemental oxygen.

30. A patient is showing early clinical manifestations of hypovolemic shock. The health care provider orders an arterial blood gas (ABG). Which ABG values does the nurse expect to see in hypovolemic shock?
    a. Increased pH with decreased Pao_2 and increased $Paco_2$
    b. Decreased pH with decreased Pao_2 and increased $Paco_2$
    c. Normal pH with decreased Pao_2 and normal $Paco_2$
    d. Normal pH with decreased Pao_2 and decreased $Paco_2$

31. The nurse finds a patient on the bathroom floor. There is a large amount of blood on the floor and on the patient's hospital gown. Which actions must the nurse take? **Select all that apply.**
    a. Elevate the patient's legs.
    b. Establish large-bore IV access.
    c. Look for the source of the bleeding.
    d. Ensure a patent airway.
    e. Apply direct pressure to the bleeding site if possible.
    f. Check vital signs at least every 30 minutes.

32. The nurse is caring for a postoperative patient who had major abdominal surgery. Which assessment finding is consistent with hypovolemic shock?
    a. Pulse pressure of 40 mm Hg
    b. A rapid, weak, thready pulse
    c. Warm, flushed skin
    d. Increased urinary output

33. Which IV therapy results in the greatest increase in oxygen-carrying capacity for a patient with hypovolemic shock?
    a. Lactated Ringer's solution
    b. Hetastarch
    c. Fresh frozen plasma (FFP)
    d. Packed red cells

34. A patient comes to the emergency department (ED) with severe injury and significant blood loss. The nurse anticipates that resuscitation will begin with which fluid?
    a. Whole blood
    b. 0.5% dextrose in water
    c. 0.9% sodium chloride
    d. Plasma protein fractions

35. Which change in the skin is an **early** indication of hypovolemic shock?
    a. Pallor or cyanosis in the mucous membranes
    b. Color changes in the trunk area
    c. Axilla and groin feel moist or clammy
    d. Generalized mottling of skin

36. A patient is in hypovolemic shock related to hemorrhage from a large gunshot wound. Which order must the nurse **question**?
    a. Establish a large-bore peripheral IV and give crystalloid bolus.
    b. Give furosemide (Lasix) 20 mg slow IVP.
    c. Insert a Foley catheter and monitor intake and output.
    d. Give high-flow oxygen via mask at 10 L/min.

37. The nurse is performing a psychosocial assessment on a patient who is at risk for shock. Which statement made by the patient is of **greatest** concern to the nurse?
    a. "Do you have any idea when I might go home? No one is feeding my cat."
    b. "Something feels wrong, but I'm not sure what is causing me to feel this way."
    c. "I live alone in my house and my family lives in a different state."
    d. "I would usually go golfing with my friends today. I hope they're not worried about me."

38. A patient at risk for hypovolemic shock has a central venous pressure (CVP) catheter in place. Which finding is a **priority** concern for the nurse?
    a. Heart rate is decreased from 120 to 110 per minute.
    b. Central venous pressure is increased from 1 to 6 mm Hg.
    c. Central venous pressure is decreased from 6 to 1 mm Hg.
    d. Heart rate is increased from 100 to 110 per minute.

39. A patient is being discharged from the same-day surgery unit to home. Which early indicators of shock will the nurse teach the patient and family member to watch for and to seek medical attention immediately if they occur? **Select all that apply.**
    a. Decreased thirst
    b. Decreased urine output
    c. Increased blood pressure
    d. Lightheadedness
    e. Sense of apprehension
    f. Cyanosis

40. A patient has a systemic infection with a fever, increased respiratory rate, and change in mental status. Which laboratory values does the nurse seek out that are considered **"hallmarks"** of sepsis?
    a. Increased white blood count and increased glucose level
    b. Increased serum lactate level and rising band neutrophils
    c. Increased oxygen saturation and decreased clotting times
    d. Decreased white blood count with increased hematocrit

41. The nurse is caring for an older adult patient at risk for shock. What is an **early** sign of shock in this patient?
    a. Cool, clammy skin
    b. Decreased urinary output
    c. Restlessness
    d. Hypotension

42. The nurse is caring for a patient with sepsis. At the beginning of the shift, the patient is in a hyperdynamic state. Several hours later, the patient has a rapid respiratory rate, decreased urine output, and altered level of consciousness. How does the nurse interpret this change?
    a. A positive response and a signal of recovery
    b. Temporary situation that is likely to normalize
    c. Worsening of the condition rather than improvement
    d. Expected response to standard therapies

43. The nurse is caring for a patient with sepsis. What is a **late** clinical manifestation of shock?
    a. Decrease in blood pressure
    b. MAP is decreased by less than 10 mm Hg
    c. Tachycardia with a bounding pulse
    d. Increased urine output

44. The nurse is caring for a patient at risk for sepsis. Why does the nurse closely monitor the patient for early signs of shock?
    a. The patient is unable to self-identify or report these early signs.
    b. Distributive shock usually begins as a bacterial or fungal infection.
    c. Prevention of septic shock is easier to achieve in the early phase.
    d. There is widespread vasodilation and pooling of blood in some tissues.

45. A patient has a localized infection. What assessment findings are considered evidence of a beneficial inflammatory response?
    a. Decreased urine output that normalizes after fluid bolus
    b. Pulse rate of 120 beats/min related to increased metabolic activity
    c. Decreased oxygen saturation that responds to supplemental O_2
    d. Redness and edema that subside in several days

46. The student nurse is assessing a patient's mental status because of the patient's risk for decreased tissue perfusion. The supervising nurse intervenes when the student nurse asks the patient which question?
    a. "What is today's date?"
    b. "Who is the president of this country?"
    c. "Where are we right now?"
    d. "Is your name Mr. John Smith?"

47. The nurse is caring for a patient at risk for septic shock from a wound infection. To prevent systemic inflammatory response syndrome, the nurse's **priority** is to monitor which factor?
    a. Patient's pulse rate and quality
    b. Patient's electrolyte imbalance
    c. Localized infected area
    d. Patient's intake and output

48. The nurse is evaluating the care and treatment for a patient in shock. Which finding indicates that the patient is having an appropriate response to the treatment?
    a. Blood pH of 7.28
    b. Arterial Po_2 of 65 mm Hg
    c. Distended neck veins
    d. Increased urinary output

49. The nurse is caring for a patient with septic shock. Which therapy specific to the management of septic shock for this patient does the nurse anticipate will be used?
    a. Inotropics
    b. Antibiotics
    c. Colloids
    d. Antidysrhythmics

50. A patient receives dopamine 20 mcg/kg/min IV for the treatment of shock. What does the nurse assess for while administering this drug?
    a. Decreased urine output and decreased blood pressure
    b. Increased respiratory rate and increased urine output
    c. Chest pain and hypertension
    d. Bradycardia and headache

51. Which laboratory value indicates the beginning of severe sepsis even before other symptoms are evident?
    a. Decreased level of activated protein C
    b. Decreased serum potassium level
    c. Increased hemoglobin level
    d. Increased aPTT level

52. The nurse is caring for a patient in septic shock. The nurse notes that the rate and depth of respirations are markedly increased. The nurse interprets this as a possible manifestation of the respiratory system compensating for which condition?
    a. Metabolic acidosis
    b. Metabolic alkalosis
    c. Respiratory acidosis
    d. Respiratory alkalosis

53. The ICU nurse observes petechiae, ecchymoses, and blood oozing from gums and other mucous membranes of a patient with septic shock. How does the nurse interpret this finding?
    a. Pulmonary emboli (PE)
    b. Acute respiratory distress syndrome (ARDS)
    c. Systemic inflammatory response syndrome (SIRS)
    d. Disseminated intravascular coagulation (DIC)

54. The nurse is reviewing the laboratory results of a patient with a systemic infection. What is the significance of a "left shift" in the differential leukocyte count?
    a. Expected finding because the patient has a serious infection
    b. Indication that the infection is progressing toward resolution
    c. Indication that the infection is outpacing the white cell production
    d. Important to watch for trends but otherwise not urgently significant

55. The ICU nurse is caring for a patient with septic shock. Which IV infusion order for this patient does the nurse **question**?
    a. Antibiotics
    b. Insulin
    c. 10% dextrose in water
    d. Synthetic activated C protein

56. The nurse is preparing a teaching session for a patient at risk for septic shock. Which topics does the nurse include in this teaching? **Select all that apply.**
    a. Wash hands frequently using antimicrobial soap.
    b. Avoid aspirin and aspirin-containing products.
    c. Avoid large crowds or gatherings where people might be ill.
    d. Do not share eating utensils.
    e. Wash toothbrushes in a dishwasher.
    f. Take temperature once a week.

57. A patient is at risk for sepsis. Which assessment finding is **most** indicative of the hyperdynamic activity that occurs in septic shock?
    a. Crackles in lung bases
    b. Weak, rapid peripheral pulses
    c. Cool, clammy, cyanotic skin
    d. Increased pulse rate with warm, pink skin

58. The home health nurse is visiting a frail older adult patient at risk for sepsis because of failure to thrive and immunosuppression. What does the nurse assess this patient for? **Select all that apply.**
    a. Signs of skin breakdown and presence of redness or swelling
    b. Cough or any other symptoms of a cold or the flu
    c. Appearance and odor of urine, and pain or burning during urination
    d. Patient's and family's understanding of isolation precautions
    e. Availability and type of facilities for handwashing
    f. General cleanliness of the patient's home

59. A postoperative hospitalized patient has a decrease in mean arterial pressure (MAP) of greater than 20 mm Hg from baseline value; elevated, thready pulse; decreased blood pressure; shallow respirations of 26/min; pale skin; moderate acidosis; and moderate hyperkalemia. The nurse recognizes that this patient is in what phase of shock?
    a. Compensatory/nonprogressive
    b. Progressive
    c. Refractory
    d. Multiple organ dysfunction

60. A 70-year-old man is admitted to the hospital with an infected finger of several days' duration. He is lethargic and confused and has a temperature of 101.3°F (38.5°C). Other assessment findings include blood pressure of 94/50 mm Hg, pulse 105 beats/min, respirations 40/min, and shallow breathing. These assessment findings indicate which type of shock?
    a. Hypovolemic
    b. Cardiogenic
    c. Anaphylactic
    d. Septic

61. The clinical manifestations in the first phase of sepsis-induced distributive shock result from the body's reaction to which factor?
    a. Leukocytes
    b. Infectious microorganisms
    c. Hemorrhage
    d. Hypovolemia

62. What factor increases an older adult's risk for distributive (septic) shock?
    a. Reduced skin integrity
    b. Diuretic therapy
    c. Cardiomyopathy
    d. Musculoskeletal weakness

63. Which patients are at risk for distributive septic shock? **Select all that apply.**
    a. Older adult with urinary tract infection
    b. Patient with ruptured aortic aneurysm
    c. Patient with pneumonia
    d. Patient receiving heparin therapy
    e. Older adult with sacral pressure ulcers
    f. Older adult scheduled for outpatient colonoscopy

64. The nurse is caring for a patient in septic shock with a serum glucose level of 280 mg/dL. What is the nurse's best interpretation of this finding?
    a. The patient is developing type 2 diabetes.
    b. The patient is developing type 1 diabetes.
    c. This finding is associated with a poor outcome.
    d. This finding is unexpected in septic shock.

65. The patient has been diagnosed with sepsis. Following the sepsis resuscitation bundle, which interventions should the nurse expect within the first 3 hours? **Select all that apply.**
    a. Obtain serum lactate level.
    b. Begin administering vasopressor drugs.
    c. Draw blood cultures.
    d. Administer broad-spectrum antibiotics.
    e. Assist with insertion of a central venous pressure line.
    f. Immediately transfer to the intensive care unit.

66. The unlicensed assistive personnel (UAP) working under supervision of an RN is checking vital signs on the patient at risk for hypovolemic shock. Which instruction must the nurse give the UAP?
    a. Report any increase in heart rate because it is an early sign of shock.
    b. Report any increased systolic pressure, which is an early sign of shock.
    c. Report any changes in body temperature, which may indicate sepsis.
    d. Report any increase in respiratory rate because of acid-base changes.

38
CHAPTER

Care of Patients with Acute Coronary Syndromes

1. The nurse is interviewing a patient who reports chest discomfort that occurs with moderate to prolonged exertion. The patient describes the pain as being "about the same over the past several months and going away with nitroglycerin or rest." Based on the patient's description of symptoms, what does the nurse suspect in this patient? **Select all that apply.**
   a. Chronic stable angina (CSA)
   b. Unstable angina
   c. Acute coronary syndrome (ACS)
   d. Acute myocardial infarction (MI)
   e. Coronary artery disease (CAD)
   f. Variant (Prinzmetal's) angina

2. A patient with a history of chronic stable angina is admitted for surgery. The patient now reports nausea and pressure in the chest radiating to the left arm and appears anxious; skin is cool and clammy, blood pressure is 150/90 mm Hg, pulse is 100, and respiratory rate is 32. What are the **priorities** of nursing care for this patient? **Select all that apply.**
   a. Relieve nausea
   b. Maintain NPO status
   c. Improve coronary perfusion
   d. Improve coronary oxygenation
   e. Relieve chest pain
   f. Draw troponin blood samples

3. A patient has been admitted for acute angina. Which diagnostic test identifies if the patient will benefit from further invasive management after acute angina or a myocardial infarction (MI)?
   a. Exercise tolerance test
   b. Cardiac catheterization
   c. Thallium scan
   d. Multigated angiogram (MUGA) scan

4. The nurse is talking to a patient with angina about resuming sexual activity. Which statement by the patient indicates a correct understanding about the effects of angina on sexual activity?
   a. "I won't be able to resume the same level of physical exertion as I did before I had chest pain."
   b. "I will discuss alternative methods with my partner since I will no longer be able to have sexual intercourse."
   c. "If I cannot walk a mile, I am not strong enough to resume intercourse."
   d. "With approval from my health care provider, I should resume sexual activity in the mornings or after a rest period."

5. A patient with angina is prescribed nitroglycerin tablets. What information does the nurse include when teaching the patient about this drug? **Select all that apply.**
   a. "If one tablet does not relieve the angina after 5 minutes, take two pills."
   b. "You can tell the pills are active when your tongue feels a tingling sensation."
   c. "Keep your nitroglycerin with you at all times."
   d. "The prescription should last about 6 months before a refill is necessary."
   e. "If the pain doesn't go away, just wait; the medication will eventually take effect."
   f. "The medication can cause a temporary headache."

6. A patient reports chest pain, and the nurse administers a sublingual nitroglycerin tablet. After 5 minutes, what is the nurse's **next** intervention for this patient?
   a. Apply oxygen at 2 to 4 L by nasal cannula.
   b. Administer morphine sulfate IV push.
   c. Recheck the patient's pain intensity and check vital signs.
   d. Notify the health care provider and administer a chewable aspirin.

7. A patient is hypertensive and continues to have angina despite therapy with beta blockers. The nurse anticipates which type of drug will be prescribed for this patient?
   a. Calcium channel blocker
   b. Potassium channel blocker
   c. Angiotensin-converting enzyme inhibitor
   d. Vasopressor

8. The nurse has just given a patient two doses of sublingual nitroglycerin for anginal pain. The patient's baseline blood pressure is 130/80 mm Hg. For which finding would the nurse **immediately** notify the health care provider?
   a. Patient reports a headache.
   b. Systolic pressure is 140 mm Hg.
   c. Systolic pressure is 90 mm Hg.
   d. Anginal pain continues but is somewhat relieved.

9. A patient is admitted for unstable angina. The patient is currently asymptomatic and all vital signs are stable. Which position does the nurse place the patient in?
   a. Any position of comfort
   b. Supine
   c. Sitting in a chair
   d. Fowler's

10. Which are characteristics of angina? **Select all that apply.**
    a. Pain is precipitated by exertion or stress.
    b. Pain occurs without cause, usually in the morning.
    c. Pain is relieved only by opioids.
    d. Pain is relieved by nitroglycerin or rest.
    e. Nausea, diaphoresis, feelings of fear, and dyspnea may occur.
    f. Pain lasts less than 15 minutes.

11. Which statement about coronary artery disease (CAD) is accurate?
    a. Ischemia that occurs with angina lasts more than 30 minutes and does not cause permanent damage of myocardial tissue.
    b. Postmenopausal women in their 70s have the same incidence of myocardial infarction (MI) as men.
    c. Many patients suffering sudden cardiac arrest die before reaching the hospital because of atrial fibrillation.
    d. Studies have shown that CAD in women manifests with the same symptoms as with men.

12. A patient is admitted for acute myocardial infarction (MI), but the nurse notes the absence of ST segment elevation in the electrocardiogram (ECG). What other evidence for acute myocardial infarction (MI) does the nurse expect to find in the patient? **Select all that apply.**
    a. Positive troponin markers
    b. Chronic stable angina
    c. Non-ST elevation MI (NSTEMI) on ECG
    d. Cardiac dysrhythmia
    e. Heart failure
    f. ST elevation in two contiguous leads

13. People should seek treatment for symptoms of myocardial infarction (MI) rather than delay because physical changes will occur approximately how many hours after an infarction?
    a. 3 hours
    b. 6 hours
    c. 12 hours
    d. 24 hours

14. The nurse is caring for a patient admitted with unstable angina and elevated lipid levels. What does the nurse include in teaching this patient about elevated lipid levels? **Select all that apply.**
    a. Begin a vigorous exercise program.
    b. Avoid trans-fatty acids.
    c. Reduce intake of saturated fats.
    d. Monitor the amount of cholesterol ingested, staying below 200 mg/day.
    e. Consider a weight loss program.
    f. Avoid adding salt to food at the table.

15. The nurse is auscultating the heart of a patient who had a myocardial infarction (MI). Which finding most strongly indicates heart failure?
    a. Murmur
    b. S_3 gallop
    c. Split S_1 and S_2
    d. Pericardial friction rub

16. The nurse administers sublingual nitroglycerin to a patient experiencing an episode of angina. How soon does the nurse expect the pain to begin to subside?
    a. 1-2 minutes
    b. 5-6 minutes
    c. 10-12 minutes
    d. 15-20 minutes

17. Which diagnostic tests are used to assess myocardial damage caused by a myocardial infarction (MI)? **Select all that apply.**
    a. Positive chest x-ray
    b. ST depression on ECG
    c. Thallium scan
    d. Troponin I isoenzyme elevation
    e. Cardiac catheterization
    f. Fasting lipid profile

18. A patient has heart failure related to myocardial infarction (MI). What intervention does the nurse plan for this patient's care?
    a. Administering digoxin 1.0 mg PO as a loading dose and then daily
    b. Infusing IV fluids to maintain a urinary output of 60 mL/hr
    c. Titrating vasoactive drugs to maintain a sufficient cardiac output
    d. Observing for such complications as hypertension and flushed, hot skin

19. Which patient has the highest risk for death because of ventricular failure and dysrhythmias related to damage to the left ventricle?
    a. Patient with an anterior wall MI (AWMI)
    b. Patient with a posterior wall MI (PWMI)
    c. Patient with a lateral wall MI (LWMI)
    d. Patient with an inferior wall MI (IWMI)

20. A patient had an inferior wall myocardial infarction (IWMI). The nurse closely monitors the patient for which dysrhythmia associated with this type of MI?
    a. Bradycardia and second-degree heart block
    b. Premature ventricular contractions
    c. Supraventricular tachycardia
    d. Atrial fibrillation

21. The nurse is giving a community presentation about heart disease. Because many sudden cardiac arrest victims die of ventricular fibrillation before reaching the hospital, which teaching point does the nurse emphasize?
    a. Controlling alcohol consumption and quitting cigarette smoking
    b. Modifying risk factors such as diet and weight, and blood pressure medication compliance
    c. Recognizing the difference between chronic stable angina and unstable angina
    d. Learning to operate the automatic external defibrillators (AEDs) in the workplace

22. The nurse is assessing a patient with heart disease for indicators of metabolic syndrome. Which are indicators of this syndrome? **Select all that apply.**
    a. Triglyceride level of 170 mg/dL
    b. HDL cholesterol level of 45 mg/dL in a male
    c. HDL cholesterol level of 45 mg/dL in a female
    d. Blood pressure of 130/86 mm Hg while taking a beta blocker
    e. Fasting blood sugar level of 120 mg/dL
    f. Waist size over 38 inches in a male

23. Which early reaction is most common in patients with the chest discomfort associated with unstable angina or myocardial infarction (MI)?
    a. Depression
    b. Anger
    c. Fear
    d. Denial

24. A patient is trying to make dietary modifications to reduce lipid levels. The patient would like information about omega-3 fatty acid food sources. What **best** source does the nurse recommend?
    a. Flaxseed
    b. Flaxseed oil
    c. Fish
    d. Walnuts

25. A patient comes to the walk-in clinic reporting left anterior chest discomfort with mild shortness of breath. The patient is alert, oriented, diaphoretic, and anxious. What is the **first priority** action for the nurse?
    a. Obtain a complete cardiac history to include a full description of the presenting symptoms.
    b. Place the patient in semi-Fowler's position and start supplemental oxygen.
    c. Instruct the patient to go immediately to the closest full-service hospital.
    d. Immediately alert the physician and establish IV access.

26. A patient reports having chest discomfort that started during exercise. The patient is currently pain-free but is "concerned." What questions must the nurse ask to assess the patient's pain episode? **Select all that apply.**
    a. "When did the pain start and how long did it last?"
    b. "What were you doing when the pain started?"
    c. "What did you do to alleviate the pain?"
    d. "How did you feel about the pain?"
    e. "Did the pain radiate to other locations?"
    f. "On a scale of 0 to 10 with 10 as the worst pain, what number would you use to categorize the pain?"

27. A patient is currently pain- and symptom-free but reports having intermittent episodes of chest pain over the past week. The nurse asks about which associated symptoms? **Select all that apply.**
    a. Nausea
    b. Diarrhea
    c. Diaphoresis
    d. Dizziness
    e. Joint pain
    f. Shortness of breath

28. The emergency department (ED) nurse is assessing an 86-year-old patient with acute confusion, increased respiratory rate, anxiety, and chest pain. The nurse finds a respiratory rate of 36/min with crackles and wheezes on auscultation. How does the nurse interpret these findings?
    a. Left ventricular heart failure
    b. Atypical angina
    c. Coronary artery disease
    d. Unstable angina

29. The nurse is assessing a middle-aged woman with diabetes who denies any history of known heart problems. Which are gender considerations for women with coronary artery disease (CAD)?
    a. Microvascular disease is a likely cause of CAD in women.
    b. Women typically have smaller coronary arteries than men.
    c. Women are often 5 to 10 years younger than men when CAD develops.
    d. Women with CAD have a lower risk of death when hospitalized than men.
    e. In postmenopausal women the incidence of CAD is equal to that of men.
    f. Women with CAD manifest with atypical signs and symptoms.

30. A middle-aged patient with no known medical problems has acute-onset chest pain and dyspnea. To rule out acute myocardial infarction (MI), the nurse obtains orders for which diagnostic tests?
    a. C-reactive protein
    b. Chest x-ray
    c. Total serum cholesterol, low-density lipoprotein, high-density lipoprotein
    d. Serial troponin T and I

31. A patient had severe chest pain several hours ago but is currently pain-free and has a normal ECG. Which statement by the patient indicates a correct understanding of the significance of the ECG results?
    a. "I'll go home and make an appointment to see my family doctor next week."
    b. "The ECG could be normal since I am currently pain-free."
    c. "A normal ECG means I am okay."
    d. "I have always had a strong heart, low blood pressure, and a normal ECG."

32. Which statement about silent myocardial ischemia is correct?
    a. In silent myocardial ischemia, the patient has no pain so there is less myocardial damage.
    b. Diabetic patients are susceptible to silent myocardial ischemia that is undiagnosed and without complications.
    c. Silent myocardial ischemia increases the incidence of new coronary events.
    d. In silent myocardial ischemia, the myocardium is oxygenated by increased collateral circulation.

33. The emergency department (ED) nurse is caring for a patient with acute pain associated with myocardial infarction (MI). What are the goals of collaborative management that address the patient's pain? **Select all that apply.**
    a. Return the vital signs and cardiac rhythm to baseline so the patient can resume activities of daily living.
    b. Prevent further damage to the cardiac muscle by decreasing myocardial oxygen demand and increasing myocardial oxygen supply.
    c. Aggressively diagnose and treat life-threatening cardiac dysrhythmias and restore pulmonary wedge pressure.
    d. Closely monitor the patient for accompanying symptoms such as nausea and vomiting or indigestion.
    e. Eliminate discomfort by providing pain relief modalities, decrease myocardial oxygen demand, and increase myocardial oxygen supply.
    f. Teach the patient about alternative therapies that can help decrease or replace the need for pain drugs.

34. The emergency department (ED) nurse, caring for a patient with severe chest pain and ECG changes, gives supplemental oxygen to the patient as ordered. Which other medications does the nurse anticipate giving to this patient? **Select all that apply.**
    a. IV nitroglycerin
    b. Beta blocker
    c. IV morphine
    d. Calcium channel blocker
    e. ACE inhibitor
    f. Aspirin

35. The nurse is caring for a hospitalized patient being treated initially with IV nitroglycerin. What intervention must the nurse include in this patient's care?
    a. Increase the dose rapidly to achieve pain relief.
    b. Restrict the patient to bedrest with bedpan use.
    c. Monitor blood pressure continuously.
    d. Elevate the head of the bed to 90 degrees.

36. During an annual physical exam, a patient receives an ECG and has an abnormal Q wave in several leads. What is the nurse's **best** interpretation of this result?
    a. The patient is experiencing a silent MI.
    b. The patient has experienced an MI in the past.
    c. The patient is having an acute MI at the moment.
    d. The patient is experiencing ischemia at the moment.

37. The home health nurse receives a call from a patient with coronary artery disease (CAD) who reports having new onset of chest pain and shortness of breath. What does the nurse instruct the patient to do?
    a. Rest quietly until the nurse can arrive at the house to check the patient.
    b. Chew 325 mg of aspirin and immediately call 911.
    c. Use supplemental home oxygen until symptoms resolve.
    d. Take three nitroglycerin tablets and have family drive the patient to the hospital.

38. A patient is newly diagnosed with cardiovascular disease. What psychosocial reactions does the nurse assess for? **Select all that apply.**
    a. Fear
    b. Anxiety
    c. Anger
    d. Suspicion
    e. Denial
    f. Depression

39. Which drug is given within 1 to 2 hours of a myocardial infarction (MI), when the patient is hemodynamically stable, to help the heart to perform more work without ischemia?
    a. Vasodilators, such as sublingual or spray nitroglycerin
    b. Beta-adrenergic blocking agents, such as metoprolol
    c. Antiplatelet agents, such as clopidogrel
    d. Calcium channel blockers, such as diltiazem

40. Which statements are true about the use of thrombolytic agents for a patient with an acute myocardial infarction (MI)? **Select all that apply.**
    a. A patient who has received a thrombolytic agent must be continuously monitored before and after the medication is given.
    b. Thrombolytic therapy is indicated for chest pain of less than 15 minutes' duration that is unrelieved by other medications.
    c. There are no contraindications to thrombolytic therapy if the patient is having an acute MI.
    d. Bleeding is a risk for patients receiving thrombolytic therapy.
    e. The nurse monitors only clotting studies of the patient who has received thrombolytic therapy.
    f. Patients who receive thrombolytics require percutaneous coronary intervention (PCI) for more definitive treatment such as stent placement.

41. The health care provider is considering use of thrombolytic therapy for a patient. What is the criterion for this therapy?
    a. Chest pain of greater than 15 minutes' duration that is unrelieved by nitroglycerin
    b. Chest pain lasting longer than 30 minutes that is unrelieved by nitroglycerin with ST segment elevation on the ECG
    c. Ventricular dysrhythmias shown on the cardiac monitor
    d. History of chronic, severe, poorly controlled hypertension

42. A patient is being evaluated for thrombolytic therapy. What are **absolute** contraindications for this procedure? **Select all that apply.**
    a. Ischemic stroke within 3 months
    b. Pregnancy
    c. Suspected aortic aneurysm
    d. Major trauma in the last 12 months
    e. Significant closed-head or facial trauma within 3 months
    f. Malignant intracranial neoplasm

43. The patient received thrombolytic therapy. Which manifestation indicates that the clot has been dissolved?
   a. The patient continues to have chest pain but the intensity is much less.
   b. There is sudden onset of nonsustained ventricular dysrhythmias.
   c. ST segment remains elevated with inverted T waves.
   d. Cardiac markers peak 3 to 4 hours after thrombolytic therapy.

44. A patient has received thrombolytic therapy for treatment of acute myocardial infarction (MI). What are **postadministration** nursing responsibilities for this treatment? **Select all that apply.**
   a. Document the patient's emotional reaction to thrombolytic therapy.
   b. Observe all IV sites for bleeding and patency.
   c. Monitor white blood cell (WBC) count and differential.
   d. Monitor clotting studies.
   e. Place all new IV lines to prevent infection.
   f. Test stools, urine, and emesis for occult blood.

45. A patient is receiving beta-blocker therapy for treatment of myocardial infarction (MI). What does the nurse monitor for in relation to this therapy? **Select all that apply.**
   a. Tachycardia
   b. Hypotension
   c. Decreased level of consciousness
   d. Chest discomfort
   e. Increased urinary output
   f. Auscultate lungs for crackles or wheezes

46. A patient is being treated with medication therapy following an acute myocardial infarction (MI). The nurse **questions** the order for which type of drug?
   a. Calcium channel blocker
   b. Beta blocker
   c. ACE inhibitor
   d. Angiotensin receptor blocker (ARB)

47. A patient with chronic stable angina is taking calcium channel blockers. For which complication does the nurse monitor with this patient?
   a. Wheezes
   b. Hypotension
   c. Tachycardia
   d. Forgetfulness

48. Which diagnostic test is performed after angina or myocardial infarction (MI) to determine cardiac changes that are consistent with ischemia, to evaluate medical interventions, and to determine whether invasive intervention is necessary?
   a. Exercise tolerance test
   b. Electrocardiogram
   c. Echocardiography
   d. Chest x-ray

49. The patient who was diagnosed with acute coronary syndrome (ACS) will be discharged soon. Which type of drug that will reduce the risk of developing recurrent myocardial infarction (MI), stroke, and mortality does the nurse expect the health care provider to prescribe prior to discharge?
   a. Stool softener
   b. High-intensity statin therapy
   c. Anti-inflammatory
   d. Central vasodilator

50. A patient has had a myocardial infarction (MI). The nurse anticipates which type of drug will be prescribed within 48 hours to prevent the development of ventricular remodeling and heart failure?
   a. Calcium channel blocker
   b. ACE inhibitor
   c. Beta blocker
   d. Diuretic

51. The nurse has identified the priority problem of activity intolerance for a patient who had an acute myocardial infarction (MI). What is the **best** expected outcome for this patient?
    a. Patient will progressively walk up to 200 feet four times a day without chest discomfort or shortness of breath.
    b. Patient will name three or four activities that will not cause shortness of breath or chest pain.
    c. Nurse will teach the patient to exercise and to take the pulse if symptoms of shortness of breath or pain occur.
    d. Nurse will assist the patient with ADLs until shortness of breath or pain resolves.

52. A patient is in the acute phase (phase 1) of cardiac rehabilitation. Which task is best to delegate to the unlicensed assistive personnel (UAP)?
    a. Assist the patient to ambulate approximately 200 feet three times a day.
    b. Assist the patient with ambulation to the bathroom.
    c. Assess heart rate, blood pressure, respiratory rate, and fatigue with each higher level of activity.
    d. Assist the patient into the bathtub.

53. A patient in a cardiac rehabilitation program is having difficulty coping with the changes in her health status. Which statement by the patient is the **strongest** indicator of ineffective or harmful coping?
    a. "I don't mind going to therapy, but I'm not sure if I'm getting any benefit from it."
    b. "I'll take the pills and just do whatever you want me to do."
    c. "I don't want to go to therapy; I had a bad experience yesterday with the therapist."
    d. "I know I need to talk about going home soon, but could we discuss it later?"

54. A post–myocardial infarction (MI) patient in phase 1 cardiac rehabilitation is encouraged to perform which activity?
    a. Range-of-motion exercises
    b. Modified weight training
    c. Stair climbing
    d. Jogging

55. The nurse is caring for a patient admitted for an inferior wall myocardial infarction (IWMI). The patient develops heart block with bradycardia. Which procedure is the nurse prepared to assist with?
    a. Temporary pacemaker
    b. Defibrillation
    c. 16-lead ECG
    d. Percutaneous intervention

56. The nurse is caring for a patient diagnosed with acute coronary syndrome (ACS). Which manifestations indicate cardiogenic shock? **Select all that apply.**
    a. Cold, clammy skin with poor peripheral pulses
    b. Urine output less than 0.5-1 mL/kg/hr
    c. Bradycardia and hypotension
    d. Systolic BP less than 90 mm Hg or 30 mm Hg less than the patient's baseline
    e. Agitation, restlessness, or confusion
    f. Tachypnea and crackles

57. The nurse is evaluating a patient with coronary artery disease (CAD). What is an expected patient outcome that demonstrates hemodynamic stability?
    a. Blood pressure and pulse are within range and adequate for metabolic demands.
    b. Urine output increases from 15 to 30 mL per hour.
    c. P waves are regular and there are no abnormal heart sounds.
    d. Patient expresses verbal understanding of risk factors and need for compliance.

58. The nurse is assessing a patient who is labeled Class I based on the Killip classification of heart failure. Which manifestation(s) does the nurse expect to find?
    a. Clear lung sounds and absence of S3
    b. Crackles in the lower half of the lung fields and possible S3
    c. Crackles more than halfway up the lung fields and frothy sputum
    d. Systolic blood pressure less than 90 mm Hg and oliguria

59. The nurse is reviewing medication orders for several cardiac patients. There is an order for beta-adrenergic blocking agent metoprolol XL once a day. According to the Killip classification, this drug order is most appropriate for which classes of patients?
    a. All classes
    b. Class I only
    c. Classes II and III
    d. Class IV only

60. The ICU nurse is caring for a patient with a diagnosis of acute coronary syndrome (ACS) who has developed left heart failure that is unresponsive to drug therapy. What intervention does the nurse expect may be next for this patient?
    a. Positive inotropic drugs IV
    b. Intra-aortic balloon pump insertion
    c. Fibrinolytic therapy
    d. Percutaneous coronary intervention (PCI)

61. The nurse is assessing a cardiac patient and finds a paradoxical pulse, clear lungs, and jugular venous distention that occurs when the patient is in a semi-Fowler's position. What are these findings consistent with?
    a. Right ventricle failure
    b. Unstable angina
    c. Coronary artery disease (CAD)
    d. Valvular disease

62. The intensive care nurse is monitoring a patient with a diagnosis of myocardial infarction (MI). The pulmonary artery wedge pressure (PAWP) reading is 30 mm Hg. What does the nurse do **next**?
    a. Increase the IV fluid rate to 200 mL/hour.
    b. Auscultate the lungs to assess for left-sided heart failure.
    c. Perform an ECG using right-sided precordial leads.
    d. Place the patient in semi-Fowler's position.

63. A patient continues to have chest pain despite compliance with medical therapy. The nurse teaches the patient about which diagnostic test?
    a. Cardiac catheterization
    b. Percutaneous transluminal coronary angioplasty (PTCA)
    c. Coronary artery bypass grafting (CABG)
    d. Stent placement in coronary artery

64. Immediate reperfusion is an invasive intervention that shows some promise for managing which disorder?
    a. Right ventricular failure
    b. Metabolic syndrome
    c. Cardiogenic shock
    d. Acute coronary syndrome

65. A patient is scheduled to have percutaneous coronary intervention (PCI). The nurse anticipates that an initial dose of which medication will be given before the procedure?
    a. Clopidogrel
    b. Nitroglycerin
    c. Isosorbide mononitrate
    d. Carvedilol

66. A patient has angina and is scheduled for percutaneous coronary intervention (PCI). Based on negative outcomes of the PCI, the nurse prepares the patient for immediate transfer to undergo which procedure?
    a. Intra-aortic balloon pump
    b. Coronary artery bypass graft (CABG)
    c. Cardiac catheterization
    d. Carotid endarterectomy

67. The nurse is caring for a patient who had percutaneous coronary intervention (PCI). Which symptom indicates acute closure of the vessel and warrants **immediate** notification of the health care provider?
    a. Chest pain
    b. Hyperkalemia
    c. Bleeding at the insertion site
    d. Cough and shortness of breath

68. Which patients may be potential candidates for coronary artery bypass graft (CABG)? **Select all that apply.**
    a. Patient with angina and greater than 50% occlusion of left main coronary artery that cannot be stented
    b. Patient with unstable angina with moderate one vessel disease appropriate for stenting
    c. Patient with valvular disease
    d. Patient with coronary vessels unsuitable for PCI
    e. Patient with acute myocardial infarction (MI) responding to therapy
    f. Patient with signs of ischemia or impending MI after angiography or PCI

69. The patient with left ventricular myocardial infarction (MI) is to have coronary artery bypass graft (CABG) surgery. Which interventions does the nurse perform to protect against sternal wound infection? **Select all that apply.**
    a. Shave the patient's body from neck to knees.
    b. Instruct the patient to shower with 4% chlorhexidine gluconate (CHG).
    c. Prepare the surgical site by clipping hair and applying CHG with isopropyl alcohol (either 0.5% or 2%).
    d. Send urine and sputum to the lab for culture and sensitivity.
    e. Administer IV antibiotics one hour prior to the surgical procedure.
    f. Wear gown, gloves, and a mask while preparing the patient for surgery.

70. A patient is having an elective coronary artery bypass graft (CABG) with a minimally invasive surgical technique. What does the nurse include in the preoperative teaching?
    a. Prevention of edema and scarring at the harvest site
    b. Protection and splinting of the chest incision while coughing
    c. Availability of analgesics if needed, but probably unnecessary
    d. Limitation of ambulation for several days after the procedure

71. A patient is having a coronary artery bypass graft (CABG) with the traditional surgical procedure. What does the nurse include in the **preoperative** teaching? **Select all that apply.**
    a. Coughing will be avoided to keep stress off the sternal incision.
    b. There will be a sternal incision.
    c. Expect one, two, or three chest tubes.
    d. An indwelling urinary catheter will be placed.
    e. An endotracheal tube will prevent talking.
    f. You will be on bedrest for up to 48 hours after the surgery.

72. The intensive care nurse is caring for a patient who has just had coronary artery bypass graft (CABG) surgery. The nurse notes that the patient has peripheral edema. To adjust fluid administration, the nurse collects which additional information and then consults the health care provider? **Select all that apply.**
    a. Blood pressure
    b. Pulmonary artery wedge pressure (PAWP)
    c. Skin turgor
    d. Cardiac output
    e. Blood loss
    f. Urine output

73. The health care provider orders potassium 80 mEq in 100 mL of IV bolus at a rate of 40 mEq/hr for a patient in the critical care unit through a central line. What does the nurse do **next**?
    a. Contact the health care provider because the order exceeds the recommended amount.
    b. Give the infusion; the order exceeds the recommended amount but is within acceptable standards of practice for critical care patients.
    c. Contact the health care provider because even though the dosage is acceptable, the rate is too fast.
    d. Consult with the pharmacist because even though the rate is acceptable, the mixture is too concentrated.

74. The intensive care nurse is caring for a patient who has just had coronary artery bypass graft (CABG) surgery. The patient has a systolic blood pressure of 80 mm Hg. What is the **primary** concern related to this patient's hypotension?
    a. It is associated with warm cardioplegia.
    b. It may result in the collapse of the graft.
    c. It will result in acute tubular necrosis.
    d. It is related to mechanical ventilation.

75. Following coronary artery bypass graft (CABG) surgery, a patient has a body temperature below 96.8°F (36°C). What measure should be used to rewarm the patient?
    a. Infuse warm IV fluids.
    b. Do not rewarm; cold cardioplegia is protective.
    c. Place the patient in a warm fluid bath.
    d. Use lights or thermal blankets.

76. The intensive care nurse is caring for a patient who has just had coronary artery bypass graft (CABG) surgery. What does the nurse do to assess for **postoperative** bleeding?
    a. Measure mediastinal and pleural chest tube drainage at least hourly and report drainage amounts over 150 mL/hr to the surgeon.
    b. Measure mediastinal and pleural chest tube drainage at least once a shift and report drainage amounts over 50 mL/hr to the surgeon.
    c. Assess the dressing over the sternal site every 4 hours and reinforce the dressing with sterile gauze as needed.
    d. Assess the donor site every 4 hours and report serous drainage and increasing pain to the surgeon.

77. Following coronary artery bypass graft (CABG) surgery, a patient in the ICU on a mechanical ventilator suddenly decompensates. The health care provider makes a diagnosis of cardiac tamponade. The nurse prepares the patient for which emergency procedure?
    a. Chest tube
    b. Sternotomy
    c. Pericardiocentesis
    d. Thoracentesis

78. The nurse is assessing a patient who had coronary artery bypass graft (CABG) surgery. Which finding is a permanent deficit that is associated with an intraoperative stroke?
    a. Decreased level of consciousness that resolves when body temperature is normal
    b. Arousal from anesthesia takes several hours
    c. Inability to speak clearly and coherently immediately after surgery
    d. Generalized seizure activity

79. A patient reports chest pain after coronary artery bypass graft (CABG) surgery. Which statement by the patient suggests that the pain is related to the sternotomy and **not** anginal in origin?
    a. "The pain goes down my arm or sometimes into my jaw."
    b. "My pain increases when I cough or take a deep breath."
    c. "The nitroglycerin helped to relieve the pain."
    d. "I feel nausea and shortness of breath when the pain occurs."

80. A patient with coronary artery bypass graft (CABG) surgery is transferred from the ICU to the intermediate care unit. Which activity does the nurse assist the patient with?
    a. Ambulating 25-100 feet three times a day as tolerated
    b. Turning the patient every 2 hours for the first 48 hours
    c. Dangling and turning every 2 hours for at least 24 hours
    d. Coughing and deep-breathing three times a day

81. A patient had coronary artery bypass graft (CABG) surgery with the radial artery used as a graft. The nurse performs which assessment **specific** to this patient?
    a. Check the blood pressure every hour on the unaffected arm or use the legs.
    b. Check the fingertips, hand, and arm for sensation and mobility every shift.
    c. Assess hand color, temperature, ulnar/radial pulses, and capillary refill every hour initially.
    d. Note edema, bleeding, and swelling at the donor site, which are expected.

82. A patient with coronary artery bypass graft (CABG) surgery has been diagnosed with mediastinitis. What information does the nurse expect to find in the patient's assessment documentation? **Select all that apply.**
    a. Fever continuing beyond the first 4 days after CABG
    b. Bogginess of the sternum
    c. Redness and drainage from suture sites
    d. Decreased white blood cell count
    e. Induration or swelling at the suture sites
    f. Anginal-type chest pain

83. A patient had coronary artery bypass graft (CABG) surgery with a vein graft. To help prevent collapse of the graft, what assessment does the nurse perform?
    a. Auscultate lung sounds.
    b. Monitor for hypotension.
    c. Assess for motion and sensation.
    d. Observe for generalized hypothermia.

84. The nurse is caring for a patient who had coronary artery bypass graft (CABG) surgery. The nurse pays close attention to which electrolyte levels for this postoperative patient? **Select all that apply.**
    a. Sodium
    b. Potassium
    c. Calcium
    d. Magnesium
    e. Phosphorus
    f. Creatinine

85. After coronary artery bypass graft (CABG) surgery, a postoperative patient suddenly has a decrease in mediastinal drainage, jugular vein distention with clear lung sounds, pulsus paradoxus, and equalizing pulmonary artery wedge pressure (PAWP) and right atrial pressure. What do these signs suggest to the nurse?
    a. Acute myocardial infarction (MI)
    b. Occlusion at the donor site
    c. Cardiac tamponade
    d. Prinzmetal's angina

86. The nurse coming on duty receives the change of shift report. Which patient must be assessed **first** by the nurse?
    a. Patient with anxiety, nausea, diaphoresis, and shortness of breath
    b. Patient with diabetes mellitus and elevated serum lipid levels
    c. Patient with a friction rub and elevated temperature
    d. Patient with fever, instability of sternum, and increased white blood cell count

87. The nurse is caring for a patient who had a minimally invasive direct coronary artery bypass (MIDCAB). Which sign/symptom prompts the nurse to **immediately** contact the health care provider?
    a. Acute incisional pain
    b. ST-segment changes on the monitor
    c. Drainage from the chest tubes
    d. Problems with coughing

88. A patient has discrete, proximal, noncalcified lesions of only one or two vessels. Which procedure is **most likely** to be recommended for this patient?
    a. Percutaneous coronary intervention (PCI)
    b. Stress test with pharmacologic agent
    c. Immediate thrombolytic reperfusion therapy
    d. Minimally invasive bypass surgery

89. The nurse is caring for a patient who had a percutaneous coronary intervention (PCI). Which postprocedure interventions are included in the care for this patient? **Select all that apply.**
    a. Monitor for acute closure of the vessel.
    b. Observe for bleeding from the insertion site.
    c. Maintain bedrest for 48 hours.
    d. Observe for hypotension, hypokalemia, and dysrhythmias.
    e. Teach about medications such as aspirin and beta blockers or ACE inhibitors.
    f. Instruct about lifestyle changes relating to CAD.

90. Treatment of hypothermia, a common problem after coronary artery bypass graft (CABG) surgery, is necessary because this condition may cause a patient to be at risk for which condition?
    a. Hypotension
    b. Hypertension
    c. Heart failure
    d. Loss of consciousness

91. Which statement is true about postpericardiotomy syndrome?
    a. It is a psychological disorder for which the patient needs emotional support.
    b. It is mild and self-limiting for all patients.
    c. It places the patient at risk for acute cardiac tamponade.
    d. It can be prophylactically managed with antibiotics.

92. The patient is scheduled to have robotic heart surgery. Which advantages of this type of surgery does the nurse teach the patient about? **Select all that apply.**
    a. Shorter (2- to 3-day) hospital stay
    b. Shorter surgical time than with traditional heart surgery
    c. Less pain due to smaller incisions
    d. Shorter time on heart-lung bypass machine
    e. Chest tubes are never needed
    f. Ability to reach otherwise inaccessible blockage sites

93. Which is the **primary** medical-surgical concept for a patient with unstable angina or myocardial Infarction?
    a. Comfort
    b. Tissue integrity
    c. Gas exchange
    d. Perfusion

94. Cardiac rehabilitation is recommended for patients after MI or CABG. What are **commonly cited** reasons that patients do not participate in cardiac rehab programs? **Select all that apply.**
    a. Lack of transportation
    b. Lack of insurance coverage
    c. Health care provider does not believe it is necessary
    d. Inability to perform the program activities
    e. Patient decision that it is not necessary
    f. Necessity of returning to work as soon as possible

95. A patient has been discharged after CABG surgery and is to start a simple walking program at home. What does the nurse teach the patient about a home walking program? **Select all that apply.**
    a. Begin by walking 400 feet twice a day at the rate of 1 mile/hr the first week after discharge.
    b. Each week increase the distance and rate as tolerated until you can walk 2 miles at 3 to 4 miles/hr.
    c. Take a break after walking each mile to avoid pain or shortness of breath.
    d. Check your pulse reading before, halfway through, and after exercise.
    e. Walk even when the weather is either hot or cold.
    f. Stop exercising if your pulse rate increases more than 20 beats per minute or if you develop dyspnea or angina.

96. Which alternative therapies may be helpful in reducing the patient's anxiety about progressive activity both in the immediate postoperative period and during the rehabilitation phase? **Select all that apply.**
    a. Progressive muscle relaxation
    b. Acupuncture
    c. Guided imagery
    d. Music therapy
    e. Herbal remedies
    f. Therapeutic touch

97. Which class of drugs has a strong FDA warning about **increased** risk for stroke or heart attack?
    a. Beta blockers
    b. Non-aspirin NSAIDs
    c. Calcium channel blockers
    d. ACE inhibitors

98. The nurse is teaching a patient diagnosed with acute coronary syndrome (ACS) about when to notify the health care provider and seek medical advice. Which precautions would the nurse teach this patient? **Select all that apply.**
    a. Call your health care provider if your heart rate remains at less than 50 after arising from bed.
    b. Notify your health care provider if you experience weight gain of 3 pounds in 1 week or 1 to 2 pounds overnight.
    c. Let your health care provider know every time you need to use nitroglycerin for angina.
    d. Be sure to tell your health care provider if you experience dizziness, faintness, or shortness of breath with activity.
    e. Have your spouse bring you to the hospital if you experience extremely severe chest or epigastric discomfort with weakness, nausea, or fainting.
    f. Notify your health care provider if your nitroglycerin produces a tingling sensation when you place it under your tongue.

39 CHAPTER

Assessment of the Hematologic System

1. The nurse is performing a hematologic assessment. Which finding would be considered a normal change in an older adult?
   a. Progressive loss of body hair
   b. Loss of nails and cuticles
   c. Irregular pattern of ecchymosis
   d. Cyanosis of the lips and earlobes

2. Which dinner selection represents the **best** choice of foods to supply the nutrients required for good cell quality and clotting function?
   a. Fried chicken breast with mashed potatoes and gravy and green beans
   b. Mixed fruit and vegetable salad, French bread with butter, and wine
   c. Small lean beef steak with cheese and hash brown potato casserole
   d. Grilled salmon with spinach salad and fresh strawberries for dessert

3. For a patient who has a dysfunction of the bone marrow, which sign/symptom is the nurse **most likely** to observe?
   a. Long bone pain
   b. Fatigue
   c. Loss of appetite
   d. Weight gain

4. What equipment would the nurse need to perform a hematologic assessment? **Select all that apply.**
   a. Gloves
   b. Otoscope
   c. Stethoscope
   d. Blood pressure cuff
   e. Penlight
   f. Cotton-tip applicator

5. The nurse knows that erythropoietin is a growth factor that is required for stem cell specialization. Which sign/symptom would the nurse observe if erythropoietin is lacking or not performing its role?
   a. Elevated body temperature
   b. Bruising and ecchymosis
   c. Swelling of lymph nodes
   d. Fatigue and exhaustion

6. Based on knowledge of albumin's role in maintaining osmotic pressure of the blood, which sign/symptom would the nurse look for if the patient has low albumin levels?
   a. Fever
   b. Edema
   c. Bruising
   d. Pain

7. During physical assessment the nurse gently palpates the patient's sternum and the patient reports tenderness to touch. Why would the nurse report this finding to the health care provider?
   a. Hematology problems increase risk for rib fractures.
   b. Pernicious anemia causes fissures in underlying structures.
   c. Elicited tenderness could signal myocardial infarction.
   d. Rib or sternal tenderness may occur with leukemia.

8. Which drug disrupts platelet action?
   a. Vitamin K
   b. Ibuprofen
   c. Penicillin V
   d. Morphine

9. The nurse is interviewing a patient who has iron deficiency anemia. Which symptom is the patient **most likely** to report?
    a. Fatigue
    b. Nights sweats
    c. Calf pain
    d. Blood in urine

10. When assessing the patient with darker skin for pallor and cyanosis, which area would the nurse examine?
    a. Chest and abdomen
    b. General appearance of face
    c. Fingertips and toes
    d. Oral mucous membranes

11. Based on knowledge of physiologic triggers for red blood cell (RBC) production, the nurse would anticipate which chronic health condition to be associated with an increase in RBC production?
    a. Diabetes mellitus
    b. Osteoarthritis
    c. Chronic obstructive pulmonary disease
    d. Chronic kidney disease

12. The patient is admitted for a chronic liver disorder and will be receiving vitamin K to address one of the problems associated with the disorder. Which clinical manifestation is the nurse **most likely** to observe before vitamin K therapy is initiated?
    a. Sore throat and a smooth tongue
    b. Bruising and bleeding at venipuncture sites
    c. Fever and increased white blood cell count
    d. Calf swelling due to deep vein thrombosis

13. The patient reports a history of splenectomy. Based on this information, what is the nurse **most likely** to assess for?
    a. Signs of bleeding
    b. Signs of infection
    c. Digestive problems
    d. Jaundice of the skin

14. Which laboratory result would indicate that the prescription for epoetin alfa is having the desired therapeutic effect?
    a. Increase in platelet count
    b. Increase in white blood cell count
    c. Increase in red blood cell count
    d. Increase in iron level

15. Venous stasis is considered to be an intrinsic factor that can result in activating which physiologic process?
    a. Increased red blood cell production
    b. Adjustment of osmotic fluid pressure
    c. Initiation of anticlotting forces
    d. Initiation of blood clotting cascade

16. A deficiency in any of the anticlotting factors, such as protein C, protein S, and antithrombin III increases the patient's risk for which disorder(s)? **Select all that apply.**
    a. Pulmonary embolism
    b. Myocardial infarction
    c. Iron deficient anemia
    d. Pernicious anemia
    e. Stroke
    f. Hemolytic anemia

17. Which organ is **most likely** to become enlarged as the result of severe anemia?
    a. Gallbladder
    b. Kidneys
    c. Colon
    d. Liver

18. The nurse notes that a 45-year-old woman has a low hemoglobin level. The nurse would perform a dietary assessment to identify a possible deficiency in which nutrient?
    a. Calcium
    b. Vitamin K
    c. Iron
    d. Vitamin D

19. In assessing the patient's hematologic status, which questions would the nurse include? **Select all that apply.**
    a. "Have you had unusual or increased fatigue?"
    b. "Have you ever had any radiation therapy?"
    c. "Have you ever donated blood or plasma?"
    d. "Do you have a personal or family history of blood disorders?"
    e. "What drugs have you used in the past 3 days?"
    f. "Have you ever had a job that exposed you to chemicals?"

20. While reviewing the patient's medication list, the nurse notes that the patient is receiving parenteral enoxaparin. Which outcome statement reflects the goal of the enoxaparin therapy?
    a. Patient shows no signs/symptoms of a blood clot.
    b. Patient reports a decrease in fatigue and dizziness.
    c. Patient shows no signs/symptoms of infection.
    d. Patient reports no shortness of breath on exertion.

21. The nurse is interviewing a patient who might be a candidate for fibrinolytic therapy for treatment of myocardial infarction. Why is determining the time of symptom onset essential for decision making?
    a. Fibrinolytic drugs will not dissolve clots that are older than 6 hours.
    b. Clots that are older than 6 hours are tightly meshed and complete.
    c. Tissue that is anoxic for more than 6 hours is unlikely to benefit.
    d. After 6 hours, the patient is more likely to have excessive bleeding.

22. The home health nurse notices that new medications were prescribed for a patient during a recent hospitalization. In addition, the patient reports taking daily low-dose aspirin, but aspirin is not on the medication reconciliation list. Because of the aspirin, the nurse is **most likely** to call the prescribing health care provider for clarification of which type of medication?
    a. Vitamin supplement
    b. Platelet inhibitor
    c. Antihypertensive
    d. Erythrocyte stimulating agent

23. A patient has a suspected hematologic problem. Which instruction is the nurse **most likely** to give to the unlicensed assistive personnel?
    a. Record urine output for the shift.
    b. Take the vital signs every 2 hours.
    c. Assess the patient for fatigue after exertion.
    d. Handle the patient gently to avoid bruising.

24. A patient is diagnosed with iron deficiency anemia. Which assessment finding is the nurse **most likely** to observe in this patient?
    a. Neck veins are distended and edema is present.
    b. Lower extremities show signs of phlebitis.
    c. Systolic blood pressure is lower than normal.
    d. Palpation of ribs or sternum elicits tenderness.

25. An experienced nurse is supervising a new nurse who is assessing a patient with a suspected hematologic problem. The experienced nurse would intervene if the new nurse performed which action?
    a. Palpated the edge of the liver in the right upper quadrant
    b. Auscultated the heart for abnormal heart sounds or irregular rhythms
    c. Used the fingertips to firmly press over the ribs or sternum
    d. Palpated the left upper quadrant to locate an enlarged spleen

26. The nurse routinely checks mental status on all patients; however, which patient has the **greatest** need for frequent neurologic assessment and checks of cognitive function?
    a. Elderly patient with chronic dementia has iron deficiency anemia due to poor diet.
    b. Younger female patient has low hemoglobin and hematocrit related to heavy menses.
    c. Older male with alcoholism sustains head injury during an episode of intoxication.
    d. Young male has fever and elevated white blood cell count related to an upper respiratory infection.

27. The nurse notes that the patient's platelet count is 400,000/mm³. What action is the nurse **most likely** to take?
    a. Immediately inform the health care provider because of possible spontaneous bleeding.
    b. Instruct unlicensed assistive personnel to handle patient gently to minimize bruising.
    c. Document the result because it is within the normal range and continue to monitor patient.
    d. Initiate protective isolation and monitor for signs/symptoms of systemic infection.

28. The nurse is caring for a patient who just had a bone marrow aspiration. Which outcome statement reflects the **priority** goal of care after the procedure?
    a. Patient will not experience excessive bleeding.
    b. Patient's pain level will be 3/10 or less.
    c. Patient will not show signs/symptoms of infection.
    d. Patient will verbalize understanding of procedure results.

40

CHAPTER

Care of Patients with Hematologic Problems

1. The nurse is assessing a patient who is newly diagnosed with anemia. Which assessment findings are typical of this disorder? **Select all that apply.**
   a. Dyspnea on exertion
   b. Systolic hypertension
   c. Intolerance to heat
   d. Concave appearance of nails
   e. Pallor of the ears
   f. Headache

2. A patient with sickle cell crisis is admitted to the hospital. Which questions does the nurse ask the patient to elicit information about the cause of the current crisis? **Select all that apply.**
   a. "Have you recently traveled on an airplane?"
   b. "Have you ever had radiation therapy?"
   c. "In the past 24 hours, has any activity made you short of breath?"
   d. "Have you recently consumed alcohol or used recreational drugs?"
   e. "Have you had any symptoms of infection, such as fever?"
   f. "Lately have you increased strenuous physical activities?"

3. A patient is scheduled to undergo diagnostic testing for sickle cell anemia. Which educational brochure is the nurse **most likely** to provide to the patient?
   a. "What to Expect During a Bone Marrow Biopsy"
   b. "How Your Doctor Interprets Your Platelet Count"
   c. "What Is a Philadelphia Chromosome Analysis?"
   d. "How Is Hemoglobin S Used to Confirm My Diagnosis?"

4. The student nurse is caring for a patient in sickle cell crisis. Which action by the student nurse warrants intervention by the supervising nurse?
   a. Turning down the thermostat to a cooler temperature
   b. Using distraction and relaxation techniques
   c. Positioning patient's painful areas with support
   d. Using therapeutic touch and aroma therapy

5. The nurse has taught the patient about dietary modifications for his vitamin B_{12} deficiency anemia. Which statement by the patient indicates that additional teaching is needed?
   a. "Dairy products are a good source of vitamin B_{12}."
   b. "Dried beans taste okay if they are prepared correctly."
   c. "Leafy green vegetables interfere with my therapy."
   d. "I like nuts, and I will gladly include them in my diet."

6. Which patient is **most likely** to have severe manifestations of sickle cell disease even when triggering conditions are mild?
   a. Mother and father both have hemoglobin S gene alleles.
   b. Mother has hemoglobin S gene alleles and father has hemoglobin A gene alleles.
   c. Mother has sickle cell trait and father has hemoglobin A gene alleles.
   d. Mother and father both have hemoglobin A gene alleles.

7. The nurse is caring for a patient in sickle cell crisis. What are the **priority** interventions for this patient? **Select all that apply.**
   a. Managing pain
   b. Managing nutrition
   c. Ensuring hydration
   d. Administering platelets
   e. Assessing oxygen saturation
   f. Monitoring for signs/symptoms of infection

8. The unlicensed assistive personnel (UAP) is assisting in the care of a patient in sickle cell crisis. Which action by the UAP requires intervention by the supervising nurse?
   a. Elevating the head of the bed to 25 degrees
   b. Helping to remove any restrictive clothing
   c. Obtaining the blood pressure with an external cuff
   d. Offering the patient a caffeine-free beverage

9. A patient admitted for sickle cell crisis is being discharged home. Which statement by the patient indicates the need for further post-discharge instruction?
   a. "I will walk rather than jog every morning."
   b. "I will visit my friends in Denver."
   c. "I will avoid the sauna at the gym."
   d. "I will not drink alcoholic beverages."

10. A patient has polycythemia vera. Which action by unlicensed assistive personnel requires intervention by the supervising nurse?
    a. Assisting the patient to floss his teeth
    b. Using an electric shaver on the patient
    c. Helping the patient with a soft-bristled toothbrush
    d. Assisting the patient to don support hose

11. Which abnormal vital sign is the nurse **most likely** to see in a patient who has polycythemia vera?
    a. Elevated temperature
    b. Decreased respiratory rate
    c. Increased blood pressure
    d. Rapid thready pulse

12. Which food should a patient with a low white blood cell count be encouraged to eat?
    a. Fresh blueberries
    b. Unpasteurized yogurt
    c. Green leaf lettuce
    d. Baked chicken

13. The nurse is caring for a patient with acute leukemia. Which signs/symptoms is the nurse **most likely** to observe during the assessment? **Select all that apply.**
    a. Hematuria
    b. Orthostatic hypotension
    c. Bone pain
    d. Joint swelling
    e. Fatigue
    f. Weight gain

14. In caring for a patient with acute leukemia, what is the **priority** collaborative problem?
    a. Protecting the patient from infection
    b. Minimizing the side effects of chemotherapy
    c. Controlling the patient's pain
    d. Assisting the patient to cope with fatigue

15. The nurse is helping a patient prepare for induction therapy for acute leukemia. What information will the nurse give to the patient?
    a. A donor is needed for hematopoietic stem cell transplantation.
    b. Prolonged hospitalization is common to protect against infection.
    c. The therapy may last from months to years to maintain remission.
    d. Success of the therapy results in remission and the intent is to cure.

16. Which factors are associated with an increased risk for non-Hodgkin's lymphoma? **Select all that apply.**
    a. Immunosuppressive disorders
    b. Chronic infection from *Helicobacter pylori*
    c. Epstein-Barr viral infection
    d. Chronic alcoholism
    e. Pesticides and insecticides
    f. Smoking cigars or cigarettes

17. Which disorder poses the **greatest** risk of infection for the patient?
    a. Sickle cell crisis
    b. Vitamin B_{12} deficiency anemia
    c. Polycythemia vera
    d. Thrombocytopenia

18. Which medication increases the risk for the patient to develop infection?
    a. Glucocorticoids
    b. Nonsteroidal anti-inflammatory agents
    c. Iron solutions
    d. Anticoagulants

19. The nurse is caring for a patient with thrombocytopenia. Which order does the nurse question?
    a. Test all urine and stool for occult blood.
    b. Avoid IM injections.
    c. Administer enemas.
    d. Apply ice to areas of trauma.

20. A patient has the signs/symptoms of hereditary hemochromatosis. The health care provider asks the nurse to immediately report **relevant** laboratory results, so the diagnosis can be confirmed. Which laboratory result is the health care provider waiting for?
    a. Complete blood count
    b. Blood ferritin level
    c. Platelet count
    d. Peripheral blood smear

21. The home care nurse is visiting a patient who had a stem cell transplant. Which observation by the nurse requires **immediate** action?
    a. The patient's grandson is visiting after receiving a measles, mumps, and rubella vaccine.
    b. The patient bumps his toe on a chair and applies pressure to the toe for 10 minutes.
    c. The patient with a platelet count of 48,000/mm³ follows platelet precautions.
    d. The patient avoids going outdoors if conditions are icy or slippery.

22. A patient has been taught how to care for his central venous catheter at home. Which statement by the patient indicates that further instruction is necessary?
    a. "I will flush the catheter with heparin once a day and after infusions."
    b. "I will change the Luer-Lok cap on each catheter every week."
    c. "I will look for and report any signs of infection."
    d. "I will wash my hands before working with the catheter."

23. The nurse has instructed a patient at risk for bleeding about techniques to manage bleeding. Which statements by the patient indicate that teaching has been successful? **Select all that apply.**
    a. "I will take a stool softener to prevent straining during a bowel movement."
    b. "I won't take aspirin or aspirin-containing products."
    c. "I won't participate in any contact sports."
    d. "I will report a headache that is not responsive to acetaminophen."
    e. "I will avoid bending over at the waist."
    f. "If I am injured, I will apply a warm compress for at least 10 minutes."

24. The new registered nurse is giving a blood transfusion to a patient. Which statement by the new nurse indicates the need for action by the supervising nurse?
    a. "I will complete the red blood cell transfusion within 6 hours."
    b. "I will check the patient verification with another registered nurse."
    c. "I will use normal saline solution to begin the blood transfusion."
    d. "I will remain with the patient for the first 15 to 30 minutes of the infusion."

25. The new registered nurse is identifying a patient for blood transfusion. Which action by the new nurse warrants intervention by the supervising nurse?
    a. Checks the health care provider's order before the blood transfusion
    b. Compares the identification name band and number to the blood component tag
    c. Cross-checks the patient's room number as a form of identification.
    d. Compares blood bag label and requisition slip to ensure compatibility of ABO and Rh.

26. A patient with lymphoma requires a hematopoietic stem cell transplant, and a donor is being sought. Which type of transplant is likely to yield the **best** results?
    a. Partially HLA-matched unrelated donor
    b. HLA-identical twin sibling
    c. HLA-matched first-degree relative
    d. HLA-matched stem cells from an umbilical cord of a related donor

27. The home health nurse is visiting a patient who was recently treated for leukemia. The patient says he feels fine and has been carefully following all discharge instructions. The patient's temperature is 1°F (or 0.5°C) above baseline. What should the nurse do?
    a. Tell the patient to recheck the temperature in 4 hours.
    b. Administer two 325 mg tablets of acetaminophen.
    c. Initiate standard infection control and call the health care provider.
    d. Document the temperature and other vital signs in the record.

28. During an employee health physical assessment, the patient reports noticing a large lymph node about a month ago. The patient states, "It doesn't hurt so I just ignored it." What questions would the nurse ask to find out if the patient has any of the constitutional symptoms of lymphoma? **Select all that apply.**
    a. "Have you had any unplanned weight loss?"
    b. "Have you had any headaches?"
    c. "Have you seen blood in your urine or stool?"
    d. "Have you noticed heavy night sweats?"
    e. "Have you had a fever ($>101.5°F$ or $>38.6°C$)?"
    f. "Have you had any problems with balance?"

29. Which hematologic disorder is **most likely** to cause the patient to have joint problems?
    a. Thrombocytopenia
    b. Aplastic anemia
    c. Hemophilia
    d. Warm antibody anemia

30. A patient is at high risk for the development of venoocclusive disease. What assessments does the nurse perform for **early** detection of this disorder? **Select all that apply.**
    a. Joint pain
    b. Weight gain
    c. Hepatomegaly
    d. Fluid retention
    e. Raynaud's-like response
    f. Increase in abdominal girth

31. Which person is **most likely** to benefit from a referral for genetic counseling?
    a. Young woman who has an older brother who has hemophilia A
    b. Young woman whose sister is being treated for iron deficiency anemia
    c. Young man whose mother had a thromboembolic event after taking thalidomide
    d. Young man whose older brother is being treated for Hodgkin's lymphoma

32. The nurse hears in report that the patient is diagnosed with autoimmune thrombocytopenic purpura. Which instruction is the nurse **most likely** to give to unlicensed assistive personnel?
    a. Handle the patient very gently to minimize bruising.
    b. Wear a mask when caring for the patient to prevent infection.
    c. Encourage the patient to drink fluids to prevent dehydration.
    d. Assist the patient to stand to prevent falls related to weakness.

33. Which patient has the **greatest** risk for developing a febrile transfusion reaction?
    a. Patient is an older adult, and transfusion was given too rapidly.
    b. Patient received an intraoperative autologous transfusion.
    c. Patient has received multiple blood transfusions for chronic bleeding.
    d. Patient sustained multiple injuries and needed an emergency transfusion.

34. Which electrolyte imbalance can occur related to a blood transfusion?
    a. Hyponatremia
    b. Hyperkalemia
    c. Hypocalcemia
    d. High blood glucose

35. A patient is receiving a red blood cell transfusion through a double-lumen peripherally inserted central catheter. The patient has two other peripheral IVs: one is capped and the other has $D_5/.45$ NS running at a rate of 50 mL/hr. What can be given concurrently through the line that is selected for the red cell transfusion?
    a. Normal saline
    b. Infusion of platelets
    c. Dextrose in water
    d. Morphine 2 mg IV push

36. Which blood product is **most likely** to have stricter monitoring policies requiring that a physician be present on the unit during administration?
    a. Packed red blood cell transfusion
    b. White blood cell transfusion
    c. Fresh frozen plasma transfusion
    d. Platelet transfusion

37. To avoid transfusion reaction, the nurse is carefully monitoring the patient during a blood transfusion. When are hemolytic reactions to blood transfusion **most likely** to occur?
    a. 1 mL is sufficient
    b. 5 mL is typical
    c. Within the first 50 mL
    d. After 100 mL

38. Which types of medications are used as premedication to prevent a reaction for patients receiving a stem cell transfusion?
    a. Vitamin K and a diuretic
    b. Aspirin and hydroxyurea
    c. Diphenhydramine and acetaminophen
    d. Hydrocortisone and an antihypertensive

39. An older patient is receiving a blood transfusion. Which signs/symptoms suggest that the patient is experiencing transfusion-associated circulatory overload?
    a. Hypertension, bounding pulse, and distended neck veins
    b. Fever, chills, and tachycardia
    c. Urticaria, itching, and bronchospasm
    d. Headache, chest pain, and hemoglobinuria

40. The nurse is performing the **immediate** post-procedure care for a bone marrow donor. What is the **priority** assessment that the nurse will perform?
    a. Monitoring for activity intolerance
    b. Monitoring for infection
    c. Monitoring for fluid loss
    d. Monitoring platelet count

41. The experienced nurse is supervising a new graduate nurse during administration of a blood product. In which circumstance would the experienced nurse intervene?
    a. New graduate nurse prepares to use blood administration tubing to infuse stems cells.
    b. New graduate nurse obtains Y-tubing with a blood filter to administer packed red blood cells.
    c. New graduate nurse uses a special shorter tubing with a smaller filter to deliver platelets.
    d. New graduate nurse rapidly delivers fresh frozen plasma through regular straight filtered tubing.

42. Which outcome statement indicates successful engraftment of transplanted cells in the patient's bone marrow?
    a. There is no evidence of graft-versus-host disease.
    b. White blood cell, red blood cell, and platelet counts are rising.
    c. Laboratory results indicate probable regressive chimerism.
    d. Laboratory results show decreasing percentage of donor cells.

43. The nurse would measure abdominal girth to monitor for which complication of hematopoietic stem cell transplantation?
    a. Failure to engraft
    b. Graft-versus-host disease
    c. Venoocclusive disease
    d. Septic shock

44. A patient reports fatigue, bone pain, and frequent bacterial infections. Further investigation reveals anemia and hypercalcemia, and x-ray findings show bone thinning with areas of bone loss that resemble Swiss cheese. The signs/symptoms and diagnostic findings are consistent with which disorder?
    a. Acute leukemia
    b. Multiple myeloma
    c. Non-Hodgkin's lymphoma
    d. Sickle cell anemia

45. A patient with acute leukemia has been receiving an erythropoiesis-stimulating agent (ESA). The nurse sees that the hemoglobin level is 10.5 mg/dL. Why does the nurse call the health care provider to have the ESA discontinued?
    a. The hemoglobin level is below normal limits, and this increases the risk for side effects.
    b. The ESA therapy is not effective, and an alternate medication should be ordered.
    c. ESAs can cause hypertension and increase the risk for myocardial infarction.
    d. The hemoglobin level of 10.5 mg/dL is the cutoff point recommended by the manufacturer.

46. The nurse has just received a handoff report and is planning care for several patients who must receive blood products during the shift. Which patient will require the **most** monitoring for the longest period of time?
    a. Young woman needs a unit of packed red blood cells for a hemoglobin of 5 mg/dL.
    b. Patient with thrombocytopenia needs pooled platelets for a platelet count of 45,000.
    c. Older patient with heart failure needs washed red blood cells for chronic bleeding.
    d. Patient with thrombotic thrombocytopenic purpura needs fresh frozen plasma.

47. What instructions would the home health nurse give to the home health aide about helping a patient who needs to conserve energy?
    a. Assist the patient to complete activities and exercises when he gets short of breath.
    b. Let the patient decide whether he has the energy to bathe every day.
    c. Encourage people not to visit to allow the patient to rest and conserve energy.
    d. Offer 4-6 small, easy-to-eat meals rather than serving three large meals.

48. The patient is diagnosed with hereditary hemochromatosis. Which therapy does the nurse expect will be prescribed for this patient?
    a. Interferon alfa therapy to control RBC production
    b. Hydration to decrease "sludging" of blood
    c. Phlebotomy to reduce overall iron load of the blood
    d. Administration of folic acid and vitamin B_{12} to prevent anemia

49. Which lab values would the nurse expect to see for a patient with sickle cell disease? **Select all that apply.**
    a. 80% hemoglobin S
    b. 90% red blood cell sickling
    c. Increased hematocrit
    d. Increased reticulocyte count
    e. Decreased total bilirubin
    f. Elevated total white blood cell count

50. What is the **first** priority intervention when the nurse recognizes that a patient is having a transfusion reaction?
    a. Stop the transfusion.
    b. Notify the Rapid Response Team.
    c. Flush the IV tubing with normal saline.
    d. Apply oxygen via face mask.

51. A patient scheduled for surgery tells the nurse that he is fearful of the possibility of needing a blood transfusion. What is the nurse's **best** response?
    a. "Have you spoken with your health care provider about a family member donating blood for your transfusion?"
    b. "With today's technology, typing and receiving blood is a very safe procedure, and there is no need to worry."
    c. "Autologous transfusion, where you donate your own blood for later transfusion, may be an option for you."
    d. "Have you had previous unpleasant experiences with blood transfusions during past surgeries?"

41 CHAPTER

Assessment of the Nervous System

1. Which situation is the **best** example of superior cerebellar function?
   a. Soprano sings an aria that the audience loves.
   b. Student recites *Hamlet* after reading it once.
   c. Downhill skier races down a steep narrow slope.
   d. Master chess player defeats all competitors.

2. The nurse is assessing the mental status of a patient. Which question **best** assesses recall memory?
   a. "How did you get to the hospital?"
   b. "What city were you born in?"
   c. "What is your mother's maiden name?"
   d. "How many children do you have?"

3. The patient diagnosed with an ischemic brainstem stroke has sustained damage to the medulla and pons area of the brain. What is the **priority** concern?
   a. Increased intracranial pressure
   b. Respiratory arrest
   c. Seizure activity
   d. Brainstem herniation

4. A patient with cerebellar dysfunction is **most likely** to need assistance in what situation?
   a. Orientation to place and time
   b. Buttoning the shirt
   c. Verbal communication
   d. Mood and pain control

5. Which patient has the **greatest** disadvantage related to the blood-brain barrier?
   a. Patient has pneumonia and needs supplemental oxygen.
   b. Patient has bacterial meningitis and needs antibiotics.
   c. Patient is dehydrated and needs IV fluids to correct fluid status.
   d. Patient needs major surgery and requires general anesthesia.

6. Which event suggests that the nursing student's reticular activating system is functioning correctly?
   a. Memorizes information and applies it during clinical practicum
   b. Walks up four flights of stairs to get some exercise
   c. Feels a little hungry, so decides to eat an energy bar
   d. Wakes up when alarm clock goes off at 6:00 AM

7. If the sympathetic nervous system is sufficiently stimulated, what would the nurse expect to observe?
   a. Increase in heart rate
   b. Myoclonus in the muscles
   c. Hyperactive deep tendon reflexes
   d. Increased salivation

8. The nurse is teaching an older adult patient about medication and healthy lifestyle. Which teaching strategy is the **best** to use with this patient?
   a. Give limited and simplified information.
   b. Provide the teaching late in the afternoon.
   c. Relate the information to recent events.
   d. Allow extra time for teaching and questions.

9. The nurse is caring for an older adult patient who is at risk for falling related to altered balance and decreased coordination. Which **initial** intervention will the nurse employ for this patient?
   a. Instruct the patient to move slowly when changing positions.
   b. Encourage the patient not to get out of bed unless he really needs to.
   c. Raise all four side rails and place the bed in the lowest position.
   d. Assign a sitter to stay with the patient and assist as needed.

10. The nurse is obtaining baseline information from an older adult patient about his ability to perform activities of daily living. He is at risk for a neurologic disorder; why does the nurse ask whether the patient is right- or left-handed?
    a. The patient may be somewhat stronger on the dominant side, which is expected.
    b. Effects of a neurologic event will be worse if the nondominant side is involved.
    c. This information is part of any standardized database for all older patients.
    d. The patient should be encouraged to strengthen and rely on the dominant side.

11. A patient sustained a head injury and multiple other injuries in an automobile accident. The health care team has addressed the ABCs (airway, breathing, and circulation). Which **priority** assessment should be addressed next?
    a. Stabilize long bone fractures.
    b. Rule out cervical spine fracture.
    c. Determine presence of a toxidrome.
    d. Check for peripheral sensation.

12. The nurse on the neurologic unit is evaluating several patients using the Glasgow Coma Scale (GCS). Which findings must be reported to the health care provider **immediately? Select all that apply.**
    a. GCS decrease of 3 points
    b. Fixed nonreactive pupils
    c. Asks for pain medication
    d. Extreme flexion of upper extremities
    e. Suddenly unable to remember where he is
    f. Arouses with supraorbital pressure

13. When performing a neurologic examination, what would the nurse do to assess cognition? **Select all that apply.**
    a. Ask the patient his name, date of birth, today's date, time, and location.
    b. Observe how well the patient follows a topic or attends to an activity.
    c. Observe the patient as he walks across the room, turns, and walks back.
    d. Show the patient a familiar object and have him state its name and purpose.
    e. Note if the patient responds quickly and relevantly to questions.
    f. Give the patient a simple command and observe how he reacts.

14. An older adult patient is brought to the clinic by the family, who reports that "Dad doesn't seem to be quite like himself." Which behavior is an **early** sign of a neurologic problem?
    a. Inability to remember a trip that he took last week
    b. Failure to remember his mother's maiden name
    c. Failure to recall where he went to high school
    d. Inability to describe his favorite hobby

15. In performing a mental status examination on a patient, the nurse asks, "What would you do if you saw a fire in the wastebasket?" Which frontal lobe function is the nurse assessing with this question?
    a. Reasoning and abstraction
    b. Access to past information
    c. Access to current sensory data
    d. Affective response to a situation

16. The emergency department nurse detects sudden one-sided loss of function and sensation while completing a neurologic assessment on a patient. What is the nurse's **first priority** action at this time?
    a. Apply oxygen at 2 L/min by nasal cannula.
    b. Order a stat computed tomography scan.
    c. Immediately notify the health care provider.
    d. Place the patient in a semi-Fowler's position.

17. What is a contraindication for sharp and dull sensory assessment?
    a. Patient is sensitive to pain and temperature changes.
    b. Patient is unable to move the affected or injured side.
    c. Patient's pulses are not palpable in the distal extremities.
    d. Patient takes anticoagulant medication and bruises easily.

18. The nurse is caring for several older adult patients in a long-term care facility. In planning care with consideration for the sensory changes related to aging, which intervention does the nurse implement?
    a. Controls environmental odors because older adults have a heightened sense of smell.
    b. Plans simple teaching sessions because of the decline in intellectual ability.
    c. Increases the ambient lighting because of the decrease in pupil size.
    d. Limits physical contact because the touch sensation increases.

19. The nurse instructs the patient to close his eyes and hold his arms perpendicular to his body with the palms up for 15-30 seconds. Which reaction indicates that the patient has a cerebral or brainstem reason for muscle weakness?
    a. Arm on the patient's weak side starts to drift with the palm turning inward.
    b. Arms, wrists, and fingers are flexed with internal rotation.
    c. There is abnormal movement with rigidity and extension of the arms.
    d. Dorsiflexion of the thumb and spreading of the other fingers occur.

20. An older adult patient is admitted to a long-term care facility, and the nurse performs a baseline physical assessment that includes neurologic and sensory function. What is the purpose of the assessment?
    a. Determine a level of function for later comparison.
    b. Show the family what problems the older adult has.
    c. Gain information on past sensory changes.
    d. Determine rehabilitation potential.

21. Which question would the nurse ask to **best** assess a patient's remote memory?
    a. "Who is your primary care provider?"
    b. "What did you have for breakfast this morning?"
    c. "What is the name of the town where you grew up?"
    d. "What is your usual bowel and bladder pattern?"

22. The nurse is assessing the sensory functions of a patient with Guillain-Barré syndrome (GBS). The nurse makes a clinical judgment to forgo assessing for light touch discrimination. Why does the nurse make this decision?
    a. Patient's pain and temperature sensations are intact.
    b. Sensory testing is done routinely every 4 hours.
    c. Only patients with spinal trauma require this assessment.
    d. Patient with GBS will be too confused to respond appropriately.

23. The nurse is testing a patient for touch discrimination by touching the patient on both shoulders. What is a normal finding for this assessment?
    a. Pointing to where each shoulder was touched
    b. Moving the shoulders against resistance
    c. Describing the touch as sharp or dull
    d. Sensing touch on the ipsilateral side

24. During neurologic assessment, which test does the nurse use to assess the patient's fine coordination?
    a. Patient walks across the room, and returns, as instructed.
    b. With arms out to the side, the patient touches the nose two to three times.
    c. Patient holds the arms perpendicular to the body with eyes closed.
    d. Patient grasps and squeezes the nurse's fingers and shows equal strength.

25. The nursing student is performing a neurologic assessment on a patient who sustained a stroke (brain attack). The nurse observes the student evaluating grip and hand strength only on the affected side. What is the nurse's **first** action?
    a. Give the student positive feedback for performing the assessment correctly.
    b. Remind the student that strength testing needs to be done bilaterally.
    c. Redo the entire assessment and instruct the student to watch the process.
    d. Suggest to the instructor that the student needs remediation for assessment.

26. A patient has injury to cervical spinal nerves at C6 and C7. What sensory changes would the nurse expect to see?
    a. Sensory changes in throat and mouth, particularly the ability to taste and swallow
    b. Sensory changes at the back of the neck and shoulders near area of C6 and C7
    c. Sensory changes in thumb, index, and middle fingers, middle of palm, and back of hand
    d. No sensory changes, because spinal nerves are only involved in motor functions

27. While assessing a patient's gait and equilibrium, the nurse observes that the patient has the Romberg sign. What is the **priority** patient problem associated with this objective data?
    a. Potential for falls related to dysfunction in awareness of body position
    b. Inability to do activities of daily living due to decreased muscle strength
    c. Functional incontinence related to inability to ambulate to bathroom
    d. Potential for falls related to inability to make good judgments

28. The nurse asks the patient, "What do you think this liquid smells like?" Which cranial nerve is the nurse testing?
    a. Cranial nerve I
    b. Cranial nerve II
    c. Cranial nerve III
    d. Cranial nerve IV

29. The nurse is attempting to assess a coma patient's response to pain. Which technique does the nurse try **first**?
    a. Gently shake the patient, similar to attempting to wake a sleeping child.
    b. Speak to the patient and call his or her name using a normal tone of voice.
    c. Face the patient and speak loudly and clearly, as with a hearing-impaired patient.
    d. Apply supraorbital pressure by placing the thumb under the orbital rim.

30. The nurse is assessing response to painful stimuli in a patient. What is the **maximum** length of time to apply the stimulus in the comatose patient?
    a. 1-2 seconds
    b. 5-10 seconds
    c. 20-30 seconds
    d. 40-60 seconds

31. Which neurologic disorder is **most likely** to require hourly sensory assessments of a patient?
    a. Parkinson disease
    b. Alzheimer's disease
    c. Guillain-Barré syndrome
    d. Huntington disease

32. The nurse is assessing several patients using the Glasgow Coma Scale (GCS). Which factors indicate the **most serious** neurologic presentation based on the GCS information?
    a. Eye opening to sound, localizes pain, confused conversation
    b. Eye opening to sound, obeys commands, inappropriate words
    c. Eye opening spontaneous, obeys commands, confused conversation
    d. Eye opening to pain, abnormal flexion, incomprehensible sounds

33. The nurse is performing neurologic checks every 4 hours for a patient who sustained a head injury. Which **early** sign indicates a decline in neurologic status?
    a. Nonreactive, dilated pupils
    b. Change in level of consciousness
    c. Decorticate posturing
    d. Loss of remote memory

34. The nurse has provided information about computerized tomography-positron emission tomography to a patient and his family. However, the patient is suspected of having early signs of Alzheimer's disease. Which statement by the patient indicates he did not understand the information?
    a. "I might have trouble with adding or subtracting numbers or remembering things during the test."
    b. "I am a little bit nervous about the idea of being blindfolded. Could you tell me about that?"
    c. "They will not give me my diabetes medication on the morning of the test."
    d. "I will get a mild medication to help me relax, so I'll just take a little nap during the test."

35. Determining functional status is a core measure that is recommended for all patients with complex chronic health conditions. Which assessment data includes three key concepts needed to meet this measure?
    a. Hearing impaired and requires a hearing aid but demonstrates difficulty caring for, adjusting, and using the device; prefers sign language
    b. Requires supplemental oxygen at night, experiences fatigue with minor exertion, requires assistance for most activities of daily living
    c. Wanders and spends most of the day pacing but is easily redirected and never becomes hostile, agitated, or angry at staff
    d. Independently ambulatory, requires prescription eyeglasses for reading, understands and follows medication regimen as ordered

36. A family member calls the nurse into the patient's room and says, "Mom seems really out of it. She doesn't seem to know who I am." What assessments does the nurse perform before notifying the health care provider about this change of mental status? **Select all that apply.**
    a. Auscultate lungs for possible pneumonia.
    b. Check for signs of urinary tract infection.
    c. Check oxygen saturation with pulse oximeter.
    d. Check blood glucose with a glucometer.
    e. Assess the patient's ability to stand and ambulate.
    f. Take a complete set of vital signs.

37. A patient is scheduled for an electroencephalogram. How does the nurse prepare the patient for this diagnostic test?
    a. Gives a sedative before bedtime
    b. Encourages extra fluids before the test
    c. Gives nothing by mouth after midnight
    d. Ensures that the hair is clean

38. A patient arrives on the unit alert and oriented after undergoing cerebral angiography. The report from the radiology nurse indicates the catheter was inserted into the left femoral artery. For which postprocedural order does the nurse call the health care provider for clarification?
    a. Keep the left leg straight and immobilized.
    b. Maintain an ice pack and pressure dressing to the insertion site for 2 hours.
    c. IV and oral fluid restrictions for a total of 1000 mL/24 hours.
    d. Call provider for change in skin color/temperature, or decreased pulses.

39. A patient is scheduled to have computed tomography with contrast media, and the nurse is reviewing the patient's laboratory results. Which laboratory result would warrant delay or cancellation of the procedure, thus prompting the nurse to notify the radiology department and the health care provider?
    a. Elevated creatinine level
    b. Decreased white blood cell count
    c. Blood glucose higher than baseline
    d. Abnormal urobilinogen level

40. The nursing student is talking to the patient and family about diagnostic testing. Which statement by the nursing student indicates the need for additional study about the diagnostic procedures?
    a. "You are scheduled for a magnetic resonance imaging. Do you have a cardiac pacemaker?"
    b. "You are scheduled for computed tomography of the head. Are you wearing hairpins?"
    c. "You will have x-rays of the skull and cervical spine. Are you allergic to iodine?"
    d. "You will have computerized tomography-positron emission tomography. Do you take diabetes medication?"

41. The nurse is teaching the patient and encourages smoking cessation to maintain or improve nervous system health. Which concept is **most** directly related to smoking cessation?
    a. Comfort
    b. Perfusion
    c. Mobility
    d. Cognition

42. The nurse reads in the patient's documentation: PERRLA. How does the nurse interpret this documentation?
    a. Parasympathetic nervous system is responsible for reproductive actions.
    b. Peripheral nervous system is reactive and responsive and activated.
    c. Pulses are equal in right arm and right leg and patient is ambulatory.
    d. Pupils are equal in size, round, regular, and react to light and accommodation.

43. The nurse hears in report that the patient has intention tremors. Which activity is the **most likely** to be problematic for this patient?
    a. Drinking from a teacup
    b. Ambulating down the hall
    c. Rolling over in bed
    d. Sitting down on the toilet

44. The patient has severely increased intracranial pressure. Which diagnostic test would the neurologist avoid performing on this patient?
    a. Magnetic resonance imaging
    b. Electroencephalography
    c. Computed tomography with contrast
    d. Lumbar puncture

45. The nurse is using the Glascow Coma Scale for a trauma patient with neurologic injuries. The patient does not follow commands and is unresponsive to voice. Which assessment does the nurse complete next?
    a. Instruct the patient to open his eyes and squeeze the nurse's hand.
    b. Check light touch at multiple points on the body bilaterally.
    c. In a loud voice, ask if the patient knows his name and where he is located.
    d. Pinch or squeeze the trapezius muscle at the angle of the shoulder and neck muscle.

CHAPTER 42

Care of Patients with Problems of the Central Nervous System: The Brain

1. The nurse is caring for a patient with stage 2 Parkinson disease. What is the **priority** concept to consider in planning care for this patient?
   a. Perfusion
   b. Cognition
   c. Comfort
   d. Mobility

2. What are signs/symptoms of a migraine headache? **Select all that apply.**
   a. Throbbing, unilateral pain
   b. Nausea
   c. Photophobia
   d. Phonophobia
   e. Recurrent episodic headaches
   f. Transient loss of consciousness

3. A patient comes to the clinic for headaches. He is irritable and impatient to receive treatment but is alert and oriented, speech is clear, and he is able and willing to answer the nurse's questions. Which questions will the nurse ask to solicit additional relevant information about this patient's headaches? **Select all that apply.**
   a. "When do the headaches occur?"
   b. "How often do the headaches occur?"
   c. "What kind of treatment would you like for your headaches?"
   d. "Can you point to the place where your head hurts the worse?"
   e. "Do you experience other symptoms with the headaches?"
   f. "Have there been any recent changes in your headaches?"

4. A patient with a history of migraine headaches reports his current headache as "my usual throbbing pain, but today it is behind my left eye." Which question does the nurse ask to elicit information about trigger factors?
   a. "Have you ever been treated for major depression?"
   b. "Did you feel short of breath before the headache started?"
   c. "Did you eat any fish or seafood before the headache started?"
   d. "Did you drink wine or coffee before the headache occurred?"

5. Which patient needs to be reminded to keep the scheduled laboratory appointments to check serum drug levels?
   a. Patient has Alzheimer's disease and takes memantine.
   b. Patient has migraine headaches and takes sumatriptan.
   c. Patient has Parkinson disease and takes levodopa-carbidopa.
   d. Patient has tonic-clonic seizures and takes fosphenytoin.

6. During a patient's last visit, the nurse instructed the patient about headaches and techniques to manage this condition. Which statement by the patient indicates teaching has been successful?
   a. "I have been keeping track of when my headaches occur."
   b. "My doctor told me that my headaches were not very serious."
   c. "My spouse knows the instructions that you gave me."
   d. "I have not had any headaches since we last talked."

7. The health care provider tells the nurse that the patient has a migraine headache with phonophobia. Which intervention is the nurse **most likely** to implement?
   a. Darken the lights in the patient's room and close the curtains.
   b. Put the patient in a quiet room; tell the staff to minimize noise.
   c. Ensure that the staff knows that the patient needs help to ambulate.
   d. Increase the amount of ambient light so that the patient can see.

8. A patient is prescribed ergotamine with caffeine for migraine headaches. Which statement by the patient indicates that she is experiencing a side effect of this drug?
   a. "My headache is initially relieved by the medication, but then it returns."
   b. "I seem to be gaining weight since I started taking this medication."
   c. "My headache seems worse in the morning when I take the medication."
   d. "I notice that I bruise more easily and my skin seems fragile and dry."

9. A patient has received a prescription for sumatriptan for the treatment of migraine headaches. The patient tells the nurse that she elected not to tell the health care provider about all her health conditions "because I just wanted treatment for my headaches and I didn't want to go into everything else." Which question(s) should the nurse ask? **Select all that apply.**
   a. "Do you have a personal or family history for glaucoma or other vision problems?"
   b. "Will you come back so we can monitor your prothrombin time and electrolytes?"
   c. "Have you been diagnosed with suspected or actual ischemic heart disease?"
   d. "Do you have hypertension or peripheral vascular disease?"
   e. "Is there any chance you could be pregnant?"
   f. "What kind of contraception do you use?"

10. In planning care for a patient with a migraine headache, what is the **priority** concept?
    a. Cognition
    b. Comfort
    c. Nutrition
    d. Perfusion

11. In report, the nurse hears that a patient with migraine headaches is frequently experiencing an aura of flashing lights and diplopia. Based on this information, which instruction would the nurse give to unlicensed assistive personnel?
    a. Draw the shades, dim the lights in the room, and close the door.
    b. Assist the patient to locate and always wear his eyeglasses.
    c. Help the patient to ambulate because he could trip or misstep.
    d. Immediately report any tremors or signs of impeding seizure activity.

12. The home health nurse reads in the patient's chart that the patient had surgery for a vagal nerve stimulating (VNS) device. Which question would the nurse ask to evaluate if the VNS device is having the desired effect?
    a. Has the VNS helped to improve your memory?
    b. Has the VNS reduced or relieved the headaches?
    c. Has the VNS controlled or reduced your seizures?
    d. Has the VNS helped to relieve your muscle rigidity?

13. During a generalized tonic-clonic seizure, the young adult patient becomes cyanotic. What should the nurse do **first**?
    a. Raise the head of the bed and apply nasal cannula oxygen.
    b. Call the provider and obtain the equipment to intubate.
    c. Suction the patient and alert the Rapid Response Team.
    d. Stay with the patient because cyanosis is usually self-limiting.

14. An elementary school teacher has just been informed that her student's brother has absence seizures. The teacher is fearful that her student may have the same types of seizures and is unsure what to expect. Which signs does the school nurse advise the teacher to look for?
    a. Brief jerking or stiffening of muscles that lasts only a few seconds
    b. Loss of consciousness and rhythmic jerking of extremities
    c. Brief loss of consciousness that may appear as daydreaming or blank staring
    d. "Blackout" that lasts 10 to 30 minutes with loss of memory and disorientation

15. What is the **priority** concern for a patient with atonic (akinetic) seizures?
    a. Potential for injury related to falls
    b. Organ ischemia related to decreased perfusion
    c. Confusion related to postictal state
    d. Limited mobility related to atonicity of muscles

16. The nurse is caring for a patient who has clonic seizures. Which seizure precaution is the **most important**?
    a. Ensure that the IV access is patent.
    b. Place patient in a side-lying position.
    c. Put a mattress on the floor beside the bed.
    d. Ensure that the call bell is in place.

17. An older adult patient is brought to the emergency department from the local mall after bystanders saw her "having a seizure." The patient is currently responsive to voice but is lethargic, confused, and unable to give an accurate history. Which aspect of this patient's health history is the **most important** to verify with the family?
    a. History of acute or chronic respiratory problems
    b. Baseline ability to answer questions accurately
    c. Date and time of day that they last saw her
    d. Name of patient's primary care provider

18. Which prescribed medication would the nurse **clarify** before administering?
    a. Diazepam rectal gel for a patient with status epilepticus
    b. Carbamazepine for a patient with tonic-clonic seizures
    c. Warfarin for a patient who takes phenytoin for seizures
    d. Gabapentin for a patient who has partial seizures

19. A patient is treated in the emergency department for status epilepticus and is awaiting transfer to the medical-surgical unit. The admission orders include seizure precautions. What equipment should be in the room before the patient's arrival?
    a. Cardiac monitor and a pulse oximeter
    b. Penlight and a neurologic assessment flow sheet
    c. Padded tongue blades and padding for side rails
    d. Oxygen and suction equipment

20. The patient reports neck stiffness, light sensitivity, noise sensitivity, headache, muscle aches, nausea, vomiting, and "feeling foggy and kind of out of it." Although the nurse recognizes that all vital signs are important, which question is the nurse **most likely** to ask to assist the health care provider to determine the diagnosis?
    a. "Do you feel like your heart is beating too fast?"
    b. "Have you had fever or chills?"
    c. "Have you been breathing hard or rapidly?"
    d. "What is your baseline blood pressure?"

21. Which people should be advised to get the meningococcal vaccine? **Select all that apply.**
    a. Healthy 12-year-old school child
    b. 25-year-old who had a splenectomy due to an auto accident
    c. Healthy 18-year-old who has enlisted in the military
    d. Healthy 20-year-old who is planning to live in a university dormitory
    e. Healthy 24-year-old who is interning with a lawyer for the summer
    f. Healthy 22-year-old who is unsure about vaccination status and plans to go to Asia

22. The nurse is caring for a patient who was admitted for a diagnosis of meningococcal meningitis. Which nursing action is **specific** to this type of meningitis?
    a. Administering an antifungal agent such as amphotericin B
    b. Observing the patient for genital lesions
    c. Placing the patient in isolation per hospital procedure
    d. Checking to see if the patient is HIV positive

23. The nurse is reviewing the electrolyte values for a patient with bacterial meningitis and notes that the serum sodium is 126 mEq/L (126 mmol/L). How does the nurse interpret this finding?
    a. Within normal limits considering the diagnosis of bacterial meningitis but warrants repeat laboratory testing for downward trends
    b. Evidence of syndrome of inappropriate antidiuretic hormone, which is a complication of bacterial meningitis
    c. A protective measure that causes increased urination and therefore reduces the risk of increased intracranial pressure
    d. An early warning sign that the electrolyte imbalances will potentiate an acute myocardial infarction or shock

24. A patient with meningitis reports a headache, and the nurse gives the appropriate IV push medication. Several hours later, the patient reports pain in the left hand; the radial pulse is very weak, the hand feels cool, and capillary refill is sluggish compared to the left. What does the nurse suspect is occurring in this patient?
    a. Stroke secondary to increased intracranial pressure resulting from meningitis
    b. Sickle cell crisis associated with an increased risk of meningitis
    c. Thrombotic or embolic complication causing vascular compromise
    d. Local phlebitis from the IV push pain medication that was given

25. A patient arrives in the emergency department reporting headache, fever, nausea, and photosensitivity. The patient has been living with two people who were diagnosed with meningitis. Which diagnostic test does the nurse anticipate the health care provider will order to rule out meningitis?
    a. X-rays of the skull
    b. Lumbar puncture
    c. Myelography
    d. Cerebral angiogram

26. The nurse is caring for a patient who has symptoms and risk factors for bacterial meningitis. For which symptom must the nurse **alert** the health care provider?
    a. Capillary refill of 3 seconds
    b. Headache with nausea and vomiting
    c. Inability to move eyes laterally
    d. Oral temperature of 101.6°F

27. The nurse is carefully monitoring a patient with a severe case of encephalitis for signs of increased intracranial pressure. What vital sign changes are associated with increased intracranial perssure?
    a. Tachycardia and shallow, rapid respirations
    b. Increased core temperature and bradycardia
    c. Decreased pulse pressure and tachypnea
    d. Widened pulse pressure and bradycardia

28. The student nurse is caring for a patient with encephalitis. Which action by the student nurse warrants intervention by the supervising nurse?
    a. Performs deep suctioning for copious secretions in the airway
    b. Elevates the head of bed to 30 degrees after a lumbar puncture
    c. Encourages and helps the patient to turn every 2 hours
    d. Performs a neurologic assessment every 2 hours

29. The nurse is assessing a patient with Parkinson disease. Which **cardinal** findings does the nurse expect to observe? **Select all that apply.**
    a. Tremors
    b. Rigidity
    c. Dementia
    d. Aphasia
    e. Postural instability
    f. Slow movements

30. A patient with Parkinson disease is prescribed selegiline, which is a selective monoamine oxidase type B (MAO-B) inhibitor. What information does the nurse include for safe medication administration?
    a. Take the medication with meals.
    b. Avoid driving or operating heavy machinery.
    c. Avoid eating aged cheese and cured meats.
    d. Take medication daily at bedtime.

31. During the nurse's assessment of a patient with Parkinson disease, the nurse notes that the patient has masklike facies. What functional assessment is now a **priority**?
    a. Ability to hear normal voice tones
    b. Ability to chew and swallow
    c. Ability to sense pain in the facial area
    d. Ability to see in a low light environment

32. The home health nurse is visiting an older adult patient with stage 1 Parkinson disease. He demonstrates some trembling and weakness in his right hand and arm and reports he occasionally gets dizzy when he first stands up. The patient is currently living by himself and has no family in the immediate area. What is the **priority** patient problem?
    a. Decreased ability for activities of daily living
    b. Feelings of isolation and loneliness
    c. Potential for injury due to falls
    d. Poor nutritional and fluid intake

33. A patient has been taking benztropine for Parkinson disease. What sign indicates that the patient may be having drug toxicity associated with this drug?
    a. Acute confusion
    b. Tremors and rigidity
    c. Choreiform movements
    d. Seizure activity

34. A patient has moderate Parkinson disease with an impaired ability to communicate related to psychomotor deficit. Which nursing intervention is the **best** to use with this patient?
    a. Speaking clearly and asking questions slowly
    b. Watching the patient's lips when he speaks
    c. Giving step-by-step instructions to the patient
    d. Providing visual cues when trying to explain

35. An older woman is brought to the clinic by her husband. She went out to do some gardening, but a neighbor found her walking aimlessly down the street. She is currently "just like herself," but the patient cannot explain what she was doing or where she was going. Which questions will the nurse ask to assess cognitive changes in this patient? **Select all that apply.**
    a. "Have you noticed any forgetfulness, for example misplacing your keys?"
    b. "Has there been any memory loss, such as not remembering a recent conversation?"
    c. "Are there any changes in ability to make judgments, such as taking a medication?"
    d. "Have you noticed any problems with walking, such as loss of balance?"
    e. "Are there any changes in abilities to do a task like balancing your checkbook?"
    f. "What were you thinking about while you were walking down the street?"

36. The home health nurse reads in the patient's chart that the patient has Alzheimer's disease and is demonstrating apraxia. Which patient behavior supports the documentation?
    a. Pushes at the food on her plate with her eyeglasses
    b. Is unable to understand or follow a simple command
    c. Sustains a burn from a heating pad, without realizing it
    d. Says she can't remember the name of her dog

37. The nurse is assessing an older adult patient with Alzheimer's disease using the Mini-Mental State Examination. What does this exam measure?
    a. Level of intelligence
    b. Functional ability
    c. Severity of cognitive impairment
    d. Alterations in communication

38. A patient has advanced Alzheimer's disease and is staying in a long-term care facility. Which intervention is the **best** to use with this patient?
    a. Repeating the date, time, and place as needed
    b. Providing puzzles, games, and hands-on activities
    c. Using memory aids such as pill reminders
    d. Reflecting the patient's feelings and concerns

39. A patient is experiencing mild memory loss, and the patient and family are hoping the nurse can offer suggestions to help stimulate and strengthen the patient's current abilities. What is the nurse's **first** action?
    a. Show the family how to stimulate the memory by repeating what the patient just said.
    b. Discuss with the family and patient any practical memory problems that are occurring.
    c. Suggest that the patient identify and reminisce about pleasant past experiences.
    d. Provide name tags for the patient, family, and friends for use during group gatherings.

40. According to current research, which patient is **more likely** to progress to Alzheimer's disease?
    a. 70-year-old male with tremors in the upper extremities that increase with stress
    b. 63-year-old female with depressive symptoms and mild cognitive impairment
    c. 25-year-old female with a history of simple partial seizures accompanied by an aura
    d. 56-year-old male with acute confusion secondary to bacterial meningitis

41. The patient with mild Alzheimer's disease lives at home with a daughter who works part time and is the primary caregiver. Which home safety precaution is appropriate for this patient?
    a. Patient has access to a cell phone and the internet.
    b. Geri-chair with a waist belt is in the patient's bedroom.
    c. Patient wears a bracelet that shows the daughter's address.
    d. Medications are carefully organized in the bathroom cabinet.

42. The nurse is caring for several patients with Alzheimer's disease in a long-term care facility. Which task is **best** to delegate to unlicensed assistive personnel?
    a. Give hygienic care to the patient who is currently exhibiting sundowning.
    b. Assist the patient who has incontinence with toileting every 2 hours.
    c. Calm the agitated patient by using soft voice tones and distraction.
    d. Follow the patient and observe for hoarding or rummaging.

43. The nurse reads in the chart that the patient has Alzheimer's disease and is displaying agnosia. What does the nurse expect to observe?
    a. Wanders around and is at risk for elopement.
    b. Is unable to remember the purpose of a fork.
    c. Is telling everyone that she is Queen Elizabeth.
    d. Does not recognize herself or members of her family.

44. The patient with dementia was just admitted to the hospital. Which strategies should the nurse use to protect the patient? **Select all that apply.**
    a. Soft restraints, especially at night
    b. Frequent surveillance
    c. Toileting every 2 hours
    d. Side rails up at all times
    e. Sitters at the bedside as needed
    f. Keep a clear path between the bed and bathroom

45. The psychologist tells the nurse that the patient with Alzheimer's disease scored a 5 on the Mini-Mental State Examination. Which intervention is the nurse **most likely** to use with the patient?
    a. Asks the patient to relate a story about her childhood
    b. Engages the patient in a simple board game
    c. Delegates hygienic care to unlicensed assistive personnel
    d. Explains the purpose of the toilet training program

43 CHAPTER

Care of Patients with Problems of the Central Nervous System: The Spinal Cord

1. The nurse is taking a history on an adult patient who reports acute back pain. Which question is the nurse **most likely** to ask to identify causative factors?
   a. "Have you had a recent fall or accident or lifted a heavy object?"
   b. "Do you have a family history for neurologic disorders?"
   c. "Are you having trouble walking or maintaining your balance?"
   d. "Are you having pain that radiates down the back of your leg?"

2. The nurse is preparing to physically assess a patient's report of paresthesia in the lower extremities. To accomplish this assessment, which assessment technique does the nurse use?
   a. Use a Doppler to locate the pedal pulse, the dorsalis pedis pulse, or the popliteal pulse.
   b. Ask the patient to identify sharp and dull sensation by using a paper clip and cotton ball.
   c. Use a reflex hammer to test for deep tendon patellar or Achilles reflexes.
   d. Ask the patient to walk across the room, and observe gait and equilibrium.

3. Which position is therapeutic and comfortable for a patient with acute lower back pain from a herniated disc?
   a. Semi-Fowler's position with a pillow under the knees to keep them flexed
   b. Supine position with arms and legs in a correct anatomical position
   c. Orthopneic position; sitting with trunk slightly forward; arms supported on a pillow
   d. Modified Sims' position with upper arm and leg supported by pillows

4. A patient has been talking to the health care provider about drugs that could potentially be used in the treatment of acute low back pain. Which statement by the patient indicates a need for additional teaching?
   a. "The doctor may prescribe a muscle relaxant, so I should not drive or operate machinery until I see how the medication will affect me."
   b. "The doctor may suggest over-the-counter ibuprofen; therefore, I should watch for and report dark or tarry stools."
   c. "The doctor may prescribe an oral steroid such as prednisone; this would be short-term therapy, and the dose would gradually taper off."
   d. "The doctor may prescribe an opioid medication, and it may cause drowsiness; I should not drive or drink alcohol when I take it."

5. A patient is scheduled for lumbar surgery. Which key points must the nurse include in a preoperative teaching plan for this patient? **Select all that apply.**
   a. Techniques for getting in and out of bed
   b. Expectations for turning and moving in bed
   c. Limitations and restrictions for home activities
   d. Restricted to bedrest for at least 48 hours
   e. Immediately report any numbness and tingling
   f. Expect difficulties moving affected leg or both legs

6. The nurse is assessing a patient who presented to the emergency department reporting acute onset of numbness and tingling in the right leg. How does the nurse document this subjective finding?
   a. Paraparesis
   b. Paresthesia
   c. Ataxia
   d. Quadriparesis

7. A patient has just undergone a spinal fusion and a laminectomy and has returned from the operating room. Which assessments are done in the first 24 hours? **Select all that apply.**
   a. Take vital signs every 4 hours and assess for fever and hypotension.
   b. Perform a neurologic assessment every 4 hours with attention to movement and sensation.
   c. Monitor intake and output and assess for urinary retention.
   d. Assess for ability and independence in ambulating and moving in bed.
   e. Observe for clear fluid on or around the dressing.
   f. Assess for and immediately report sudden onset of headache.

8. The nurse is caring for several patients on an orthopedic surgical unit. Which patient has the **greatest** risk for fat embolism syndrome?
   a. 66-year-old who had laser-assisted laparoscopic lumbar diskectomy
   b. 46-year-old who had a spinal fusion for spine stabilization
   c. 52-year-old who had a laminectomy to relieve back pain
   d. 62-year-old who had minimally invasive surgery

9. A patient has just undergone a laminectomy and returned from surgery at 1300 hours. At 1530 hours, the nurse is performing the change of shift assessment. Which postoperative finding is **immediately** reported to the surgeon?
   a. Some serosanguineous drainage
   b. Pain along the incision site
   c. Swelling or bulging at the operative site
   d. Reluctance or refusal to cough and breathe deeply

10. A patient has just undergone spinal fusion surgery and returned from the operating room 12 hours ago. Which task is best to **delegate** to unlicensed assistive personnel?
    a. Assist the nurse to log-roll the patient every 2 hours.
    b. Help the patient dangle the legs.
    c. Assist the patient to put on a brace.
    d. Help the patient ambulate to the bathroom.

11. The nurse reviews the discharge and home care instructions with a patient who had conventional open back surgery. Which statement by the patient indicates further teaching is needed?
    a. "I will drive myself to my doctor's office next week."
    b. "I guess my wife will have to walk the dog for 6 more weeks."
    c. "I will try to increase fruits and vegetables and decrease fats."
    d. "I plan to get a new ergonomic chair at work."

12. A patient had an anterior cervical diskectomy with fusion and has returned from the recovery room. What is the **priority** assessment?
    a. Assess for gag reflex and ability to swallow own secretions.
    b. Check for bleeding and drainage at the incision site.
    c. Monitor vital signs and check neurologic status.
    d. Assess for patency of airway and respiratory effort.

13. The patient with chronic back pain is receiving ziconotide by intrathecal (spinal) infusion with a surgically implanted pump. The patient develops hallucinations. What is the nurse's **best first** action?
    a. Request a psychiatric evaluation.
    b. Notify the health care provider.
    c. Assess level of consciousness.
    d. Decrease the dose of medication.

14. A teenager dove head first into a rock quarry pond and is brought the emergency department by emergency medical services (EMS). Which questions will the nurse ask the EMS? **Select all that apply.**
    a. What were the location and position of the patient immediately after injury?
    b. Were there problems extricating the patient from the water?
    c. Have the parents been notified to get permission for treatment?
    d. What symptoms were reported by bystanders and noted en route?
    e. What changes occurred at the scene or en route?
    f. What treatments were given at the scene or en route?

15. The nurse is caring for a patient with a spinal cord injury who is experiencing neurogenic shock. The patient has a dopamine drip, but the systolic blood pressure is 88 mm Hg. There is a new order to infuse 500 mL of dextran-40 over 4 hours. At what rate does the nurse set the infusion pump?
    a. 75 mL/hr
    b. 100 mL/hr
    c. 125 mL/hr
    d. 150 mL/hr

16. A patient who was involved in a high-speed motor vehicle accident sustained multiple injuries. He is transported to the emergency department by emergency medical services with immobilization devices in place. There is a high probability of cervical spine fracture; the patient has altered mental status and extremities are flaccid. What is the **priority** assessment for this patient?
    a. Check the mental status using the Glasgow Coma Scale.
    b. Assess the respiratory pattern and ensure a patent airway.
    c. Observe for intraabdominal bleeding and hemorrhage.
    d. Assess for loss of motor function and sensation.

17. The nurse is caring for a patient who is experiencing spinal shock. What are expected findings that occur with this condition?
    a. Temporary loss of motor, sensory, reflex, and autonomic functions
    b. Stridor, garbled speech, or inability to clear airway
    c. Hypotension and a decreased level of consciousness
    d. Bradycardia and decreased urinary output

18. Which neurologic assessment technique does the nurse use to test a patient for sensory function?
    a. Touch the skin with a clean paper clip and ask whether it feels sharp or dull.
    b. Ask the patient to elevate both arms off the bed and extend wrists and fingers.
    c. Have the patient close the eyes and move toes up or down, while identifying the positions.
    d. Have the patient sit with the legs dangling; use a reflex hammer to test reflex responses.

19. Assessment of a patient with a lower spinal cord injury confirms that the patient has paralysis of the bilateral lower extremities. How does the nurse document this finding?
    a. Paraparesis
    b. Paraplegia
    c. Quadriparesis
    d. Quadriplegia

20. Which symptoms indicate that a patient with a spinal cord injury is experiencing autonomic dysreflexia? **Select all that apply.**
    a. Flaccid paralysis
    b. Hypertension
    c. Tachypnea
    d. Severe headache
    e. Blurred vision
    f. Loss of reflexes below the injury

21. The nurse is assessing a patient with a spinal cord injury that occurred several months ago. The nurse recognizes that the patient is experiencing autonomic dysreflexia. What is the nurse's **first priority** action?
    a. Check for bladder distention.
    b. Raise the head of the bed.
    c. Administer an antihypertensive medication.
    d. Notify the primary health care provider.

22. Which patient behavior is **most likely** to occur with spinal shock?
    a. Demonstrates restlessness and is easily agitated
    b. Displays inability or difficulty moving extremities
    c. Is disoriented to person, place, and time
    d. Reports severe pain that radiates down the spine

23. The nurse is preparing a patient with quadriplegia for discharge and has taught the spouse to assist the patient with a "quad cough" to prevent respiratory complications. Which observation indicates that the spouse has understood what has been taught?
    a. Spouse assists the patient into a wheelchair or chair and coaches him to do deep coughing.
    b. Spouse places her hands below the patient's diaphragm and pushes upward as the patient exhales.
    c. Spouse places her hands on the patient's lateral chest and pushes inward as the patient exhales.
    d. Spouse assists the patient into a high Fowler's position and encourages him to take deep breaths.

24. The nurse is caring for a patient with a recent spinal cord injury (SCI). Which interventions does the nurse use to target and prevent the potential SCI complication of autonomic dysreflexia? **Select all that apply.**
    a. Frequently perform passive range-of-motion exercises.
    b. Loosen or remove any tight clothing.
    c. Monitor stool output and maintain a bowel program.
    d. Keep the patient immobilized with neck or back braces.
    e. Monitor urinary output and check for bladder distention.
    f. Maintain stable environmental temperature.

25. What is a potential adverse outcome of autonomic dysreflexia in a patient with a spinal cord injury?
    a. Heatstroke
    b. Paralytic ileus
    c. Hypertensive stroke
    d. Aspiration and pneumonia

26. The home health nurse reads in the patient's chart that he has spinal cord injury and has developed heterotopic ossification of the right hip. What would the nurse expect to observe while assessing the hip?
    a. Redness, warmth, and decreased range of motion
    b. Obvious deformity, with protrusion of the hip joint
    c. Pronounced muscle atrophy and wasting of the femur
    d. Poor skin turgor, with fragility and possible skin tears

27. The nurse and the nursing student are working together to bathe and reposition a patient who is in a halo fixator device. Which action by the nursing student causes the supervising nurse to intervene?
    a. Uses the log-roll technique to clean the patient's back and buttocks
    b. Turns the patient by grasping the top of the halo device
    c. Positions the patient with the head and neck in alignment
    d. Supports the head and neck area during the repositioning

28. The nurse is caring for several patients who have spinal cord injuries. Which task is best to **delegate** to unlicensed assistive personnel?
    a. Encourage use of incentive spirometry; evaluate the patient's ability to use it correctly.
    b. Log-roll the patient; maintain proper body alignment and place a bedpan for toileting.
    c. Check for skin breakdown under the immobilization devices during bathing.
    d. Insert an indwelling catheter and report the amount and color of the urine.

29. A patient with an spinal cord injury has paraplegia and paraparesis. The nurse assesses the calf area of both legs for swelling, tenderness, redness, or pain. This assessment is specific to the patient's **increased** risk for which condition?
    a. Contractures of joints
    b. Bone fractures
    c. Pressure ulcers
    d. Venous thromboembolism

30. The nurse is caring for a patient who has been in a long-term care facility for several months following a spinal cord injury. The patient has had problems with urinary retention and subsequent overflow incontinence, and a bladder retraining program was recently initiated. What is an expected outcome of the training program?
    a. Does not experience a urinary tract infection
    b. Catheterizes himself independently
    c. Controls incontinence by decreasing fluid intake
    d. Takes initiative to call for help when needed

31. The patient with a spinal cord injury has a heart rate of 42/minute. Which drug does the nurse expect to administer?
    a. Methylprednisolone
    b. Dextran
    c. Atropine
    d. Dopamine

32. The nurse is planning care for a 66-year-old patient with spinal cord injury. Based on the nurse's knowledge of the **most likely** complication and cause of death for this patient, what would the nurse recommend?
    a. Increase calcium intake and exercise against resistance.
    b. Ensure influenza and pneumococcus vaccinations are current.
    c. Drink adequate liquids and eat a high-fiber diet.
    d. Practice meticulous skin care, including frequent repositioning.

33. An adolescent patient has quadriplegia as a result of a diving accident. The unlicensed assistive personnel reports that the patient started yelling and spitting at her while she was trying to bathe him. He is angry and hostile, stating, "Nobody is going to do anything else to me! I'm going to get out of this place!" What is the **priority** patient problem?
    a. Noncompliance with treatment plan
    b. Self-care deficit for hygiene
    c. Difficulties with situational coping
    d. Feelings of hopelessness

34. The nurse is giving home care instructions to a patient who will be discharged with a halo device. What does the nurse instruct the patient to **avoid**?
    a. Going out in the cold
    b. Driving
    c. Sexual activity
    d. Bathing in the bathtub

35. Which disorder could have a similar clinical presentation to multiple sclerosis?
    a. Amyotrophic lateral sclerosis
    b. Spinal cord tumor
    c. Guillain-Barré
    d. Quadriplegia

36. A patient reports increased fatigue and stiffness of the extremities. These symptoms have occurred in the past, but they resolved and no medical attention was sought. Which questions does the nurse ask to assess whether the symptoms may be associated with multiple sclerosis? **Select all that apply.**
    a. "Are you having persistent headaches that occur with stress?"
    b. "Do you have a persistent sensitivity to temperature?"
    c. "Do you ever have slurred speech or trouble swallowing?"
    d. "Are you having trouble breathing with minor exertion?"
    e. "Has anyone in your family been diagnosed with multiple sclerosis?"
    f. "Do you have spasms at night that wake you from your sleep?"

37. A patient tells the nurse, "I have the symptoms of multiple sclerosis [MS], and I have been dealing with them for so long! Why won't anyone help me?" Which intervention should the nurse employ **first**?
    a. Help the patient to locate and make an appointment with a specialist.
    b. Ask the patient to describe the symptoms and past treatments.
    c. Encourage the patient to verbalize feelings and frustrations.
    d. Give the patient a brochure about the diagnosis and treatment of MS.

38. The home health nurse sees in the patient's record that he takes riluzole. Which question is the nurse **most likely** to ask?
    a. When were you first diagnosed with amyotrophic lateral sclerosis?
    b. Has the medication relieved any of the symptoms caused by multiple sclerosis?
    c. Has your acute back pain returned to the more familiar chronic pain?
    d. Have you always had neurogenic bladder problems since your spinal cord injury?

39. A patient with multiple sclerosis is prescribed oral fingolimod. Which **key** point must the nurse teach the patient about this drug?
    a. "You must be carefully monitored for allergic reactions because the drug tends to build up in the body."
    b. "We need to teach you how to monitor your pulse rate because this drug can cause a slow heart rate."
    c. "This drug will decrease the frequency of clinical relapses, but there is an increased risk for stroke."
    d. "The medication will improve your ability to walk, but it also increases the risk for seizure activity."

40. The nurse has provided teaching to the husband of a 33-year-old woman who was recently diagnosed with multiple sclerosis. Which statement by the patient's husband indicates he needs additional teaching on the course of the illness?
    a. "She could fall because she may lose her balance and have poor coordination."
    b. "Eventually she will not be able to drive because of vision problems."
    c. "She will probably have a decreased libido and diminished orgasm."
    d. "As the disease progresses, she could have intermittent short-term memory loss."

41. The nurse is teaching a patient with multiple sclerosis and her family about her exercise program. Which points must the nurse include? **Select all that apply.**
    a. Range-of-motion exercises are an important component.
    b. Stretching should precede rigorous activity.
    c. Increased body temperature can lead to increased fatigue.
    d. Steadily increasing walking distances can lead to jogging.
    e. Stretching and strengthening exercises will be part of your program.
    f. Take your pain medication at least 30 minutes prior to exercise.

42. The patient with multiple sclerosis has dysarthria. What assessment would the nurse perform to monitor for a likely coexisting complication?
    a. Watch the patient walk and note smoothness of movement.
    b. Check the patient's gag reflex and ability to swallow.
    c. Ask the patient to use a pencil to write a sentence.
    d. Have the patient stand and close eyes, and observe the patient for sway.

43. The patient with multiple sclerosis states she is bothered by diplopia. Which intervention does the nurse expect to implement?
    a. Obtain an order for consultation or referral for corrective lenses
    b. Teach the patient scanning techniques, moving her head from side to side
    c. Application of an eye patch alternating from eye to eye every few hours
    d. Prophylactic bilateral patches to both eyes at night

44. The nurse is participating in a committee to decrease back injuries among the staff. What recommendations should the nurse suggest? **Select all that apply.**
    a. Assign committee members to review OSHA guidelines for the prevention of back injuries.
    b. Develop policies and procedures for the therapeutic use of patient handling equipment.
    c. Train all staff and family caregivers in the safe operation of all ergonomic-appropriate equipment.
    d. Assign all patients the responsiblity for learning how to use assistive equipment.
    e. Develop competency-based assessments that demonstrate proficiency in patient handling.
    f. Encourage quality improvement projects and research that support safe and effective patient handling.

45. The home health nurse reads in the patient's chart that he has a spinal cord stimulator. What question would the nurse ask to evaluate the efficacy of the treatment?
    a. "Has the device helped you to gain control over the urinary incontinence?"
    b. "Does the device allow you to have sexual arousal that is satisfying?"
    c. "Have you been able to program the device to achieve maximum comfort?"
    d. "Have you programmed the device to achieve various levels of mobility?"

Care of Patients with Problems of the Peripheral Nervous System

1. The nurse is assessing a patient with a diagnosis of Guillain-Barré syndrome. Which signs and symptoms would the nurse expect to observe? **Select all that apply.**
   a. Bilateral sluggish pupil response
   b. Sudden onset of weakness in the legs
   c. Muscle atrophy of the legs
   d. Change in level of consciousness
   e. Double vision
   f. Uncoordinated movements

2. During shift report, the nurse hears that a patient with Guillain-Barré syndrome has a decrease in vital capacity that is less than two-thirds of normal, and there is a progressive inability to clear and cough up secretions. The health care provider has been notified and is coming to evaluate the patient. What intervention is the nurse prepared to implement for this patient?
   a. Frequent oral suctioning
   b. Rigorous chest physiotherapy
   c. Elective intubation
   d. Elective tracheostomy

3. A patient with Guillain-Barré syndrome is identified as having poor dietary intake secondary to dysphagia. A feeding tube is prescribed. How does the nurse monitor this patient's nutritional status?
   a. Check skin turgor and urinary output
   b. Give enteral feedings via feeding tube
   c. Review weekly serum prealbumin level
   d. Review potassium and sodium levels

4. A patient with Guillain-Barré syndrome has been intubated for respiratory failure. The nurse must suction the patient. In assessing the risk for vagal nerve stimulation, what does the nurse **closely** monitor the patient for?
   a. Tachypnea
   b. Atrial fibrillation
   c. Cyanosis
   d. Bradycardia

5. A patient is admitted for a probable diagnosis of Guillain-Barré syndrome but needs additional diagnostic testing for confirmation. Which test does the nurse anticipate will be ordered for this patient?
   a. Electroencephalography
   b. Cerebral blood flow
   c. Electrophysiologic study
   d. Electrocardiogram

6. The nurse is reviewing the cerebral spinal fluid (CSF) results for a patient with probable Guillain-Barré syndrome, who has been having symptoms for several weeks. Which abnormal finding is **most likely** to be seen at this time?
   a. Increase in CSF protein level
   b. Increase in CSF glucose level
   c. Cloudy appearance of CSF
   d. Elevation of lymphocyte count in CSF

7. An ambulatory patient has sought treatment for symptoms of Guillain-Barré syndrome. IV immunoglobulin therapy has been prescribed. Which precaution does the nurse expect with this therapy?
   a. IV immunoglobulin is given concurrently with plasmapheresis.
   b. A shunt must be placed prior to beginning the therapy.
   c. IV immunoglobulin is slowly infused when it is started.
   d. Three or four treatments are given 1 to 2 days apart.

8. The patient with Guillain-Barré syndrome is at risk for aspiration. Which precautions must the nurse initiate to prevent aspiration? **Select all that apply.**
   a. Elevate the head of the bed at least 45 degrees.
   b. Assess for dysphagia prior to giving oral fluids or medications.
   c. Teach coughing and deep-breathing exercises.
   d. Have suctioning equipment available at the bedside.
   e. Turn the patient from side to side at least every 2 hours.
   f. Restrict food and fluids until exacerbation resolves.

9. What is the nursing concept that underlies the etiology and the pathophysiology of Guillain-Barré syndrome?
   a. Sensory perception
   b. Mobility
   c. Gas exchange
   d. Immunity

10. A patient with Guillain-Barré syndrome is receiving IV immunoglobulin. The nurse monitors for which **major** potential complication of this drug therapy?
    a. Ventricular fibrillation
    b. Hypertensive crisis
    c. Anaphylaxis
    d. Malignant hyperthermia

11. The nurse is monitoring a patient with Guillain-Barré syndrome undergoing plasmapheresis. The patient reports dizziness and has a heart rate that has dropped to 48 beats per minute. The nurse notifies the primary care provider. Which order does the nurse anticipate?
    a. Atropine IV push
    b. Epinephrine IV push
    c. Continue to monitor
    d. Defibrillate the patient

12. A patient has been newly diagnosed with Guillain-Barré syndrome. The nurse is teaching the patient and family about the condition. Which statement by the family indicates a need for additional teaching?
    a. "He could recover in 4 to 6 months."
    b. "He'll never be able to walk again."
    c. "He will receive medication for pain."
    d. "He will be monitored for breathing problems."

13. Which strategies should be incorporated in the plan of care to provide emotional support for a patient with Guillain-Barré syndrome? **Select all that apply.**
    a. Limit information provided to the patient and family.
    b. Encourage the patient to verbalize feelings.
    c. Teach the patient and family about the condition.
    d. Explain all procedures and tests.
    e. Allow regularly scheduled rest periods.
    f. Assess previous coping skills.

14. What is the **priority** expected outcome in a patient with Guillain-Barré syndrome?
    a. Maintain airway patency and gas exchange.
    b. Promote communication.
    c. Manage pain and discomfort.
    d. Prevent complications of immobility.

15. The nurse is reviewing the admission and history notes for a patient admitted for Guillain-Barré syndrome (GBS). Which medical condition is **most likely** to be present before the onset of GBS?
    a. Diabetes mellitus
    b. Recent bacterial infection
    c. Peripheral vascular disease
    d. Addison disease

16. The patient has Guillain-Barré syndrome with ascending paralysis. What would the nurse expect to observe?
    a. Motor weakness that starts in legs and then spreads to arms and upper body
    b. Extensive paralysis similar to quadriplegia, but sensory function is retained
    c. Motor weakness and fatigue that progressively worsens throughout the day
    d. Paralysis that is worse in the upper body, particularly the arms and hands

17. To maintain mobility for the patient with Guillain-Barré syndrome, which intervention is **best** for the nurse to delegate to unlicensed assistive personnel?
    a. Perform passive range of motion every 2 to 4 hours.
    b. Turn the patient every 2 hours and assess for skin breakdown.
    c. Ask the patient if he feels strong enough to go to physical therapy.
    d. Assist the patient to ambulate in the hall several times during the shift.

18. The patient with Guillain-Barré syndrome is immobile and shows evidence of malnutrition. What is the **priority** concern related to immobility and nutritional status?
    a. Respiratory failure
    b. Constipation
    c. Risk for pressure ulcers
    d. Cardiac dysrhythmias

19. For a patient with Guillain-Barré syndrome, what is the expected and desired outcome of plasmapheresis?
    a. Decreases the symptoms
    b. Puts patient into remission
    c. Cures almost all patients
    d. Slows progression of disease

20. The nurse is caring for a patient who has undergone plasmapheresis. Which laboratory tests must the nurse monitor in relation to this therapy? **Select all that apply.**
    a. Complete blood count
    b. Coagulation studies
    c. Serum protein electrophoresis
    d. Arterial blood gases
    e. Electrolytes
    f. Cerebral spinal fluid results

21. The nurse is caring for a patient who is slowly recovering from Guillain-Barré syndrome with ascending paralysis. Which sign of physical recovery would the nurse expect to see **first**?
    a. Respiratory effort improves
    b. Gross motor of arms improves
    c. Fine motor of fingers returns
    d. Movement of lower legs returns

22. The nurse asks a patient with Guillain-Barré syndrome to smile, frown, whistle, and drink from a straw. Which cranial nerve is the nurse assessing?
    a. Cranial nerve I
    b. Cranial nerve II
    c. Cranial nerve VII
    d. Cranial nerve X

23. To assess the hypoglossal nerve (cranial nerve XII), what will the nurse ask the patient to do?
    a. Blink eyelids and raise eyebrows.
    b. Read an eye chart or newspaper.
    c. Demonstrate a deep cough.
    d. Stick the tongue straight out.

24. The nurse is assessing a patient with myasthenia gravis. Which manifestations can the nurse expect to observe? **Select all that apply.**
    a. Ptosis
    b. Diplopia
    c. Delayed pupillary responses to light
    d. Ocular palsies
    e. Decreased pupillary accommodation
    f. Fatigue

25. The nurse reads in the patient's chart that he has myasthenia gravis with bulbar involvement. Which intervention is the nurse **most likely** to use?
    a. Administer medication 45-60 minutes before meals.
    b. Assess for bowel and bladder function after meals.
    c. Assist the patient to comb hair and don shirt.
    d. Use pillows to prop patient upright when sitting.

26. What can be one cause of a cholinergic crisis?
    a. Withdrawal from anticholinesterase drugs
    b. Too many anticholinesterase drugs
    c. Some type of bacterial infection
    d. Allergic reaction to anticholinesterase drugs

27. What diagnostic test is used to differentiate a cholinergic crisis from a myasthenic crisis?
    a. Electrophysiologic studies
    b. Repetitive nerve stimulation
    c. Tensilon challenge testing
    d. Cerebral spinal fluid protein level

28. The nurse is caring for a patient with myasthenia gravis. What problem does the nurse expect the patient to have?
    a. Patient has more trouble with mobility when he is fatigued.
    b. Patient has difficulty sleeping, and wakes around 3:00 AM.
    c. Patient is disorientated in the late afternoon.
    d. Patient has pain that interferes with activities of daily living.

29. The most common symptoms of myasthenia gravis are related to involvement of the levator palpebrae or extraocular muscles. Which assessment technique would the nurse use?
    a. Use a penlight and check for pupil size and response.
    b. Stand to the patient's side and observe for protrusion of the eyeballs.
    c. Check accommodation by moving the finger toward the patient's nose.
    d. Face the patient and instruct to open and close the eyelids.

30. What is the **priority** nursing assessment for a patient with myasthenia gravis?
    a. Presence of pain in the extremities
    b. Loss of bowel and bladder function
    c. Ability to chew and swallow
    d. Quality and volume of the voice

31. A patient with myasthenia gravis and the nurse are having a long discussion about plans for the future. After an extended conversation, what does the nurse anticipate will occur in this patient?
    a. Speech will be slurred and difficult to understand.
    b. Voice may become weaker or exhibit a nasal twang.
    c. Voice quality will become harsh and strident.
    d. Voice will become toneless and affect will be flat.

32. A patient with myasthenia gravis reports having difficulty climbing stairs, lifting heavy objects, and raising arms over the head. What is the underlying pathophysiology of this patient's symptoms?
    a. Limb weakness is more often proximal.
    b. Spinal nerves are affected.
    c. Large muscle atrophy is occurring.
    d. Demyelination of neurons is occurring.

33. The nurse is planning activities for a patient with myasthenia gravis. Which factor does the nurse consider to promote self-care, yet prevent excessive fatigue?
    a. Time of day
    b. Severity of symptoms
    c. Medication times
    d. Sleep schedule

34. A patient is suspected of having myasthenia gravis, and a Tensilon challenge test has been ordered. What does the nurse do to prepare the patient for the test?
    a. Ensure that the patient has a patent IV access.
    b. Draw a blood sample and send it for baseline analysis.
    c. Withhold food and fluids after midnight.
    d. Have the patient void before the beginning of the test.

35. The nurse is caring for a patient recently diagnosed and admitted with myasthenia gravis. During the morning assessment, the nurse notes some abnormal findings. Which symptom is cause for the **greatest** concern?
    a. Diarrhea
    b. Fatigue
    c. Inability to swallow
    d. Difficulty opening eyelids

36. What is considered a positive diagnostic finding of a Tensilon challenge test?
    a. 60 minutes after the cholinesterase inhibitor is administered, there are no observable changes in muscle strength or tone.
    b. Within 30-60 seconds after receiving the cholinesterase inhibitor, there is increased muscle tone that lasts 4-5 minutes.
    c. Within 30 minutes of receiving the cholinesterase inhibitor, there is improved muscle strength that lasts for several weeks.
    d. After the cholinesterase inhibitor is first administered, the patient will experience muscle weakness and then return to baseline.

37. Although an adverse reaction during the Tensilon challenge test is considered rare, which medication should be readily available to give as an antidote in case a patient should experience complications?
    a. Protamine sulfate
    b. Naloxone
    c. Atropine sulfate
    d. Phentolamine mesylate

38. The nurse is caring for a patient newly diagnosed with myasthenia gravis. The nurse is alert for complications related to both myasthenic crisis and cholinergic crisis. What is the **priority** nursing assessment for this patient?
    a. Monitor cardiac rate and rhythm.
    b. Assess respiratory status and function.
    c. Monitor fatigue and activity levels.
    d. Perform neurologic checks every 2-4 hours.

39. The nurse is performing patient and family teaching about myasthenia gravis and medications. What important information does the nurse give during the teaching session?
    a. If a dose of cholinesterase is missed, a double dose is taken the next day.
    b. Antibiotics such as kanamycin synergize cholinesterase inhibitors.
    c. Medications must be taken on an empty stomach with a full glass of water.
    d. Drugs containing morphine or sedatives can increase muscle weakness.

40. A patient with myasthenia gravis demonstrates a weak cough. Auscultation of the lungs reveals coarse crackles throughout the lung fields. The nurse identifies the patient is unable to cough effectively enough to clear the airway of secretions. Which intervention is **best** for this patient?
    a. Low flow oxygen therapy
    b. Chest physiotherapy
    c. Endotracheal suction
    d. Elective intubation

41. A patient with myasthenia gravis is experiencing cholinergic crisis. What is the **major** concern when caring for this patient?
    a. Brainstem herniation
    b. Respiratory failure
    c. Renal failure
    d. Hypertensive crisis

42. A patient with myasthenia gravis has generalized weakness and fatigue and is limited in the ability to perform activities of daily living (ADLs). Which nursing action is **best** to help this patient avoid excessive fatigue?
    a. Schedule activities after medication administration.
    b. Schedule activities during the late afternoon or early evening.
    c. Encourage ambulation during periods of maximal strength.
    d. Instruct unlicensed assistive personnel to assist with all ADLs.

43. The nurse is reviewing medication orders for a patient with myasthenia gravis. The patient is scheduled to receive pyridostigmine on a daily basis. What does the nurse expect regarding this drug?
    a. Noting daily dosage change related to presenting symptoms
    b. Administering medication 30 minutes after an antacid
    c. Monitoring for 60 minutes for a cholinergic crisis
    d. Gradual tapering and weaning off the drug

44. The nurse is caring for a patient receiving cholinesterase inhibitor drugs for myasthenia gravis. Which symptoms does the nurse **immediately** report to the health care provider?
    a. Increasing loss of motor function
    b. Ineffective nonproductive cough
    c. Dyspnea and difficulty swallowing
    d. Gastrointestinal side effects

45. During the shift report, the nurse learns that a patient with myasthenia gravis deteriorated toward the end of the shift and the health care provider was called. Tensilon challenge test indicated that the patient was having a myasthenic crisis. What is the **priority** problem for this patient?
    a. Potential for inadequate oxygenation
    b. Potential for decreased ability to do self-care
    c. Potential for aspiration pneumonia
    d. Potential for increase in blood pressure

46. A patient with myasthenia gravis has been referred to a surgeon for a procedure that may improve the patient's symptoms. Which brochure would the nurse prepare for the patient?
    a. "What Is Percutaneous Stereotactic Rhizotomy?"
    b. "How to Prepare for Your Surgical Thymectomy"
    c. "Expected Outcomes for Microvascular Decompression"
    d. "Stereotactic Radiation Treatments by Gamma Knife"

47. A patient with myasthenia gravis experienced a cholinergic crisis and is currently being maintained on a ventilator. The patient received several 1-mg doses of atropine IV. What does the nurse closely monitor for?
    a. Increasing muscle weakness
    b. Increased salivation
    c. Ventricular fibrillation
    d. Development of mucus plugs

48. The nurse is performing teaching for the family of a patient with myasthenia gravis about fatigue and activities of daily living. Which statement by a family member indicates a need for additional teaching?
    a. "Rest is critical because increased fatigue can precipitate a crisis."
    b. "We should do hygienic care for her to avoid undue frustration and fatigue."
    c. "Activities should be done after we give her the medication."
    d. "The physical therapist will be able to recommend some energy-saving devices."

49. A patient with myasthenia gravis is experiencing impaired communication related to weakness of the facial muscles. Which interventions are **best** in assisting the patient to communicate with the staff and family? **Select all that apply.**
    a. Instruct patient to speak slowly.
    b. Use short, simple sentences.
    c. Ask yes or no questions.
    d. Use system of eye blinking.
    e. Have patient use a picture, letter, or word board.
    f. Face patient and speak clearly.

50. A patient with myasthenia gravis is having difficulty maintaining an adequate intake of food and fluid because of difficulty chewing and swallowing. Which task for this patient is **best** to delegate to unlicensed assistive personnel?
    a. Perform daily weights.
    b. Monitor calorie counts.
    c. Ask about food preferences.
    d. Evaluate intake and output.

51. Which intervention is appropriate to protect a patient with myasthenia gravis from corneal abrasions?
    a. Instruct the patient to keep the eyes closed.
    b. Apply an eye patch to both eyes after breakfast.
    c. Apply lubricant gel and shield to the eyes at bedtime.
    d. Place a clean moist washcloth over the patient's eyes.

52. A patient is receiving a cholinesterase inhibitor drug for the treatment of myasthenia gravis. What is a nursing implication for this medication that relates to patient safety?
    a. Monitor for orthostatic hypotension.
    b. Take the patient's apical pulse prior to administration.
    c. Feed meals 45-60 minutes after administration.
    d. Encourage at least 8 glasses of water each day.

53. The nurse is caring for a patient with myasthenia gravis who had a thymectomy. The patient demonstrates restlessness and reports chest pain and shortness of breath. What are the **priority** nursing interventions? **Select all that apply.**
    a. Instruct to use the incentive spirometry.
    b. Administer oxygen.
    c. Raise the head of the bed 45 degrees.
    d. Place in supine position to encourage rest.
    e. Notify the Rapid Response Team.
    f. Prepare to administer atropine.

54. The nurse is teaching the patient and family about factors that predispose the patient to episodes of exacerbation of myasthenia gravis. Which factors does the nurse mention? **Select all that apply.**
    a. Infection
    b. Stress
    c. Sedatives
    d. Any physical exercise
    e. Enemas
    f. Strong cathartics

55. The nurse is caring for a patient who has a shunt for plasmapheresis. Which intervention related to the shunt does the nurse perform?
    a. Assess for bruit or thrill every 2-4 hours.
    b. Flush the shunt with sterile normal saline.
    c. Wrap the shunt with a protective gauze dressing.
    d. Ensure that IV fluid is infusing at prescribed rate.

56. Which patient has the **highest** risk factors for restless leg syndrome?
    a. Obese patient with renal failure
    b. 65-year-old woman who routinely jogs
    c. 43-year-old man with hypertension
    d. Underweight teenager who smokes

57. A patient is diagnosed with restless leg syndrome. What nonpharmacologic interventions does the nurse suggest for this patient? **Select all that apply.**
    a. Limit caffeine intake.
    b. Quit smoking.
    c. Take a warm bath before going to bed.
    d. Take naps during the day.
    e. Apply ice packs and elevate legs.
    f. Walk and perform stretching exercises.

58. A patient is prescribed ropinirole for restless leg syndrome. What nursing implication is related to this medication?
    a. Medication is taken with or immediately after meals.
    b. Medication is taken in divided doses throughout the day.
    c. Medication should be taken at bedtime.
    d. Medication is contraindicated in Parkinson disease.

59. A patient reports "excruciating, sharp, shooting" unilateral facial pain that lasts from seconds to minutes and describes a reluctance to smile, eat, or talk because of fear of precipitating an attack. This patient's description of symptoms is consistent with the symptoms of which disorder?
    a. Peripheral nerve trauma
    b. Trigeminal neuralgia
    c. Bell's palsy
    d. Eaton-Lambert syndrome

60. What is the **priority** concern in caring for a patient with trigeminal neuralgia?
    a. Pain management
    b. Promoting communication
    c. Maintaining nutrition
    d. Providing psychosocial support

61. A patient is diagnosed with trigeminal neuralgia. Which therapy is the **first-line** choice for this patient?
    a. Antiepileptic such as carbamazepine
    b. Muscle relaxant such as baclofen
    c. Percutaneous stereotactic rhizotomy
    d. Microvascular decompression

62. A patient has had percutaneous stereotactic rhizotomy to relieve the pain of trigeminal neuralgia. What is included in the postoperative care of this patient? **Select all that apply.**
    a. Apply an ice pack to the operative site on the cheek and jaw for 3-4 hours.
    b. Perform a focused cranial nerve assessment.
    c. Discourage the patient from chewing on the affected side until paresthesias resolve.
    d. Instruct the patient to avoid rubbing the eye on the affected side.
    e. Teach that dental procedures require extra anesthesia for pain control.
    f. Instruct to wear an eye patch and gel lubricant at night.

63. Which strategies will the nurse teach a patient with Bell's palsy to use in managing pain and paralysis? **Select all that apply.**
    a. Massage
    b. Opioid pain medications
    c. Application of warm, moist heat
    d. Chew on the affected side of the mouth
    e. Facial exercises
    f. Elevate head of bed

64. A patient is diagnosed with Bell's palsy, and the right side of the face is affected. Related to the patient's right eye, which nursing intervention is essential?
    a. Check the pupil size and reaction using a penlight.
    b. Check the patient's visual acuity in both eyes.
    c. Teach the patient to instill artificial tears throughout the day.
    d. Teach the patient to prevent eye strain by resting eyes periodically.

65. The patient tells the nurse that he is waiting for results of repetitive nerve stimulation testing. While waiting for the test results, the nurse is vigilant for signs and symptoms of which disorder?
    a. Guillain-Barré syndrome
    b. Myasthenia gravis
    c. Restless leg syndrome
    d. Trigeminal neuralgia

45
CHAPTER

Care of Critically Ill Patients with Neurologic Problems

1. Which clinical finding could help the health care team differentiate a transient ischemic attack from a stroke?
   a. Patient has a unilateral facial droop.
   b. Patient has slurred speech.
   c. Symptoms resolve in 30-60 minutes.
   d. Electrocardiogram is normal.

2. The nurse is preparing to discharge a patient with transient ischemic attacks. What topics does the nurse include in discharge teaching? **Select all that apply.**
   a. Reduction of high blood pressure
   b. Drug teaching for aspirin or other antiplatelet drug
   c. Lifestyle changes such as smoking cessation
   d. Self-care for managing chronic conditions, such as diabetes
   e. Increased risk for stroke and signs/ symptoms
   f. Benefits of taking vitamin supplements

3. The home health nurse is assessing a patient who had a stroke that affected the right hemisphere. What would the nurse expect to observe?
   a. Patient is overly anxious and cautious when asked to do a new task.
   b. Patient is euphoric and smiling but disoriented to person, place, and time.
   c. Patient is depressed and expresses ongoing worries about the future.
   d. Patient has a flat affect but is able to answer most questions appropriately.

4. The nurse is assessing a patient who was brought to the emergency department for altered mental status. In the absence of family members or witnesses to give a history, what does the nurse do to identify two conditions that could mimic emergent neurologic conditions?
   a. Check skin turgor and perform a bladder scan.
   b. Check blood glucose and oxygen saturation.
   c. Observe for jugular vein distention and pitting edema.
   d. Observe for jaundice and abdominal distention.

5. Following a left cerebral hemisphere stroke, the patient has expressive (Broca's) aphasia. Which intervention is **best** to use when communicating with this patient?
   a. Repeat the names of objects on a routine basis.
   b. Face the patient and speak slowly and clearly.
   c. Obtain a whiteboard with an erasable marker.
   d. Use a picture board that displays objects and activities.

6. The nurse is caring for a patient with right cerebral hemisphere damage. The patient demonstrates disorientation to time and place and neglect of the left visual field, and he has poor depth perception. Which task is **best** delegated to unlicensed assistive personnel?
   a. Move the patient's bed so that his affected side faces the door.
   b. Teach the patient to wash both sides of his face.
   c. Ensure a safe environment by removing clutter.
   d. Suggest to the family that they bring familiar family photos.

7. A patient with a right cerebral hemisphere stroke may have safety issues related to which factor?
   a. Poor impulse control
   b. Alexia and agraphia
   c. Loss of language and analytical skills
   d. Slow and cautious behavior

8. A stroke patient is at risk for increased intracranial pressure and is receiving oxygen 2 L via nasal cannula. The nurse is reviewing arterial blood gas (ABG) results. Which ABG value is of **greatest** concern for this patient?
   a. pH 7.32
   b. $Paco_2$ of 60 mm Hg
   c. Pao_2 of 95 mm Hg
   d. HCO_3^- of 28 mEq/L

9. What is the **priority** concept for the interdisciplinary care and treatment of a patient who is suspected of having a stroke?
   a. Pain
   b. Cognition
   c. Perfusion
   d. Sensory perception

10. The preferred administration time for intravenous (systemic) fibrinolytic therapy is generally within what time frame of stroke symptom onset?
    a. 30-60 minutes
    b. 3-4.5 hours
    c. 6-8 hours
    d. 24-30 hours

11. A patient who had a stroke several years ago continues to have the potential for aspiration. Which intervention is **best** to delegate to unlicensed assistive personnel?
    a. Monitor the patient for and notify the charge nurse of any occurrence of coughing, choking, or difficulty breathing.
    b. Elevate the head of the bed and slowly feed small spoonfuls of pudding, pausing between each spoonful.
    c. Check for swallow reflex by placing index finger and thumb on the Adam's apple and palpating during swallowing.
    d. Give the patient a glass of water before feeding solid foods, and have oral suction ready at the bedside.

12. A patient is diagnosed with an ischemic stroke. Unlicensed assistive personnel (UAP) reports that the patient's blood pressure (BP) is 150/100 mm Hg. The patient's BP prior to the stroke was normally around 120/80 mm Hg. What action does the nurse take **first**?
    a. Immediately report BP to the health care provider because there is a danger of rebleeding.
    b. Ask UAP to repeat the BP measurement in the other extremity with a manual cuff.
    c. Check the health care provider's orders to see if BP is within the acceptable parameters.
    d. Document BP and continue to monitor because an elevated BP is necessary for cerebral perfusion.

13. A patient with an ischemic stroke is placed on a cardiac monitor. Which cardiac dysrhythmia places the patient at risk for emboli?
    a. Sinus bradycardia
    b. Atrial fibrillation
    c. Sinus tachycardia
    d. First-degree heart block

14. The nurse is caring for a patient receiving medication therapy to prevent recurrence of stroke. Which medication is pharmacologically appropriate for this purpose?
    a. Enteric-coated aspirin
    b. Gabapentin
    c. Alteplase
    d. Acetaminophen

15. A patient sustained a stroke that affected the right hemisphere of the brain. The patient has visual spatial deficits and deficits of proprioception. After assessing the safety of the patient's home, the home health nurse identifies which environmental feature that represents a potential safety problem for this patient?
    a. The handrail that borders the bathtub is on the right-hand side.
    b. The patient's favorite chair faces the front door of the house.
    c. The patient's bedside table is on the left-hand side of the bed.
    d. Family has relocated the patient to a ground-floor bedroom.

16. The patient reports a sudden, severe headache, with nausea and vomiting. He says, "This is the worst headache of my life." What condition does the nurse suspect?
    a. Brain tumor
    b. Migraine headache
    c. Cerebral aneurysm
    d. Ischemic stroke

17. A patient presents to the advanced stroke center with signs and symptoms of an ischemic stroke. What is the **priority** factor when considering fibrinolytic therapy?
    a. Age less than 80 years
    b. History of stroke
    c. Recent surgery
    d. Time of onset of symptoms

18. A patient received alteplase for the treatment of ischemic stroke. Following drug administration, the nurse monitors for which adverse effect?
    a. Severe headache and hypertension
    b. Hypotension secondary to anaphylaxis
    c. Respiratory depression and low O_2 saturation
    d. Elevated hematocrit or hemoglobin

19. The nurse notices that a patient seems to be having trouble swallowing. Which intervention does the nurse employ for this patient?
    a. Limit the diet to clear liquids given through a straw.
    b. Withhold food and fluids until swallowing is assessed.
    c. Monitor the patient's weight and compare trends to baseline.
    d. Observe the patient while eating and note problematic foods.

20. The nurse is working on a medical-surgical unit, and unlicensed assistive personnel tells the nurse that a patient who was dressing to go home suddenly developed slurred speech and left-sided weakness. What does the nurse do **first**?
    a. Instruct the patient to wait and initiate neuro checks every 2 hours.
    b. Call health care provider to obtain a delay in the discharge order.
    c. Assess the patient within 10 minutes for signs/symptoms of a stroke.
    d. Instruct the patient to follow up tomorrow with his primary care provider.

21. A patient with increased intracranial pressure is to receive IV mannitol. Which assessment would the nurse perform to prevent complications in a body system other than the nervous system?
    a. Assess for cardiac dysthymias.
    b. Assess for gastric bleeding.
    c. Assess for respiratory distress.
    d. Assess for acute renal failure.

22. The nurse is talking to the family of a stroke patient about home care measures. Which topics does the nurse include in this discussion? **Select all that apply.**
    a. Need for caregivers to plan for routine respite care and protection of own health
    b. Evaluation for potential safety risks such as throw rugs or slippery floors
    c. Awareness of potential patient frustration associated with communication
    d. Avoidance of independent transfers by the patient because of safety issues
    e. Access to health resources such as publications from the American Heart Association
    f. Referral to hospice and encouragement of family discussion of advance directives

23. Which patients are at increased risk for stroke? **Select all that apply.**
    a. 66-year-old man with diabetes mellitus
    b. 43-year-old healthy woman who uses oral contraceptives
    c. 47-year-old woman who exercises regularly
    d. 35-year-old man with history of multiple transient ischemic attacks
    e. 25-year-old woman with Bell's palsy
    f. 53-year-old man with chronic alcoholism

24. The nurse hears in report that the patient with a stroke had a score of 25 on the National Institutes of Health Stroke Scale when assessed in the emergency department. After therapy and treatment, the most recent score is 20. How does the nurse interpret this information?
    a. Patient's condition can only be interpreted by trending several scores.
    b. Patient should be carefully monitored for life-threatening symptoms.
    c. Patient is possibly a little worse, but change is insignificant.
    d. Patient is showing improvement and has fewer neurologic deficits.

25. Which interventions does the nurse use for a patient with a left cerebral hemisphere stroke? **Select all that apply.**
    a. Teach the patient to wash both sides of the face.
    b. Place pictures and familiar objects around the patient.
    c. Reorient the patient frequently.
    d. Repeat names of commonly used objects.
    e. Approach the patient from the affected side.
    f. Establish a structured routine for the patient.

26. The nursing student has just studied about carotid artery angioplasty with stenting. Which statement by the student indicates an understanding of the purpose of the procedure?
    a. "The stent opens the blockage enough to establish blood flow."
    b. "The stent occludes the abnormal artery to prevent bleeding."
    c. "The stent bypasses the blockage for collateral circulation."
    d. "The stent catches any debris, particularly embolic clots."

27. The nurse is providing discharge teaching to a patient following carotid stent placement. The nurse would tell the patient to **immediately** report which symptoms to the health care provider? **Select all that apply.**
    a. Weight gain
    b. Drowsiness or new-onset confusion
    c. Muscle weakness or motor dysfunction
    d. Severe neck pain
    e. Neck swelling
    f. Hoarseness or difficulty swallowing

28. The nurse is caring for a patient at risk for increased intracranial pressure related to ischemic stroke. For what purpose does the nurse place the patient's head in a midline neutral position?
    a. Provide comfort for the patient.
    b. Protect the cervical spine.
    c. Facilitate venous drainage from brain.
    d. Maintain presence of cerebrospinal fluid.

29. In planning care for a patient with increased intracranial pressure (ICP), what does the nurse do to minimize ICP?
    a. Gives the bath, changes the linens, does passive range of motion (ROM) to hands/fingers, and then allows the patient to rest
    b. Gives the bath, allows rest, changes linens, allows rest, and then performs passive ROM exercises to hands/fingers
    c. Gives the bath; defers the linen change and passive ROM exercises until the danger of increased ICP has passed
    d. Contacts the health care provider for specific orders about activities related to patient care that might cause increased ICP

30. The nurse is caring for a patient at risk for increased intracranial pressure (ICP). Which sign is **most likely** to be the **first** indication of increased ICP?
    a. Decline of level of consciousness
    b. Increase in systolic blood pressure
    c. Change in pupil size and response
    d. Abnormal posturing of extremities

31. The stroke patient is prescribed a stool softener every morning. What is the purpose of this drug specific to **this patient**?
    a. Stimulates peristaltic action to aid defecation
    b. Increases frequency of bowel movements
    c. Decreases fluid and fiber content of stool
    d. Prevents Valsalva maneuver during defecation

32. Which patient handling situation has the **greatest** potential to lead to a subdural hematoma?
    a. Sudden vertical elevation of head of the bed of an older patient
    b. Log-rolling a patient who has a possible cervical spine injury
    c. Pulling on the affected flaccid arm of an older stroke patient
    d. Keeping patient flat and alternating side-lying position every 2 hours

33. The nurse is caring for a patient who has decreased level of consciousness with the medical diagnosis of epidural hematoma. During the shift, the patient becomes lucid and is alert and talking. The family reports this is her baseline mental status. What is the nurse's **next** action?
    a. Stay with the patient and have the charge nurse alert the health care provider because this is an ominous sign for the patient.
    b. Document the patient's exact behaviors, compare to previous nursing entries, and continue the neurologic assessments every 2 hours.
    c. Point out to the family that the dangerous period has passed, but encourage them to leave so the patient does not become overly fatigued.
    d. Monitor the patient for the next 48 hours to 2 weeks because a subacute condition may be slowly developing.

34. What are the **most** common symptoms of stroke? **Select all that apply.**
    a. Sudden dizziness, trouble walking, or loss of balance or coordination
    b. Sudden numbness or weakness of the face, arm, or leg
    c. Sudden trouble seeing in one or both eyes
    d. Sudden shortness of breath or trouble breathing
    e. Sudden confusion or trouble speaking or understanding others
    f. Sudden severe headache with no known cause

35. A patient has been diagnosed with a large lesion of the parietal lobe and demonstrates loss of sensory function. Which nursing intervention is applicable for this patient?
    a. Play music for the patient for at least 30 minutes each day.
    b. Teach the patient to test the water temperature used for bathing.
    c. Position the patient reclining in bed or in a chair for meals.
    d. Show a picture of the spouse and ask patient to identify the person.

36. A patient has been diagnosed with subarachnoid hemorrhage. Which drug does the nurse anticipate will be ordered to control cerebral vasospasm?
    a. Nimodipine
    b. Phenytoin
    c. Dexamethasone
    d. Clopidogrel

37. The home health nurse reads in the patient's chart that he has a mild hemiparesis and ataxia that are residual from a stoke that occurred several years ago. Based on this information, the nurse would assess for functionality and availability of what type of adaptive equipment for this patient?
    a. Walker and wheelchair for mobility and handrails in the bathroom
    b. Picture boards, flash cards, or other methods of communication
    c. Cell phone, computer with internet access, or medical alert device
    d. Hearing aid, corrective eyeglasses, dentures, and orthotic devices

38. The nurse is caring for a patient who had a stroke in the right cerebral hemisphere, and the patient demonstrates unilateral body neglect syndrome. Based on this information, which behavior would the nurse expect to observe?
    a. Patient uses a pencil and fingers to eat food from the meal tray.
    b. Patient combs hair on the unaffected side but not on the affected side.
    c. Patient tells the nurse that bathing and hygiene should be done next month.
    d. Patient generally looks disheveled and disorganized but is always pleasant.

39. The neurologist tells the nurse that the stoke patient has some deficits associated with cranial nerves V, VII, IX, X, and XII. Which intervention is the nurse **most likely** to initiate?
    a. Prevention of Valsalva maneuver
    b. Fall precautions
    c. Prevention of corneal abrasions
    d. Aspiration precautions

40. Following a stroke, a patient demonstrates emotional lability. What is the family **most likely** to report?
    a. "He is so depressed all of the time that he hardly even eats anything."
    b. "He will laugh loudly and then suddenly start crying for no apparent reason."
    c. "He seems really cheerful, almost giddy and euphoric most of the time."
    d. "He is starting to behave and interact with us like he did before the stroke."

41. The nurse is caring for a patient with an ischemic stroke. Which concept underlies the rationale for placing the patient in a supine position with a low head-of-bed elevation?
    a. Comfort
    b. Perfusion
    c. Gas exchange
    d. Mobility

42. The patient with a traumatic brain injury is receiving mechanical ventilation. Why does the health care provider order ventilator settings to maintain a partial pressure of arterial carbon dioxide ($Paco_2$) at 35-38 mm Hg?
    a. Lower levels of arterial carbon dioxide are essential for gas exchange.
    b. Carbon dioxide is a vasodilator that can cause increased intracranial pressure.
    c. Carbon dioxide is a waste product that must be eliminated from the body.
    d. Lower levels of arterial carbon dioxide facilitate brain oxygenation.

43. The nurse is caring for a patient who had a craniotomy. What interventions should the nurse use to prevent respiratory complications of atelectasis and pneumonia?
    a. Turn frequently and encourage frequent deep breaths.
    b. Perform deep suction frequently to keep airway patent.
    c. Place in a high Fowler's position and apply oxygen.
    d. Coach to perform deep coughing to expectorate secretions.

44. Which Glasgow Coma Scale (GCS) data set indicates the **most** severe injury for a patient with traumatic brain injury and loss of consciousness?
    a. GCS of 13 with loss of consciousness for 5 minutes
    b. GCS of 9 with loss of consciousness for 30 minutes
    c. GCS of 12 with loss of consciousness for 15 minutes
    d. GCS of 8 with loss of consciousness for 60 minutes

45. The nurse is assessing a patient who was struck in the head several times with a baseball bat. There is clear fluid that appears to be leaking from the nose. What action does the nurse take **first**?
    a. Ask the patient to gently blow the nose; observe the nasal discharge for blood clots.
    b. Immediately report the finding to the health care provider and document the observation.
    c. Place a drop of the fluid on a white absorbent background and look for a yellow halo.
    d. Assist patient to wipe his nose, but no other action is needed; he has probably been crying.

46. Which determination must be made **first** in assessing a patient with traumatic brain injury?
    a. Presence of spinal injury
    b. Hypovolemia with hypotension
    c. Patency of airway
    d. Glasgow Coma Score

47. A patient is admitted for a closed head injury sustained during a fall down the stairs. The patient has no history of respiratory disease and no apparent respiratory distress. However, the health care provider orders oxygen 2 L via nasal cannula. What is the nurse's **best** action?
    a. Use pulse oximeter and apply the oxygen if the saturation level drops below 90%.
    b. Question the order because oxygen is unnecessary and therefore an extra cost to the patient.
    c. Deliver oxygen as ordered because hypoxemia may increase intracranial pressure.
    d. Apply nasal cannula as ordered and wean from oxygen when patient is discharged.

48. The nurse is conducting a presentation to a group of students on the prevention of head injuries. Which statement by a student indicates a need for additional teaching?
    a. "Drinking, driving, and speeding contribute to the risk for injury."
    b. "Males are more likely to sustain head injury compared to females."
    c. "Young people are less likely to get injured because of faster reflexes."
    d. "Following game rules and not 'goofing around' can prevent injuries."

49. The nurse is taking a history on a teenager who was involved in a motor vehicle accident with friends. The patient has an obvious contusion of the forehead, seems confused, and is laughing loudly and yelling, "Ruby! Ruby!" What is the **best** question for the nurse to ask the patient's friends?
    a. "Where and why did the accident occur?"
    b. "How can we notify the family for consent for treatment?"
    c. "Was the patient using drugs or alcohol prior to the accident?"
    d. "Who is Ruby, and why is the patient calling for her?"

50. The nurse is assessing a patient who had a traumatic brain injury and observes that the patient's right pupil appears more ovoid in shape compared to the left and to previous assessments. What is the clinical significance of this observation?
    a. Ovoid pupil is not significant unless the nurse observes severe hypertension, change of mental status, or respiratory distress.
    b. Ovoid pupil is assumed to signal brain herniation in progress with a poor prognosis until proven otherwise.
    c. Ovoid pupil is considered a normal variation for a small percentage of patients who sustain minor head injuries.
    d. Ovoid pupil is regarded as midstage between a normal pupil and a dilated pupil and should be reported immediately.

51. The nurse is performing discharge teaching for the family and patient who had prolonged hospitalization and rehabilitation therapy for severe craniocerebral trauma after a motorcycle accident. What important points does the nurse include? **Select all that apply.**
    a. Review seizure precautions.
    b. Stimulate the patient with frequent changes in the environment.
    c. Develop a routine of activities with consistency and structure.
    d. Attend follow-up appointments with therapists.
    e. Encourage the family to seek respite care if needed.
    f. Encourage the patient to wear a helmet when riding.

52. A patient has sustained a major head injury, and the nurse is assessing the patient's neurologic status every 2 hours. What **early** sign of increased intracranial pressure does the nurse monitor for?
    a. Change in level of consciousness
    b. Cheyne-Stokes respirations
    c. Cushing's triad
    d. Dilated and nonreactive pupils

53. The emergency department (ED) nurse is giving discharge instructions to the mother of a child who bumped his head on a table. Which statement by the mother indicates an understanding of the instructions?
    a. "I should not let him fall asleep today or during the early evening."
    b. "There's really nothing to worry about. It was just a bump on the head."
    c. "I should take him back to the ED for weakness or slurred speech."
    d. "He can run and play as he usually does, as long as he doesn't climb."

54. The nurse is caring for an intubated patient with increased intracranial pressure (ICP). If the patient needs to be suctioned, which nursing action does the nurse take to **avoid** further aggravating the increased ICP?
    a. Manually hyperventilate with 100% oxygen before passing the catheter.
    b. Maintain strict sterile technique when performing endotracheal suctioning.
    c. Perform oral suctioning frequently, but do not perform endotracheal suctioning.
    d. Obtain an order for an arterial blood gas before suctioning the patient.

55. A patient has sustained a traumatic brain injury. Which nursing intervention is **best** for this patient?
    a. Assess vital signs every 8 hours.
    b. Position to avoid extreme flexion of neck.
    c. Increase fluid intake for the first 48 hours.
    d. Restrict visitors until cognition improves.

56. The nurse is assessing a patient who sustained a relatively minor head injury after a bump to the head. The nurse has the **greatest** concern about which symptom?
    a. Headache
    b. Nausea and vomiting
    c. Unequal pupils
    d. Dizziness

57. The emergency department nurse is caring for a trauma patient. The spinal board has been removed, but the health care provider indicates that spinal precautions should be maintained. What is included? **Select all that apply.**
    a. Bedrest with bathroom privileges
    b. No neck flexion with a pillow or roll
    c. No thoracic or lumbar flexion with head of bed elevation/bed controls
    d. No reverse Trendelenburg positioning
    e. Manual control of the cervical spine anytime the rigid collar is removed
    f. "Log-roll" procedure to reposition the patient

58. The nurse is caring for a patient who had a craniotomy. Which intervention targets the **primary** concern of postoperative care in the first 4-6 hours after this procedure?
    a. Monitoring for periorbital edema and ecchymosis around eyes
    b. Assessing neurologic and vital signs every 15-30 minutes
    c. Monitoring complete blood count, electrolyte levels, and osmolarity
    d. Orienting the patient to person, place, and time

59. A patient had an infratentorial craniotomy. Which position does the nurse use for this patient?
    a. High Fowler's position, turned to the operative side
    b. Head of bed at 30 degrees, turned to the nonoperative side
    c. Flat in bed, except elevate head of bed for meals and medications
    d. Flat and positioned side-lying, alternating sides every 2 hours

60. The nurse is caring for a patient who sustained a traumatic brain injury and is intubated. To prevent increased intracranial pressure, what would the nurse use to quickly detect hypercarbia?
    a. Pulse oximeter
    b. Capnography
    c. Arterial blood gas
    d. Glasgow Coma Scale

61. What are key features of a brainstem tumor? **Select all that apply.**
    a. Vomiting unrelated to food intake
    b. Facial pain or weakness
    c. Nystagmus
    d. Headache
    e. Hearing loss
    f. Hoarseness

62. A patient who had a craniotomy develops the postoperative complication of syndrome of inappropriate antidiuretic hormone. The patient's sodium level is 117 mEq/L, and the serum osmolality is decreased. In light of this development, which intervention would the nurse **question**?
    a. Encourage oral fluids
    b. Slow IV infusion of hypertonic sodium
    c. Strict intake and output
    d. Daily weights

63. A patient had a brain tumor removed. Which position does the nurse place the patient in?
    a. Place on operative side to protect the unaffected side of the brain.
    b. Place flat and repositioned on either side to decrease tension on the incision.
    c. Do not reposition unless specific positions are ordered by the surgeon.
    d. Reposition every 2 hours but do not turn the patient onto the operative side.

64. A patient is admitted to the critical care unit after a craniotomy to debulk a grade 3 astrocytoma. What is the **priority** patient problem?
    a. Risk for infection leading to septic shock
    b. Risk for memory loss and confusion
    c. Risk for increased intracranial pressure
    d. Risk for multi-organ failure

65. The nurse observes that a patient who had surgery for a benign hemangioblastoma has bilateral periorbital edema and ecchymosis. Because this patient's care is based on the general principles of caring for the patient with a craniotomy, what is the nurse's **first** action?
    a. Immediately inform the surgeon.
    b. Apply cold compresses.
    c. Check the pupillary response.
    d. Perform a full neurologic assessment.

66. What is **best** practice for managing increased intracranial pressure in a patient who experienced a stroke?
    a. Restrict visitors until level of consciousness improves.
    b. Keep the environment cheerful and stimulating.
    c. Obtain an order for a low-fat and low-sodium diet.
    d. Position head of the bed to less than 25 degrees.

67. The nurse is teaching a patient who will receive a disc-shaped wafer (carmustine) as part of the treatment for a brain tumor. Which statement by the patient indicates understanding of how the wafer works?
    a. "I'll place the wafer under my tongue and allow it to dissolve."
    b. "The wafer will be taped to my chest, and the drug will be absorbed."
    c. "The wafer will be placed directly into the cavity during the surgery."
    d. "The wafer is to be dissolved in water and taken with meals."

68. The oncoming intensive care nurse is told that the patient with a traumatic brain injury manifested Cushing's triad several minutes ago, just before shift change. Which intervention does the oncoming nurse anticipate?
    a. Helping family to prepare for imminent death
    b. Assisting with arrangements for hospice care
    c. Aggressive administration of osmotic diuretics
    d. Emergency transfer to the operating room

69. Which patient is demonstrating an **early** indicator of change in level of consciousness?
    a. Middle-aged patient with a brain tumor wanders naked in the halls.
    b. Older patient who had a stroke several days ago is snoring loudly.
    c. Elderly patient is restless and irritable after a fall and bump to the head.
    d. Adolescent patient is difficult to arouse after drinking and fighting.

70. The health care provider orders therapeutic hypothermia for a patient with a traumatic brain injury. What is the **priority** assessment during the rewarming process?
    a. Assess for change of mental status.
    b. Monitor for cardiac dysthymias.
    c. Watch for rebound elevation of temperature.
    d. Observe for hypovolemic shock.

71. The nurse is providing postoperative care for a patient who had a craniotomy. The nurse would **immediately** notify the surgeon of which assessment finding?
    a. Drainage via Jackson-Pratt of 45 mL/8 hours
    b. Intracranial pressure of 15 mm Hg
    c. Pco_2 level of 35 mm Hg
    d. Serum sodium of 119 mEq/L

72. The nurse is performing discharge teaching for a patient who underwent a craniotomy for a brain tumor. What instructions does the nurse include? **Select all that apply.**
    a. Suggestions to make the environment safe, such as removing scatter rugs
    b. Seizure precautions and what to do if seizure occurs
    c. Information about drugs such as dose, administration, and side effects
    d. Doing regular physical exercise within limits of disability
    e. Advice about which over-the-counter products are safe to use
    f. Referral to a resource such as the American Brain Tumor Association

46

Assessment of the Eye and Vision

1. Light waves pass through each of the eye structures listed below to reach the retina. Place them in sequence using the numbers 1 through 5, with number 1 being the outermost structure and number 5 being the innermost structure.
   _____ a. Vitreous humor
   _____ b. Aqueous humor
   _____ c. Lens
   _____ d. Cornea
   _____ e. Retina

2. An older patient reports a sensation of eye dryness. The nurse would teach the patient to use saline eye drops and to increase the humidity in the house to **reduce** the risk for which eye disorder?
   a. Corneal abrasion
   b. Presbyopia
   c. Hyperopia
   d. Yellowing of the sclera

3. If the superior rectus muscle is damaged or not functioning properly, the patient would have difficulty with which eye movement?
   a. Looking upwards
   b. Looking downwards
   c. Gazing inwards to the nose
   d. Gazing outwards to the ear

4. The nurse asks the patient to open and close his eyelids. Which cranial nerve is the nurse assessing?
   a. Cranial nerve II (optic)
   b. Cranial nerve III (oculomotor)
   c. Cranial nerve V (trigeminal)
   d. Cranial nerve VII (facial)

5. One of the expected changes of the eyes associated with aging is the decreased ability of the iris to dilate. How will this affect the patient's eyes or vision?
   a. Difficulty with tear production resulting in dry eyes
   b. Decreased ability to see objects that are close
   c. Difficulty distinguishing blues, greens, or violets
   d. Increased difficulty seeing in dark environments

6. A 29-year-old patient tells the nurse that he spends a great deal of time in the sun and rarely wears sunglasses. The patient's behavior **increases** the risk for which eye disorder?
   a. Hyperopia
   b. Ptosis
   c. Ocular melanoma
   d. Exophthalmos

7. A 45-year-old patient has diabetes mellitus. Which information about vision protection does the nurse include in the teaching plan?
   a. People with diabetes mellitus have an increased incidence of ocular melanoma.
   b. Fluctuating blood glucose levels are undesirable but do not cause vision problems.
   c. Use over-the-counter eye drops every day to flush potential infective organisms.
   d. Annual eye examinations are recommended for patients with diabetes mellitus.

8. The nurse reads in the patient's chart that he has anisocoria. Which assessment of the eye will reveal this variation that is considered normal in 5% of the population?
   a. Corneal assessment
   b. Scleral assessment
   c. Pupillary assessment
   d. Eye movement assessment

9. A patient reports not being able to see objects in his peripheral vision. Which method is used to evaluate this symptom?
   a. Jaeger card
   b. Six cardinal positions of gaze
   c. Confrontation test
   d. Corneal light reflex test

10. A patient who works in a machine shop has a suspected metal foreign body in the eye. Which test is **contraindicated** for this patient?
    a. Corneal staining
    b. Computed tomography scan
    c. Magnetic resonance imaging
    d. Ultrasonography

11. The nurse needs to assess the patient for color blindness. Which assessment tool will the nurse use?
    a. Ishihara chart
    b. Confrontation test
    c. Snellen chart
    d. Rosenberg Pocket Vision Screener

12. The nurse reads in the patient's chart that the patient's visual acuity is 20/40. What is the correct interpretation of this documentation?
    a. Patient has 50% of the ideal 20/20 visual acuity.
    b. Patient stood 40 feet from the chart rather than 20 feet from the chart.
    c. Patient sees at 20 feet from the chart what a healthy eye sees at 40 feet.
    d. Patient stood 20 feet from the chart and sees 40% of the letters.

13. The patient underwent a fluorescein angiography. What postprocedure instructions will the nurse give the patient?
    a. You may see a yellow haze for several days.
    b. Use over-the-counter artificial tears to flush the eye.
    c. Drink fluids to help eliminate the dye from the body.
    d. Wear bilateral eye patches for 24 hours to rest eyes.

14. What is included in the correct procedure for instilling ophthalmic drops in a patient's eyes? **Select all that apply.**
    a. Check the name, strength, and expiration date of the solution.
    b. Have the patient tilt the head backward and look down.
    c. Release drops into the conjunctival pocket.
    d. Avoid contaminating the tip of the bottle.
    e. Rest the wrist holding the bottle against the patient's cheek.
    f. After instilling a drop, tell patient to tightly close eyelids.

15. Why might the health care provider order a computed tomography scan to examine the eye?
    a. To validate the function of extraocular muscles
    b. To verify intraocular pressure
    c. To determine the degree of peripheral vision
    d. To detect an ocular tumor in the orbital space

16. What would be included in the procedure for using an ophthalmoscope?
    a. The nurse comes toward the patient's eye from 6 inches away.
    b. The test should be done in a brightly lit room to enhance visibility.
    c. Have an assistant firmly hold a confused patient during the examination.
    d. The nurse stands on the same side as the eye being examined.

17. A patient is diagnosed with arcus senilis. Which intervention will the nurse use in caring for this patient?
    a. Assist the patient in activities that require near vision.
    b. Teach the patient how to instill the prescribed eye drops.
    c. Reassure the patient that the vision is not affected.
    d. Instruct that consistent use of sunglasses prevents worsening.

18. Which assessment findings of the eye are normal? **Select all that apply.**
    a. Presbyopia in a 45-year-old woman
    b. Ptosis of the eyelids
    c. Yellow sclera with small pigmented dots in a dark-skinned person
    d. Pupil constriction in response to accommodation
    e. Pupil constriction within 1 minute in response to light
    f. Nystagmus in the far lateral gaze

19. Which method is used to measure intraocular pressure?
    a. Corneal staining
    b. Tonometry
    c. Slit lamp examination
    d. Electroretinography

20. The patient has an intraocular pressure greater than 21 mm Hg. The patient's use of which over-the-counter product should be brought to the **immediate** attention of the ophthalmologist?
    a. Aspirin
    b. Antihistamine
    c. Vitamin supplement
    d. Artificial tear eye drops

21. What is the pathophysiology that underlies the development of glaucoma?
    a. Pressure on retinal vessels decreases blood flow so photoreceptors and nerve fibers become hypoxic.
    b. Decreased muscle tone reduces ability to keep the gaze focused on a single object.
    c. Cornea flattens, and the surface becomes irregular with worsening of astigmatism and blurred vision.
    d. The lens hardens, shrinks, and loses elasticity, and cataracts begin to form.

22. Which medications can adversely affect the eyes and vision? **Select all that apply.**
    a. Heparin
    b. Decongestants
    c. Oral contraceptives
    d. Acetaminophen
    e. Corticosteroids
    f. Antibiotics

23. Which conditions or diseases can adversely affect a patient's eyes and vision? **Select all that apply.**
    a. Pregnancy
    b. Inflammatory bowel disease
    c. Diabetes
    d. Hypertension
    e. Osteoarthritis
    f. Thyroid problems

24. Which activity is **most likely** to be very difficult for the patient if the visual function of accommodation is not working correctly?
    a. Reading a newspaper
    b. Playing tennis
    c. Watching a sunset
    d. Walking in a dark hallway

25. Which intervention would be **best** to use for a patient with presbyopia?
    a. Encouragement to get a prescription for reading glasses
    b. Administration of the prescribed eye medications
    c. Reinforcement to wear sunglasses for protection against UV light
    d. Reminder to have annual examination for early detection of glaucoma

26. Which patient has the **greatest** risk for cataracts and needs an annual eye examination?
    a. 25-year-old who was treated for an episode of eye infection
    b. 16-year-old who was struck in the face by a basketball
    c. 57-year-old with no history of eye problems or vision changes
    d. 35-year-old who is pregnant with her first child

27. A neighbor calls the nurse for advice because he thinks he may have got some metal shavings in his eye while working on a home improvement project. What advice should the nurse give?
    a. Rinse the eye with water and then don protective eyewear.
    b. Immediately notify his health care provider or ophthalmologist.
    c. Mention the incident during the annual eye examination.
    d. Resting the eye is sufficient unless there is pain or loss of vision.

28. Which food would the nurse recommend, that would be particularly good for eye health?
    a. Whole-grain cereal
    b. Low-fat milk
    c. Raw almonds
    d. Fresh tomatoes

29. Although the older patient denies any problems with his vision, the nurse frequently observes that he closes one eye when trying to look at his meal tray or personal items on the bedside table. What does the nurse suspect?
    a. Patient has arcus senilis.
    b. Patient has double vision.
    c. Patient has dry eye syndrome.
    d. Patient has a small cataract.

30. Which method would the nurse use to perform a corneal assessment?
    a. Inspect the corneas to determine if they are equal distance from the nose.
    b. Quickly and unexpectedly bring a hand toward the patient's cornea.
    c. Use a penlight and direct the light on the cornea from the side.
    d. Ask the patient to open and close eyelids, and observe the cornea.

31. The nurse reads PERRLA in the patient's chart as noted by the nurse who worked the previous shift. What does the nurse do to determine if the patient still displays PERRLA or if the patient's status has changed?
    a. Assesses for presence, relief, or reduction of pain
    b. Checks pupils, retina, and light refraction
    c. Assesses the size, shape, and reactivity of pupils
    d. Checks for signs of presbyopia or retinal detachment

32. The nurse is assessing a patient who is unable to see the 20/400 characters on the Snellen chart. Which assessment will the nurse try **first**?
    a. Ask the patient to detect stationary, left-right, or up-down hand movements.
    b. Ask the patient to count the number of fingers held up in front of the eyes.
    c. Ask the patient to report "on" or "off" when detecting light in a darkened room.
    d. Ask the patient to self-select a distance from Snellen chart where 20/400 is visible.

33. The home health nurse is interviewing a patient and discovers that there may be a previously undiagnosed vision problem. The nurse does not have a Jaeger card available at the patient's house to assess the suspected problem. Which item would serve as the **best** temporary substitute for a Jaeger card?
    a. Flashlight
    b. Ophthalmoscope
    c. Snellen chart
    d. Newspaper

34. In assessing the corneal light reflex of the older patient's eye, the nurse notes an asymmetric reflex. What is the clinical significance of this assessment finding?
    a. This is a normal finding for an older adult.
    b. Eye is deviating because of possible muscle weakness.
    c. The reflex is asymmetrical because of a cataract.
    d. Eye strain and eye fatigue can alter the reflex.

35. What would be an important point to include in the documentation of a patient's intraocular pressure (IOP)?
    a. Patient's body position during the IOP measurement
    b. IOP measurement performed in a darkened room
    c. Type and time of IOP measurement
    d. Time of mydriatic drops and response to IOP measurement

47 CHAPTER

Care of Patients with Eye and Vision Problems

1. What is an **early** sign of primary open-angle glaucoma?
   a. Sudden severe pain around the eyes
   b. Gradual loss of visual fields
   c. Seeing halos around lights
   d. Brow pain with nausea and vomiting

2. Which patient behavior would prompt the nurse to suggest that the patient should see an ophthalmologist about the possible development of a cataract?
   a. Patient frequently wipes a creamy white, dry, crusty drainage from the eyelids.
   b. Patient has tearing and a reddened sclera after instilling prescribed eye drops.
   c. Patient frequently removes eyeglasses and repeatedly cleans the lenses.
   d. Patient rubs eyelids because of itching, mild swelling, and irritation.

3. Age is important because cataracts are most prevalent in the older adult. In addition, the nurse would ask about which predisposing factors? **Select all that apply.**
   a. Exposure to radioactive materials, x-rays, or UV light
   b. Family history of cataracts
   c. Family history of rheumatoid arthritis
   d. Systemic disease (e.g., diabetes mellitus, hypoparathyroidism)
   e. Recent or past trauma to the eye
   f. Prolonged use of corticosteroids, chlorpromazine, beta blockers, or miotic drugs

4. The nurse is working at an ophthalmology specialty center and has just received a handoff report. Which patient needs to be assessed and managed **first**?
   a. Patient needs postprocedural care after phacoemulsification.
   b. Patient was just diagnosed with primary angle-closure glaucoma.
   c. Patient requires therapy for exudative macular degeneration.
   d. Patient is resting quietly, with probable retinal detachment.

5. The home health nurse is visiting an older patient who was discharged to home yesterday after cataract surgery. The patient reports pain during the evening with nausea and vomiting that started this morning. The home health nurse decides to contact the health care provider for suspicion of which complication?
   a. Dry eye syndrome
   b. Tissue graft rejection
   c. Corneal infection
   d. Increased intraocular pressure

6. The patient is being treated for an eye infection. The drug therapy may continue for 3 or more weeks; eye drops are required at night, and the patient is not allowed to wear contact lenses for weeks to months until the infection is completely cleared. Which patient statement indicates that the patient understands the goal of therapy?
   a. "Stopping the infection can save the vision in my infected eye."
   b. "I'll never have to worry about cataracts once this infection clears."
   c. "Antibiotic drops are easier than surgery, so I guess I'll use them."
   d. "Three weeks is a long time, but I have a spare pair of eyeglasses."

7. What is the nursing care **priority** for a deceased patient who is a corneal donor?
   a. Instill saline solution into the eyes.
   b. Instill antibiotic drops into the eyes.
   c. Lay the deceased in a flat supine position.
   d. Apply loose patches moistened with saline.

8. The nurse is providing the immediate postoperative care for a patient who had a keratoplasty. Which assessment will the nurse perform to identify the **most likely** complication?
   a. Assess for bleeding.
   b. Assess for photosensitivity.
   c. Monitor for respiratory depression.
   d. Monitor for hypotension.

9. For a patient who had a keratoplasty, which discharge instruction will the nurse give?
   a. Sleep on the operative side to reduce intraocular pressure.
   b. Keep eye covered for 1 week with the initial dressing and shield.
   c. Wear the shield at night for the first month after surgery.
   d. Apply a small cloth-covered ice pack to reduce swelling.

10. What is an **early** sign/symptom of a cataract?
    a. Double vision
    b. Photophobia
    c. Decreased depth perception
    d. Decreased color perception

11. The nurse is using an ophthalmoscope to examine the lens of a patient with a mature cataract. Which finding does the nurse expect to see?
    a. Dilated pupil
    b. Yellow tinge to sclera
    c. Enlarged retina
    d. Bluish-white pupil

12. What is an **early** sign/symptom of macular degeneration?
    a. Mild blurring
    b. Decreased tear production
    c. Loss of central vision
    d. Difficulty with activities of daily living

13. A 46-year-old patient calls the clinic and reports sudden "floating dark spots" in her vision. What should the nurse say to the patient?
    a. Advise the patient to immediately call her ophthalmologist.
    b. Advise the patient that this is normal for her age.
    c. Ask the patient if the spots were accompanied by pain.
    d. Tell the patient to mention this during her annual eye appointment.

14. A patient has had cataract surgery and is ready to go home. During the discharge education, what does the nurse tell the patient about activities?
    a. Driving in the daylight is okay, but do not drive at night.
    b. Meal preparation and doing dishes are acceptable activities.
    c. Vacuuming and mopping are okay, but do not bend over to scrub.
    d. Exercises, such as jogging or swimming, can be done at a slow pace.

15. Which signs and symptoms should a patient who has had cataract surgery report to the health care provider? **Select all that apply.**
    a. Sharp, sudden pain in the eye
    b. Decreased vision
    c. Mild eye itching
    d. Green or yellow thick discharge
    e. Flashes of light
    f. Lid swelling

16. In caring for a patient who was recently diagnosed with dry age-related macular degeneration, which teaching point would the nurse emphasize?
    a. Importance of adhering to the exact schedule for eye drops
    b. Dietary modifications to slow progression of vision loss
    c. Avoiding activities that cause rapid or jerking head movements
    d. Good handwashing and keeping the tip of the eyedropper clean

17. After a scleral buckling procedure, which aspect of postoperative care is affected if gas or oil has been placed in the eye?
    a. Type of eye patch
    b. Position of the head
    c. Eye drop schedule
    d. Effects of anesthesia

18. After a scleral buckling procedure, the patient is advised to avoid reading, writing, or close work, such as sewing. What is the rationale for avoiding these activities?
    a. They cause increased intraocular pressure.
    b. Close, fine work is likely to cause pain.
    c. They cause rapid eye movement.
    d. Close work or fine print will be blurry.

19. Which sign/symptom is the most common **early** clinical manifestation of retinitis pigmentosa?
    a. Cataracts
    b. Night blindness
    c. Headache
    d. Vitamin A deficiency

20. A patient with myopia tells the nurse that he forgot to bring his glasses to the hospital and that his wife will bring them later when she comes to see him. Which activity is the patient **most likely** to have difficulty with while he is waiting for his glasses?
    a. Eating his lunch
    b. Looking at a brochure
    c. Using his cell phone
    d. Watching television

21. A young patient was hit in the left eye with a baseball. There is discoloration around the eye. Which treatment does the nurse expect to give this patient?
    a. Eye patch to rest the eye
    b. Warm, moist compresses
    c. Small ice application to area
    d. Bedrest in semi-Fowler's position

22. Which traumatic injury is **most likely** to cause loss of vision in the injured eye?
    a. Metal shavings on the cornea
    b. Contusion to periorbital soft tissue
    c. Laceration to the margin of the eyelid
    d. Wood splinter embedded in eyeball

23. During mealtimes, the nursing student is assisting an older patient who has reduced vision. When would the nursing instructor intervene to help the student to improve the quality of care?
    a. Student opens sealed packages and removes lids from cups and bowls.
    b. Student describes food placement on the plate in terms of a clock face.
    c. Student asks the charge nurse how much assistance the patient needs during meals.
    d. Student places meal tray on a table and tells the patient to call for help as needed.

24. A 23-year-old athlete suffered a traumatic eye injury and enucleation was required. The nurse is trying to do discharge teaching, but the patient verbalizes anger and hopelessness, saying, "What's the point of learning about how to take care of this stupid empty hole in my face?" What is the nurse's **first** response?
    a. "Let's just take things one step at a time. I'll come back later."
    b. "Would you like information about joining a support group?"
    c. "Preventing infection will prevent further disfigurement and problems."
    d. "You are frustrated. Tell me how this accident will affect your life."

25. What is the **priority** for a patient with impaired vision?
    a. Self-care
    b. Communication
    c. Mobility
    d. Safety

26. The nurse is teaching a patient about self-medication with eye drops for glaucoma. Which intervention does the nurse suggest to prevent systemic absorption of the medication?
    a. Wait 15 minutes between instilling different eye drops.
    b. Place pressure on the corner of the eye near the nose.
    c. Place all eye medications in one eye and then the other.
    d. Blink rapidly after instilling drops and keep head upright.

27. The patient is diagnosed with bilateral eye infection and receives a prescription for two bottles of the same antibiotic solution. What instructions should the nurse give to the patient?
    a. Obtain one bottle from the pharmacy and return for the second if the infection does not clear.
    b. Obtain and use one bottle for both eyes; the second bottle is not necessary.
    c. Obtain both bottles and label one for the right eye and the other for the left eye.
    d. Obtain both bottles but save the second one because the infection will probably recur.

28. The nurse hears in shift report that the patient will have phacoemulsification for treatment of an eye problem. What does the nurse anticipate in the care of this patient?
    a. Patient will be discharged within an hour of surgery.
    b. Patient is likely to mourn the loss of the body part.
    c. Patient will need opioid medication for severe pain.
    d. Patient should be closely observed for postoperative bleeding.

29. The older patient has reduced visual sensory perception and is newly admitted to the medical-surgical unit. What instructions should the nurse give to unlicensed assistive personnel about assisting the patient with activities of daily living?
    a. "When entering and exiting the room, be very quiet so the patient is not disturbed."
    b. "Put personal belongings in the closet so the patient knows where they are."
    c. "During mealtimes, sit with the patient and explain how he should eat and drink."
    d. "When walking with the patient, offer your arm and walk a step ahead."

30. The patient tells the nurse that he had LASIK (laser in-situ keratomileusis) surgery several years ago. Which question is the nurse **most likely** to ask?
    a. "What was the intraocular pressure prior to having LASIK performed?"
    b. "Did you have LASIK for nearsightedness, farsightedness, or astigmatism?"
    c. "In addition to LASIK, are you getting sufficient antioxidants, vitamin B_{12}, and carotenoids?"
    d. "After LASIK, did you see 'shooting stars' or thin 'lightning streaks' or 'floaters'?"

48

CHAPTER

Assessment and Care of Patients with Ear and Hearing Problems

1. What questions would the nurse ask to assess auditory sensory perception? **Select all that apply.**
   a. "Do you have a hearing problem now?"
   b. "Have you ever had any ear trauma or surgery?"
   c. "What kind of music does you like to listen to?"
   d. "Have you ever been exposed to loud noises?"
   e. "Have you had problems with excessive earwax?"
   f. "Are you having any pain or itching in your ears?"

2. Which cranial nerve is the nurse testing when performing a bedside hearing test?
   a. V
   b. VI
   c. VIII
   d. IX

3. A patient who works on the tarmac at a busy airport is being seen for a routine examination. What protection measures for hearing does the nurse suggest to the patient?
   a. Wear cotton ball ear inserts.
   b. Listen to music to mask noise.
   c. Wear a hat with ear covers.
   d. Wear an over-the-ear headset.

4. Which factors can decrease blood supply to the ear in an older patient? **Select all that apply.**
   a. Osteoporosis
   b. Diabetes
   c. Smoking
   d. Heart disease
   e. Hypertension
   f. Cerumen

5. Sequentially order the events that allow for hearing. Use 1 for the first step and 6 for the final step.
   _____ a. Sound waves are transferred to the malleus.
   _____ b. Sound waves are transferred to the incus and the stapes.
   _____ c. Vibrations are transmitted to the cochlea.
   _____ d. Neural impulses are conducted by the auditory nerve.
   _____ e. Sound waves strike the mastoid and the movable tympanic membrane.
   _____ f. Sound is processed and interpreted by the brain.

6. A sensorineural hearing loss results from impairment of which structure?
   a. Mobility of bony ossicles
   b. First cranial nerve
   c. Patency of external canal
   d. Eighth cranial nerve

7. An adult patient is having problems with hearing. Which of the patient's medications is ototoxic?
   a. Vitamin B_{12}
   b. Digoxin
   c. Furosemide
   d. Levothyroxine

8. What changes in the ear are related to aging? **Select all that apply.**
   a. Tympanic membrane may appear dull and retracted.
   b. Pinna becomes shorter and thickened.
   c. Cerumen is drier and impacts more easily.
   d. Cochlear nerve cells degenerate.
   e. High-frequency sounds are lost first.
   f. Hair in the canal is very sparse or absent.

9. Which technique would the nurse use to perform otoscopic assessment?
   a. The patient's head should be tilted slightly toward the nurse.
   b. The nurse holds the otoscope upside down, like a large pen.
   c. The pinna is pulled downwards and backwards.
   d. The internal ear is visualized while the speculum is slowly inserted.

10. On the figure below, locate the tympanic membrane and describe what the normal tympanic membrane looks like when assessed with an otoscope.

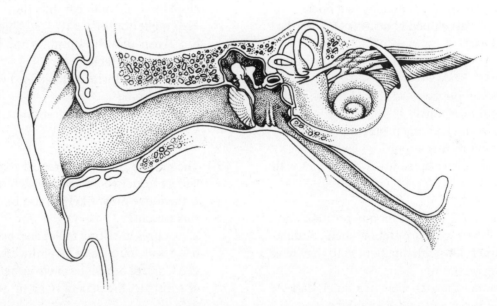

_____

_____

11. The nurse is on a camping trip, and one of the camper's reports, "I think there is an insect in my ear. I can hear it and feel it moving around inside my ear canal." What should the nurse try **first**?
    a. Shine a flashlight in the canal and try to coax the insect to come out.
    b. Instill cooking oil into the ear to suffocate the insect, then flush the canal with water.
    c. Apply a thin coating of antibiotic ointment to the external canal and pinna.
    d. Instruct the camper to tilt head downwards and vigorously shake the head.

12. Before performing a physical examination, what assessments related to the patient's hearing can be done while observing the patient? **Select all that apply.**
    a. Observe the patient's clothes and hygiene.
    b. Observe the patient's body posture and position.
    c. Observe if the patient is anxious or overly talkative.
    d. Notice if the patient asks for questions to be repeated.
    e. Notice whether the patient tilts the head toward the examiner.
    f. Notice patient's response when not looking in direction of sound.

13. The nurse gently taps over the patient's mastoid process, and the patient reports tenderness. This finding may indicate which condition?
    a. Excessive cerumen
    b. Hyperacusis
    c. Ruptured eardrum
    d. Inflammatory process

14. During the physical assessment, the nurse identifies a defect of the patient's external ear. Based on knowledge of embryonic development, which question will the nurse ask to identify potential problems in a body system that developed concurrently with the external ear?
    a. "Have you ever had problems with your heart?"
    b. "Do you notice shortness of breath with minor exertion?"
    c. "Have you had any problems with your kidneys or urination?"
    d. "Do you have episodes of headaches with confusion?"

15. How would the nurse use body position and the surrounding environment when conducting an interview with a patient who may have a hearing problem?
    a. Conduct the interview in a quiet, darkened room without distractions.
    b. Sit beside the patient and speak directly into the patient's ear.
    c. Sit directly in front of the patient in a room with adequate lighting.
    d. Stand over the patient and use hand motions for emphasis.

16. Which disorder of the ear/hearing is more commonly found among men aged 20-50 years old?
    a. Ménière's disease
    b. Otosclerosis
    c. Excessive cerumen
    d. Labyrinthitis

17. Which person has the **highest** risk for developing hearing problems related to occupation?
    a. Nurse who works night shift in an emergency department
    b. Coach who instructs a high school swim team
    c. Bus driver who picks up elementary school children
    d. Bartender who works in a nightclub with live music

18. Which child is **most likely** to develop hearing loss in adulthood?
    a. 1-year-old with ear infections related to "night bottles"
    b. 2-year-old who stumbles and bumps his head on a table
    c. 5-year-old who is diagnosed with Down syndrome
    d. 10-year-old with a grandparent who has hearing problems

19. The nurse hears in shift report that a patient suffers from hyperacusis. Which intervention is the nurse **most likely** to use in the care of this patient?
    a. Supply a writing tablet and pen.
    b. Speak loudly and carefully enunciate.
    c. Control or reduce environmental noise.
    d. Instruct the patient to sit up slowly.

20. The nurse is assisting an inexperienced health care provider who is trying to perform an otoscopic examination on an older patient who is being treated for delirium caused by infection. What should the nurse do?
    a. Quietly talk to the patient to distract him as the provider inserts the speculum.
    b. Gently hold the patient's head to prevent movement during the examination.
    c. Suggest that the otoscopic examination be deferred until the delirium resolves.
    d. Suggest using a Rinne tuning fork test instead of the otoscopic examination.

21. The home health nurse is visiting the patient for the first time. The nurse notices that the patient frequently tilts his head and gives odd answers to simple questions. The nurse has a stethoscope, a digital watch, a pen, and a blood pressure cuff in her supply bag. Which method would the nurse use to test hearing during this visit?
    a. Hold the watch about 5 inches from each ear and ask the patient what he hears.
    b. Stand 2 feet away, have patient block one ear, whisper a sentence, and ask patient to repeat it.
    c. Apply the blood pressure cuff and ask if patient can hear the separation of the Velcro fastener.
    d. Have the patient don the stethoscope and listen to and count his own heartbeat.

22. The nurse reads in the patient's chart that the Weber tuning fork test showed that the patient had lateralization to the right. Based on this information, what would the nurse do while caring for the patient?
    a. Instruct the patient to turn his head to the right if he is having trouble hearing.
    b. Ask the patient in which ear the sound is louder, because the test is inconclusive.
    c. Position self to the patient's right, so that voice travels directly to the right ear.
    d. Lateralization indicates normal hearing, so the nurse would perform routine care.

23. Which patient is the **most likely** candidate to benefit from the Rinne tuning fork test?
    a. Patient requires differentiation of hearing by air conduction versus bone conduction.
    b. Patient has a mental disability and is unable to follow instructions for audiometry or other tests.
    c. Patient has a family history of sensorineural hearing loss and genetic mutation in gene GJB2.
    d. Patient is unable to identify and report which ear has the greater hearing loss.

24. The results of an audiometry test indicate that the patient hears about 50% of the time at 0 decibels. Based on these results, which action is the nurse **most likely** to take?
    a. Prepare a brochure about different types of hearing aids.
    b. Explain the purpose and procedure of caloric testing.
    c. Use normal conversation speech when speaking to the patient.
    d. Ask the patient which ear is better and direct voice toward that side.

25. Which patient is **most likely** to have the lowest threshold for hearing tones and speech?
    a. 25-year-old patient with no previous hearing problems
    b. 76-year-old patient with significant hearing loss
    c. 43-year-old patient who is well adapted to a hearing aid
    d. 60-year-old patient with no known health problems

26. For a person who is just beginning to notice some hearing loss, which sounds would be the **most** difficult to clearly hear?
    a. Woman singing in the soprano range
    b. Toddler who is angry and screaming
    c. Cell phone ringing with low-frequency tones
    d. Gunfire shots on a television show

27. What is a **contraindication** for a patient having electronystagmography (ENG)?
    a. Dental problems
    b. Previous ENG
    c. Prosthetic hip
    d. Pacemaker

28. A patient is having problems with speech discrimination. What is the nurse **most likely** to observe?
    a. Patient speaks very loudly during a conversation.
    b. Patient can hear high tones but not low tones.
    c. Patient cannot accurately repeat two-syllable words.
    d. Patient repeats back "say" when the nurse says "stay."

29. Tympanometry is helpful in distinguishing which disorder?
    a. Middle ear infections
    b. External ear infections
    c. Hearing loss for low-pitched tones
    d. Indurated lesions on the pinna

30. What is the normal response to caloric testing?
    a. Vertigo and nystagmus within 20-30 seconds
    b. Vertigo and nystagmus immediately
    c. Vertigo and nystagmus within 5 minutes
    d. Nystagmus with no vertigo

31. The health care provider asks the nurse to obtain a pneumatic otoscope so that the external canal can be inspected. What **specific** assessment finding is this instrument used for?
    a. To detect infection or inflammation
    b. To gently elicit pain or discomfort
    c. To detect mobility of the eardrum
    d. To verify the patency of the eardrum

32. Which treatments are used for external otitis? **Select all that apply.**
    a. Application of heat
    b. Oral analgesics
    c. Topical antibiotics
    d. Myringotomy
    e. Minimizing head movements to reduce pain
    f. Ear irrigation with warm water

33. During physical assessment of an older patient, the nurse notes a small, crusted ulceration on the pinna. What should the nurse do **first**?
    a. Ask the patient how long the sore has been there.
    b. Teach the patient how to clean the ears to prevent infection.
    c. Ask the health care provider to check the ear for cancer.
    d. Document the finding and mention it at shift change.

34. The nurse uses irrigating fluid that is 98.6°F (37°C) to irrigate a patient's ear to remove cerumen. What is the **best** rationale for using fluid at this temperature?
    a. Evidence-based practice guides the selection of temperature.
    b. It reduces the chance of stimulating the vestibular sense.
    c. It is less painful than hotter or colder temperatures.
    d. It potentiates the melting and mobilization of cerumen.

35. An adult patient has external otitis. After the inflammation resolves, which action should the patient **avoid**?
    a. Using earplugs during swimming or other water sports
    b. Dropping diluted alcohol in the ear to prevent recurrence
    c. Inserting cotton-tipped applicator into ears after bathing
    d. Using analgesics and warm compresses for pain relief

36. Which patient has the **greatest** risk for potential life-threatening complications?
    a. Patient with diabetes mellitus needs treatment for external otitis.
    b. Patient who is immunosuppressed develops necrotizing otitis.
    c. Patient who is homeless has limited opportunities for hygiene and has tinnitus.
    d. Patient who works as a lifeguard frequently has problems with "swimmer's ear."

37. An adult patient has otitis media. What does the nurse expect the patient's **main** concern to be?
    a. Ear pain
    b. Rhinitis
    c. Drainage
    d. Swelling

38. A patient underwent electronystagmography, and results showed failure of nystagmus to occur with cerebral stimulation. Which action is the nurse **most likely** to take because of the test results?
    a. Initiate fall precautions.
    b. Use a whiteboard as needed.
    c. Give an antiemetic medication.
    d. Speak slowly to patient.

39. An adult patient with a history of otitis media states that his left ear pain is better. Now, the patient has noticed some pus with blood in the affected ear. What does the nurse suspect has happened?
    a. Antibiotics are resolving the infection.
    b. The eardrum has perforated.
    c. The infection has worsened.
    d. The ear is permanently damaged.

40. Which step is a correct part of the procedure for instilling eardrops?
    a. Gently irrigate the ear if the membrane is not intact.
    b. Place the bottle of eardrops in a bowl of hot water for 10 minutes.
    c. Tilt the patient's head in the opposite direction of the affected ear.
    d. Perform hand hygiene and use sterile gloves during the procedure.

41. A 30-year-old patient has cerumen in the left ear. When irrigating the ear, the nurse uses which amount of fluid?
    a. 10-30 mL
    b. 50-70 mL
    c. 60-100 mL
    d. 150-200 mL

42. The nurse immediately stops irrigating the ear if the patient reports which symptom?
    a. Persistent pain
    b. Sensation of fullness
    c. Tingling sensation
    d. Feelings of fatigue

43. What are the nurse's instructions to a patient after a myringotomy? **Select all that apply.**
    a. Report excessive drainage to your health care provider.
    b. Avoid washing hair for 1 week.
    c. Use a straw for drinking liquids.
    d. Leave ear dressing in place until the next office visit.
    e. Blow the nose gently with the mouth open.
    f. Stay away from people with respiratory infections.

44. Lymph node tenderness is **most likely** to be a symptom of which disorder?
    a. Ménière's disease
    b. Mastoiditis
    c. Otosclerosis
    d. Cerumen impaction

45. Which patient is **most likely** to benefit by having music playing during sleeping hours?
    a. Patient has frequent episodes of acute otitis media.
    b. Patient reports an odd sensation of "whirling in space."
    c. Patient has a hearing aid and reports excessive background noise.
    d. Patient reports tinnitus that contributes to emotional disturbance.

46. Tinnitus may be caused by which factors? **Select all that apply.**
    a. Tophi of the pinna
    b. Otosclerosis
    c. Continuous exposure to loud noise
    d. Medications
    e. Ménière's disease
    f. Excessive cleaning of ears

47. The patient tells the nurse that he has unpredictable episodes of vertigo. What instructions are the **most important** to give to the unlicensed assistive personnel who is assisting the patient with activities of daily living?
    a. "Face the patient directly whenever speaking to him."
    b. "There is a high risk for falls, so use a gait belt during ambulation."
    c. "Noise from the television or hallway should be minimized."
    d. "Patient's pain is likely to escalate, so report any discomfort."

48. The patient is taking meclizine. Which question will the nurse ask to determine if the medication is having the desired therapeutic effect?
    a. "On a scale of 1 to10, which number represents your current level of pain?"
    b. "Do you feel the medication helped to relieve the dizziness and nausea?"
    c. "Do you feel the medication decreased the buzzing sound that you reported?"
    d. "Do you think that your hearing has improved after completing the medication?"

49. For a patient with Ménière's disease, what is the purpose of the recommended nutrition therapy?
    a. To ensure an adequate intake of nutrients to slow progression of the disease
    b. To reduce harmful lipid accumulation in the acoustic-vestibular system
    c. To improve general overall health and strengthen the immune system
    d. To stabilize body fluid and prevent excess endolymph accumulation

50. An adult patient has been diagnosed with Ménière's disease. Which points does the nurse include in the teaching plan for this patient? **Select all that apply.**
    a. Move or turn head very slowly.
    b. Reduce the intake of salt.
    c. Stop smoking.
    d. Take vitamin supplements.
    e. Avoid caffeine.
    f. Irrigate ears frequently to decrease cerumen.

51. The health care provider tells the nurse that the patient was informed about the diagnosis of acoustic neuroma and was also given information about the prognosis, treatment, and possible complications. Which patient statement indicates that the patient understood the information?
    a. "The tumor is benign, so I am not going to worry about it."
    b. "I am not sure if I want chemotherapy and radiation."
    c. "The tumor is benign, but neurologic damage sounds scary."
    d. "Hearing loss in one ear is not too bad, if that's the worst complication."

52. Which precautions does the nurse instruct a patient to take after having ear surgery? **Select all that apply.**
    a. Avoid air travel for 5-7 days.
    b. Stay away from people with colds.
    c. Do not drink through a straw for 2-3 weeks.
    d. Keep your ear dry for 6 weeks.
    e. Avoid straining when having a bowel movement.
    f. Avoid rapidly moving head, bouncing, or bending over for 2-3 days.

53. Which condition requires extra caution when patients are prescribed ototoxic drugs?
    a. Chronic heart failure
    b. Chronic pancreatitis
    c. Chronic glomerulonephritis
    d. Chronic obstructive pulmonary disease

54. What should the nurse teach a patient who is learning to use a hearing aid?
    a. Soak the hearing aid in a solution of mild soap and water.
    b. Plug the hearing aid into an electrical source when not in use.
    c. Avoid exposing the hearing aid to extreme temperatures.
    d. Adjust volume to the highest setting to maximize hearing.

55. Which action could prevent ear trauma?
    a. Holding the nose when sneezing to reduce pressure
    b. Not using small objects to clean the external ear canal
    c. Occluding one nostril when blowing the nose
    d. Not using soap or water around the external ear and canal

56. For which ear condition might a myringotomy be recommended?
    a. Labyrinthitis
    b. Acoustic neuroma
    c. Otitis media
    d. Presbycusis

57. The nurse is assessing a patient who was admitted to the unit after undergoing a stapedectomy. The patient's face has an asymmetric appearance, and there is drooping of features on the affected side. What should the nurse do **first**?
    a. Tell the patient that this is a temporary condition related to anesthesia.
    b. Ask the patient about sensations of taste and touch on the affected side.
    c. Notify the surgeon because it is likely that there is cranial nerve damage.
    d. Call the Rapid Response Team because the patient may be having a stroke.

58. What is the nurse **most likely** to notice if the patient has problems with auditory sensory perception?
    a. Patient frequently looks away when being spoken to.
    b. Patient feigns disinterest or annoyance when spoken to.
    c. Patient frequently asks speaker to repeat statements.
    d. Patient often seeks out others for assistance.

59. What interventions can the nurse use to enhance communication with a hearing-impaired patient? **Select all that apply.**
    a. Have conversations in a quiet room with minimal distractions.
    b. Use appropriate hand motions.
    c. Stand in front of a bright light or a window.
    d. Get the patient's attention before speaking.
    e. Face the patient while speaking.
    f. Sit side by side to access the patient's better ear.

Assessment of the Musculoskeletal System

CHAPTER 49

1. Which ethnic group has the **lowest** risk for developing osteoporosis?
   a. African American
   b. European American
   c. Asian American
   d. Hispanic American

2. Which patient is **most likely** to be at risk for osteoporosis related to cultural differences and nutritional intake?
   a. Older African-American male who is a vegetarian
   b. Young Chinese American female who has anorexia nervosa
   c. Middle-aged Native American female who has type 2 diabetes
   d. Young white Irish American male who is overweight

3. Which patient has sustained a fracture of a bone that would normally function to protect vital organs?
   a. Has tibia-fibula fracture that occurred during a skateboarding accident
   b. Has sternal fracture secondary to being thrown from a motorcycle
   c. Has spiral fracture of the wrist that happened during a climbing accident
   d. Has compound femur fracture related to falling from a roof

4. Which clinical manifestation typifies the **priority** concept for patients who have disorders of the musculoskeletal system?
   a. Pain in the knee joint that worsens after jogging
   b. Mild dehydration and dark urine after being in the sun
   c. Exertional dyspnea after attempting to climb stairs
   d. Lightheadedness when standing up too quickly

5. Which clinical finding **most strongly** suggests that the patient is having a dysfunction of the musculoskeletal system?
   a. Oxygen saturation is low.
   b. Red cell count is low.
   c. Temperature is elevated.
   d. Blood pressure is elevated.

6. A patient is at risk for a parathyroid hormone imbalance related to a recent surgical procedure. Based on this information, which blood level must the nurse monitor?
   a. Blood glucose
   b. Serum calcium
   c. Serum potassium
   d. Serum magnesium

7. Which food would be the **best** choice to supply a vitamin that plays a key role in bone health?
   a. Carrots
   b. Apples
   c. Milk
   d. Whole grain bread

8. The nurse is caring for an adult patient with a recent increase in growth hormone that has resulted in acromegaly. In assessing this patient, what does the nurse expect to find?
   a. Bone and soft-tissue deformities
   b. Pain that increases when flexing joints
   c. Unusually tall height for ethnic background
   d. Marked lateral curvature of the spine

9. What is an example of a pivot joint?
   a. Knee joint
   b. Radioulnar area
   c. Shoulder joint
   d. Cranial area

10. A patient is experiencing inflammatory arthritis accompanied by synovitis. Based on the nurse's knowledge of anatomy and physiology, which diarthrodial joint is involved?
    a. Vertebral joint
    b. Cranial joint
    c. Pelvis joint
    d. Elbow joint

11. The nurse would ask the patient to perform extension and flexion to assess full range of motion for which joint?
    a. Elbow joint
    b. Pelvis area
    c. Hip joint
    d. Cervical area

12. The nurse is assessing a patient's shoulder joint. What would be considered a normal finding?
    a. Patient can perform slight rotation and full flexion and extension.
    b. Patient can freely move the joint in any direction.
    c. Patient has motion in one plane of flexion and extension.
    d. Patient demonstrates rotation only without discomfort.

13. A decrease in the body's vitamin D level can result in which disorder of the musculoskeletal system?
    a. Acromegaly
    b. Osteomalacia
    c. Muscular dystrophy
    d. Polymyositis

14. An athletic young adult man broke his leg several weeks ago and is now having his cast removed for the first time. Upon seeing the appearance of the leg, he is stunned. What is the nurse's **best** response to this patient's surprise?
    a. "Don't worry; it looks crusty and withered, but the strength and function are normal."
    b. "The cast compresses the tissue, but your leg will look normal in a couple of days."
    c. "Let's just wash off the dead skin, and you will see that it is not as bad as it seems."
    d. "Without regular exercise, muscles atrophy; strength can be restored with use."

15. A 55-year-old woman with a small frame is aware of her increased risk for osteoporosis and loss of bone mass. She currently has no pain or loss of function. She asks the nurse to recommend an exercise designed to counteract the risk. What does the nurse suggest?
    a. Swimming and water aerobics
    b. Deep-breathing and isometric exercise
    c. Walking with arm weights
    d. Meditation and yoga

16. The nurse is assessing an older construction worker who tells the nurse that he developed osteoarthritis as a result of his work duties. Which joints is the nurse **most likely** to assess to detect this disorder?
    a. Knees and lumbar spine
    b. Fingers and toes
    c. Shoulders and pelvis
    d. Wrists and thoracic spine

17. The nurse is assessing an older woman who has osteoporosis. Which assessment findings would the nurse expect? **Select all that apply.**
    a. Swelling in the finger joints
    b. Postural changes
    c. Gait changes
    d. Inability to bear weight
    e. Muscle atrophy
    f. History of fractures

18. Which group has the **greatest** risk for trauma resulting in injuries to muscles and bones?
    a. Older adult men as a result of occupational injuries
    b. Young men as a result of motor vehicle accidents
    c. Young women as a result of sports injuries
    d. Children who are not supervised during play

19. The nurse observes that the older adult has kyphosis. Which topic does the nurse select to address this assessment finding?
    a. Isometric exercises
    b. Weight-bearing exercises
    c. Proper body mechanics
    d. Use of warm, moist heat

20. The patient is a construction worker in his early 30s who was treated with oral antibiotics after stepping on a nail. The wound does not appear to be responding to antibiotic treatment as expected, despite the patient's compliance. The nurse suspects the patient may have a family history of which disorder?
    a. Nephritis
    b. Crohn's disease
    c. Skin cancer
    d. Diabetes mellitus

21. The nurse sees that a patient has an elevated alkaline phosphatase (ALP). What is the clinical significance of this result?
    a. The concentration of ALP increases with bone or liver damage.
    b. An increased ALP indicates progressive muscular dystrophy.
    c. An above normal ALP value suggests patient may have acromegaly.
    d. An elevated ALP indicates that patient is ingesting too much calcium.

22. A patient had an arthroscopy in the right leg. In assessing the patient's neurovascular status of the extremity, what does the nurse evaluate? **Select all that apply**.
    a. Presence of pain
    b. Gait and balance
    c. Distal pulses
    d. Capillary refill
    e. Sensation
    f. Temperature of skin

23. For which circumstance is the nurse or rehabilitation therapist **most likely** to use a goniometer?
    a. Older patient had knee surgery and is undergoing physical therapy.
    b. Older patient is undergoing therapy to correct difficulties with balance and gait.
    c. Young woman had a wrist cast removed and arm muscles appear atrophied.
    d. Teenager had surgery for scoliosis and is undergoing physical therapy.

24. Which assessment finding of the musculoskeletal system indicates an abnormality?
    a. Symmetry in the upper extremities and equal muscle mass
    b. Gait balance and a smooth and regular stride
    c. Flexion, extension, and rotation of the neck
    d. Opposition of three of four fingers to the thumb

25. Which outcome statement indicates that calcitonin is performing its intended function?
    a. Calcium level is within normal limits.
    b. Muscle mass is improving with exercise.
    c. Growth of healthy bone tissue is occurring.
    d. White cell blood count is within normal range.

26. The nurse is reviewing the laboratory results and sees that the patient has hypercalcemia. Which laboratory result does the nurse expect because of the inverse relationship to calcium?
    a. Low level of sodium
    b. Low level of phosphorus
    c. High level of thyroxine
    d. High level of insulin

27. Which hormones affect bone growth? **Select all that apply**.
    a. Glucocorticoids
    b. Renin
    c. Thyroxine
    d. Estrogens
    e. Androgens
    f. Catecholamines

28. Which laboratory result may indicate liver damage or metastatic cancer of the bone?
    a. Serum calcium 9.5 mg/dL
    b. Aspartate aminotransferase 15 units/L
    c. Lactate dehydrogenase 185 units/L
    d. Alkaline phosphatase 140 units/L

29. Which substances affect bone growth and metabolism? **Select all that apply.**
    a. Chloride
    b. Calcium
    c. Vitamin C
    d. Phosphorus
    e. Vitamin D
    f. Sodium

30. A patient reports pain in the left lower ankle. Which questions does the nurse ask to elicit relevant information about this patient's musculoskeletal problem? **Select all that apply.**
    a. "Do you eat foods that supply iron and protein?"
    b. "What seems to make the pain worse?"
    c. "What measures help alleviate the symptoms?"
    d. "What did your family doctor tell you?"
    e. "When did your pain start?"
    f. "Do you have a history of diabetes mellitus?"

31. The nurse is assessing a patient's posture and gait and notes that the patient has a lurch and shifts his shoulders from side to side while walking. What is the clinical significance of this finding?
    a. Muscles in the buttocks and/or legs are too weak to allow weight change from one foot to the other.
    b. Patient has a prosthetic device, such as an artificial hip that is limiting motion and flexibility.
    c. Part of one leg is painful, so the patient shortens the stance phase on the affected side.
    d. One leg is much shorter than the other, and this causes asymmetric body movement.

32. In assessing a patient's functional ability and range of motion (ROM), the patient is unable to actively move a joint through the expected ROM. Which technique does the nurse use to assess joint mobility?
    a. Patient relaxes the muscles while the nurse moves the joint through ROM.
    b. Nurse holds one hand above and one hand below the joint and allows passive ROM.
    c. Patient moves the joint through ROM while the nurse applies gentle resistance.
    d. Patient moves the joint to the best of ability while the nurse palpates for crepitus.

33. What is the **most** common musculoskeletal assessment finding in patients who have abdominal obesity?
    a. Scoliosis
    b. Crepitus
    c. Lordosis
    d. Kyphosis

34. Which activity does the nurse ask a patient to perform when assessing range of motion in the patient's hands?
    a. Wave the hand as though waving goodbye.
    b. Grip the nurse's hand as hard as possible.
    c. Rapidly move hands from palm up to palm down.
    d. Make a fist and then appose each finger to thumb.

35. A patient has an effusion of the right knee. Which assessment finding does the nurse expect to assess in this patient?
    a. Limitations in movement and accompanying pain
    b. Poor alignment as in genu valgum
    c. Crepitus and difficulty bearing weight
    d. Obvious redness and skin breakdown

36. The nurse notices that an older patient has gait changes with decreased coordination and muscle strength. What is the **priority** goal for the shift?
    a. Encourage mobility.
    b. Prevent falls.
    c. Increase strength.
    d. Avoid worsening.

37. The nurse is reviewing laboratory results for a patient who was involved in an accident. There is no evidence of fracture or bone damage, but multiple soft tissue injuries were sustained. Which muscle enzymes are expected to be elevated because of the injuries? **Select all that apply.**
    a. Creatine kinase
    b. Aspartate aminotransferase
    c. Alkaline phosphatase
    d. Lactic dehydrogenase
    e. Aldolase
    f. Lipase

38. For which circumstance is the nurse **most likely** to use a Doppler during patient assessment?
    a. Patient has progressive decreased flexion and extension of the wrist related to a contracture.
    b. Blood pressure cannot be obtained because patient has bilateral arm casts.
    c. Distal peripheral pulses of the affected extremity are difficult to locate and palpate.
    d. Patient refuses to do active range of motion (ROM) or allow passive ROM because of pain.

39. Which patient has the **greatest** risk for developing chronic osteomyelitis?
    a. Stepped on a rusty nail 30 years ago
    b. Has recurrent diabetic foot ulcer
    c. Has osteopenia and is noncompliant with therapy
    d. Performs heavy manual labor

40. The patient admits to drinking excessive alcohol. What additional assessment should the nurse perform to identify how the patient's intake of alcohol may be interfering with musculoskeletal health?
    a. Perform a neurologic assessment.
    b. Assess muscle strength against resistance.
    c. Perform a dietary assessment.
    d. Assess mobility of weight-bearing joints.

41. Which person has the **greatest** risk for developing a soft tissue injury?
    a. Middle-aged adult runs 5 miles every day.
    b. Older adult does water aerobics 3 times a week.
    c. Teenager spends 7 hours a day using a computer.
    d. College student rides a bicycle 2-3 times every week.

42. The nurse is caring for a patient who just had a bone biopsy. What is the **priority** nursing action?
    a. Administer pain medication
    b. Assess for bleeding
    c. Review test results
    d. Assess for infection

43. The nurse hears in report that the patient has chronic muscle weakness in the upper extremities. Which question is the nurse **most likely** to ask the off-going nurse?
    a. "How often did the patient ask for prn pain medication?"
    b. "Do they know what is causing the weakness?"
    c. "How much assistance is required for activities of daily living?"
    d. "Is the family going to come in and bathe the patient?"

44. What instructions would the home health nurse give to the home health aide about assisting an older patient who has a shoulder injury?
    a. Feed the patient
    b. Select clothing for the patient
    c. Wash the patient's hair
    d. Brush the patient's teeth

50
CHAPTER

Care of Patients with Musculoskeletal Problems

1. Which patient has the **most** risk factors associated with osteoporosis?
   a. Male over 50 years of age, European heritage
   b. Female, white, menopausal, thin, lean, immobilized
   c. Older adult with vitamin B deficiency, insufficient exposure to sunlight
   d. Adult who usually exercises and has moderate alcohol intake

2. Which lunch tray contains the **most** nutritional elements required for healthy bones?
   a. Processed lunch meat on whole-grain bread, apple juice, chips, and salsa
   b. Green leafy vegetable salad with cheese wedges and low-fat milk
   c. Fruit salad, iced tea, and a whole-grain muffin with butter and jam
   d. Pasta with red tomato sauce, garlic toast, seltzer water, and ice cream

3. A patient is at high risk for a vertebral compression fracture. Which activity should the patient be instructed to avoid?
   a. Walking
   b. Climbing stairs
   c. Jogging
   d. Swimming

4. The nurse is conducting an assessment on a patient with osteoporosis. Which factors and/or patient data may be associated with osteoporosis? **Select all that apply.**
   a. Muscle cramps
   b. Sedentary lifestyle
   c. Back pain relieved by rest
   d. Fracture
   e. Urinary or renal stones
   f. High cholesterol diet

5. The nurse is interviewing a patient to help the health care provider determine the patient's risk for osteomalacia. Which assessment is the nurse **most likely** to perform?
   a. Typical 24-hour dietary intake
   b. Usual patterns for rest and sleep
   c. Type and frequency of exercise
   d. Presence of pain and pain management

6. During physical assessment, the nurse notes that the patient has kyphosis. Which question is the nurse **most likely** to ask?
   a. "Have you had any pain in your lower extremities?"
   b. "Have you ever had any diagnostic testing for osteoporosis?"
   c. "Lately, have you had a fever or any signs of infection?"
   d. "Are you having any discomfort associated with your shoes?"

7. The nurse is reviewing T-scores for a 68-year-old woman. The patient has a T-score of 2.5. How does the nurse interpret this data?
   a. The patient has osteopenia.
   b. The patient has osteoporosis.
   c. This is a normal score for the patient's age.
   d. There is osteoblastic activity.

8. Which patient is at risk for regional osteoporosis?
   a. Patient who has been in a long leg cast for 10 weeks
   b. Patient on long-term corticosteroid therapy
   c. Patient with a history of hyperparathyroidism
   d. Patient in menopause with a history of falls

9. Which patients are at risk for osteoporosis because of nutritional issues? **Select all that apply.**
   a. Older female patient who drinks five cups of coffee daily
   b. Patient who is overweight for height
   c. Patient who is on the high-protein Atkins diet
   d. Patient who prefers to drink diluted powdered milk
   e. Patient who drinks a carbonated soda every day
   f. Older male patient with chronic alcoholism

10. The nurse is assessing an older adult patient at risk for osteoporosis. Which task can be delegated to unlicensed assistive personnel?
    a. Inspect the vertebral column.
    b. Take height and weight measurements.
    c. Compare observations to previous findings.
    d. Ask if the patient has gained or lost weight.

11. A patient with osteoporosis moves slowly and carefully with voluntary restriction of movement. The lower thoracic area is tender on palpation. How does the nurse interpret this assessment data?
    a. Vertebral compression fracture
    b. Kyphosis of the dorsal spine
    c. Osteopenia related to immobility
    d. Increased osteoblastic activity

12. The home health nurse is visiting an older adult patient with osteoporosis and severe kyphosis. When the nurse asks about activities she has been doing, the patient replies, "I used to be very active and beautiful when I was younger." What is the nurse's **best** response?
    a. "You are still very beautiful."
    b. "Activity can help to prevent fractures."
    c. "Tell me what you used to do."
    d. "Let's discuss age-appropriate exercises."

13. A patient is scheduled to have a dual x-ray absorptiometry. What information does the nurse give to the patient about preparing for the test?
    a. "Leave metallic objects such as jewelry, coins, and belt buckles at home."
    b. "Have someone come with you to drive you home after the test."
    c. "You will be asked to give a urine specimen prior to the test."
    d. "Bring a comfortable loose nightgown without buttons or snaps."

14. A patient is lactose intolerant and would like suggestions about food sources that supply adequate calcium and vitamin D. In addition to a generally well-balanced diet, what foods does the nurse suggest?
    a. Fresh apples and pears
    b. Whole-grain bread and pasta
    c. Fortified soy or rice products
    d. Prune or cranberry juice

15. A patient has been advised by the health care provider that exercising may help prevent osteoporosis. Which exercise does the nurse recommend to the patient?
    a. Swimming 10-15 laps 3-5 times a week
    b. Running for 20 minutes 4 times a week
    c. Bowling for 60 minutes 3 times a week
    d. Walking for 30 minutes 3-5 times a week

16. The health care provider is considering calcitonin for a patient to treat her osteoporosis. Which information should be relayed to the health care provider prior to the prescription of calcitonin?
    a. Patient hesitates over periodic subcutaneous injections.
    b. Patient is 5 years postmenopausal.
    c. Patient has a history of allergy to salmon.
    d. Patient has a T-score lower than −2.5.

17. The nurse sees that the patient has been prescribed raloxifene. Which information, specific to the medication, should be brought to the attention of the prescribing health care provider?
    a. Patient has a family history of osteoporosis.
    b. Patient has had recurrent venous thromboembolism.
    c. Patient has had previous episodes of hypoglycemia.
    d. Patient has a history of iron deficiency anemia.

18. What are potential adverse reactions of alendronate? **Select all that apply.**
    a. Difficulty swallowing
    b. Drowsiness
    c. Esophagitis
    d. Constipation
    e. Esophageal ulcers
    f. Gastric ulcers

19. Why do men develop osteoporosis after the age of 50?
    a. Older men have decreased testosterone levels.
    b. Older men are prescribed more medications.
    c. In older men hyperparathyroidism causes osteoporosis.
    d. After age 50, men are much less active.

20. The nurse is reviewing the prescriptions for a patient receiving drug therapy for the prevention of osteoporosis. The patient also has hypertension and heart disease. Which prescription order does the nurse question?
    a. Calcium supplements
    b. Hormone replacement therapy
    c. Alendronate
    d. Zoledronic acid (IV)

21. The nurse is palpating the back and spinal area of a patient who has advanced osteoporosis. The nurse is especially gentle at which area of the spine because it is the **most** common site for vertebral compression fractures?
    a. Between C1 and C5
    b. Between T1 and T5
    c. Between T8 and L3
    d. Between L4 and L5

22. A patient tells the nurse that he has "soft bones." What additional information supports the likelihood of osteomalacia in this patient?
    a. Recent immigration from a country where famine is common
    b. Taking hormone replacement therapy for a prolonged time
    c. Unable to perform a prescribed exercise regimen
    d. History of recent episode of venous thromboembolism

23. Although any person can develop fallophobia, which person is **most likely** to have this condition?
    a. Toddler who has fallen several times and bumped her head
    b. Woman who recently had a fasciectomy for Dupuytren's contracture
    c. Man who has severe pain in the foot arch when getting out of bed
    d. Postmenopausal woman who fell recently and broke her wrist

24. The nurse is teaching a community group about osteoporosis. What information would the nurse give about routine laboratory testing?
    a. Serum calcium and phosphorus levels should be routinely monitored biannually for postmenopausal women who are at a high risk for the disease.
    b. Serum calcium and vitamin D_3 levels should be routinely monitored annually for all women and for men older than 50 years who are at a high risk for the disease.
    c. Serum calcium and estrogen levels should be routinely monitored every 5 years for younger women and annually for women over the age of 50.
    d. Serum calcium and vitamin D_3 levels should be routinely monitored every 2-3 years for all women and for men older than 50 years who are at a high risk for the disease.

25. The nurse is working in a clinic that uses serum and urinary bone turnover markers in the care of patients with osteoporosis. Which outcome statement reflects the purpose of using these markers?
    a. Patient is noncompliant with medications.
    b. Patient is able to walk without discomfort.
    c. Patient's bone density is maintained.
    d. Patient's height and weight are maintained.

26. Magnetic resonance imaging and magnetic resonance spectroscopy are more reliable and offer more information about bone change than bone mineral density measurements alone. What is the current barrier for using these tests to diagnose and evaluate osteoporosis?
    a. Many health care providers are not aware of the value of these procedures.
    b. Radiation exposure is excessive for the purpose of annual screening.
    c. These tests are expensive, and third parties do not recognize the value to reimburse costs.
    d. Many facilities do not have the specialized equipment to perform these tests.

27. The nurse is volunteering at a community health fair. A 56-year-old woman has just had a peripheral dual-energy x-ray absorptiometry (pDXA) and comments to the nurse, "I'm happy with these results. I guess I won't have to worry about my bones for the next few years." What is the nurse's **best** response?
    a. "Yep, you're good to go! Thanks for taking the time to stop and have the pDXA."
    b. "Your results are good, but the pDXA is not as precise as the tests that your doctor can order."
    c. "You should have the peripheral quantitative ultrasound densitometry (pQUS) to verify results."
    d. "We are offering the pDXA at next year's health fair. Be sure to stop by to have it repeated."

28. According to the clinical guidelines outlined by the National Osteoporosis Foundation, vertebral imaging is indicated for which groups? **Select all that apply.**
    a. Women aged 65 to 69 and men aged 70 to 79 if bone mineral density (BMD) is less than or equal to 1.5
    b. Women aged 70 and older and men aged 80 and older if BMD is less than or equal to a T-score of 1.0
    c. Men aged 50 and older with significant height loss and history of low-trauma fracture or being on long-term corticosteroids
    d. Postmenopausal women with significant height loss, history of low-trauma fracture, or history of being on long-term corticosteroids
    e. Men aged 40 or younger with significant weight gain, history of high-impact trauma fractures, or history of being on long-term steroids for bodybuilding
    f. Women aged 40 or older who have never been pregnant, history of irregular menses, or history of being on long-term oral contraceptives

29. Which outcome statement indicates that the goal has been achieved in preventing the **most** common complication of osteoporosis?
    a. Patient has avoided fractures by preventing falls and managing her risk factors.
    b. Patient has not developed jaw osteonecrosis secondary to medication therapy.
    c. Patient has not developed kyphosis of the dorsal spine ("dowager's hump").
    d. Patient understands how to avoid esophagitis associated with bisphosphonates.

30. The physical therapist has instructed the patient about several exercises to perform for the prevention and management of osteoporosis. Which exercise is **most** directly related to the concept of mobility?
    a. Abdominal muscle tightening
    b. Focused deep-breathing exercise
    c. Pectoral muscle tightening
    d. Range-of-motion exercise

31. A 40-year-old patient is admitted for acute osteomyelitis of the left lower leg. What does the nurse expect to find documented in the patient's admitting assessment?
    a. Temperature greater than 101°F, swelling, tenderness, erythema, and warmth of area
    b. Ulceration resulting with sinus tract formation, localized pain, and drainage
    c. Aching pain, poorly described, deep, and worsened by pressure and weight bearing
    d. Shortening of the extremity with pain during weight bearing or palpation

32. The nurse is caring for a patient with osteomyelitis. Which laboratory results are of **primary** concern for this disorder?
    a. Bone-specific alkaline phosphatase and osteocalcin
    b. Serum calcium level and alkaline phosphatase
    c. White blood cell count and erythrocyte sedimentation rate
    d. Thyroid function tests and uric acid levels

33. Which patient is the **most likely** to be a candidate for hyperbaric oxygen therapy?
    a. Patient with osteomalacia related to poverty
    b. Patient with an advanced case of osteosarcoma
    c. Patient with chronic, unremitting osteomyelitis
    d. Patient with osteoporosis and recurrent fractures

34. A patient comes to the emergency department after accidentally puncturing his hand with an automatic nail gun. Which disorder is this patient **primarily** at risk for?
    a. Osteoporosis
    b. Osteomyelitis
    c. Osteomalacia
    d. Dupuytren's contracture

35. Which person is following the recommendations for healthy bones related to alcohol consumption?
    a. Slender young woman drinks less than 5 ounces per day.
    b. Obese older woman has 3 drinks on Friday, Saturday, and Sunday.
    c. Older man has 2 drinks on weekdays and 5-6 on the weekend.
    d. Young man drinks 60 ounces or more but only on Saturday nights.

36. The nurse is teaching a patient about antibiotic therapy for osteomyelitis. What information does the nurse give to the patient?
    a. Single-agent therapy is the most effective treatment for acute infections.
    b. Chronic osteomyelitis may require 1 month of antibiotic therapy.
    c. Patients usually remain hospitalized to complete the full course of antibiotic therapy.
    d. The infected wound may be irrigated with one or more types of antibiotic solutions.

37. The patient has a low-grade fever. How is this fact sometimes **misinterpreted** by the health care team in trying to evaluate musculoskeletal disorders?
    a. Osteoporosis is misdiagnosed for osteomalacia.
    b. Ewing's sarcoma is thought to be osteomyelitis.
    c. Osteoporosis is thought to be osteopenia.
    d. Osteosarcoma is mistaken for secondary metastasis.

38. Which patient has the **greatest** risk for acute hematogenous osteomyelitis?
    a. Older man with a catheter-related urinary tract infection
    b. Older patient in intensive care with poor dental hygiene
    c. Older woman with a methicillin-resistant *Staphylococcus aureus* infection
    d. Young patient with a leg fracture who has external skeletal pins

39. In older adults, what is the **most** common cause of contiguous osteomyelitis?
    a. Malignant external otitis media
    b. Slow-healing foot ulcers
    c. Periodontal infections
    d. Gastrointestinal salmonella infections

40. Compared to acute osteomyelitis, which characteristic is **more** associated with chronic osteomyelitis?
    a. Fever
    b. Swelling
    c. Erythema
    d. Sinus tract formation

41. The patient is admitted for acute osteomyelitis of the right lower leg with severe vascular compromise. Upon assessment, the patient denies pain or discomfort in the leg. Based on the concept of perfusion, how does the nurse interpret the patient's response?
    a. Vascular compromise may be severe, but the distal tissue is still being perfused.
    b. An order for Doppler flow studies should be obtained to validate lack of perfusion.
    c. Patient has sustained extensive nerve damage because of inadequate perfusion.
    d. Patient's current position in bed is allowing for adequate perfusion to distal tissues.

42. A patient is being seen in the clinic for dull pain and swelling of the proximal femur over 2-3 months. Which type of malignant bone tumor is associated with these symptoms?
    a. Ewing's sarcoma
    b. Chondrosarcoma
    c. Fibrosarcoma
    d. Osteosarcoma

43. A 49-year-old man comes to the clinic for left mid-tibia tenderness for the past 3 months. The nurse notes a small palpable mass. What type of malignant bone tumor is associated with these signs/symptoms?
    a. Chondrosarcoma
    b. Ewing's sarcoma
    c. Fibrosarcoma
    d. Osteosarcoma

44. What is the **most** common type of malignant bone tumor?
    a. Ewing's sarcoma
    b. Chondrosarcoma
    c. Fibrosarcoma
    d. Osteosarcoma

45. Which assessment finding in a patient who has undergone a bone graft for a tumor does the nurse report to the health care provider **immediately**?
    a. Skin distal to the operative site is warm and pink.
    b. Cast over the operative site is cool to the touch.
    c. Distal pulses are decreased and difficult to palpate.
    d. Pain is present in the operative extremity.

46. A patient with a bone tumor is grieving and anxious. The nurse includes which psychosocial interventions? **Select all that apply.**
    a. Allow the patient to verbalize feelings.
    b. Offer to call the patient's spiritual or religious adviser.
    c. Prepare the patient for death.
    d. Share stories of personal losses.
    e. Redirect the patient to more cheerful topics.
    f. Listen attentively while the patient talks.

47. A patient is being evaluated for bone pain in the lower extremity. Which laboratory result would suggest a malignant bone tumor?
    a. Elevated serum alkaline phosphatase
    b. Decreased serum calcium level
    c. Low vitamin D level
    d. Decreased erythrocyte sedimentation rate

48. A patient with bone sarcoma had surgery to salvage an upper limb. The nurse has identified that the patient has impaired physical mobility related to musculoskeletal impairment. Which intervention does the nurse perform in the **early** postoperative period?
    a. Encourage the patient to use the opposite hand to achieve forward flexion and abduction of the affected shoulder.
    b. Encourage the patient to emphasize strengthening the quadriceps muscles by using passive and active motion.
    c. Instruct unlicensed assistive personnel to perform all hygiene until the patient expresses readiness to do self-care.
    d. Evaluate the patient's and family's readiness to use the continuous passive motion machine in the home setting.

49. A patient with bone cancer has had the right lower leg surgically removed. The patient has been brave and uncomplaining, but the nurse recognizes that the patient is likely to experience grieving. What is the nurse's **most** important role?
    a. Act as a patient advocate to promote the surgeon-patient relationship.
    b. Encourage the patient to talk to the family and complete an advance directive.
    c. Be an active listener and encourage the patient and family to verbalize feelings.
    d. Help the patient and family cope with and resolve grief and loss issues.

50. Which type of benign tumor is commonly located in the hands and feet?
    a. Chondroma
    b. Giant cell tumor
    c. Osteochondroma
    d. Fibrogenic tumor

51. The nurse is caring for a patient who had an allograft for a large bone defect that resulted from tumor removal. Which findings need to be reported **immediately** to the health care provider? **Select all that apply.**
    a. Pain at the surgical site
    b. Signs of infection
    c. Hemorrhage
    d. Fracture
    e. Difficulty ambulating
    f. Loss of muscle tone

52. A patient who is a long-distance runner reports severe pain in the arch of the foot, especially when getting out of bed and with weight bearing. What does the nurse suspect in this patient?
    a. Hypertrophic ungual labium
    b. Plantar fasciitis
    c. Hammertoe
    d. Hallux valgus deformity

53. The nurse observes that an older patient has flexion contractures of the fourth and fifth fingers. The patient reports that he had a similar problem on the other hand and had a fasciectomy, which improved the function. What condition does the patient have?
    a. Dupuytren's contracture
    b. Ganglion cyst
    c. Bunion
    d. Volkmann's contracture

54. A patient is diagnosed with plantar fasciitis. What instruction does the nurse give to the patient about self-care for this condition?
    a. Use rest, elevation, and warm packs.
    b. Perform gentle jogging exercises.
    c. Strap the foot to maintain the arch.
    d. Wear loose or open shoes, such as sandals.

55. The nurse is caring for several patients on an orthopedic unit. Which patient is **most likely** to need blood cultures?
    a. Patient is 2 days postop for limb salvage surgery.
    b. Patient is admitted for acute osteomyelitis of right leg.
    c. Patient has osteoporosis and sustained a left hip fracture.
    d. Patient has osteosarcoma that has metastasized to the lungs.

1. Which signs/symptoms represent the **priority** concepts for musculoskeletal trauma?
   a. Patient notes mild shortness of breath and palpitations with minor exertion.
   b. Patient describes discomfort in knee and hip joints that is worse in the morning.
   c. Patient reports decreased range of motion and pain in leg that is unrelieved by medication.
   d. Patient has problems getting adequate calcium and vitamin D because of lactose intolerance.

2. The nurse is caring for several patients on an orthopedic trauma unit. Which conditions pose a high risk for development of acute compartment syndrome? **Select all that apply.**
   a. Lower legs caught between the bumpers of two cars
   b. Massive infiltration of IV fluid into forearm
   c. Bivalve cast on the lower leg
   d. Multiple insect bites to lower legs
   e. Daily use of oral contraceptives
   f. Severe burns to the upper extremities

3. A patient has a fracture of the right wrist. What is an **early** sign that indicates this patient may be having a complication?
   a. Patient loses ability to wiggle fingers without pain.
   b. Fingers are cold and pale; pulses are impalpable.
   c. Pain is severe and seems out of proportion to injury.
   d. Patient reports a subjective numbness and tingling.

4. The nurse is assessing a patient for severe pain in the right wrist after falling off a step stool. How does the nurse assess this patient's motor function?
   a. Performs passive range of motion for the wrist.
   b. Asks the patient to move the fingers.
   c. Has the patient flex and extend the elbow.
   d. Instructs the patient to rotate the wrist.

5. A patient in traction reports severe pain from a muscle spasm. What is the nurse's **priority** action?
   a. Assess the patient's body alignment.
   b. Give the patient a prn pain medication.
   c. Notify the health care provider.
   d. Remove some of the traction weights.

6. The nurse is reviewing the orders for a patient who was admitted for 24-hour observation of a leg fracture. A cast is in place. Which order does the nurse question?
   a. Elevate lower leg above the level of the heart.
   b. Perform neurovascular assessments every 8 hours.
   c. Apply ice pack for 24 hours.
   d. Provide regular diet as tolerated.

7. A patient with a leg cast denies pain; toes are pink, capillary refill is brisk and toes move freely, and the leg is elevated with an ice pack. Six hours later, the patient reports worsening pain unrelieved by medication. The patient's toes are cool, and pulse is difficult to detect. What does the nurse suspect is occurring with this patient?
   a. Crush syndrome
   b. Fat embolism syndrome
   c. Acute compartment syndrome
   d. Fasciitis

8. What is the **priority** concept related to changes that occur during the ischemia-edema cycle?
   a. Comfort
   b. Mobility
   c. Tissue integrity
   d. Perfusion

9. An older adult has been admitted with a hip fracture. Approximately 20 hours after injury, the patient develops a sign/symptom that the nurse recognizes as an **early** indicator of fat embolism syndrome. Which sign/symptom is the patient displaying?
   a. Severe respiratory distress
   b. Significantly increased pulse rate
   c. Change in mental status
   d. Petechial rash over the neck

10. The student nurse is assessing a patient with a probable fractured tibia-fibula. What assessment technique used by the student nurse causes the nursing instructor to intervene?
   a. Inspects the fracture site for swelling or deformity.
   b. Instructs the patient to wiggle the toes.
   c. Assesses bilateral dorsalis pedis pulses.
   d. Pushes on the leg to elicit pain response.

11. The nurse is caring for several orthopedic patients who are in different types of traction. What should the nurse do to assess the traction equipment? **Select all that apply**.
   a. Inspect all ropes, knots, and pulleys once every 24 hours.
   b. Inspect ropes and knots for fraying or loosening every 8 to 12 hours.
   c. Check the amount of weight being used against the prescribed weight.
   d. Observe the traction equipment for proper functioning.
   e. Check if the ropes have been changed or cleaned within the past 48 hours.
   f. Reduce or adjust the weights if the patient is having excessive pain.

12. A patient was put into traction at 0800 hours. Hourly neurovascular checks were ordered for the first 24 hours and then every 4 hours thereafter. At what time can the nursing staff start performing the 4-hour checks?
   a. 2000 hours same day
   b. 0000 hours next day
   c. 0800 hours next day
   d. 1200 hours next day

13. The nurse is educating a patient who will have external fixation for treatment of a compound tibial fracture. What information does the nurse include in the teaching session?
   a. "The device allows for early ambulation."
   b. "The device is sterile; there is no danger of infection."
   c. "The device is a substitute therapy for a cast."
   d. "The advantage of the device is rapid bone healing."

14. The nurse is helping to evaluate several patients to determine candidacy for the Ilizarov external fixation device. Which patient is the **best** candidate?
   a. Older woman who lives alone with a fracture of nonunion
   b. Child with a congenital bone deformity whose mother is a nurse
   c. Teenager with an open fracture and bone loss of the left lower leg
   d. Middle-aged man with a new comminuted fracture of the dominant forearm

15. An older adult patient has a fractured humerus. The health care provider is considering the use of electrical bone stimulation and asks the nurse to obtain a medical history on the patient. Which question does the nurse ask to identify if the patient has a contraindication for this therapy?
    a. "Are you taking any medication for seizures?"
    b. "Do you have a cardiac pacemaker?"
    c. "Have you ever been treated for a stroke?"
    d. "Do you have a surgically implanted metallic device?"

16. A patient is prescribed low-intensity pulsed ultrasound treatments for a very slow-healing fracture of the right lower leg. What information does the nurse give this patient related to the treatment?
    a. Test for pregnancy before the therapy, and use birth control until treatment is complete.
    b. The treatment is experimental, but there are no known adverse effects.
    c. The device is implanted directly into the fracture site, and there is no external apparatus.
    d. Expect to dedicate approximately 20 minutes each day for a treatment.

17. The nursing student is assisting with the care of a patient with musculoskeletal pain related to soft tissue injury and bone disruption. The student sees that the patient has a prn (as-needed) order for pain medication. What does the student do **first** to decide when to give the pain medication?
    a. Ask the health care provider to give specific parameters.
    b. Ask the primary nurse or the charge nurse for advice.
    c. Ask the patient about types of activities that increase the pain.
    d. Ask the nursing instructor for help interpreting the order.

18. A patient is receiving scheduled and prn opioids for severe pain related to a musculoskeletal injury. The nurse finds that the patient's abdomen is distended and bowel sounds are hypoactive. Because the nurse suspects that the patient is having a medication side effect, which question does the nurse ask the patient?
    a. "Are you having nausea and vomiting?"
    b. "When was your last bowel movement?"
    c. "Does your abdomen hurt?"
    d. "Are you having diarrhea or loose stool?"

19. A patient comes into the emergency department after falling off his four-wheeler. Assessment of his lower leg reveals bleeding and bone fragments protruding from the skin. What type of fracture does this patient **most likely** have?
    a. Impacted
    b. Open
    c. Pathologic
    d. Displaced

20. A patient comes to the emergency department after slipping on some chalk in her classroom. She "did not have a hard fall" and was able to walk with the assistance of one of her students. What type of fracture is this patient **most likely** to have?
    a. Compression
    b. Displaced
    c. Impacted
    d. Incomplete

21. A female patient with osteoporosis comes to the emergency department after falling suddenly while opening her car door. She said it felt as though her "leg gave way" and caused her to fall. What type of fracture is this patient **most likely** to have?
    a. Pathologic
    b. Colles'
    c. Impacted
    d. Compound

22. The nurse is caring for a patient with an open fracture. Which intervention does the nurse perform to prevent infection of the fracture?
    a. Use aseptic technique for dressing changes and wound irrigations.
    b. Culture the wound and an obtain an order for antibiotics.
    c. Place the patient in contact isolation and wear sterile gloves.
    d. Place the patient on neutropenic precautions and perform hand hygiene.

23. The nurse must adjust a pair of crutches to properly fit a patient. Which description illustrates correct crutch adjustment?
    a. Axilla rests lightly on the top of the crutch when the crutch is moved forward.
    b. Patient can easily use the crutch without subjective complaints.
    c. Elbow is flexed no more than 30 degrees when the palm is on the handle.
    d. Adult patient is of average height, and the crutches are medium-sized.

24. An older patient's family is trying to find an appropriate cane for the patient to use because of chronic pain in the right ankle. The nurse instructs the family to purchase which type of cane?
    a. One with top that is parallel to greater trochanter of the femur
    b. One that creates about 45 degrees of flexion of the elbow
    c. One that is adequate to safely support the patient's weight
    d. One with padding on the handle grip to ensure safety

25. Which member of the health care team is responsible for teaching the patient about proper use of the cane?
    a. Occupational therapist
    b. Physical therapist
    c. Orthopedic surgeon
    d. Home health aide

26. The home health nurse reads in the documentation that the patient has Volkmann's contracture that occurred several years ago. Which assessment is the nurse **most likely** to perform to assess this condition?
    a. Ability to do activities of daily living
    b. Presence of distal pulses
    c. Ability to climb the stairs
    d. Need for pain medication

27. An older patient with a hip fracture has prolonged immobility related to difficulties in performing the prescribed weight-bearing exercises. Based on fracture pathophysiology and the patient's abilities, which condition could the patient develop?
    a. Osteomyelitis
    b. Internal derangement
    c. Neuroma
    d. Pulmonary embolism

28. The home health nurse is reviewing environmental safety of an older patient who was discharged to her own home after surgery for a hip fracture. Which observation indicates a need for additional teaching?
    a. Patient's bed has been moved to the ground floor level.
    b. There are handlebars around the toilet and tub.
    c. Floors are clean and shiny and covered with throw rugs.
    d. Patient's walker is close to the patient's bedside.

29. The nurse is reviewing the laboratory results of a patient who may have fat embolism syndrome. Which abnormal laboratory findings accompany this condition? **Select all that apply.**
    a. Decreased Pao_2 level (often below 60 mm Hg)
    b. Increased erythrocyte sedimentation rate
    c. Decreased serum calcium levels
    d. Decreased red blood cell and platelet counts
    e. Increased serum level of lipids
    f. Increased serum potassium levels

30. A 25-year-old patient sustained a crush injury to his right upper extremity and right lower extremity when heavy equipment fell on him. Signs and symptoms of hypovolemia and compartment syndrome are present. Management of care for this patient will focus on preventing which complication?
    a. Acute liver failure
    b. Ischemic heart failure
    c. Respiratory failure
    d. Myoglobinuric renal failure

31. Which patient has the **greatest** risk for developing avascular necrosis?
    a. "Little person" with a congenital bone deformity
    b. Woman with osteoporosis and a Colles' fracture
    c. Older adult with a hip fracture
    d. Teenager with a dislocated shoulder

32. A 30-year-old patient who is hospitalized for repair of a fractured tibia and fibula reports shortness of breath. Which complication related to the injury might the patient be experiencing?
    a. Acute renal failure
    b. Fat embolism
    c. Acute compartment syndrome
    d. Pneumonia

33. The older patient has a fracture that has failed to heal. Which fracture complication **best** describes this situation?
    a. Malunion
    b. Avascular necrosis
    c. Nonunion
    d. Crush syndrome

34. A patient who tripped and fell down several stairs reports hearing a popping sound and fears that she has broken her ankle. How does the nurse **initially** assess for fracture in this patient?
    a. Measures the circumference of the distal leg
    b. Gently moves the ankle through full range of motion
    c. Inspects for crepitus and skin color
    d. Observes for deformity or misalignment

35. The nurse is assessing an adolescent patient with an injury to the shoulder and upper arm that occurred during wrestling practice. What is the **best** position for this patient's assessment?
    a. Supine so that the extremity can be elevated
    b. Low Fowler's on an exam table for patient comfort
    c. Sitting to observe for shoulder droop
    d. Slow ambulation to observe for natural arm movement

36. The nurse is caring for a patient with skeletal pins that have been placed for traction. What does the nurse expect in the **first** 48 hours?
    a. Clear fluid drainage weeping from the pin insertion site
    b. Some bloody drainage at the site but very minimal
    c. Swelling at the site with tenderness to gentle touch
    d. Dressings around the pin sites to be dry and intact

37. In older adults, what potential adverse effect can occur with the use of meperidine?
    a. Hypertension
    b. Angina
    c. Kidney failure
    d. Seizures

38. The unlicensed assistive personnel (UAP) is assisting the orthopedic cast technician to cut a window in a patient's cast. What does the nurse instruct the UAP to do?
    a. Check the distal pulses after the window is cut.
    b. Clean up and dispose of all casting debris.
    c. Inform the patient that the procedure is painless.
    d. Save the cutout cast piece so it can be taped in place.

39. The nurse is caring for a patient in Buck's (skin) traction. Which task is **best** to delegate to unlicensed assistive personnel (with supervision)?
    a. Turning and repositioning
    b. Inspecting heels and sacral area
    c. Asking the patient about muscle spasms
    d. Adjusting the weights on the apparatus

40. The nurse is instructing a teenage patient who has a tibia-fibula fracture that was treated with internal fixation and a long leg cast. He is anxious to know when the cast will be removed so that he can resume football practice. Which statement by the patient indicates a need for additional teaching?
    a. "There's a possibility that the cast could be removed in 4 weeks."
    b. "The plates and screws reduce the length of time I'll be in the cast."
    c. "The cast could remain in place as long as 6 weeks."
    d. "I'll use crutches for 2 weeks, and then the cast will be removed."

41. In the emergency care of a patient with a fracture, which action does the nurse implement **first**?
    a. Check the neurovascular status of the area distal to the injury: temperature, color, sensation, movement, and distal pulses. Compare affected and unaffected limbs.
    b. Remove or cut the patient's clothing to inspect the affected area while supporting the injured area above and below the injury.
    c. Elevate the affected area on pillows, apply an ice pack that is wrapped to protect the skin, and obtain an order for pain medication.
    d. Immobilize the extremity by splinting; include joints above and below the fracture site. Recheck circulation after splinting.

42. The nurse is planning interventions for a patient with a family history of osteoporosis. What action does the nurse take?
    a. Ask the patient's age and assess for weight loss.
    b. Review the patient's dietary intake of calcium.
    c. Assess the patient for kyphoscoliosis or other deformities.
    d. Assess the patient for occult fractures of the long bones.

43. The nurse's neighbor comes running over because her husband "cut his finger off with a power saw." What is the **priority** nursing action?
    a. Examine the amputation site.
    b. Assess for airway or breathing problems.
    c. Elevate the hand above the heart.
    d. Assess the severed finger.

44. A man who severed a finger while working on his car comes to the emergency department. The bleeding from the site is well controlled, and the patient is alert and stable. What does the nurse do with the severed finger?
    a. Place it directly into a bag of ice and then put the bag into a refrigerator.
    b. Wrap it in moist sterile gauze and ensure that it stays with the patient.
    c. Wrap it in dry gauze, place it in a waterproof bag, and put the bag in ice water.
    d. Carefully clean it with sterile saline, and then place it in a sterile container.

45. Which nursing intervention is **best** to prevent increased pain in a patient experiencing phantom limb pain?
    a. Handle the residual limb carefully when assessing the site or changing the dressing.
    b. Advise the patient that the sensation is temporary and will diminish over time.
    c. Remind the patient that the part is not really there, so the pain is not real.
    d. Encourage the patient to mourn the loss of the body part and express grief.

46. A young high school athlete had a great toe amputated because of severe injury. The patient is depressed and withdrawn after the health care provider tells him that the amputation will affect balance and gait. What should the nurse do **first**?
    a. Explain the role of physical therapy exercises that help with balance and gait.
    b. Involve the parents and patient in a discussion about rehabilitation programs.
    c. Encourage verbalization of feelings and thoughts related to the situation.
    d. Explore how the patient has coped and handled stressful situations in the past.

47. The patient is a middle-aged man with a history of uncontrolled diabetes. His right foot is a dark brownish-purple color, and there is no palpable dorsalis pedis or posterior tibial pulse. The nurse prepares the patient for which diagnostic test?
    a. X-ray of the foot and ankle
    b. Doppler ultrasound
    c. Electromyelogram
    d. Arthrogram

48. Which patients with fractures have factors that put them at risk for developing venous thromboembolism? **Select all that apply.**
    a. Has type 2 diabetes mellitus
    b. Had hip surgery that took several hours
    c. Is obese and smokes 2 packs per day
    d. Takes oral contraceptives
    e. Takes steroid medication
    f. Was bedridden prior to sustaining fracture

49. A patient injured a lower extremity and has been placed in running traction. What instructions does the nurse give to unlicensed assistive personnel?
    a. Support the weights when turning the patient every 2 hours.
    b. Ask the patient to turn and move himself, so that he is in control of painful stimuli.
    c. Defer hygienic care and moving the patient until traction is removed.
    d. Do not move the patient or the bed because the countertraction can be altered.

50. The nurse is caring for a patient with an above-the-knee amputation. To prevent hip flexion contractures, how does the nurse position the patient?
    a. Supine position with the residual limb elevated on a pillow
    b. Prone position every 3-4 hours for 20- to 30-minute periods
    c. Supine position with an abduction pillow placed between the legs
    d. Head of the bed elevated 30 degrees with bandage snug around the limb

51. The nurse applies bandages to a patient's residual limb to help shape and shrink the limb for a prosthesis. What is the proper technique for the nurse to use?
    a. Reapply the bandages every 8 hours or more often if they become loose.
    b. Use a proximal-to-distal direction when wrapping.
    c. Use soft, flexible bandage material and pad the area with gauze.
    d. Use a figure-eight wrapping method to prevent restriction of blood flow.

52. An older patient is discharged to home following an orthopedic injury. Which mobilization device would be preferred if the patient is having trouble with balance?
    a. Crutches
    b. Cane
    c. Walker
    d. Wheelchair

53. The nurse is interviewing an older adult with a history of osteoporosis who reports falling and catching her weight on her outstretched dominant hand. This patient is **most likely** to have sustained what type of fracture?
    a. Carpal scaphoid fracture
    b. Phalanges fracture
    c. Humeral fracture
    d. Colles' wrist fracture

54. Which factor presents the **greatest** risk for hip fracture?
    a. Decreased visual acuity
    b. Joint stiffness
    c. Osteoporosis
    d. Cardiac drug regimen

55. An older adult patient has skin traction in place for a hip fracture. Which outcome statement reflects that the goal of the therapy is successful?
    a. Patient reports a decrease in painful muscle spasms.
    b. X-ray indicates that the fracture shows signs of healing.
    c. Patient can perform activities of daily living with some assistance.
    d. There are no signs/symptoms of compression syndrome.

56. The nurse is caring for a patient who had hemiarthroplasty and is at risk for hip dislocation. The nurse ensures that the hip is maintained in which position?
    a. Adduction
    b. Anatomically neutral
    c. Abduction
    d. Extended

57. A patient reports dramatic changes in color and temperature of the skin over the left foot with intense burning pain, sensitive skin, excessive sweating, and edema. The health care provider makes a preliminary medical diagnosis of complex regional pain syndrome. What is the **priority** for nursing care?
    a. Patient education
    b. Prevention of skin breakdown
    c. Management of pain
    d. Assessment of circulation

58. A teenager is brought to the emergency department by a group of excited friends. He is dazed and unable to answer questions. The nurse observes deformity to the right forearm and ecchymosis over the right lateral chest and abdomen. What is the **most** important reason to ask the friends about mechanism of injury?
    a. To determine if the teenagers were using drugs or alcohol
    b. To make a judgment about whether to call the police
    c. To assist the health care provider to complete the history
    d. To aid in making the diagnosis of other types of injuries

59. A patient who was involved in a motor vehicle accident is brought to the emergency department by emergency medical services. He is on a backboard, C-collar is in place, and there is a splint on the left leg. **Place the assessment steps in the order of priority.**
    _____ a. Assess mental status and orientation.
    _____ b. Determine if the airway is clear.
    _____ c. Check for signs of bleeding.
    _____ d. Observe respiratory effort.
    _____ e. Make bilateral comparison of legs for the 6 Ps.

60. A patient arrives in the emergency department reporting pain and immobility of the right shoulder. The patient reports a history of recurrent dislocations of the same shoulder. Which additional sign/symptom would the nurse assess for a dislocation injury?
    a. Bone fragments protruding from skin
    b. Deviation in length of the extremity
    c. Muscle atrophy with weakness
    d. Mottled skin discoloration

61. The nurse is reviewing the laboratory results of a patient who was beaten into unconsciousness by an unknown assailant. Which laboratory result would accompany extensive tissue damage and the expected inflammatory response?
    a. Decreased hemoglobin and hematocrit
    b. Increased serum calcium level
    c. Increased serum phosphorus level
    d. Elevated erythrocyte sedimentation rate

62. The nurse is caring for patients on an orthopedic unit who are being treated with a variety of therapies, including immobilization with a bandage, a splint, a cast, specialized orthopedic shoe, and traction. What is the **priority** nursing concern for all of these patients?
    a. Assessment and prevention of neurovascular dysfunction and compromise
    b. Assessment and management of pain and discomfort
    c. Assessment of abilities to do activities of daily living after discharge
    d. Assessment and intervention for concerns related to disability and immobility

63. The health care provider tells the nurse that a patient has a mild first-degree sprain to the ankle. What instructions does the nurse give to the patient about the treatment for the injury? **Select all that apply.**
    a. Rest the injured part; immobilize the joint above and below the injury by applying a splint if needed.
    b. Apply ice intermittently for the first 4-6 hours.
    c. Apply a compression bandage for the first 24-48 hours.
    d. Elevate the foot to decrease swelling.
    e. Perform range-of-motion exercises every 4 hours.
    f. Use crutches until the swelling resolves.

64. A patient is informed by the health care provider that a fiberglass cast must be applied to the lower extremity. What does the nurse teach the patient about the procedure before the cast is applied?
    a. "The stockinette should be changed once a week."
    b. "The cast material will dry and become rigid in a few minutes."
    c. "The cast will increase your risk for skin breakdown."
    d. "The fiberglass is not waterproof, so avoiding getting it wet."

65. The nurse is caring for a patient with a plaster splint applied to the ankle. The patient received oral pain medication at 0900. At 1100, the patient reports that the pain is getting worse, not better. What is the nurse's **priority** action?
    a. Give the patient IV pain medication.
    b. Reposition the extremity on a pillow and place an ice pack.
    c. Assess the pulses and skin temperature distal to the splint.
    d. Call the health care provider to report the increasing pain.

66. The nurse is supervising a nursing student who is caring for a patient with a cast to the lower leg who reports pain that is worsening despite medication, with decreased movement and skin sensation. The nurse would intervene if the student performed which action?
    a. Instructs the patient to move the toes
    b. Places an extra pillow underneath the cast
    c. Checks for dorsalis pedis pulse
    d. Checks agency protocol to see who may cut the cast

67. The nurse is providing teaching for a patient with a forearm cast. What information does the nurse give to the patient?
    a. "Forearm should be in an anatomical position when resting."
    b. "Use an ice pack for the first 6-8 hours, and cover the pack with a towel."
    c. "Sling should distribute weight over a large area of the shoulders and trunk."
    d. "Limit movement of the fingers or wrist joints to prevent pain."

68. The patient has a musculoskeletal injury that resulted from excessive stretching of a muscle or tendon. Which type of injury has this patient sustained?
    a. Dislocation
    b. Sprain
    c. Strain
    d. Subluxation

69. A patient with a lower extremity injury is being treated with external fixation. Which nursing assessment is of particular concern in the care of a patient with this type of system?
    a. Maintaining a 30-degree flexed position of the knee
    b. Measuring the weights used for counter-traction
    c. Observing the patient's ability to adjust the clickers
    d. Observing the points of entry of the pins and wires

70. The nurse is caring for a patient who had a kyphoplasty. What is included in the postoperative care of this patient? **Select all that apply.**
    a. Monitor and record vital signs.
    b. Perform frequent neurologic assessments.
    c. Apply a warm pack to the puncture site if needed to relieve pain.
    d. Assess pain level and compare it to the preoperative level.
    e. Give opioid analgesics to maintain comfort level.
    f. Monitor for bleeding at the puncture site.

71. A patient in a cast reports a painful "hot spot" underneath the cast, and the nurse notices an unpleasant odor. Which intervention is the nurse **most likely** to perform **first**?
    a. Offer the patient a prn pain medication.
    b. Help the patient with hygiene around the cast.
    c. Take the patient's temperature and other vital signs.
    d. Call the orthopedic technician to change the cast.

72. A patient with a long leg cast that was applied in the emergency department is being admitted to the orthopedic unit. Which task is **best** for the nurse to delegate to unlicensed assistive personnel?
    a. Obtain a fracture pan and use caution to prevent spillage on the cast.
    b. Assist the patient to stand and bear weight when the cast is dry.
    c. Check flexion/extension and color of the toes.
    d. Turn the patient every 4-6 hours to allow the cast to dry.

73. A patient who has sustained a traumatic amputation of the left leg expresses grief and loss. What resources could the nurse recommend to help the patient adjust to his lost limb? **Select all that apply.**
    a. Chaplain
    b. Psychiatric social worker
    c. Physical therapist
    d. Orthopedic surgeon
    e. National Amputation Foundation
    f. Other spiritual leaders

Assessment of the Gastrointestinal System

1. What is the name of the first 12 inches of the small intestine?
   a. Jejunum
   b. Ileum
   c. Duodenum
   d. Esophagus

2. Which structure is involved in the protective function of the liver?
   a. Sphincter of Oddi
   b. Gallbladder
   c. Pancreas
   d. Kupffer cells

3. The pancreas performs which functions? **Select all that apply**.
   a. Breaks down amino acids
   b. Secretes enzymes for digestion from the exocrine part of the organ
   c. Breaks down fatty acids and triglycerides
   d. Produces glucagon from the endocrine part of the organ
   e. Produces enzymes that digest carbohydrates, fats, and proteins
   f. Detoxifies potentially harmful compounds

4. Which statements about intrinsic factor are correct? **Select all that apply.**
   a. It is produced by the parietal cells.
   b. It is essential to fat emulsification.
   c. It aids in the absorption of vitamin B_{12}.
   d. It forms and secretes bile.
   e. Its absence causes pernicious anemia.
   f. It causes the stomach to secrete hydrochloric acid.

5. Which statements about Kupffer cells are true? **Select all that apply.**
   a. They are located in the epithelial cell layer lining in the GI tract.
   b. They are found in the liver.
   c. They phagocytize harmful bacteria.
   d. They are part of the substance that aids in the absorption of vitamin B_{12}.
   e. They are part of the body's reticuloendothelial system.
   f. They aid in the metabolism of proteins.

6. Which substances predispose a patient to peptic ulcer disease and gastrointestinal (GI) bleeding? **Select all that apply.**
   a. Nonsteroidal anti-inflammatory drugs
   b. Anticoagulants
   c. Aspirin
   d. Lasix
   e. Digitalis
   f. Caffeine

7. Which gastrointestinal problem is related to anorexia?
   a. Heartburn
   b. Constipation
   c. Steatorrhea
   d. Loss of appetite

8. Dyspepsia is characterized by which factors? **Select all that apply.**
   a. Indigestion associated with eating
   b. Loss of appetite for food
   c. Malabsorption of fats
   d. Heartburn associated with eating
   e. Vomiting that occurs after eating
   f. Unintentional weight loss

9. The nurse is caring for a patient with abdominal pain. While assessing the patient, which questions will the nurse ask the patient? **Select all that apply.**
   a. "Is the pain burning, gnawing, or stabbing?"
   b. "Can you point to where you feel the pain?"
   c. "Do you have a family history of cancer?"
   d. "When did you first notice the pain?"
   e. "Have you gained weight since the pain began?"
   f. "Does the pain spread anywhere?"

10. When beginning an abdominal assessment, the nurse would begin in which quadrant?
    a. Right lower quadrant (RLQ)
    b. Left lower quadrant (LLQ)
    c. Left upper quadrant (LUQ)
    d. Right upper quadrant (RUQ)

11. When examining the abdomen, which technique for abdominal assessment is used second?
    a. Inspection
    b. Percussion
    c. Palpation
    d. Auscultation

12. The nurse is performing an abdominal assessment on a patient. For which finding does the nurse alert the health care provider immediately?
    a. Borborygmus
    b. Blumberg's sign
    c. Bulging, pulsating mass
    d. Cullen's sign

13. The nurse is auscultating a patient's abdomen. Which technique should the nurse use?
    a. Place the diaphragm of the stethoscope lightly on the abdominal wall.
    b. Place the bell of the stethoscope lightly on the abdominal wall.
    c. Hold the diaphragm of the stethoscope firmly on the abdominal wall.
    d. Hold the bell of the stethoscope firmly on the abdominal wall.

14. The nurse auscultates a patient's abdomen and hears high-pitched, loud, musical sounds in an air-filled abdomen. How does the nurse **best** describe this finding?
    a. Bruits
    b. Tympanic
    c. Dull
    d. Medium-pitched

15. While performing an abdominal assessment on a patient with abdominal pain, the nurse performs inspection of the abdomen. Which inspection findings should the nurse be sure to document? **Select all that apply.**
    a. Overall shape of the abdomen
    b. Presence of discoloration or scarring
    c. Size of percussed abdominal organs
    d. Symmetry or asymmetry of the abdominal contour
    e. Family history of abdominal illnesses
    f. Distention of the abdomen

16. A patient reports decreased appetite over the past month along with simultaneous decreased intake or oral nutrition as well as episodes of nausea. What priority information should the nurse inquire about **next**?
    a. Favorite foods
    b. Bowel pattern
    c. Patient weight
    d. Vital signs

17. The nurse discovers that a patient has a recent change in bowel habits. What important information must the nurse gather from this patient? **Select all that apply.**
    a. Color and appearance of urine
    b. Occurrence of diarrhea or constipation
    c. Presence of abdominal distention or gas
    d. Intentional weight gain
    e. Occurrence of bloody or tarry stools
    f. Current pattern of bowel movements

18. When the nurse assesses a patient after abdominal surgery, assessment reveals diminished, hypoactive bowel sounds. What is the nurse's **best** action?
    a. Notify the surgeon immediately.
    b. Document the finding and continue to monitor.
    c. Place an NG (nasogastric) tube.
    d. Obtain a stat abdominal x-ray.

19. What is the **most** reliable method of assessing the return of peristalsis?
    a. Auscultate and count the number of bowel sounds over 30 seconds.
    b. Administer a laxative as ordered by the health care provider.
    c. Monitor and document all oral intake of food and fluids.
    d. Assess whether the patient has passed flatus or a stool.

20. The patient reports episodes of diarrhea for the past 2 days. What types of bowel sounds does the nurse expect to auscultate when assessing this patient?
    a. Increased loud and gurgling sounds
    b. Decreased soft and diminished sounds
    c. Increased in the left lower quadrant only
    d. Decreased in the right upper quadrant only

21. The nurse is supervising a student during assessment of the abdomen. When must the nurse intervene with the student?
    a. The nursing student inspects the patient's abdomen for symmetry.
    b. The nursing student auscultates for bowel sounds in an organized manner.
    c. The nursing student performs light palpation for areas of discomfort.
    d. The nursing student performs deep palpation for a pulsing midline mass.

22. Which are **most** likely laboratory values for a patient with liver disease? **Select all that apply.**
    a. Increased prothrombin time
    b. Increased aspartate transaminase (AST)
    c. Increased albumin levels
    d. Decreased ammonia levels
    e. Increased unconjugated bilirubin
    f. Decreased alanine aminotransferase (ALT)

23. Laboratory values for a patient with acute pancreatitis may show which abnormal findings? **Select all that apply.**
    a. Increased hemoglobin
    b. Decreased serum amylase
    c. Increased serum lipase
    d. Decreased urine nitrates
    e. Increased serum amylase
    f. Increased cholesterol

24. The patient presents with abdominal discomfort and a history of gastrointestinal cancer. Which cancer-specific laboratory studies does the nurse expect will be ordered by the health care provider?
    a. Oncofetal antigens (CA19-9 and CEA)
    b. Conjugated (direct) bilirubin and unconjugated (indirect) bilirubin
    c. Aspartate aminotransferase (AST) and alanine aminotransferase (ALT)
    d. Serum amylase and lipase

25. Why is patient compliance higher with the fecal immunochemical test (FIT) than with the traditional fecal occult blood test (FOBT)?
    a. Anticoagulants, such as warfarin, and NSAIDs should be discontinued for 7 days before FIT testing begins.
    b. Drugs and food do not interfere with the FIT test results.
    c. Raw fruits and vegetables and red meat must be avoided before the FIT test.
    d. Vitamin C–rich foods, juices, and tablets must also be avoided before the FIT test.

26. The patient is scheduled for a plain abdominal x-ray in the morning. What preprocedure teaching does the nurse provide?
    a. "Wear a hospital gown and remove any jewelry or belts."
    b. "You will receive nothing by mouth from midnight until after the procedure."
    c. "We will place a nasogastric tube before the procedure to decompress your stomach."
    d. "A laxative will be given to move stool out of your bowel before the procedure."

27. A patient being seen the emergency department (ED) has been vomiting blood for the past 12 hours. What test will likely be ordered for the patient?
    a. Endoscopic retrograde cholangiopancreatography (ERCP)
    b. Upper GI radiographic series
    c. Esophagogastroduodenoscopy (EGD)
    d. Barium enema

28. The nurse is providing care for a patient after an esophagogastroduodenoscopy (EGD). What is the **first priority** action after this diagnostic study?
    a. Monitor vital signs.
    b. Auscultate breath sounds.
    c. Keep patient NPO until gag reflex returns.
    d. Keep accurate intake and output.

29. The nurse is caring for a patient who received a barium swallow with a small bowel follow-through. What key points must the nurse include in teaching this patient after the procedure? **Select all that apply.**
    a. "Drink lots of fluids."
    b. "Depending on the results, you may need a colonoscopy."
    c. "You will be on bedrest for about 6-8 hours."
    d. "A laxative will be provided to help remove the barium."
    e. "Your stools will be chalky white for 1-3 days."
    f. "Be sure to tell the health care provider if you are allergic to seafood or iodine."

30. Which diagnostic test does the nurse expect the health care provider to order to visually examine a patient's liver, gallbladder, bile ducts, and pancreas to identify the cause and location of an obstruction?
    a. Esophagogastroduodenoscopy (EGD)
    b. Upper GI radiographic series
    c. Percutaneous transhepatic cholangiography (PTC)
    d. Endoscopic retrograde cholangiopancreatography (ERCP)

31. The nurse is caring for a patient scheduled for a colonoscopy in 3 days after discharge. What does the nurse teach the patient about preparations for this diagnostic test? **Select all that apply.**
    a. "Take only clear liquids the day before your colonoscopy."
    b. "Drink lots of red, orange, or purple (grape) beverages the day before the test."
    c. "You should take nothing by mouth for 4-6 hours before the test."
    d. "Do not take aspirin, NSAIDs, or anticoagulants for several days before the test."
    e. "After you drink the bowel-cleansing solution, you may develop constipation in 1-2 days."
    f. "You will have an IV placed to receive medication to help you relax during the procedure."

32. The nurse is monitoring a patient after endoscopy. Vital signs are stable, and the patient tells the nurse that he is very thirsty. What is the nurse's **best** action?
    a. Administer a small amount of ice chips only.
    b. Give the patient small sips of water through a straw.
    c. Check to see if the patient's gag reflex has returned.
    d. Keep the patient NPO for at least 4 hours.

33. Which diagnostic test is a noninvasive imaging procedure that can get multidimensional views of the entire colon?
    a. Abdominal ultrasound
    b. Virtual colonography
    c. Colonoscopy
    d. Sigmoidoscopy

34. Mild gas pain and flatulence may be experienced because of air instilled into the rectum during the examination, and if a biopsy specimen is obtained, a small amount of bleeding may be observed. Which endoscopic procedure is this follow-up care describing?
    a. Colonoscopy
    b. Proctosigmoidoscopy
    c. Enteroscopy
    d. Endoscopic retrograde cholangiopancreatography (ERCP)

35. A feeling of fullness, cramping, and passage of flatus can be expected for several hours after the test, and a small amount of blood may be in the first stool after the test if a biopsy specimen is taken or a polypectomy is performed. Vital signs should be checked every 15 minutes, the patient should be monitored for signs of perforation or hemorrhage, and excessive bleeding should be reported immediately. Which procedure is this follow-up care describing?
    a. Esophagogastroduodenoscopy (EGD)
    b. Enteroscopy
    c. Small bowel series
    d. Colonoscopy

36. A patient is given midazolam hydrochloride before receiving a colonoscopy procedure. What is the **priority** assessment for the nurse during this procedure?
    a. Monitor rate and depth of respirations.
    b. Auscultate for bowel sounds in all 4 quadrants.
    c. Place on a cardiac monitor and watch for dysrhythmias.
    d. Suction secretions to prevent aspiration.

37. Following an endoscopic retrograde cholangiopancreatography (ERCP), the nurse would include which postprocedure follow-up care interventions in the plan of care? **Select all that apply.**
    a. Observe for cholangitis, perforation, sepsis, and pancreatitis.
    b. Assess for nausea and vomiting.
    c. Tell the patient to report any abdominal pain.
    d. Assess for return of gag reflex.
    e. Provide ice chips to moisten throat.
    f. Insert a nasogastric tube (NG) for excessive nausea.

38. Following an esophagogastroduodenoscopy, the nurse should instruct the patient in which activity?
    a. Avoid all strenuous activity for 2 weeks.
    b. Maintain high-fat, low-protein diet after procedure.
    c. Use incentive spirometry for 24 hours after procedure.
    d. Avoid driving for 12 hours postprocedure.

39. Which body structures are located in the RUQ of the abdomen? **Select all that apply.**
    a. Duodenum
    b. Liver
    c. Stomach
    d. Spleen
    e. Gallbladder
    f. Pancreas head

40. Which gastrointestinal changes occur in older adults? **(Select all that apply.)**
    a. Increased hydrochloric acid secretion
    b. Decreased absorption of iron and vitamin B_{12}
    c. Decreased peristalsis may cause constipation
    d. Increased cholesterol synthesis
    e. Decreased lipase with decreased fat digestion
    f. Increased risk for constipation or impaction

41. The nurse is taking a GI health history from a newly admitted patient. Which questions would the nurse include in the interview? **Select all that apply.**
    a. "Have you lost or gained weight recently?"
    b. "Have you had any recent cardiac or respiratory surgeries?"
    c. "Do you wear dentures, and if so, how do they fit you?"
    d. "Do you have difficulty chewing or swallowing?"
    e. "Have you traveled in the USA recently, and where?"
    f. "What is your usual bowel elimination pattern?"

42. The patient's potassium level is 3.1 mEq/L. Which condition would cause this value?
    a. Malabsorption
    b. Gastric suctioning
    c. Acute pancreatitis
    d. Kidney failure

43. The patient tells the nurse that she is experiencing emotional stress related to concerns about her children and husband and whether she will be able to return to her job. Which GI condition is she at increased risk for?
    a. Exacerbation of irritable bowel syndrome
    b. Nausea accompanied with vomiting
    c. Esophageal ulcers
    d. Hiatal hernia

44. During abdominal assessment, the nurse detects a loud bruit near midline. What must the nurse do?
    a. Measure the circumference of the patient's abdomen just under the diaphragm.
    b. Check the patient's record for a history of stomach ulcers.
    c. Avoid palpation or percussion of the abdomen.
    d. Ask the patient about nausea and gastric reflux.

45. A patient is scheduled for an abdominal CT scan with contrast. What preprocedural teaching should the nurse give this patient? **Select all that apply.**
    a. "You will have an IV placed for injection of the contrast."
    b. "You may experience the presence of borborygmus."
    c. "You may feel warm and flushed or experience a metallic taste after the injection."
    d. "The CT technician may ask you to hold your breath while a series of images are taken."
    e. "If you are claustrophobic, we can give you a mild sedative before the procedure."
    f. "The test takes 30-45 minutes."

53 CHAPTER

Care of Patients with Oral Cavity Problems

1. Which patients are **commonly** affected by oral cavity disorders? **Select all that apply.**
   a. Patients who are homeless or live in institutions
   b. Patients who work in coal mines
   c. Patients who are developmentally disabled
   d. Patients who regularly use tobacco or alcohol
   e. Patients who have sexually transmitted diseases
   f. Patients who eat too much of an unhealthy diet

2. When a patient has an oral cavity disorder, what is the patient's **priority** medical-surgical concept?
   a. Nutrition
   b. Gas exchange
   c. Tissue integrity
   d. Comfort

3. Which are examples of primary stomatitis? **Select all that apply.**
   a. Chemotherapy-induced stomatitis
   b. Aphthous stomatitis
   c. Herpes simplex stomatitis
   d. Bacterial stomatitis
   e. Traumatic ulcers
   f. Viral stomatitis

4. What statement is true about the *Candida albicans* form of stomatitis?
   a. It is a common type of primary stomatitis.
   b. *Candida albicans* is a bacterial infection.
   c. This infection is uncommon in patients who are immunocompromised.
   d. Patients on steroid therapy often experience this infection.

5. The nurse has provided teaching to a patient on ways to prevent the recurrence of aphthous ulcers. Which statement by the patient indicates teaching has been effective?
   a. "I will rinse with the tetracycline syrup for 2 minutes and then swallow the syrup."
   b. "Potatoes have nothing to do with the development of the ulcers."
   c. "I will continue to eat peanut butter and jelly sandwiches."
   d. "It doesn't matter what types of foods I eat as long as I brush my teeth after every meal."

6. When caring for a patient with stomatitis, what is the **most** important priority for the nurse to assess?
   a. Nutritional status
   b. Level of pain
   c. Self-care abilities
   d. Airway status

7. The nurse is performing an oral assessment on a patient and notes white plaque-like lesions on the tongue, palate, pharynx, and buccal mucosa. When the patches are wiped away, the underlying surface is red and sore. What disorder does the nurse suspect the patient has?
   a. Leukoplakia
   b. *Candida albicans*
   c. Erythroplakia
   d. Kaposi's sarcoma

8. The unlicensed assistive personnel (UAP) is providing care to a patient with stomatitis. Which intervention by the UAP illustrates correct care for this patient?
   a. Using a hard-bristled toothbrush to thoroughly clean the oral cavity
   b. Rinsing the mouth with a commercial mouthwash
   c. Using a warm saline, hydrogen peroxide, or sodium bicarbonate solution to rinse the mouth
   d. Rinsing the mouth frequently with cold tap water and vinegar solution

9. The unlicensed assistive personnel (UAP) reports to the nurse that a patient being fed experienced coughing and choking when swallowing. The patient states that "It feels like the food is stuck in my throat." What does the nurse suspect is happening with this patient?
   a. The patient is aspirating food.
   b. The patient is having dysphagia.
   c. The UAP is feeding the patient too quickly.
   d. The patient has an airway obstruction.

10. What is the drug of choice for the treatment of a fungal mouth infection?
    a. Nystatin
    b. Acyclovir
    c. Minocycline
    d. Benzocaine

11. Which statement by the student nurse indicates the need for a better understanding of the care of patients with oral cavity problems?
    a. "I will use lemon-glycerin swabs to clean the patient's mouth."
    b. "The patient should eat a soft, bland diet."
    c. "Dentures should be removed."
    d. "Gauze may be used for oral care."

12. A patient is in the clinic for a nonhealing sore on the lower left corner of her bottom lip and right side of her tongue. The lesions are red, raised, and have erosions. After taking a history, the nurse suspects the patient may have which type of oral cancer?
    a. Basal cell carcinoma
    b. Kaposi's sarcoma
    c. Squamous cell carcinoma
    d. Erythroplakia

13. The health care provider prescribes "magic mouthwash" for a patient experiencing oral pain from cancer treatments. What is the nurse's best response when the patient asks, "What ingredients are in this concoction?" **Select all that apply.**
    a. Lidocaine
    b. Benadryl
    c. Maalox
    d. Tetracycline
    e. Nystatin
    f. Carafate

14. Which statement by a patient indicates the need for **additional** teaching about oral care?
    a. "I will use a soft-bristled toothbrush to clean my teeth and gums."
    b. "I will brush my teeth with a toothpaste with sodium lauryl sulfate."
    c. "I will rinse my mouth with a sodium bicarbonate solution."
    d. "I will read the labels of mouthwash bottles for alcohol content."

15. A patient has a Kaposi's sarcoma lesion on his hard palate. How is this lesion described? **Select all that apply.**
    a. Small raised lesion
    b. Dark-yellow nodule
    c. Painful lesion
    d. Purplish-brown nodule
    e. Usually not painful
    f. Appears off-white and raised

16. Which type of oral cavity tumor appears as a red, velvety lesion on the tongue, palate, floor of the mouth, or mandibular mucosa?
    a. Leukoplakia
    b. Erythroplakia
    c. Basal cell carcinoma
    d. Kaposi's sarcoma

17. Which question would the nurse be sure to ask a patient with suspected leukoplakia?
    a. "Do you smoke, dip, or chew tobacco products?"
    b. "How much alcohol do you drink each day?"
    c. "Do you eat a lot of fast food meals?"
    d. "How often do you have dental checkups?"

18. Which oral cavity lesion is associated with progression of human immunodeficiency virus (HIV) to acquired immunodeficiency syndrome (AIDS)?
    a. Erythroplakia
    b. Squamous cell carcinoma
    c. Oral hairy leukoplakia
    d. Basal cell carcinoma

19. Which are recommended prevention strategies for oral cancer? **Select all that apply.**
    a. Minimize sun exposure.
    b. Stop using tobacco.
    c. Avoid intake of fatty foods.
    d. Decrease alcohol intake.
    e. Exercise 3-5 days per week.
    f. Avoid use of tanning beds.

20. Which oral cavity tumor appears as a raised scab, primarily on the lips, and evolves to an ulcer with a raised pearly border?
    a. Leukoplakia
    b. Erythroplakia
    c. Basal cell carcinoma
    d. Kaposi's sarcoma

21. A patient is scheduled for multiple tests to evaluate an oral tumor. The patient asks the nurse which of the tests is the **best** to determine if the tumor is cancerous. What is the nurse's **best** response?
    a. "All of the tests need to be looked at together because no single test can tell if you have cancer."
    b. "Magnetic resonance imaging is the only diagnostic test that will need to be done."
    c. "Biopsy is the definitive method for diagnosing oral cancer."
    d. "An aqueous solution of toluidine blue 1% can be applied to the oral lesion. If the lesion is malignant it will not absorb the solution."

22. During an assessment of a patient with an oral tumor, the nurse notes that the patient develops stridor. What functional assessment is the **least** important for the nurse to complete at this time?
    a. Ability to speak
    b. Gag reflex
    c. Quality of respirations
    d. Pain rating

23. Which operative procedure includes excision of a segment of the mandible with the oral lesion, and radical neck dissection?
    a. Oropharyngeal resection
    b. Glossectomy
    c. Mandibulectomy
    d. Commando procedure

24. The nurse is teaching a patient who will have a radical neck dissection. The nurse will teach the patient that what structures will be removed during this procedure? **Select all that apply.**
    a. Sternocleidomastoid muscle
    b. Removal of the jaw
    c. Excision of cervical lymph nodes on the affected side
    d. Cranial nerve XI
    e. Excision of the tongue
    f. Internal jugular vein

25. After a patient has undergone a radical neck dissection, what is the **priority** nursing intervention?
    a. Manage the patient's pain.
    b. Maintain fluid and electrolyte balance.
    c. Maintain the patient's airway.
    d. Enhance the patient's ability to communicate.

26. Which interventions prevent or minimize the risk factors in patients at risk for aspiration? **Select all that apply.**
    a. Requesting medications in pill form
    b. Providing liquids with a thickening agent
    c. Positioning the patient upright at 90 degrees
    d. Keeping the head of bed elevated for 5 minutes after eating
    e. Keeping suction equipment nearby
    f. Feeding the patient small bites

27. After receiving implantation of radioactive substances (brachytherapy) in the floor of the mouth, the nurse will place the patient on radiation transmission precautions that include which of the following key elements? **Select all that apply.**
    a. Place the patient in a private room with lead-lined walls.
    b. Visitors may stay only less than 30 minutes a day.
    c. Pregnant women and children can visit for only 10 minutes a day.
    d. Anything that goes into the patient's room may not come out.
    e. A tracheostomy may be needed for edema and increased secretions.
    f. The patient will be expected to consume foods high in iron content.

28. How is xerostomia characterized?
    a. Reduction of taste sensation
    b. Inflammation of a salivary gland
    c. Excessive mouth dryness
    d. Inflammation of the mouth

29. Which are considered acute effects of radiation therapy? **Select all that apply.**
    a. Excessive drooling
    b. Stomatitis
    c. Herpes simplex
    d. Treatment-related mucositis
    e. Alteration in taste
    f. Xerostomia

30. The unlicensed assistive personnel (UAP) is providing oral care for a patient after resection of an oral tumor. Which would the nurse instruct the UAP to report **immediately**?
    a. There was unusual odor from the patient's mouth.
    b. Oral care was provided every 4 hours.
    c. The suture site appears to be intact.
    d. The patient's secretions were thick before oral care was given.

31. The unlicensed assistive personnel (UAP) is caring for a patient undergoing radiation therapy to the neck. Which action by the UAP requires intervention by the supervising nurse?
    a. Reminding the patient to avoid sun exposure when he goes home
    b. Shaving the patient with an electric razor
    c. Using of alcohol-based aftershave lotion
    d. Using gentle nondeodorant soap to wash the patient

32. Which patient is at **lowest** risk for development of acute sialadenitis?
    a. Patient with Sjögren's syndrome
    b. Patient with HIV infection
    c. Patient with anemia
    d. Patient prescribed phenothiazine drugs

33. When assessing a patient with a salivary gland tumor, the nurse pays particular attention to the facial nerve. Which requests by the nurse are likely to determine if the tumor has affected the facial nerve? **Select all that apply.**
    a. "Puff out your cheeks."
    b. "Wrinkle your nose."
    c. "Cough."
    d. "Raise your eyebrows."
    e. "Turn your head back and forth."
    f. "Pucker your lips."

34. The nurse has taught a patient with acute sialadenitis to use sialagogues to stimulate saliva. The patient demonstrates teaching has been effective when the patient states he will eat which food?
    a. Lemon slices
    b. Apple slices
    c. Bananas
    d. Bread

35. Which patients are at **higher** risk for development of oral cavity disorders? **Select all that apply.**
    a. Homeless veteran
    b. Overweight adult with type 2 diabetes
    c. Older adult living in a long-term care facility
    d. Middle-aged smoker who is alcoholic
    e. Underweight teen with anorexia
    f. Middle-aged adult with history of working outdoors for over 20 years

36. The nurse is assessing a patient's mouth for lesions. Which actions will the nurse implement? **Select all that apply.**
    a. Wear clean gloves.
    b. Assure adequate lighting with a penlight.
    c. Ask the patient to say "ahh."
    d. Use a tongue blade.
    e. Instruct the patient to perform the Valsalva maneuver.
    f. Assess for lesions, coatings, and cracking.

54 CHAPTER

Care of Patients with Esophageal Problems

1. Which physiologic factor contributes to gastroesophageal reflux disease (GERD)?
   a. Accelerated gastric emptying
   b. Irritation from reflux of stomach contents
   c. Competent lower esophageal sphincter
   d. Increased esophageal clearance

2. Which statement is true about Barrett's epithelium in the patient with gastroesophageal reflux disease (GERD)?
   a. It is considered premalignant and is associated with higher risk for cancer.
   b. This new tissue is less resistant to acid so it must be removed.
   c. Barrett's epithelium is resistant to the development of cancer.
   d. Esophageal strictures are less likely to occur with this type of epithelium.

3. Which statements about gastroesophageal reflux disease (GERD) are correct? **Select all that apply.**
   a. Overweight and obese patients are at an increased risk.
   b. Thin and underweight patients are at an increased risk.
   c. It is a common disorder in the Asian and Hispanic populations.
   d. There is a high incidence in patients who eat mostly hot and spicy foods.
   e. It is a common upper gastrointestinal disorder in the United States.
   f. Eating large meals predisposes a patient to reflux.

4. Which are the **two most** common manifestations of gastroesophageal reflux disease (GERD)? **Select all that apply.**
   a. Dyspepsia
   b. Eructation
   c. Water brash
   d. Regurgitation
   e. Odynophagia
   f. Flatulence

5. The patient with gastroesophageal reflux disease (GERD) describes painful swallowing. Which symptom does the nurse identify?
   a. Dyspepsia
   b. Regurgitation
   c. Odynophagia
   d. Dysphagia

6. A patient with severe gastroesophageal reflux disease (GERD) tells the nurse that she has pain after each meal that lasts for 45 minutes and is worse when she lies down. What interventions should the nurse teach this patient? **Select all that apply.**
   a. Drink fluids.
   b. When you lie down, try lying on your side.
   c. Take an antacid as prescribed by your health care provider.
   d. Eat something bland such as a slice of white bread.
   e. Maintain an upright position for at least 1 hour after you eat.
   f. Try pressing over your abdomen to mobilize the food in your stomach.

7. A patient is scheduled to have several diagnostic tests to verify the medical diagnosis of gastroesophageal reflux disease (GERD). Which diagnostic test is the **most** accurate method of diagnosing this disorder?
   a. Esophagogastroduodenoscopy (EGD)
   b. Ambulatory pH monitoring examination
   c. Esophageal manometry
   d. Motility testing

8. The nurse has provided teaching to a patient with gastroesophageal reflux disease (GERD). Which statement by the patient indicates the teaching has been effective?
   a. "I will eat three meals a day."
   b. "I will not snack 1 hour before I go to bed."
   c. "I will stay up for at least 15-30 minutes after eating dinner before going to bed."
   d. "I won't lift heavy objects."

9. A patient with gastroesophageal reflux disease (GERD) is on a medication that raises the pH of gastric contents. Which drug does the nurse expect to administer?
   a. Ranitidine
   b. Mylanta
   c. Gaviscon
   d. Omeprazole

10. A patient who has been prescribed famotidine is being discharged home. Which statement by the patient indicates a need for further discharge teaching by the nurse?
    a. "I will double up on the dose if I begin to feel increased heartburn."
    b. "I will avoid all alcohol."
    c. "I will call the health care provider if I continue to have heartburn."
    d. "This drug is available over the counter."

11. Which statement is true about the drug rabeprazole for treatment of gastroesophageal reflux disease (GERD)?
    a. It is rapidly released into the body after it is administered.
    b. The tablets are large and may be crushed if the patient has difficulty swallowing them.
    c. It is a histamine receptor antagonist.
    d. If once-a-day dosing does not control symptoms, it may be taken twice a day.

12. Which group of drugs is the main treatment for severe gastroesophageal reflux disease (GERD)?
    a. Antacids
    b. Histamine receptor agonists
    c. Proton pump inhibitors
    d. Gaviscon preparations

13. The nurse is teaching a patient with gastroesophageal reflux disease (GERD) about lifestyle changes. Which key points would the nurse include? **Select all that apply.**
    a. Consume 4-6 large meals per day.
    b. Limit or eliminate alcohol and tobacco.
    c. Eat slowly and chew food thoroughly.
    d. Elevate the head of your bed 3-5 inches using wooden blocks.
    e. Do not wear restrictive clothing.
    f. Reduce or eliminate spicy foods that cause increased gastric acid.

14. By which actions do drugs used to treat gastroesophageal reflux disease (GERD) help to decrease the pain and discomfort the patient experiences? **Select all that apply.**
    a. Inhibition of gastric acid production
    b. Blocking of pain sensation in the CNS
    c. Accelerating gastric emptying
    d. Decreasing lower esophageal sphincter pressure
    e. Protecting the gastric mucosa
    f. Destroying *H. pylori* bacteria

15. An older adult with gastroesophageal reflux disease (GERD) is prescribed omeprazole. What **priority** teaching point must the nurse instruct the patient about while taking this drug?
    a. Older adults taking this drug may be at increased risk for hip fracture because it interferes with calcium absorption.
    b. Because of this drug's effect of decreasing potassium, the patient may be prescribed a potassium supplement.
    c. This drug causes sodium retention so the patient may be prescribed a sodium restriction.
    d. A heart monitor may be needed because of changes in magnesium that can lead to life-threatening dysrhythmias.

16. A patient has returned to the unit after a Stretta procedure for gastroesophageal reflux disease (GERD). Which action by the student nurse requires the supervising nurse to intervene?
    a. The patient is offered clear liquids in the early postprocedure period.
    b. The patient's routine 81 mg of aspirin is held.
    c. A proton pump inhibitor is administered.
    d. A nasogastric tube is prepared for insertion.

17. Which lifestyle adjustment may a patient have to make to **best** control gastroesophageal reflux disease (GERD)?
    a. Sleep in the Trendelenburg position.
    b. Attain and maintain ideal body weight.
    c. Wear snug-fitting belts and waistbands.
    d. Engage in strenuous exercise such as weightlifting.

18. Which statements will the nurse include when providing health teaching for a patient with hiatal hernia? **Select all that apply.**
    a. "Elevate the head of your bed at least 6 inches for sleeping at night."
    b. "Remain in the upright position for several hours after eating."
    c. "Avoid straining or excessive vigorous exercise."
    d. "After surgery, you will have no dietary restriction."
    e. "Avoid wearing clothing that is tight around the abdomen."
    f. "Avoid eating in the late evening."

19. What diagnostic test **best** identifies a hiatal hernia?
    a. Esophagogastroduodenoscopy (EGD)
    b. 24-hour ambulatory pH monitoring
    c. Esophageal manometry
    d. Barium swallow study with fluoroscopy

20. Which statements about Barrett's esophagus are accurate? **Select all that apply.**
    a. It is considered to be a premalignant condition.
    b. It is associated with excessive intake of fresh fruits and vegetables.
    c. It results from exposure to acid and pepsin.
    d. It is associated with pickled and fermented foods.
    e. Normal cells undergo dysplasia to become cancerous.
    f. It is more common in younger adults.

21. The nurse has provided postoperative teaching for a patient who underwent a laparoscopic Nissen fundoplication. Which statement by the patient indicates a need for additional teaching?
    a. "I will walk every day."
    b. "I will no longer need the anti-reflux drugs after the surgery."
    c. "I will report a fever above 101°F."
    d. "I'll remove the gauze dressing 2 days after surgery and shower."

22. What is the **primary** focus of care after conventional surgery for hiatal hernia?
    a. Prevention of respiratory complications
    b. Pain management
    c. Management of fluid balance
    d. Teaching the patient self-care activities

23. Uncontrolled gastroesophageal reflux disease (GERD) can be a cause of which adult-onset disorders? **Select all that apply.**
    a. Dental decay
    b. Aspiration pneumonia
    c. Laryngitis
    d. Diverticulitis
    e. Asthma
    f. Cardiac disease

24. The nurse is assessing a patient's nasogastric drainage following a conventional fundoplication procedure. How does the nurse expect the drainage to appear in the first 8 hours after surgery?
    a. Dark brown
    b. Bright red mixed with brown
    c. Yellowish to green
    d. Green to clear

25. The nurse is giving discharge instructions to a patient after a fundoplication procedure. The patient is instructed to **avoid** which activities? **Select all that apply.**
    a. Drinking carbonated beverages
    b. Beginning clear liquids when peristalsis has returned
    c. Drinking with a straw
    d. Eating gas-producing foods
    e. Eating soft foods that are easy to swallow
    f. Chewing gum

26. A patient is prescribed pantoprazole. What does the nurse tell the patient is the **major** action of this medication?
    a. It produces a coating on the stomach lining.
    b. It neutralizes gastric acid.
    c. It heals esophageal irritation.
    d. It inhibits gastric acid secretion.

27. In the postoperative period, following an open fundoplication repair for a paraesophageal (rolling) hernia, the nurse notes that with oral feedings, the patient has continuous dysphagia. What is the nurse's **best** interpretation of this finding?
    a. The fundoplication is too tight, and dilation may be required.
    b. The patient is not ready for any nutrition other than clear liquids.
    c. The health care provider will need to prescribe a stool softener.
    d. The patient needs a nasogastric tube placed to decompress the stomach.

28. A patient is undergoing a workup for carcinoma of the esophagus. What are the two **primary** risk factors associated with the development of this carcinoma?
    a. High-fat, low-fiber diet and tobacco use
    b. Tobacco use and obesity
    c. Sedentary lifestyle and family history of squamous cell carcinoma
    d. Heavy alcohol intake and high-fat, low-fiber diet

29. What is the **most** common symptom of esophageal cancer reported by patients?
    a. Productive cough
    b. Reflux especially at night
    c. Difficulty with swallowing
    d. Shortness of breath

30. The patient describes experiencing a dull and steady substernal pain, especially after drinking cold liquids. Which manifestation of esophageal cancer does the nurse recognize?
    a. Angina
    b. Aspiration
    c. Dysphagia
    d. Odynophagia

31. The **definitive** diagnosis for esophageal cancer is made with which procedure?
    a. Barium swallow
    b. Esophageal manometry
    c. Esophageal ultrasound with fine needle aspiration
    d. Esophagogastroduodenoscopy (EGD)

32. Nonsurgical treatment options for cancer of the esophagus can include which therapies? **Select all that apply.**
    a. Swallowing therapy
    b. Chemoradiation
    c. Targeted therapies
    d. Smoking cessation programs
    e. Photodynamic therapy
    f. Endoscopic therapies

33. For which patient is radiation therapy **contraindicated**?
    a. Patient with lung cancer
    b. Patient with esophageal tumor
    c. Patient with sliding hernia
    d. Patient with tracheoesophageal fistula

34. Which procedure would the health care provider recommend for immediate relief of dysphagia?
    a. Photodynamic therapy
    b. Esophageal dilation
    c. Targeted therapy
    d. Chemoradiation therapy

35. The patient with esophageal cancer has an excess of HER2 protein on the cell surface. What therapy does the nurse expect will be ordered for this patient?
    a. Targeted therapy with IV trastuzumab
    b. Chemoradiation with chemotherapy during the first and fifth weeks
    c. Radiation therapy alone to shrink the tumor
    d. Nutrition and swallowing therapy to prevent malnutrition

36. The nurse is collaborating with the speech-language pathologist to assist the patient with oral exercises to improve swallowing (swallowing therapy) and with the occupational therapist for feeding therapy. Which key points must be included when teaching this patient? **Select all that apply.**
    a. Ask the patient to suck on a lollipop to enhance tongue strength.
    b. Teach the patient to reach for food particles on the lips or chin using the tongue.
    c. Instruct the patient to place food at the front of the mouth.
    d. In preparation for swallowing, remind the patient to position the head in forward flexion (chin tuck).
    e. Monitor the patient for sealing of the lips and for tongue movements while eating.
    f. Check for pocketing of food under the tongue after swallowing.

37. Which therapy may be used as a cure for patients who have **small localized** tumors?
    a. Chemotherapy
    b. Photodynamic therapy
    c. Nutrition therapy
    d. Radiation therapy

38. The nurse is caring for a patient with esophageal cancer who is scheduled to undergo an esophagogastrostomy with a section of the jejunum to replace the esophagus. Which procedure does the nurse expect to perform preoperatively?
    a. Complete bowel preparation
    b. Abdominal shave
    c. Urinary catheter placement
    d. Nasogastric tube placement for feeding

39. After an esophagectomy, what is the nurse's **priority** for patient care?
    a. Wound care
    b. Nutrition care
    c. Respiratory care
    d. Hydration care

40. Which instruction would the nurse be sure to give to the unlicensed assistive personnel (UAP) who will be assisting a patient with an esophageal tumor to eat?
    a. Feed the patient as fast as you can because there are three more patients who will need help.
    b. Position the patient in a high Fowler's position before feedings.
    c. Always suction the patient between bites to avoid aspiration.
    d. Remind the patient to cough and deep-breathe between bites of food.

41. The nurse is caring for a postoperative patient after esophageal surgery. On assessment, the nurse discovers that the patient's temperature is 101°F (38.3°C), heart rate is 120/minute, and respiratory rate is 32/minute. Lung sounds include bilateral crackles. What is the nurse's **priority first** action?
    a. Raise the head of the patient's bed.
    b. Call the Rapid Response Team.
    c. Apply oxygen at 2 L per nasal cannula.
    d. Administer IV normal saline at 75 mL/hour.

42. The nurse is supervising a senior nursing student in the care of a patient after esophageal surgery. For which action by the student must the nurse intervene?
    a. Student secures the NG tube to prevent dislodgment.
    b. Student prepares to irrigate NG tube.
    c. Student provides mouth care every 2-4 hours.
    d. Student elevates the head of the patient's bed.

43. The postoperative patient who had esophageal surgery has an NG tube in place. What intervention should the nurse delegate to the unlicensed assistive personnel (UAP)?
    a. Check the NG tube for proper placement.
    b. Teach the patient about the purpose of the NG tube.
    c. Assess the patient's lungs for the presence of abnormal breath sounds.
    d. Provide the patient with thorough mouth and nasal care every 2-4 hours.

44. What manifestations are expected when a patient has esophageal diverticula?
    Select all that apply.
    a. Halitosis
    b. Dysphagia
    c. Swelling with difficulty breathing
    d. Nocturnal cough
    e. Regurgitation
    f. Pain radiating to the right arm

45. Which statement about esophageal trauma caused by chemical injury is accurate?
    a. Alkaline substances tend to affect the superficial mucosal lining.
    b. Acid burns cause deep penetrating injuries.
    c. Strong alkalis can cause full perforation of the esophagus within 1 minute.
    d. Chemical injuries damage the mouth and esophagus over a period of several hours.

55

CHAPTER

Care of Patients with Stomach Disorders

1. Which are pathologic changes associated with acute gastritis? **Select all that apply.**
   a. Vascular congestion
   b. Severe mucosal damage and ruptured vessels
   c. Autodigestion
   d. Acute inflammatory cell infiltration
   e. Increased cell production in the superficial epithelium of the stomach lining
   f. Edema

2. Which are possible complications of chronic gastritis? **Select all that apply.**
   a. Pernicious anemia
   b. Thickening of the stomach lining
   c. Gastric cancer
   d. Decreased gastric acid secretion
   e. Peptic ulcer disease
   f. Local irritation from radiation therapy

3. Which statements about gastritis are accurate? **Select all that apply.**
   a. The diagnosis of gastritis is made solely on clinical symptoms.
   b. The onset of infection with *Helicobacter pylori* can result in acute gastritis.
   c. Long-term use of acetaminophen is a high-risk factor for acute gastritis.
   d. Atrophic gastritis is a form of chronic gastritis that is seen most in older adults.
   e. Type B chronic gastritis affects the glands in the antrum but may affect all the stomach.
   f. Type A chronic gastritis involves erosion in the fundus of the stomach.

4. The nurse is teaching a patient about health promotion and maintenance to prevent gastritis. Which information does the nurse include? **Select all that apply.**
   a. "A balanced diet can help prevent gastritis."
   b. "To prevent gastritis, you should limit your intake of salt."
   c. "If you stop smoking, there is less of a chance that you will develop gastritis."
   d. "Yoga has been found to be effective in preventing gastritis."
   e. "Although regular exercise is good for you, it has not been found to influence the prevention of gastritis."
   f. "To prevent gastritis, alcohol should be avoided."

5. A patient with chronic gastritis is being admitted. Which sign/symptom does the nurse identify as being associated with this patient's condition?
   a. Pernicious anemia
   b. Gastric hemorrhage
   c. Hematemesis
   d. Dyspepsia

6. When teaching a patient about pernicious anemia, which statement does the nurse include?
   a. "Patients with pernicious anemia are not able to digest fats."
   b. "Pernicious anemia results from a deficiency of vitamin B_{12}."
   c. "All patients with gastrointestinal bleeding will eventually develop pernicious anemia."
   d. "Oral iron supplements are an effective treatment for pernicious anemia."

7. A patient comes to the emergency department (ED) reporting rapid onset of epigastric pain with nausea and vomiting. The patient says the pain is worse than any heartburn he has had, and that he has not had an appetite for the past day. What does the nurse suspect this patient has?
   a. Peritonitis
   b. *H. pylori* infection
   c. Duodenal ulcer
   d. Acute gastritis

8. Which diagnostic test is the gold standard for diagnosing gastritis?
   a. Esophagogastroduodenoscopy (EGD) with biopsy
   b. Computed tomography (CT) scan
   c. Upper gastrointestinal (GI) series
   d. Cholangiogram

9. The nurse is teaching a patient about ranitidine (Zantac) prescribed for gastritis. Which statement by the patient indicates effective teaching by the nurse?
   a. "The drug will heal the areas of my stomach that are sore."
   b. "This drug will block the secretions of my stomach."
   c. "Zantac will coat the inside of my stomach to protect it from acid."
   d. "This pill kills the bacterial infection I have in my stomach."

10. A patient with acute gastritis is receiving treatment to block and buffer gastric acid secretions to relieve pain. Which drug does the nurse identify as an antisecretory agent (proton pump inhibitor)?
    a. Sucralfate
    b. Ranitidine
    c. Mylanta
    d. Omeprazole

11. The nursing student caring for a patient with a duodenal ulcer is about to administer a proton pump inhibitor (PPI). Which statement about this medication is true?
    a. These drugs should not be used for a prolonged period because they may contribute to osteoporotic-related fractures.
    b. PPIs may not be given via feeding tube.
    c. These drugs help prevent stress-induced ulcers.
    d. PPIs work by coating the stomach with a protective barrier.

12. The nurse is teaching a patient being discharged home about taking prescribed medications that include sucralfate. Which statement by the patient indicates teaching has been effective?
    a. "The main side effect of sucralfate is diarrhea."
    b. "I will take sucralfate with meals."
    c. "I will take sucralfate along with the antacid medication I take."
    d. "Sucralfate works to heal my ulcer."

13. Which types of ulcers are included in peptic ulcer disease? **Select all that apply.**
    a. Esophageal ulcers
    b. Gastric ulcers
    c. Pressure ulcers
    d. Duodenal ulcers
    e. Stress ulcers
    f. Colon ulcers

14. Which type of gastric ulcer does the nurse expect may occur when caring for a patient with extensive burns?
    a. Curling's ulcer
    b. Cushing's ulcer
    c. Stress ulcer
    d. Ischemic ulcer

15. Which type of nonsteroidal anti-inflammatory (NSAID) drug is less likely to cause mucosal damage to the stomach?
    a. Ibuprofen
    b. Aspirin
    c. Acetaminophen
    d. Celecoxib

16. The nurse is caring for a patient who vomited coffee-ground emesis. Where does the nurse suspect the patient is bleeding?
    a. Colon
    b. Rectum
    c. Small intestine
    d. Upper GI system

17. The patient with a gastric ulcer suddenly develops sharp constant epigastric pain that spreads over the entire abdomen. What complication has the patient **most** likely developed?
    a. Hemorrhage
    b. Gastric erosion
    c. Perforation
    d. Gastric cancer

18. The patient with a gastric ulcer presents with a rigid, tender, and painful abdomen. He prefers lying in a knee-chest (fetal) position. What is the nurse's **priority** action at this time?
    a. Notify the health care provider.
    b. Administer opioid pain medication.
    c. Reposition the patient supine.
    d. Measure the abdominal circumference.

19. Which simple noninvasive tests can be used to detect *H. pylori* in a patient with peptic ulcer disease (PUD)? **Select all that apply.**
    a. Echocardiogram
    b. Serologic testing for antibodies
    c. Urea breath test
    d. Stool antigen test
    e. CT scan
    f. MRI

20. Drug therapy for peptic ulcer disease (PUD) is implemented for which purposes? **Select all that apply.**
    a. Pain relief
    b. Rebuild the mucosal lining of the stomach
    c. Eliminate *H. pylori* infection
    d. Heal ulcerations
    e. Prevent recurrence
    f. Control bleeding

21. Which is the **most** commonly reported symptom associated with peptic ulcer disease (PUD)?
    a. Rebound pain
    b. Indigestion
    c. Bleeding
    d. Diarrhea

22. Which peptic ulcer disease drug is useful to protect patients against NSAID-induced ulcers?
    a. Magnesium hydroxide
    b. Omeprazole
    c. Esomeprazole
    d. Misoprostol

23. The patient develops abdominal bloating along with nausea and vomiting. Which complication of peptic ulcer disease (PUD) does the nurse recognize?
    a. Perforation
    b. Hemorrhage
    c. Pyloric obstruction
    d. Intractable PUD

24. Which statement about the use of antacids in the treatment of gastric ulcers is true?
    a. Antacids should be administered with meals.
    b. Patients should take calcium carbonate.
    c. The patient should take antacids on an empty stomach.
    d. Avoid using antacids with phenytoin.

25. A patient with peptic ulcer disease is receiving Maalox. Which actions does the nurse take when administering this medication? **Select all that apply.**
    a. Give the medication 2 hours after the patient's meal.
    b. Instruct the patient to lie on the left side after taking an antacid.
    c. Assess the patient for a history of renal disease before giving Maalox.
    d. Assess the patient for a history of heart failure before giving Maalox.
    e. Observe the patient for the side effect of constipation.
    f. Do not give other drugs within 1-2 hours of antacids.

26. The nurse has provided instruction for a patient prescribed sucralfate to treat a gastric ulcer. Which statement by the patient indicates that teaching has been effective?
    a. "This drug will stop the secretion of acid in my stomach."
    b. "I will take this drug on an empty stomach."
    c. "I will not be able to take ranitidine (Zantac) with this drug."
    d. "The main side effect of this drug that I can expect is diarrhea."

27. An older adult patient is admitted with an upper GI bleed. Which finding does the nurse expect to assess in the patient?
    a. Decreased pulse
    b. Increased hemoglobin and hematocrit
    c. Dizziness
    d. Increased blood pressure

28. A patient develops an active upper GI bleed. Which are the **priority** actions the nurse takes in caring for this patient? **Select all that apply.**
    a. Provide oxygen.
    b. Start 1-2 large-bore IV lines.
    c. Prepare to infuse 0.9% normal saline solution.
    d. Monitor serum electrolytes.
    e. Prepare for nasogastric (NG) tube insertion.
    f. Monitor hematocrit and hemoglobin.

29. When performing an assessment on a patient with an active upper GI bleed, which conditions does the nurse identify as common causes of upper GI bleeding? **Select all that apply.**
    a. Esophageal cancer
    b. Esophageal varices
    c. Gastroesophageal reflux disease
    d. Duodenal ulcer
    e. Gastritis
    f. Gastric cancer

30. The student nurse is performing a gastric lavage on a patient with an active upper GI bleed. Which action by the student requires intervention by the supervising nurse?
    a. Using an ice-cold solution to perform lavage of the stomach
    b. Instilling the lavage solution in volumes of 200-300 mL
    c. Continuing the lavage until the solution returned is clear or light pink without clots
    d. Positioning the patient on his left side during the procedure

31. Which drug would the health care provider prescribe to treat *H. pylori* infection?
    a. Ranitidine
    b. Omeprazole
    c. Clarithromycin
    d. Pantoprazole

32. The health care provider has prescribed quadruple therapy for a patient with PUD due to *H. pylori* infection. Which drugs will the nurse expect to administer? **Select all that apply.**
    a. A proton pump inhibitor (PPI)
    b. Sucralfate
    c. Two antibiotics
    d. A histamine H2 antagonist
    e. Bismuth
    f. Two antacids

33. The nurse is caring for several patients with gastric and duodenal ulcers. Which differential features of gastric ulcers compared to duodenal ulcers does the nurse identify? **Select all that apply.**
    a. In gastric ulcers, there is normal secretion or hyposecretion.
    b. Gastric ulcers are relieved by ingestion of food.
    c. Hematemesis is more common than melena.
    d. No gastritis is present.
    e. Most often, the patient has type O blood.
    f. Pain occurs 30-60 minutes after a meal and at night.

34. The nurse is taking a history from a patient with peptic ulcer disease. Which factor indicates the largest risk for stomach cancer?
    a. History of GERD for 6 weeks
    b. History of hiatal hernia
    c. History of gastritis
    d. History of infection with *H. pylori*

35. The patient tells the nurse that he is fearful of developing stomach cancer, which caused his father's death. Which foods should the nurse teach the patient to **avoid**?
    a. Foods that cause reflux
    b. Pickled and processed foods
    c. Large and heavy meals
    d. Heavily spiced foods

36. The nurse is assessing a patient who has had a total gastrectomy today and notes bright-red blood in the nasogastric (NG) tube and abdominal distention. What does the nurse do **next**?
    a. Irrigate the NG tube.
    b. Reposition the NG tube.
    c. Inform the surgeon of these findings.
    d. Remove the NG tube.

37. Which are symptoms of **early** dumping syndrome? **Select all that apply.**
    a. Tachycardia
    b. Confusion
    c. Desire to lie down
    d. Syncope
    e. Occurs 30 minutes after eating
    f. Palpitations

38. What is the cause of **late** dumping syndrome?
    a. Rapid emptying of food into the small intestine
    b. Shift of fluids into the gut leading to abdominal distention
    c. Release of an excessive amount of insulin
    d. Rapid entry of high-protein foods into the jejunum

39. Which strategies does the nurse expect to implement in the management of dumping syndrome? **Select all that apply.**
    a. Provide more frequent smaller meals.
    b. Provide a high-carbohydrate diet.
    c. Eliminate liquids ingested with meals.
    d. Increase protein and fat in the diet.
    e. Administer acarbose to decrease carbohydrate absorption.
    f. Subcutaneous octreotide (Sandostatin) 2-3 times a day, 30 minutes before meals as prescribed.

40. The nurse is caring for a patient who underwent gastric resection. On assessment, the nurse notes that the patient's tongue is smooth and shiny and appears "beefy." What does the nurse suspect has occurred?
    a. Vitamin B_{12} deficiency
    b. Anemia
    c. Hypovolemia
    d. Inadequate nutrition

41. The nurse is teaching a patient with dumping syndrome about diet. Which statement by the patient indicates that teaching has been effective?
    a. "I will use sugar-free gelatin with caution."
    b. "I will avoid rice in my diet."
    c. "Meat in my diet will consist of a total of 8 ounces a day."
    d. "I will limit fluids with my meals to 8 ounces."

42. Which statement about general principles of diet therapy for patients with dumping syndrome is true?
    a. Patients with dumping syndrome should have liquids between meals only.
    b. Patients with dumping syndrome should be encouraged to eat a diet high in roughage.
    c. Patients with dumping syndrome should eat a high-carbohydrate diet.
    d. The diet for a patient with dumping syndrome must be low in fat and protein.

43. The nurse is providing discharge teaching for a patient after a gastrectomy. Which teaching points will the nurse include to help the patient **minimize** dumping syndrome? **Select all that apply.**
    a. "Eat small frequent meals."
    b. "Drink an 8-ounce glass of water with each meal."
    c. "Eliminate alcohol and caffeine from your diet."
    d. "Lie flat for a short time after eating."
    e. "Take B$_{12}$ injections as prescribed by your health care provider."
    f. "Begin a smoking cessation program."

44. The nurse is teaching a patient with dumping syndrome. Which foods should the patient be instructed are permitted and encouraged? **Select all that apply.**
    a. White bread, rolls, and crackers
    b. Sweetened juice or fruit
    c. Cooked vegetables
    d. Carbonated drinks
    e. Fish, poultry, beef, or pork
    f. Butter and salad dressings

45. Which is a **key** feature in advanced gastric cancer?
    a. Feeling of fullness
    b. Indigestion
    c. Epigastric, back, or retrosternal pain
    d. Progressive weight loss

Care of Patients with Noninflammatory Intestinal Disorders

1. The patient has a diagnosis of irritable bowel syndrome (IBS). Which forms can IBS take? **Select all that apply.**
   a. Diarrhea (IBS-D)
   b. Constipation (IBS-C)
   c. Bloating (IBS-B)
   d. Alternating diarrhea and constipation (IBS-A)
   e. Mix of constipation and diarrhea (IBS-M)
   f. Uncertain (IBS-U)

2. Which test may be used in diagnosing IBS?
   a. Erythrocyte sedimentation rate
   b. Stool sample for ova and parasites
   c. Hydrogen breath test
   d. Blood cultures for infection

3. The patient with IBS reports abdominal distention and feeling bloated to the nurse. The patient states she had a bowel movement that morning. What drug treatment does the nurse expect the health care provider to order?
   a. Loperamide
   b. Psyllium hydrophilic mucilloid
   c. Lubiprostone
   d. Rifaximin

4. What action of darifenacin makes it suitable for treatment of IBS?
   a. Inhibits intestinal motility
   b. Decreases abdominal distention
   c. Eliminates constipation
   d. Increases fluid in the intestines

5. Which medication is the drug of choice for the treatment of IBS when pain is the predominant symptom?
   a. Amitriptyline
   b. Fesoterodine
   c. Loperamide
   d. Psyllium hydrophilic mucilloid

6. The nurse is teaching a patient with IBS about complementary and alternative therapies for the disease. Which patient statements indicate that teaching has been effective? **Select all that apply.**
   a. "Hydrotherapy may help decrease symptoms."
   b. "Probiotics can help decrease bacteria and decrease my IBS symptoms."
   c. "Peppermint oil has been used to expel gas and relax spastic intestinal muscles."
   d. "Regular exercise will help decrease stress and lead to regular bowel movements."
   e. "Ginkgo can be used for abdominal discomfort and to expel gas."
   f. "Meditation may help decrease stress and help with GI symptoms."

7. The patient has an abdominal hernia with a sac that can be returned into the abdominal cavity by gentle pressure. Which type of hernia does the nurse recognize?
   a. Incisional
   b. Irreducible
   c. Indirect inguinal
   d. Reducible

8. The nurse assesses a patient with a hernia and finds that the patient's symptoms include abdominal distention, nausea, vomiting, and pain. The patient's heart rate is 118/minute and temperature is 101°F (38.3°C). Which type of hernia does the nurse suspect?
   a. Incisional
   b. Incarcerated
   c. Strangulated
   d. Umbilical

9. The nurse is performing an abdominal assessment on a patient suspected of having an abdominal hernia. The nurse auscultates the abdomen and determines the absence of bowel sounds. What does the nurse suspect in this patient?
   a. Peritonitis
   b. IBS
   c. Obstruction and strangulation
   d. Low intraabdominal pressure

10. Which are true statements about caring for a patient with a truss? **Select all that apply.**
   a. A surgical binder holds the truss in place.
   b. The truss is removed only for bathing.
   c. The truss is only used after the hernia has been reduced by the health care provider.
   d. The truss is applied before the hernia is reduced to decrease pain.
   e. Powder should be applied to the skin under the truss daily.
   f. The patient should apply the truss on waking.

11. Which activity does the nurse tell the patient to **avoid** after surgery for a hernia repair?
   a. Ambulating
   b. Turning
   c. Coughing
   d. Deep-breathing

12. The nurse would include which intervention in the plan of care for a male patient who has had an inguinal herniorrhaphy?
   a. Apply a warm pack to the scrotum.
   b. Elevate the scrotum on a pillow.
   c. Encourage use of a bedpan to void.
   d. Decrease fluid intake to decrease bladder emptying.

13. The nurse is providing teaching about ways to reduce the risk for colorectal cancer. Which dietary suggestions will the nurse be sure to include in the teaching? **Select all that apply.**
   a. Low fat
   b. Low protein
   c. High fiber
   d. High in red meat
   e. Low in refined carbohydrates
   f. High in brassica vegetables

14. Which are the most common signs of colorectal cancer (CRC)? **Select all that apply.**
   a. Change in stool consistency
   b. Absent bowel sounds
   c. Abdominal cramping
   d. Anemia
   e. Rectal bleeding
   f. Gas pains

15. Which test is definitive for the diagnosis of colorectal cancer (CRC)?
   a. Carcinoembryonic antigen (CEA)
   b. Barium swallow
   c. Colonoscopy with biopsy
   d. Fecal occult blood test (FOBT)

16. After colostomy surgery, which intervention does the nurse employ?
   a. Cover the stoma with a dry, sterile dressing.
   b. Apply a pouch system as soon as possible.
   c. Make a hole in the pouch for gas to escape.
   d. Watch for the colostomy to start functioning on day 1.

17. Which discharge instruction does the nurse include for a patient after abdominoperitoneal (AP) resection?
   a. "Use a soft pillow to sit on whenever you sit down."
   b. "Lie on your back when you are resting in bed."
   c. "Use a rubber doughnut device for sitting on when in the car."
   d. "Sit in a chair for at least 4 consecutive hours a day."

18. Which findings does the nurse expect for a postoperative colostomy patient? **Select all that apply.**
    a. Reddish-pink, moist stoma
    b. Small amount of bleeding
    c. Large amount of stoma swelling
    d. Mucocutaneous separation
    e. Smooth, intact peristomal skin
    f. Excoriation immediately around the stoma

19. Which findings for a patient with a new colostomy will the nurse report to the surgeon? **Select all that apply.**
    a. A dark-red, dry stoma
    b. Stoma protruding about 2 cm from the abdominal wall
    c. Mucocutaneous separation
    d. A slight amount of edema in the initial postoperative period
    e. Large amount of bleeding
    f. Moist pink stoma

20. The nurse is teaching a patient about what kind of stool to expect after a descending colon colostomy. The nurse tells the patient to expect to have what kind of stool?
    a. Similar to stool expelled from the rectum
    b. Thick and paste-like
    c. Thin and gelatin-like
    d. Watery

21. Which sign/symptom is a patient who had an AP resection instructed to report to the health care provider **immediately**?
    a. Serosanguineous drainage from the wound
    b. Sensations of having a bowel movement
    c. Constant perineal odor and pain
    d. Occasional perineal pain and itching

22. The nurse is teaching a patient about colostomy care. Which information does the nurse include in the teaching plan?
    a. The stoma will enlarge within 6-8 weeks of surgery.
    b. Use a moisturizing soap to cleanse the area around the stoma.
    c. Place the colostomy bag on the skin when the skin sealant is still damp.
    d. An antifungal cream or powder can be used if a fungal rash develops.

23. A patient with a colostomy may safely include which food item in the diet?
    a. Burritos
    b. Yogurt
    c. Cabbage
    d. Carbonated beverages

24. The nurse is teaching a patient about how to control gas and odor from a colostomy. Which information does the nurse include?
    a. Placing a breath mint in the pouch can help.
    b. Place an aspirin in the colostomy.
    c. Do not consume buttermilk.
    d. Do not eat parsley.

25. Which are examples of mechanical bowel obstructions? **Select all that apply.**
    a. Paralytic ileus
    b. Adhesions
    c. Tumors
    d. Absent peristalsis
    e. Fecal impaction
    f. Hernias

26. Which acid-base abnormality results from a bowel obstruction high in the small intestine?
    a. Respiratory acidosis
    b. Respiratory alkalosis
    c. Metabolic acidosis
    d. Metabolic alkalosis

27. Which description best defines intussusception of the intestine?
    a. Twisting of the intestine
    b. Fecal constipation or impaction
    c. Telescoping of a segment of the intestine within itself
    d. Adhesions forming scar tissue

28. The nurse is assessing a patient newly admitted with obstipation and failure to pass flatus. Which condition is the **most likely** cause of this patient's symptoms?
    a. Complete obstruction
    b. Partial obstruction
    c. Colorectal cancer
    d. Crohn's disease

29. Which key feature does the nurse most likely find when performing a physical assessment on a patient with a small bowel obstruction?
    a. Visible peristaltic waves in the upper and middle abdomen
    b. Minimal or no vomiting
    c. No major fluid and electrolyte imbalances
    d. Metabolic acidosis

30. What nursing care does a patient with a nasogastric (NG) tube require? **Select all that apply.**
    a. Assess proper placement at least every 12 hours.
    b. Keep patient in a semi-Fowler's position.
    c. Confirm NG tube placement by x-ray if it is repositioned.
    d. Monitor contents of the NG tube.
    e. Irrigate the tube with 30 mL of normal saline as ordered.
    f. Instruct the patient that feelings of nausea are due to tube placement.

31. Which NG tubes can be connected to low continuous suction?
    a. Salem sump
    b. Levin
    c. Anderson
    d. Carney

32. The nurse providing care for a patient with a bowel obstruction notes that the patient has started passing flatus and had a small bowel movement. What has occurred with this patient?
    a. Blockage is complete.
    b. Peristalsis has returned.
    c. Peritonitis has occurred.
    d. The patient is rehydrated.

33. Which intervention applies to the nursing care of an older patient with heart failure and hypovolemia related to an intestinal obstruction?
    a. Provide frequent mouth care with lemon-glycerin swabs.
    b. Offer ice chips to suck on before surgery.
    c. Offer a small glass of water.
    d. Assess for crackles in the lungs.

34. The nurse is to administer alvimopan to a patient with postoperative ileus. What is the action of this drug?
    a. Increases gastrointestinal (GI) motility
    b. Laxative promotes bowel movement
    c. Antibiotic prevents infection
    d. Prevents nausea and vomiting

35. Which observation of a patient with an intestinal obstruction does the nurse report immediately?
    a. Urinary output of 1000 mL in an 8-hour period
    b. The patient's request for something to drink
    c. Abdominal pain changing from colicky to constant discomfort
    d. The patient is changing positions frequently

36. Which discharge information does the nurse include for the patient who has had an intestinal obstruction caused by fecal impaction?
    a. Encourage the patient to report abdominal distention, nausea or vomiting, and constipation.
    b. Provide the patient a written description of a low-fiber diet.
    c. Remind the patient to limit activity.
    d. Remind the patient to decrease fluid intake.

37. Which nursing care actions should the nurse delegate to the unlicensed assistive personnel (UAP) for an older patient with a bowel obstruction? **Select all that apply.**
    a. Administer analgesics as needed.
    b. Provide mouth care every 2 hours.
    c. Assess abdomen for distention.
    d. Teach the patient about surgical procedures.
    e. Provide the patient with a few ice chips.
    f. Record intake and output.

38. Why does the nurse place a patient with a bowel obstruction in semi-Fowler's position? **Select all that apply.**
    a. To promote increased peristalsis
    b. To alleviate the pressure of abdominal distention on the chest
    c. To decrease the likelihood of nausea and vomiting
    d. To facilitate breathing
    e. To prevent aspiration
    f. To relieve pressure on the back

39. The nurse is providing care for a patient who had a minimally invasive inguinal hernia repair (MIIHR) through a laparoscope. What must the nurse be sure to include during discharge teaching? **Select all that apply.**
    a. "Avoid strenuous activity for several days before returning to work and normal activity."
    b. "Limit your fluid intake to 1000 to 1200 mL per day."
    c. "Take your prescribed stool softener to prevent constipation."
    d. "You will need to learn how to insert a straight catheter for the first week after surgery."
    e. "Observe your incisions for signs of infection or increased pain and report these immediately."
    f. "This procedure is fairly painless, so you should not need any pain drugs."

40. Which significant factors contribute to increased intraabdominal pressure (IAP)? **Select all that apply.**
    a. Obesity
    b. Daily exercise
    c. Pregnancy
    d. Heavy lifting
    e. Constipation
    f. Hernia formation

41. Which statement about intraabdominal pressure (IAP) is correct?
    a. The normal IAP for adults is 15-20 mm Hg.
    b. Patients with high IAP have bradycardia.
    c. High IAP leads to elevated systemic and portal venous pressure.
    d. Patients with high IAP are hypertensive.

42. Which are potential complications of polyps? **Select all that apply.**
    a. Gross rectal bleeding
    b. Colorectal cancer
    c. Intestinal obstruction
    d. Septic shock
    e. Intussusception
    f. Bowel strangulation

43. Which information does the nurse include when teaching a patient with new-onset hemorrhoids about prevention of hemorrhoid flare-up? **Select all that apply.**
    a. "Increase the fiber in your diet to prevent constipation."
    b. "Do not participate in any physical exercise."
    c. "Maintain a healthy weight."
    d. "Increase your amount of fluid intake."
    e. "Prolonged sitting or standing will not affect the development of hemorrhoids."
    f. "Avoid stimulant laxatives."

44. Which intervention is contraindicated in the nonsurgical management of hemorrhoids?
    a. Diets low in fiber and fluids
    b. Dibucaine ointment
    c. Warm sitz baths three or four times a day
    d. Cleansing the anal area with moistened cleaning tissues

45. Which statement by a patient indicates an understanding of surgical management of hemorrhoids?
    a. "It will take 10-14 days for the rubber band used on the hemorrhoid to fall off."
    b. "My first bowel movement after the surgery may be very painful."
    c. "After surgery, I will need to eat a low-fiber, low-fluid diet."
    d. "Stool softeners and laxatives are avoided after hemorrhoid surgery."

46. What is the classic symptom of malabsorption syndrome?
    a. Unintentional weight loss
    b. Decreased libido
    c. Bloating with flatus
    d. Chronic diarrhea

47. Which laboratory results are expected with malabsorption syndrome resulting in hypochromic microcytic anemia? **Select all that apply.**
    a. Low mean corpuscular hemoglobin (MCH)
    b. High serum vitamin A level
    c. Elevated fecal fat content
    d. Increased mean corpuscular volume (MCV)
    e. Decreased serum cholesterol level
    f. Low mean corpuscular hemoglobin concentration (MCHC)

48. Which diagnostic test measures urinary excretion of vitamin B_{12} for diagnosis of pernicious anemia and other malabsorption syndromes?
    a. Bile acid breath test
    b. Schilling test
    c. Hydrogen breath test
    d. D-xylose absorption test

49. What are the major focus areas for interventions aimed at treating malabsorption syndromes? **Select all that apply.**
    a. Avoiding substances that aggravate malabsorption
    b. Use of complementary and alternative therapies
    c. Supplementation of nutrients
    d. Assessment and supplementation of coping strategies
    e. Curative radiation therapy
    f. Chemotherapy to prevent cancer

50. Which is an example of an environmental factor that can lead to IBS?
    a. Pseudomonas aeruginosa
    b. Dairy products
    c. Pro-inflammatory interleukins
    d. Mental stress

51. Which tasks for patient care of a male with an inguinal hernia repair should the nurse **delegate** to the UAP? **Select all that apply.**
    a. Record all patient intake and output.
    b. Perform an intermittent catheterization if the patient is unable to urinate.
    c. Remind the patient to consume at least 1500 mL per day.
    d. Assist the patient to stand while urinating.
    e. Assess the patient's level of pain.
    f. Teach the patient to keep the wound dry and clean it with antibacterial soap and water.

52. Which signs and symptoms suggest to the nurse that a patient is experiencing a small bowel obstruction? **Select all that apply.**
    a. Intermittent lower abdominal cramping
    b. Epigastric abdominal distention
    c. Nausea with profuse vomiting
    d. Metabolic acidosis
    e. Fluid and electrolyte imbalances
    f. Pain with visible peristaltic waves

53. The patient with malabsorption syndrome is experiencing liquid stools. Which drug does the nurse expect will be prescribed?
    a. Dicyclomine hydrochloride
    b. Docusate
    c. Atropine sulfate
    d. Penicillin

54. The patient with malabsorption syndrome is prescribed IV fluids of one liter 0.9 saline to infuse over 8 hours for hydration. At what rate does the nurse set the IV pump in mL/hr to infuse this fluid as ordered?
    a. 100 mL/hr
    b. 110 mL/hr
    c. 120 mL/hr
    d. 125 mL/hr

55. Which is a **priority** concept for a patient with a noninflammatory intestinal disorder?
    a. Elimination
    b. Nutrition
    c. Fluid and electrolyte balance
    d. Comfort

56. The nurse is teaching a group of older adults how to prevent fecal impaction. Which are key teaching points? **Select all that apply.**
    a. Include plenty of raw fruits and vegetables and whole-grain products in your diet.
    b. Take your prescribed laxative every morning as directed.
    c. Walking every day is an excellent exercise for increasing bowel motility.
    d. Take bulk-forming products, such as Metamucil, to provide fiber.
    e. Use a bedpan instead of a commode or toilet for bowel movements.
    f. Drink lots of fluids, especially water.

57
CHAPTER

Care of Patients with Inflammatory Intestinal Disorders

1. The patient comes to the emergency department (ED) with right lower quadrant pain. What does the ED nurse suspect?
   a. Gastroenteritis
   b. Ulcerative colitis
   c. Appendicitis
   d. Crohn's disease

2. The nurse is caring for the patient with acute appendicitis. Which interventions will the nurse perform? **Select all that apply.**
   a. Maintain the patient on NPO status.
   b. Administer IV fluids as prescribed.
   c. Apply warm compresses to the right lower abdominal quadrant.
   d. Maintain the patient in the supine position.
   e. Administer laxatives.
   f. If tolerated, maintain the patient in a semi-Fowler's position.

3. The patient has been diagnosed with acute appendicitis. Based on this diagnosis, which intervention does the nurse perform?
   a. Start a bowel cleansing program.
   b. Prepare the patient for surgery.
   c. Apply a heating pad to the lower abdomen.
   d. Assess the patient's knowledge about dietary modifications.

4. The nurse on the surgical unit is expecting to admit the patient who has had an appendectomy with abscess. What does the nurse anticipate care for this patient will include? **Select all that apply.**
   a. Clear liquids
   b. Wound drains
   c. IV antibiotics
   d. Nonsteroidal anti-inflammatory drugs (NSAIDs) for pain control
   e. Nasogastric (NG) tube care
   f. Prescribed opioid pain drugs

5. Which laboratory finding does the nurse expect may occur with a diagnosis of appendicitis?
   a. Decreased hematocrit and hemoglobin
   b. Increased coagulation time
   c. Decreased potassium
   d. Increased WBC count

6. Which statements about peritonitis are true? **Select all that apply.**
   a. Peritonitis is caused by contamination of the peritoneal cavity by bacteria or chemicals.
   b. Continuous ambulatory peritoneal dialysis (CAPD) can cause peritonitis.
   c. White blood cell counts are often decreased with peritonitis.
   d. Abdominal wall rigidity is a classic finding in patients with peritonitis.
   e. Chemical peritonitis is caused by leakage of pancreatic enzymes or gastric acids.
   f. Respiratory problems can be caused by increased abdominal pressure against the diaphragm.

7. The fluid shift that occurs in peritonitis may result in which of the following events?
   a. Intracellular fluid moving into the peritoneal cavity
   b. Significant increase in circulatory volume
   c. Decreased circulatory volume and hypovolemic shock
   d. Increased bowel motility caused by increased fluid volume

8. The respiratory problems that may accompany peritonitis are a result of which factor?
   a. Associated pain interfering with ventilation
   b. Decreased pressure against the diaphragm
   c. Fluid shifts to the thoracic cavity
   d. Decreased oxygen demands related to the infectious process

9. Which nursing intervention is part of nonsurgical management for a patient with peritonitis?
    a. Monitor weekly weight and intake and output.
    b. Insert a nasogastric tube to decompress the stomach.
    c. Order a breakfast tray when the patient is hungry.
    d. Administer NSAIDs for pain.

10. What key assessment data would the nurse expect to find in a patient with peritonitis?
    a. Fever and headache
    b. Dizziness with nausea and vomiting
    c. Abdominal pain, distention, and tenderness
    d. Nausea and loss of appetite

11. Which intervention does the nurse **delegate** to the unlicensed assistive personnel (UAP) when caring for a postoperative patient with peritonitis?
    a. Measure intake and output.
    b. Assess wound drainage.
    c. Administer IV antibiotics.
    d. Teach patient about wound care.

12. The nurse is instructing a patient about home care after an exploratory laparotomy for peritonitis. Which statement by the patient indicates that teaching has been effective?
    a. "It is normal for the incision site to be warm."
    b. "I will stop taking the antibiotics if diarrhea develops."
    c. "I will call the health care provider for a temperature greater than 101°F (38.3°C)."
    d. "I will resume activity with my bowling league this week for exercise."

13. The patient with gastroenteritis due to infection with the norovirus asks the nurse how this illness occurred. Which statement by the patient indicates correct understanding of the nurse's teaching?
    a. "I got this infection from being around my grandchildren when they had respiratory illnesses."
    b. "It is likely that I got this illness from either contaminated water or food."
    c. "I may have gotten sick when I was travelling last month."
    d. "It's really important that everything I eat is cooked until it is well done."

14. Which interventions are useful in preventing spread of gastroenteritis? **Select all that apply**.
    a. Careful handwashing
    b. Sanitizing all surfaces that may be contaminated
    c. Prophylactic use of antibiotics
    d. Easily accessible hand sanitizers
    e. Testing all food preparation employees
    f. Proper food and beverage preparation

15. The nurse is assessing a patient with viral gastroenteritis. Which data is the nurse **most** concerned about?
    a. Orthostatic blood pressure changes
    b. Poor skin turgor
    c. Dry mucous membranes
    d. Rebound tenderness

16. What is the **priority** nursing concern for a patient with gastroenteritis?
    a. Nutrition therapy
    b. Fluid replacement
    c. Skin care
    d. Drug therapy

17. Which are common manifestations in a 28-year-old patient with dehydration secondary to gastroenteritis? **Select all that apply.**
    a. Peripheral edema
    b. Elevated temperature
    c. Dry mucous membranes
    d. Hypertension
    e. Oliguria
    f. Poor skin turgor

18. As part of the routine treatment plan for a patient with bacterial gastroenteritis, which drugs does the nurse anticipate the patient will **most likely** be prescribed?
    a. Anticholinergics
    b. Antiemetics
    c. Antiperistaltic drugs
    d. Antibiotics

19. The nurse is caring for a patient with gastroenteritis who has frequent stools. Which task is **best** to delegate to the unlicensed assistive personnel (UAP)?
    a. Teach the patient to avoid use of toilet paper and harsh soaps.
    b. Instruct the patient on how to take a sitz bath.
    c. Use a warm washcloth to remove stool from the skin.
    d. Dry the skin with absorbent cotton.

20. Which characteristics pertain to Crohn's disease (CD)? **Select all that apply.**
    a. It begins in the rectum and proceeds in a continuous manner toward the cecum.
    b. Fistulas commonly develop.
    c. There are five to six soft, loose, nonbloody stools per day.
    d. There is an increased risk of colon cancer.
    e. Some patients experience extraintestinal manifestations such as migratory polyarthritis, ankylosing spondylitis, and erythema nodosum.
    f. There is a cobblestone appearance of the internal intestine.

21. A patient is suspected to have ulcerative colitis (UC). Which diagnostic tests does the nurse expect the patient to undergo to confirm the diagnosis? **Select all that apply.**
    a. Sigmoidoscopy
    b. C-reactive protein
    c. Albumin levels
    d. Erythrocyte sedimentation rate
    e. Magnetic resonance enterography (MRE)
    f. Clotting studies

22. A patient is prescribed sulfasalazine for the treatment of ulcerative colitis (UC). Which patient statement indicates the patient is experiencing a side effect of this drug?
    a. "My skin is covered with a rash."
    b. "My knees hurt."
    c. "My appetite has increased."
    d. "I wake up at night sweating sometimes."

23. Which statement is true about the medical treatment of ulcerative colitis (UC)?
    a. Infliximab is approved as a first-line therapy.
    b. Immunomodulators are not thought to be effective; however, in combination with steroids, they may offer a synergistic effect.
    c. When a therapeutic level of glucocorticoids is reached, the dosage of the drug stays the same to maintain the therapeutic effect.
    d. The method of action for the aminosalicylates is interruption of the pain pathway.

24. A patient with ulcerative colitis (UC) who has had an ileostomy is being discharged home. Which statements by the patient indicate the discharge teaching has been effective? **Select all that apply.**
    a. "I will avoid foods that cause gas."
    b. "I will call the health care provider if I have a fever over 101°F (38.3°C)."
    c. "I will change the adhesive for the appliance daily."
    d. "I know the pouch needs emptying when I feel pain in that area."
    e. "I will call the health care provider if I feel like my heart is beating fast."
    f. "I will include adequate amounts of salt and water in my diet because an ileostomy causes their loss."

25. Which statement is true about drug therapy for Crohn's disease (CD) or ulcerative colitis (UC)?
    a. Infliximab is used to manage episodes of diarrhea with CD.
    b. Sulfasalazine is the first aminosalicylate approved for UC.
    c. Metronidazole has been helpful in patients with fistulas and UC.
    d. Adalimumab is a glucocorticoid approved for the treatment of CD.

26. A patient with Crohn's disease (CD) has a fistula. Which assessment finding indicates possible dehydration?
    a. Weight gain of 2 pounds in one day
    b. Abdominal pain
    c. Foul-smelling urine
    d. Decreased urinary output

27. In caring for a patient with Crohn's disease (CD), the nurse observes for which complications? **Select all that apply.**
    a. Peritonitis
    b. Small bowel obstruction
    c. Nutritional and fluid imbalances
    d. Presence of fistulas
    e. Appendicitis
    f. Severe nausea and vomiting

28. A patient returns to the unit following a total proctocolectomy with a permanent ileostomy. The nurse understands that which organs were removed during this procedure?
    a. All of the small intestine
    b. Distal colon and rectum
    c. Colon, rectum, and anus
    d. Colon, rectum, and anus, with surgical closure of the anus

29. Which type of diet has been implicated in the formation of diverticula?
    a. High-fat diet
    b. Low-protein diet
    c. High-cholesterol diet
    d. Low-fiber diet

30. What is the nature of pain associated with diverticulitis?
    a. Intermittent becoming progressively steady
    b. Sharp and continuous
    c. Localized to the right upper quadrant
    d. Severe and incapacitating

31. The nurse is assessing an older adult patient with abdominal pain. Assessment findings include generalized abdominal pain with rigidity, nausea and vomiting, temperature 101.2°F (38.4°C), heart rate 122/minute, and chills. The patient is also somewhat confused and does not know where he is. What does the nurse suspect with this patient?
    a. Crohn's disease
    b. Ulcerative colitis
    c. Diverticulitis
    d. Peritonitis

32. Which drug is often used in older patients for pain management of moderate to severe diverticulitis?
    a. An NSAID drug
    b. An acetaminophen-based drug
    c. An aspirin-based drug
    d. An opioid analgesic drug

33. Which statement about diverticular disease is true?
    a. Most diverticula occur in the sigmoid colon.
    b. Diverticula are uncomfortable even when not inflamed.
    c. High-fiber diets contribute to diverticula occurrence.
    d. Diverticula form where intestinal wall muscles are weak.

34. The nurse would teach the patient about what preventive measure for diverticular disease?
    a. Excluding whole-grain breads from the diet
    b. Avoiding fresh apples, broccoli, and lettuce
    c. Taking bulk agents such as psyllium hydrophilic mucilloid
    d. Taking routine anticholinergics to reduce bowel spasms

35. Which type of stoma will a patient with diverticulitis most likely have postoperatively?
    a. Ileostomy
    b. Jejunostomy
    c. Colostomy
    d. Cecostomy

36. Which interventions does the nurse expect to implement when caring for a patient with diverticulitis? **Select all that apply.**
    a. Laxative and enemas as ordered
    b. IV fluids to prevent dehydration
    c. Broad-spectrum antibiotics
    d. Teaching the patient to refrain from lifting or straining
    e. Keeping the patient NPO if symptoms are severe
    f. Administering diuretics to prevent fluid overload

37. Which description best defines an anal fissure?
    a. Perianal tear that can be very painful
    b. Duct obstruction and infection
    c. Communicating tract
    d. Localized area of induration with pus

38. The nurse is providing teaching for a patient with an anal fissure as a complication of Crohn's disease (CD). Which statement by the patient indicates the need for further teaching?
    a. "I will use warm sitz baths."
    b. "A diet that is low in bulk-producing agents is best for me."
    c. "Hydrocortisone cream may be helpful to decrease discomfort."
    d. "Topical anti-inflammatory agents will help if I am uncomfortable."

39. Which parasitic infection is manifested by diarrhea and occurs most commonly in immunosuppressed patients, especially those with human immunodeficiency virus (HIV)?
    a. *Entamoeba histolytica*
    b. *Cryptosporidium*
    c. *Giardia lamblia*
    d. *Escherichia coli*

40. Which statements does the nurse include while providing discharge instructions for a patient with giardiasis? **Select all that apply.**
    a. "Avoid contact with stool from dogs and beavers."
    b. "All household and sexual partners should have stool examinations for parasites."
    c. "Treatment will most likely consist of metronidazole (Flagyl)."
    d. "The infection can be transmitted to others until the amebicides kill the parasites."
    e. "Stools are examined 6 days after treatment to assess for eradication."
    f. "Be sure to bathe or shower at least every other day."

41. The emergency department nurse is assessing a patient admitted with frequent, liquid, foul-smelling stools containing mucus and blood. Assessment findings include temperature 103.8° F (39.9°C), tenesmus, abdominal tenderness, and vomiting. Which additional laboratory test(s) does the nurse expect to collect?
    a. Serial stool samples
    b. Urine culture
    c. Throat culture
    d. Sputum culture

42. The patient recovering from surgery for peritonitis tells the nurse that he is experiencing abdominal pain and has developed foul-smelling drainage from his wound, and his incision is red and swollen. What is the nurse's **best first** action?
    a. Clean and dress the incision.
    b. Measure the patient's abdominal girth.
    c. Notify the health care provider.
    d. Place the patient on bedrest in semi-Fowler's position.

43. The patient who had an ileostomy asks the nurse about how to choose the best ostomy pouching system. Which guidelines best describe an effective system? **Select all that apply.**
    a. The adhesive barrier lasts 1-2 days.
    b. The system protects the patient's skin.
    c. The pouch system contains the drainage and reduces odor.
    d. The ostomy pouch system is relatively inexpensive.
    e. The pouch remains securely attached to the skin for a dependable period of time.
    f. A large pouch is best because it holds more stools.

44. The patient comes to the Urgent Care Unit and describes symptoms of diarrhea, abdominal pain, and low-grade fever. She states she has constant abdominal pain in the right lower quadrant and has lost 25 pounds in the past month. What diagnosis does the nurse suspect?
    a. Ulcerative colitis
    b. Diverticulitis
    c. Peritonitis
    d. Crohn's disease

45. Which action should the nurse delegate to the unlicensed assistive personnel (UAP) when providing care for a patient with Crohn's disease?
    a. Check the patient's daily weight.
    b. Instruct the patient about the importance of adequate nutrition.
    c. Assess the patient's skin for areas of breakdown.
    d. Provide the patient with information about the disease process.

58 CHAPTER

Care of Patients with Liver Problems

1. A patient with decompensated cirrhosis is at risk for which complications? **Select all that apply.**
   a. Jaundice
   b. Esophageal varices
   c. Coagulation defects
   d. Hepatitis A virus (HAV)
   e. Spontaneous bacterial peritonitis
   f. Ascites

2. What is the most common cause for Laennec's cirrhosis?
   a. Hepatitis C virus (HPC)
   b. Chronic biliary obstruction
   c. Autoimmune disorders
   d. Chronic alcoholism

3. The nurse is assessing a patient with massive ascites. What related complication must the nurse monitor for with this patient?
   a. Bleeding due to fragile, thin-walled veins
   b. Hematemesis due to absence of clotting factors
   c. Increased ascites due to sodium and water retention
   d. Bruising due to low platelet count

4. When admitting the patient with cirrhosis, the nurse assesses for which conditions related to splenomegaly as possible complications of the disease?
   a. Thrombocytopenia
   b. Bleeding esophageal varices
   c. Hepatorenal syndrome
   d. Portal hypertensive gastropathy

5. Patients with cirrhosis are susceptible to bleeding and easy bruising because there is a decrease in the production of bile in the liver, preventing the absorption of which vitamin?
   a. Vitamin A
   b. Vitamin D
   c. Vitamin E
   d. Vitamin K

6. Which key points does the nurse include when teaching the patient with cirrhosis and his family about drug therapy before discharge? **Select all that apply.**
   a. "Do not take over-the-counter medications unless approved by your health care provider."
   b. "The beta-blocker called propranolol will cause your heart rate to increase."
   c. "The lactulose syrup should cause you to have two to three bowel movements every day."
   d. "Take your furosemide early in the day so that it does not keep you up at night."
   e. "Report any muscle weakness or lightheadedness to your health care provider right away."
   f. "Your health care provider may prescribe a potassium supplement to replace losses."

7. The nurse identifies which laboratory value as the **usual** indication of hepatic encephalopathy?
   a. Elevated sodium level
   b. Elevated ammonia level
   c. Increased blood urea nitrogen (BUN)
   d. Increased clotting time

8. The nurse is assessing a male patient with cirrhosis. Which **male-specific** characteristics does the nurse expect to find? **Select all that apply.**
   a. Gynecomastia
   b. Testicular atrophy
   c. Ascites
   d. Impotence
   e. Spider angiomas
   f. Petechiae

9. Which assessment finding indicates neurologic function deterioration in a patient with stage II cirrhosis?
   a. Fetor hepaticus
   b. Asterixis
   c. Palmar erythema
   d. Icterus

10. Which intervention should the nurse delegate to the unlicensed assistive personnel (UAP) when caring for a patient with cirrhosis experiencing pruritus?
    a. Apply lotion to soothe the patient's skin.
    b. Use lots of soap and hot water to cleanse the skin.
    c. Assess the patient for signs of skin infection.
    d. Encourage the patient to use distraction to avoid scratching.

11. Which elevated laboratory test results indicate hepatic cell destruction? **Select all that apply.**
    a. Elevated serum aspartate aminotransferase (AST)
    b. Elevated serum alanine aminotransferase (ALT)
    c. Elevated lactate dehydrogenase (LDH)
    d. Decreased serum total bilirubin
    e. Increased fecal urobilinogen
    f. Increased International Normalized Ratio (INR)

12. A patient is scheduled for a procedure to place a stent in the biliary tract. For which procedure does the nurse provide patient teaching?
    a. Esophagogastroduodenoscopy (EGD)
    b. Endoscopic retrograde cholangiopancreatography (ERCP)
    c. Upper gastrointestinal (GI) series
    d. Cholangiogram

13. The nurse is teaching a patient with cirrhosis about nutrition therapy. Which statement by the patient indicates teaching has been effective?
    a. "I will only use table salt with my dinner meal."
    b. "I will read the sodium content labels on all food and beverages."
    c. "I will avoid the use of vinegar."
    d. "I will not take vitamin supplements."

14. When preparing a patient for paracentesis, what does the nurse do? **Select all that apply.**
    a. Ask the patient to void before the procedure.
    b. Place the patient in the supine position.
    c. Weigh the patient before the procedure.
    d. Obtain the patient's heart rate.
    e. Assess the patient's respiratory rate.
    f. Obtain the patient's blood pressure.

15. A patient will undergo an abdominal paracentesis. Which factor provides an additional safety measure?
    a. The procedure is performed using ultrasound.
    b. The procedure is performed at the bedside.
    c. A trocar is inserted into the peritoneal cavity.
    d. General anesthesia is administered.

16. The student nurse is caring for a patient with cirrhosis. Which action by the student nurse causes the supervising nurse to intervene?
    a. Uses a straight-edge razor to shave the patient.
    b. Monitors for orthostatic changes of blood pressure.
    c. Avoids intramuscular injections.
    d. Uses a toothette for oral care.

17. The nurse who is assessing a patient with portal-systemic encephalopathy finds that the patient has fetor hepaticus, a positive Babinski's sign, and seizures, but no asterixis. The nurse identifies the patient as being in which stage of portal-systemic encephalopathy?
    a. Stage I prodromal
    b. Stage II impending
    c. Stage III stuporous
    d. Stage IV comatose

18. Which statements about a patient with cirrhosis and esophageal varices are accurate? **Select all that apply.**
    a. All patients with cirrhosis should be screened for esophageal varices to detect them before they bleed.
    b. Bleeding esophageal varices are a medical emergency.
    c. Esophageal balloon tamponade is often used to control bleeding esophageal varices.
    d. A nonselective beta blocker such as propranolol is prescribed to prevent varices from bleeding.
    e. Bleeding esophageal varices can be managed by use of endoscopic variceal ligation.
    f. The bleeding appears as dark coffee grounds in emesis or stool.

19. The nurse is teaching a patient with cirrhosis about lactulose therapy. Which statement by the patient indicates the teaching has been effective?
    a. "This therapy will promote the removal of ammonia in my stool."
    b. "Constipation is a frequent side effect of this therapy."
    c. "I will know the therapy is working when I am less itchy."
    d. "The drug tastes bitter and is watery."

20. How is neomycin sulfate used to treat patients with cirrhosis?
    a. It treats the current infection the patient has.
    b. It prevents future infections of the liver.
    c. It restores normal function to the liver cells.
    d. It decreases the rate of ammonia production.

21. The patient with liver cancer will be discharged with a tunneled ascites drain. What statements by the patient indicate an understanding of the purpose of this device? **Select all that apply.**
    a. "I will have this drain until I am able to get the tumor removed."
    b. "I will not remove more than 2000 mL of fluid at a time."
    c. "The drain will make breathing more comfortable for me after some fluid is removed."
    d. "After I drain off the extra fluid, I can remove the drain."
    e. "This drain will be useful to remove fluid from my belly when there is too much."
    f. "I will flush the tunneled ascites drain twice a day with normal saline."

22. Which statements about hepatitis are accurate? **Select all that apply.**
    a. Hepatitis D is the leading cause of cirrhosis and liver failure in the U.S.
    b. Hepatitis A is spread through the fecal-oral route.
    c. Hepatitis B can be transmitted through unprotected sexual intercourse.
    d. Hepatitis carriers have chronic obvious signs of hepatitis B.
    e. Hepatitis C is transmitted by casual contact or intimate household contact.
    f. Hepatitis D only occurs with hepatitis B to cause viral replication.

23. When teaching a group of adult patients about measures for preventing hepatitis A (HAV), which information does the nurse include? **Select all that apply.**
    a. Perform proper handwashing, especially after handling shellfish.
    b. Receive immune globulin within 14 days if exposed to the virus.
    c. Receive the HAV vaccine before traveling to Mexico or the Caribbean.
    d. After exposure, HAV symptoms always let the patient know something is wrong.
    e. Receive the vaccine if working in a long-term care facility.
    f. Avoid unprotected sex with a person who has HAV.

24. Which people need immunization against hepatitis B (HBV)? **Select all that apply.**
    a. People who have unprotected sex with more than one partner
    b. Men who have sex with men
    c. Any patient scheduled for a surgical procedure
    d. Firefighters
    e. Health care providers
    f. Patients prescribed immunosuppressant drugs

25. What is the **major** source of hepatitis B transmission to health care workers?
    a. Improper handwashing
    b. Needle sticks
    c. Touching contaminated surfaces
    d. Contact with infected stool

26. How many vaccine injections does a health care worker usually need to be protected with the hepatitis B vaccine?
    a. 1
    b. 2
    c. 3
    d. 4

27. Which actions will help prevent viral hepatitis in health care workers? **Select all that apply.**
    a. Wash hands before and after each patient.
    b. Use needleless systems.
    c. Use contact and respiratory precautions.
    d. After exposure to hepatitis A, get immunoglobulin (Ig).
    e. Report all cases of hepatitis to the health department.
    f. Wear gloves during all patient contacts.

28. Which laboratory test result indicates permanent immunity to hepatitis A?
    a. Immunoglobulin G (IgG) antibodies
    b. Immunoglobulin M (IgM) antibodies
    c. A positive enzyme-linked immunosorbent assay (ELISA)
    d. The presence of anti-HAV antibodies

29. Which antiviral drugs are given to patients with chronic hepatitis B virus? **Select all that apply.**
    a. Lamivudine
    b. Entecavir
    c. Tenofovir
    d. Oral ribavirin
    e. Adefovir
    f. Telaprevir

30. Which conditions place a patient at high risk for the development of fatty liver (steatosis)? **Select all that apply.**
    a. Hypertension
    b. Diabetes mellitus
    c. Obesity
    d. Elevated lipid profile
    e. Alcohol abuse
    f. Hepatitis A

31. In performing an assessment on a patient with liver trauma, what does the nurse expect to find? **Select all that apply.**
    a. Right upper quadrant pain
    b. Increased blood pressure
    c. Guarding of the abdomen
    d. Bradypnea
    e. Kehr's sign
    f. Abdominal rigidity

32. The nurse is assessing a patient with liver trauma and finds that the patient is confused, with a blood pressure of 86/50 mm Hg, heart rate of 128/minute, and cool, clammy skin. What does the nurse suspect?
    a. Septic shock
    b. Liver hemorrhage
    c. Liver cancer
    d. GI bleeding

33. What test result is the tumor marker for cancers of the liver?
    a. Decreased alkaline phosphatase
    b. Increased serum ammonia
    c. Decreased serum total bilirubin
    d. Increased alpha-fetoprotein (AFP)

34. Which treatment offers the patient with liver cancer the possibility of long-term survival?
    a. Chemotherapy
    b. Selective internal radiation therapy
    c. Liver transplantation
    d. Hepatic arterial embolization

35. What is the **priority** focus in caring for a patient with advanced liver cancer?
    a. Hospice and end-of-life care
    b. Getting placed on the liver transplant list
    c. Hepatic arterial infusion of chemotherapy
    d. Cryotherapy to freeze and destroy liver tumors

36. Administration of which drug has greatly improved the success of organ transplants?
    a. Telaprevir
    b. Entecavir
    c. Tenofovir
    d. Cyclosporine

37. The patient who had a liver transplant develops a heart rate of 134/minute, temperature of 102°F (38.8°C), jaundiced skin, and right upper quadrant pain. What does the nurse suspect?
    a. Liver infection
    b. Hypovolemic shock
    c. Liver transplant rejection
    d. Liver trauma from the transplant surgery

38. Which procedure uses energy waves to heat cancer cells and kill them?
    a. Cryotherapy
    b. Selective internal radiation therapy (SIRT)
    c. Hepatic artery embolization
    d. Radiofrequency ablation (RFA)

39. Which patients **would not** be considered candidates for a liver transplant? **Select all that apply.**
    a. Patient with metastatic tumors
    b. Patient with type 2 diabetes
    c. Patient with severe respiratory disease
    d. Patient with chronic liver disease
    e. Patient with advanced cardiac disease
    f. Patient who is unable to follow instructions

40. The nurse is teaching a patient with cirrhosis about nutrition therapy. Which key points must the nurse include? **Select all that apply.**
    a. Do not use table salt.
    b. Adding salt when cooking is acceptable.
    c. Eat small frequent meals.
    d. Drink supplemental liquids such as Ensure.
    e. Be sure to take a multivitamin every day.
    f. Avoid foods that are rich in vitamin K.

41. The patient with cirrhosis is prescribed furosemide 60 mg orally each morning. Which patient care concept is at risk for this patient?
    a. Comfort
    b. Cellular regulation
    c. Immunity
    d. Fluid and electrolyte balance

42. Which factors may lead to hepatic encephalopathy in patients with cirrhosis? **Select all that apply.**
    a. High-protein diet
    b. Hypervolemia
    c. Infection
    d. Constipation
    e. Hyperkalemia
    f. Use of illicit drugs

43. The nurse is teaching a young woman about cirrhosis prevention by limiting alcohol intake. What is the nurse's **best** advice?
    a. "As few as two or three drinks per day over 10 years can lead to cirrhosis."
    b. "You should be all right as long as you drink less than five drinks per day."
    c. "Binge drinking, rather than drinking every day, reduces your risk for hepatitis or fatty liver."
    d. "The amount of alcohol that causes cirrhosis does not vary by gender."

44. The nurse is providing care for a patient with cirrhosis who has massive ascites and has developed hepatopulmonary syndrome. Which elements of nursing care are appropriate for this patient? **Select all that apply.**
    a. Auscultate lungs every 4-8 hours for crackles.
    b. Monitor the patient's oxygen saturation.
    c. Elevate the head of the bed 15 degrees.
    d. Apply oxygen therapy.
    e. Weigh the patient every day.
    f. Lower the patient's legs and feet.

45. The patient who needs a liver transplant asks the nurse where the livers come from. What is the nurse's **best** response?
    a. "Most commonly they come from family members."
    b. "Often they are harvested from cadavers."
    c. "Trauma victims are where most donor livers come from."
    d. "It is best if the liver comes from a blood relative."

46. The patient who just had a liver transplant develops oozing around two IV sites as well as some new bruising. What is the nurse's **best** first action?
    a. Apply pressure to the IV sites.
    b. Measure the size of the bruises.
    c. Document these findings as the only action.
    d. Notify the surgeon immediately.

47. The nurse is caring for a patient with acute viral hepatitis. What is the **major** care concern at this time?
    a. Providing three small meals a day
    b. Alternating periods of activity with periods of rest
    c. Monitoring for the development of jaundiced skin
    d. Teaching the patient the importance of avoiding alcohol intake

59 CHAPTER

Care of Patients with Problems of the Biliary System and Pancreas

1. A patient is admitted with obstructive jaundice. Which sign/symptom does the nurse expect to find upon assessment of the patient?
   a. Pruritus
   b. Pale urine in increased amounts
   c. Pink discoloration of sclera
   d. Dark, tarry stools

2. The daughter of a patient with cholelithiasis has heard that there is a genetic disposition for cholelithiasis. The daughter asks the nurse about the risk factors. How does the nurse respond?
   a. "There is no evidence that first-degree relatives have an increased risk for this disease."
   b. "Cholelithiasis is seen more frequently in patients who are underweight."
   c. "Hormone replacement therapy has been associated with increased risk for cholelithiasis."
   d. "Patients with diabetes mellitus are at increased risk for cholelithiasis."

3. Which patient would the nurse assess as **low risk** for the development of gallbladder disorders?
   a. Patient with sickle cell anemia
   b. Patient who is Mexican American
   c. Patient who is 20 years old and male
   d. Patient with a history of prolonged parenteral nutrition

4. The nurse on a medical-surgical unit is caring for several patients with acute cholecystitis. Which task is **best** to delegate to the unlicensed assistive personnel (UAP)?
   a. Obtain the patients' vital signs.
   b. Determine if any foods are not tolerated.
   c. Assess what measures relieve the abdominal pain.
   d. Ask the patients to describe their daily activity or exercise routines.

5. Which are common manifestations of acute cholecystitis? **Select all that apply.**
   a. Anorexia
   b. Ascites
   c. Eructation
   d. Steatorrhea
   e. Jaundice
   f. Rebound tenderness

6. The nurse is assessing a patient with acute cholecystitis whose abdominal pain is severe. The patient is pale, is diaphoretic, and describes extreme fatigue. Vital signs are: heart rate of 118/minute, BP 95/70, respirations 32/min, temperature 101°F (38.33°C). What is the nurse's **priority** action at this time?
   a. Instruct the unlicensed assistive personnel (UAP) to reposition the patient for comfort.
   b. Auscultate the patient's abdomen in all four quadrants.
   c. Notify the patient's health care provider.
   d. Administer the ordered opioid analgesic.

7. The health care provider has assessed a patient's abdomen and found rebound tenderness on deep palpation. What does the nurse recognize?
   a. Steatorrhea
   b. Eructation
   c. Biliary colic
   d. Blumberg's sign

8. A patient is scheduled for tests to verify the medical diagnosis of cholecystitis. For which diagnostic test does the nurse provide patient teaching?
   a. Extracorporeal shock wave lithotripsy (ESWL)
   b. Ultrasonography of the right upper quadrant
   c. Endoscopic retrograde cholangiopancreatography (ERCP)
   d. Serum level of aspartate aminotransferase (AST)

9. Which type of drug is used to treat acute severe biliary pain?
   a. Acetaminophen
   b. Nonsteroidal antiinflammatory drugs (NSAIDs)
   c. Antiemetics
   d. Opioids

10. The nurse is administering ketorolac to a 78-year-old patient for mild to moderate biliary pain management. Which assessment finding indicates the patient is experiencing a side effect of this drug?
    a. Gastrointestinal upset
    b. Ventricular cardiac dysrhythmias
    c. Decreased urinary output
    d. Jaundice

11. The nurse is caring for an older adult patient with acute biliary pain. Which drug order does the nurse question?
    a. Ketorolac
    b. Meperidine
    c. Morphine
    d. Hydromorphone

12. Which factor renders a patient the least likely to benefit from extracorporeal shock wave lithotripsy (ESWL) for the treatment of gallstones?
    a. Height 5 feet 10 inches, 325 lbs
    b. Cholesterol-based stones
    c. Height 5 feet 7 inches, 138 lbs
    d. Small gallstones

13. Which statements are true regarding laparoscopic cholecystectomy? **Select all that apply.**
    a. Laparoscopic cholecystectomy is considered the "gold standard" and is performed far more often than the traditional open approach.
    b. Patients with chronic lung disease or heart failure who are unable to tolerate the oxygen used in the laparoscopic procedure are examples of patients who have the open surgical approach (abdominal laparotomy).
    c. Removing the gallbladder with the laparoscopic technique reduces the risk of wound complications.
    d. Patients who have their gallbladders removed by the laparoscopic technique should be taught the importance of early ambulation to promote absorption of carbon dioxide.
    e. Use of laparoscopic cholecystectomy puts the patient at increased risk for bile duct injuries.
    f. After a laparoscopic cholecystectomy, assess the patient's oxygen saturation level frequently until the effects of the anesthesia have passed.

14. Which statement about the care of a patient with a Jackson-Pratt (JP) drain after a traditional cholecystectomy is true?
    a. The patient is maintained in the prone position.
    b. When the patient is allowed to eat, the JP drain is clamped continuously.
    c. The JP drain is irrigated every hour for the first 24 hours.
    d. Serosanguineous drainage stained with bile is expected for 24 hours.

15. A female patient is to have her gallbladder removed by natural orifice transluminal endoscopic surgery. What does the nurse teach about this surgery?
    a. The surgeon will use powerful shock waves to break up the gallstones.
    b. The surgeon will insert a transhepatic biliary catheter to open blocked bile ducts.
    c. The surgeon will use a vaginal approach to remove the gallbladder.
    d. The surgeon will inject ursodeoxycholic acid to dissolve any remaining gallstone fragments.

16. After removal of the gallbladder, a patient experiences abdominal pain with vomiting for several weeks. What does the nurse recognize?
    a. Chronic cholecystitis
    b. Recurrence of acute cholecystitis
    c. Unremoved gallstones
    d. Postcholecystectomy syndrome

17. The patient with acute cholecystitis has a pacemaker. Which diagnostic test is **contraindicated**?
    a. Extracorporeal shock wave lithotripsy (ERCP)
    b. Magnetic resonance cholangiopancreatography (MRCP)
    c. Ultrasonography of the right upper quadrant
    d. Hepatobiliary (HIDA) scan

18. The nurse is evaluating electrolyte values for a patient with acute pancreatitis and notes that the serum calcium is 6.8 mEq/L. How does the nurse interpret this finding?
    a. Within normal limits considering the diagnosis of acute pancreatitis
    b. A result of the body not being able to use bound calcium
    c. A protective measure that will reduce the risk of complications
    d. Full compensation of the parathyroid gland

19. Disseminated intravascular coagulation (DIC) is a complication of pancreatitis. What pathophysiology leads to this complication?
    a. Hypovolemia
    b. Peritoneal irritation and seepage of pancreatic enzymes
    c. Disruption of alveolar-capillary membrane
    d. Consumption of clotting factors and formation of microthrombi

20. The patient with acute pancreatitis experiences abdominal pain. What is the **best** intervention to begin managing this pain?
    a. IV opioids by means of patient-controlled analgesia (PCA)
    b. Oral opioids such as morphine sulfate given as needed
    c. Intramuscular opioids given every 6 hours
    d. Oral hydromorphone (Dilaudid) given twice a day

21. The patient comes to the emergency department (ED) with severe abdominal pain in the midepigastric area. The patient states that the pain began suddenly, is continuous, radiates to his back, and is worst when he lies flat on his back. What condition does the nurse suspect?
    a. Acute cholecystitis
    b. Pancreatic cancer
    c. Acute pancreatitis
    d. Pancreatic pseudocyst

22. Which diagnostic test is the **most** accurate in verifying a diagnosis of acute pancreatitis?
    a. Trypsin
    b. Lipase
    c. Alkaline phosphatase
    d. Alanine aminotransferase

23. A patient with acute pancreatitis is at risk for the development of paralytic (adynamic) ileus. Which action provides the nurse with the **best** indication of bowel function?
    a. Observing contents of the nasogastric drainage
    b. Weighing the patient every day at the same time
    c. Asking the patient if he or she has passed flatus or had a stool
    d. Obtaining a computed tomography (CT) scan of the abdomen with contrast medium

24. Which condition is **most** likely to be treated with antibiotics?
    a. Cancer of the gallbladder
    b. Acute cholelithiasis
    c. Chronic pancreatitis
    d. Acute necrotizing pancreatitis

25. The nurse has instructed a patient in the recovery phase of acute pancreatitis about diet therapy. Which statement by the patient indicates that teaching has been successful?
    a. "I will eat the usual three meals a day that I am used to."
    b. "I am eating tacos for my first meal back home."
    c. "I will avoid eating chocolate and drinking coffee."
    d. "I will limit the amount of protein in my diet."

26. The nursing student is caring for a patient with chronic pancreatitis who is receiving pancreatic enzyme replacement therapy. Which statement by the student indicates the need for further study concerning this therapy?
    a. "The enzymes will be administered with meals."
    b. "The patient will take the drugs with a glass of water."
    c. "If the patient has difficulty swallowing the enzyme preparation, I will crush it and mix it with foods."
    d. "The effectiveness of pancreatic enzyme treatment is monitored by the frequency and fat content of stools."

27. Which statements about pancreatic cancer are accurate? **Select all that apply.**
    a. Venous thromboembolism (VTE) is a common complication of pancreatic cancer.
    b. Pancreatic cancer often presents in a slow and vague manner.
    c. Severe pain is an early feature of this disease.
    d. There are no specific blood tests to diagnose pancreatic cancer.
    e. Chemotherapy is the treatment of choice for pancreatic cancer.
    f. Chronic pancreatitis predisposes a patient to pancreatic cancer.

28. The nurse detects an epigastric mass while assessing a patient with acute pancreatitis. The patient describes epigastric pain that radiates to his back. What does the nurse suspect?
    a. Liver cirrhosis
    b. Pancreatic pseudocyst
    c. Gallstones
    d. Chronic pancreatitis

29. The nurse is caring for a patient with pancreatic cancer who had a Whipple procedure. Which interventions and assessments does the nurse implement? **Select all that apply.**
    a. Place the patient in semi-Fowler's position.
    b. Place the NG tube on intermittent suction.
    c. Monitor NG drainage, which should be bile-tinged and contain blood.
    d. Keep the patient NPO.
    e. Check blood glucose often.
    f. Monitor for signs of hypovolemia to prevent shock.

30. What is the **most** common and serious complication after a Whipple procedure?
    a. Diabetes mellitus
    b. Wound infection
    c. Fistula development
    d. Bowel obstruction

31. Which are manifestations of pancreatic cancer? **Select all that apply.**
    a. Light-colored urine and dark-colored stools
    b. Anorexia and weight loss
    c. Splenomegaly
    d. Ascites
    e. Leg or calf pain
    f. Weakness and fatigue

32. The nurse is teaching a patient and family how to prevent exacerbations of chronic pancreatitis. Which teaching point does the nurse include?
    a. Moderation in the use of caffeinated beverages
    b. Avoidance of alcohol and nicotine
    c. Consume a bland, high-fat, low-protein diet
    d. Regular exercise, emphasizing aerobic activities

33. The patient is to continue pancreatic enzyme replacement therapy (PERT) after discharge. Which statement indicates that the patient understands teaching about this therapy?
    a. "I will take the enzymes before meals with a full glass of water."
    b. "I will take the enzymes after I take my ranitidine."
    c. "I will mix the enzymes with chopped meat."
    d. "I will chew the capsules before swallowing the enzymes."

34. Which are potential cardiovascular complications for a patient after surgery for a Whipple procedure? **Select all that apply.**
    a. Thrombophlebitis
    b. Pulmonary embolism
    c. Myocardial infarction
    d. Heart failure
    e. Renal failure
    f. Hemorrhage at anastomosis sites with hypovolemia

35. Which abnormal laboratory findings are cardinal findings in acute pancreatitis? **Select all that apply.**
    a. Elevated serum lipase
    b. Increased serum amylase
    c. Decreased serum trypsin
    d. Elevated serum elastase
    e. Decreased serum glucose
    f. Elevated bilirubin

36. Which are advantages of minimally invasive surgery (MIS) laparoscopic cholecystectomy? **Select all that apply.**
    a. Complications are uncommon.
    b. The mortality is similar to traditional cholecystectomy.
    c. Patients recovery more rapidly.
    d. Postoperative pain is less severe.
    e. Bile duct injuries are rare.
    f. IV antibiotics are never needed because of decreased infection rates

37. What is one of the main advantages of cholecystectomy by the natural orifice transluminal endoscopic surgery (NOTES) procedure?
    a. Very small visible incisions
    b. Jackson-Pratt drain removes excess fluid
    c. No visible incision lines
    d. Resumption of normal activities the day of surgery

38. Which is a key feature of pancreatic cancer?
    a. Anorexia
    b. Weight gain
    c. Pale urine
    d. Dark-colored stools

39. The patient with acute necrotizing pancreatitis experiences a temperature spike to 104°F (40°C). What does the nurse suspect?
    a. Pancreatic pseudocyst
    b. Pancreatic abscess
    c. Chronic pancreatitis
    d. Pancreatic cancer

40. The nurse is collaborating with the dietitian to provide diet teaching for a patient with chronic pancreatitis and his family. Which are important teaching points for this teaching plan? **Select all that apply.**
    a. The patient will need increased calorie intake (4000-6000) per day to maintain weight.
    b. Be sure to include foods that are high in fat because they are essential for healing.
    c. Alcohol intake should be avoided.
    d. Provide a bland diet with frequent meals.
    e. Avoid irritating substances such as caffeinated beverages which stimulate the GI system.
    f. Add rich foods to the diet to help meet the caloric requirements.

60 CHAPTER

Care of Patients with Malnutrition: Undernutrition and Obesity

1. The nurse is assisting a patient who follows a lactovegetarian diet to fill out a menu. Based on this diet, which foods could the patient select for breakfast? **Select all that apply.**
   a. Milk
   b. Scrambled eggs
   c. Toast
   d. Sausage
   e. Cereal
   f. String cheese

2. The nurse is assisting a patient who follows a lacto-ovovegetarian diet to fill out a menu. Based on this diet, which foods could the patient select for breakfast? **Select all that apply.**
   a. Milk
   b. Scrambled eggs
   c. Toast
   d. Sausage
   e. Cereal
   f. Tuna fish

3. When caloric energy is inadequate, what does the body use for energy?
   a. Carbohydrates
   b. Proteins
   c. Glucose
   d. Fats

4. Which statement by the new graduate nurse about nutritional assessment requires clarification by the student's mentor?
   a. "A complete nutritional assessment must be done for every patient admitted to the hospital."
   b. "A nutritional screening must be completed on every patient admitted to the hospital."
   c. "An intentional weight loss of 10% within a 6-month period should be evaluated."
   d. "Measurement of height and weight are part of the nutritional assessment."

5. Which activity of a nutritional screening can be delegated to the unlicensed assistive personnel (UAP)?
   a. Review of the patient's nutritional history
   b. Review of the patient's laboratory data
   c. Obtaining the patient's height and weight
   d. Psychosocial assessment of the patient

6. Which signs/symptoms in an older adult can be an indication of "failure to thrive"? **Select all that apply.**
   a. Weakness
   b. Slow walking speed
   c. Decreased meal enjoyment
   d. Low physical activity
   e. Unintentional weight loss
   f. Exhaustion

7. The nurse is providing teaching about the risk factors for malnutrition for a group of older adults. What factors does the nurse emphasize in the teaching plan? **Select all that apply.**
   a. Poor dental health
   b. Hypersecretion of saliva
   c. Depression
   d. Chronic diarrhea
   e. Lack of transportation
   f. Acute or chronic pain

8. What is the **priority** nursing intervention for a patient who is malnourished?
   a. Determine the patient's food preferences.
   b. Provide the patient with high-calorie, high-protein food.
   c. Weigh the patient.
   d. Offer the patient snacks.

9. The nurse is caring for three patients who have undergone bariatric surgery. Which activity is **most** appropriate for the nurse to delegate to the unlicensed assistive personnel (UAP)?
   a. Give analgesics about 1 hour before mealtimes.
   b. Document the percentage of food eaten at mealtimes.
   c. Assess the patient's food preferences.
   d. Teach the patient about portion control.

10. After the unlicensed assistive personnel (UAP) tells the nurse that an older patient will not eat dinner, the nurse enters the patient's room to assess the situation. Which factors likely contribute to the patient's lack of desire to eat? **Select all that apply.**
    a. An emesis basin is on the bedside table.
    b. The volume of the television is loud.
    c. The food is cold.
    d. Housekeeping staff is in the room disinfecting the bathroom.
    e. Cartons and packages are opened, and food has been cut into bite-sized pieces.
    f. The patient's roommate has two adults and three children visiting.

11. The nurse is teaching a male patient about the 2015 Dietary Guidelines for Americans. Which statement by the patient indicates a need for additional teaching?
    a. "I'll follow a healthy eating pattern across my life span."
    b. "I'll limit my alcohol intake to 5 drinks per day."
    c. "I'll increase my intake of fruits and vegetables."
    d. "I'll limit added sugar and salt in my diet."

12. Which manifestation(s) would the nurse expect to see in a patient with a vitamin D deficit?
    a. Swollen, bleeding gums
    b. Hepatomegaly
    c. Osteomalacia, bone pain, rickets
    d. Xerosis of conjunctiva

13. The patient has alopecia. Which nutritional deficiency is the likely cause?
    a. Zinc
    b. Vitamin A
    c. Riboflavin
    d. Vitamin C

14. What is the **most** reliable indicator of fluid status?
    a. Intake and output
    b. Trends in weight
    c. Skin turgor
    d. Edema

15. The nurse hears the unlicensed assistive personnel (UAP) instructing a new UAP about obtaining patients' weights. Which statements by the UAP indicate a need for clarification? **Select all that apply.**
    a. "It is best to weigh the patients before breakfast."
    b. "Just ask the patients how much they weigh."
    c. "You can weigh the patients whenever you have time during your shift."
    d. "Weigh the patients while they are in minimal clothing and no shoes."
    e. "Ambulatory patients can be weighed on the upright scales."
    f. "Bedridden patients are weighed using a bed scale."

16. Which is the **most** accurate way to obtain a height measurement for a patient who cannot stand?
    a. Review the patient's old chart.
    b. Ask the patient's family member.
    c. Estimate height based on the patient's position in bed.
    d. Use a sliding blade knee height caliper.

17. Which statements about body mass index (BMI) measurements are accurate? **Select all that apply.**
    a. It is a measure of nutritional status that varies according to frame size.
    b. It is based on a formula using height and weight.
    c. Health risks are associated with BMIs > (greater than) 25.
    d. It indirectly estimates total fat scores.
    e. There are no health risks associated with a low BMI.
    f. Older adults should have a BMI between 23 and 27.

18. The nurse is providing discharge instructions to the family of an older female patient who was admitted for failure to thrive. The patient has a history of osteoarthritis, stroke, and dementia. What information does the nurse include to promote nutritional intake? **Select all that apply.**
    a. Do not allow her to get out of bed while eating.
    b. Withhold analgesics prior to meals.
    c. Be sure she has her glasses and hearing aid on.
    d. Encourage self-feeding as much as possible.
    e. Keep environmental noise to a minimum.
    f. Ask the patient about food likes and dislikes.

19. The nurse is assessing a patient with acquired immune deficiency syndrome (AIDS) who has muscle wasting related to poor nutrition. How does the nurse interpret this finding?
    a. Cachexia
    b. Candidiasis
    c. Protein catabolism
    d. Positive nitrogen balance

20. Which characteristics are consistent with bulimia nervosa? **Select all that apply.**
    a. It is self-induced starvation.
    b. There are episodes of binge eating.
    c. Binge eating is followed by purging.
    d. It is most often seen in older adults.
    e. It is most often seen in teens and young adults.
    f. It results from a strong fear of becoming fat.

21. The nurse assesses for which potential complications in a patient who is malnourished? **Select all that apply.**
    a. Poor wound healing
    b. Intolerance to heat
    c. Infection
    d. Lethargy
    e. Edema
    f. Increased activity tolerance

22. Which intervention does the nurse delegate to the unlicensed assistive personnel (UAP) to promote nutritional intake for an older patient?
    a. Feed the patient even if he/she is able to self-feed.
    b. Assess which foods the patient likes to eat.
    c. Administer analgesic medication before meals.
    d. Assist the patient to sit up in a chair for meals.

23. Which laboratory test is a sensitive indicator of protein deficiency in a malnourished patient?
    a. Cholesterol
    b. Total lymphocyte count (TLC)
    c. Serum albumin
    d. Prealbumin

24. Which lab value is usually low in patients with malabsorption, liver disease, pernicious anemia, terminal cancer, and sepsis?
    a. Cholesterol
    b. Hematocrit
    c. Hemoglobin
    d. Albumin

25. The nurse is providing discharge instructions to a patient who is malnourished and will be taking iron supplements at home. Which statement by the patient indicates a correct understanding of the instructions?
    a. "These supplements may cause me to have diarrhea."
    b. "I will take these supplements before or with my meals."
    c. "I will limit my fiber intake from now on."
    d. "I will limit my fluid intake from now on."

26. Total enteral nutrition (TEN) is contraindicated for which patient?
    a. Older adult receiving chemotherapy
    b. Patient who has had a stroke and has dysphagia
    c. Patient who has had extensive jaw and mouth surgery
    d. Patient with intestinal obstruction that has progressed to diffuse peritonitis

27. The patient is receiving intermittent feedings of a specified amount at specified times through a feeding tube. Which type of feeding is the patient receiving?
    a. Bolus feeding tube
    b. Continuous feeding tube
    c. Cycle feeding tube
    d. Gravity tube feeding

28. What is the **most** reliable method to confirm initial placement of nasoduodenal or nasogastric (NG) tube placement?
    a. Auscultation
    b. X-ray
    c. Capnometry
    d. Testing pH of gastric contents

29. After initial placement of nasoduodenal and NG tubes is confirmed, how often must the placement be checked? **Select all that apply.**
    a. Before intermittent feeding
    b. Before medication administration
    c. Every 4-8 hours during feeding
    d. It is not necessary to recheck placement.
    e. According to facility policy
    f. Check every 12 hours after flush with saline.

30. The nurse is using capnometry testing to check NG tube placement prior to medication administration and the capnometry test is positive for carbon dioxide. What action does the nurse take?
    a. Administer the medication orally.
    b. Remove the NG tube.
    c. Administer the medication through the NG tube.
    d. Verify placement by auscultation.

31. The nurse is caring for a patient receiving a continuous feeding through an NG tube. Which position is **best** to prevent aspiration?
    a. Semi-Fowler's
    b. Trendelenburg
    c. Supine
    d. Sims'

32. Which interventions are necessary to provide safe, quality care to a patient receiving enteral tube feeding? **Select all that apply.**
    a. Check the residual volume every 4-6 hours.
    b. Change the feeding bag and tubing every 12 hours.
    c. Keep the head of the bed elevated at least 30 degrees.
    d. Use clean technique when changing the feeding system.
    e. Allow closed system containers to hang for 24 hours.
    f. Monitor for complications especially constipation.

33. A patient is receiving a tube feeding. Which action by the student nurse requires intervention by the supervising nurse?
    a. Weighing the patient
    b. Placing food coloring in the tube feeding to assess for aspiration
    c. Discarding any unused open cans of feeding solution after 24 hours
    d. Monitoring the patient for the development of diarrhea

34. Which statement about a patient with a tube feeding indicates **best** practice for patient safety and quality care?
    a. If the tube becomes clogged, use 30 mL of water for flushing, while applying gentle pressure with a 50-mL piston syringe.
    b. Use cranberry juice to flush the tube if it is clogged.
    c. When administering medications, use cold water to dissolve the drug before administering it.
    d. Administer drugs down the feeding tube without flushing first, but flush the feeding tube after the drug is given.

35. A patient in a starvation state has been started on enteral feedings. The nurse assesses the patient and finds shallow respirations, weakness, acute confusion, and oozing from the IV site. What does the nurse suspect is happening in this patient?
    a. Septicemia
    b. Hypoglycemia
    c. Aspiration
    d. Refeeding syndrome

36. Which statement describes the correct method of testing the pH of gastrointestinal (GI) contents at the bedside?
    a. The tube is in the stomach if the pH reading is 8.0.
    b. Before aspirating the GI contents, flush the tube with 10 mL of air.
    c. If the patient takes certain medications such as H2 blockers, the pH of the stomach is usually 2.0.
    d. Wait at least 1 hour after drug administration before assessing the pH of GI contents.

37. A patient receiving intravenous fat emulsions should be monitored closely for which manifestations of fat overload syndrome? **Select all that apply.**
    a. Increased triglycerides
    b. Clotting problems
    c. Fever
    d. Multisystem organ failure
    e. Excessive weight gain
    f. Infection

38. The nurse is assessing a patient receiving total parenteral nutrition (TPN) at 100 mL/hour. The TPN solution has 50 mL left in the bag. The nurse looks for the next bag of TPN, but it is not on the unit. When the pharmacy is called, the nurse is told it will take at least 1 hour for the next bag of TPN solution to be delivered. What does the nurse do?
    a. Call the health care provider.
    b. Administer 10% dextrose/water (D/W) until the TPN is available.
    c. Prepare to treat the patient for hyperglycemia.
    d. Cap the TPN line until the next TPN solution is available.

39. Which definition **best** describes morbid obesity?
    a. Weight that has a severely negative effect on health
    b. Excessive amount of body fat when compared to lean body mass
    c. Increase in body weight for height as compared to a standard
    d. Excessive amount of body weight requiring surgical intervention

40. Which statements about obesity are accurate? **Select all that apply.**
    a. Waist-to-hip ratio (WHR) is a strong predictor of colon cancer.
    b. Obesity is the second-leading cause of preventable deaths in the United States.
    c. Genetics have been found to have no role in obesity.
    d. Drug therapy is the first-line treatment for obesity.
    e. Waist circumference is a stronger predictor of coronary artery disease than is BMI.
    f. Obese adults weigh at least 20% above the upper limit of the normal range for ideal body weight.

41. The nurse is performing an admission assessment on a morbidly obese patient. Which common complications of obesity does the nurse assess for? **Select all that apply.**
    a. Type 1 diabetes mellitus
    b. Metabolic syndrome
    c. Urinary incontinence
    d. Gout
    e. Early osteoarthritis
    f. Decreased would healing

42. Which prescribed drugs can contribute to weight gain when they are taken on a long-term basis? **Select all that apply.**
    a. Estrogens
    b. Acetaminophen
    c. Corticosteroids
    d. Nonsteroidal antiinflammatory drugs (NSAIDs)
    e. Antiepileptics
    f. Antidepressants

43. Which drugs are available for long-term treatment of obesity? **Select all that apply.**
    a. Phentermine-topiramate
    b. Lorcaserin
    c. Sibutramine
    d. Orlistat
    e. Diethylpropion
    f. Phentermine hydrochloride

44. The nurse is caring for a patient after bariatric surgery. What is the nursing **priority** for postoperative care for this patient?
    a. Nutritional intake
    b. Pain management
    c. Prevention of infection
    d. Airway management

45. Which criteria make a patient a candidate for surgical treatment of obesity? **Select all that apply.**
    a. Repeated failure with nonsurgical interventions
    b. Waist circumference greater than 40 inches
    c. A BMI greater than or equal to 40
    d. Waist-to-hip ratio of greater than 0.95
    e. Weight more than 100% above ideal body weight
    f. BMI of 35 or greater along with additional risk factors

46. A patient comes to the clinic after having bariatric surgery and says, "After I eat, I feel really funny. My heart races, I feel nauseated, and my abdomen cramps up. I even have diarrhea." What does the nurse suspect is happening with this patient?
    a. Hyperglycemia
    b. Intestinal obstruction
    c. Peritonitis
    d. Dumping syndrome

47. The nurse is assessing a patient after bariatric surgery. The patient has increased back pain, is restless, has a heart rate of 126/minute, and has only 15 mL of urine output for the past hour. What does the nurse suspect?
    a. Anastomotic leak
    b. Hypovolemic shock
    c. Bowel obstruction
    d. Hemorrhage

48. After bariatric surgery, which interventions does the nurse implement to prevent complications? **Select all that apply.**
    a. Apply an abdominal binder.
    b. Place the patient in semi-Fowler's position.
    c. Keep the patient on bedrest for 24 hours.
    d. Monitor oxygen saturation.
    e. Apply sequential compression stockings.
    f. Observe skinfolds for redness and excoriation.

49. The nurse is preparing discharge instructions for a patient after bariatric surgery. Which key teaching points will the nurse be sure to include? **Select all that apply.**
    a. Diet progression, importance of vitamin supplements and hydration
    b. Taking analgesics every 4 hours whether there is pain or not
    c. Restrictions on activities such as heavy lifting
    d. Following the health care provider's instructions for progression of activity
    e. Covering the wound during bath or shower
    f. Reporting signs of infection to the health care provider immediately

50. The patient who had bariatric surgery and is to be discharged asks the nurse when to expect the panniculectomy surgery. What is the nurse's **best** response?
    a. Usually in 6-8 months
    b. Usually in 12-18 months
    c. Usually in 18-24 months
    d. When your weight stabilizes

51. The nurse understands that a patient loses weight under which circumstance?
    a. The patient takes in more calories than are used.
    b. The patient takes in as many calories as are needed.
    c. The patient takes in fewer calories than are used.
    d. The patient takes in enough calories for daily activity

52. The nurse is assisting a vegan patient to complete a lunch menu. Which food would the nurse suggest?
    a. Black beans over rice
    b. Baked beans with bacon
    c. Tuna fish casserole
    d. Green salad with olive oil dressing

53. What dietary advice does the nurse give a patient to prevent constipation while maintaining good nutrition?
    a. "Have a cup of coffee every morning with your breakfast."
    b. "Drink eight glasses of water and eats lots of fiber."
    c. "Get at least 30 minutes of exercise every day."
    d. "Consume a protein source with each meal."

54. The nurse is providing care for a patient receiving total enteral nutrition (TEN). The patient has severe diarrhea with a foul odor. What does the nurse suspect?
    a. Dehydration
    b. Excessive residual
    c. Infection around the feeding tube
    d. Infection with *Clostridium difficile*

55. Which adipokine hormone is known as the hunger hormone?
    a. Ghrelin
    b. Cholecystokinin
    c. Leptin
    d. Resistin

56. The patient with obesity asks the nurse about the benefits of exercise. Which benefits should the nurse teach about? **Select all that apply.**
    a. Increased lean muscle
    b. Increased body fat
    c. Decreased body weight
    d. Lower death rates at any age
    e. Increased cardiovascular health
    f. Improved psychological well-being

57. Which surgical procedure is **not** appropriate for a patient with morbid obesity?
    a. Gastric restriction
    b. Liposuction
    c. Roux-en-Y gastric bypass
    d. Panniculectomy

Assessment of the Endocrine System

1. Which glands are parts of the endocrine system? **Select all that apply.**
   a. Thyroid
   b. Occipital
   c. Parathyroid
   d. Adrenal
   e. Pituitary
   f. Frontal

2. What is the name of the substance secreted by the endocrine glands?
   a. Vasoactive amines
   b. Chemotaxins
   c. Hormones
   d. Cytotoxins

3. Which mechanism is used to transport substances produced by the endocrine glands to their target tissue?
   a. Lymph system
   b. Bloodstream
   c. Direct seeding
   d. Gastrointestinal system

4. Which hormones are secreted by the posterior pituitary gland? **Select all that apply.**
   a. Testosterone
   b. Oxytocin
   c. Growth hormone (GH)
   d. Antidiuretic hormone (ADH)
   e. Cortisol
   f. Prolactin (PRL)

5. Which hormones are secreted by the thyroid gland? **Select all that apply.**
   a. Calcitonin
   b. Somatostatin
   c. Glucagon
   d. Thyroxine (T_4)
   e. Aldosterone
   f. Triiodothyronine (T_3)

6. A patient has a low serum cortisol level. Which hormone would the nurse expect will be secreted to correct this?
   a. Thyroid-stimulating hormone (TSH)
   b. Adrenocorticotropic hormone
   c. Parathyroid hormone
   d. Antidiuretic hormone

7. The target tissue for antidiuretic hormone (ADH) is which organ?
   a. Hypothalamus
   b. Thyroid
   c. Ovary
   d. Kidney

8. Which statements about hormones and the endocrine system are accurate? **Select all that apply.**
   a. There are specific normal blood levels of each hormone.
   b. Hormones exert their effects on specific target tissues.
   c. Each hormone can bind with multiple receptor sites.
   d. The endocrine system works independently to regulate homeostasis.
   e. More than one hormone can be stimulated before the target tissue is affected.
   f. Endocrine disorders are always related to an excess of one or more hormones.

9. The binding of a hormone to a specific receptor site is an example of which endocrine process?
   a. "Lock and key" manner
   b. Negative feedback mechanism
   c. Neuroendocrine regulation
   d. "Fight-or-flight" response

10. What are tropic hormones?
    a. Hormones that trigger female and male sex characteristics.
    b. Hormones that have a direct effect on final target tissues
    c. Hormones produced by the anterior pituitary gland that stimulate other endocrine glands
    d. Hormones that are synthesized in the hypothalamus and stored in the posterior pituitary gland

11. Which hormone is directly suppressed when circulating levels of cortisol are **above** normal?
    a. Corticotropin-releasing hormone (CRH)
    b. Antidiuretic hormone (ADH)
    c. Adrenocorticotropic hormone (ACTH)
    d. Growth hormone–releasing hormone (GH-RH)

12. The maintenance of internal body temperature at approximately 98.6°F (37°C) is an example of which endocrine process?
    a. "Lock and key" manner
    b. Neuroendocrine regulation
    c. Positive feedback mechanism
    d. Stimulus-response theory

13. Which statements about the pituitary gland are correct? **Select all that apply.**
    a. The main role of the anterior pituitary is to secrete tropic hormones.
    b. The posterior pituitary gland stores hormones produced by the hypothalamus.
    c. The anterior pituitary is connected to the thalamus gland.
    d. The anterior pituitary releases stored hormones produced by the hypothalamus.
    e. The anterior pituitary gland secretes gonadotropins.
    f. The pituitary gland releases hormones in response to diet, lifestyle and drugs.

14. The anterior pituitary gland secretes tropic hormones in response to which hormones from the hypothalamus?
    a. Releasing hormones
    b. Target tissue hormones
    c. Growth hormones
    d. Demand hormones

15. Which statement about pituitary hormones is correct?
    a. Adrenocorticotropic hormone (ACTH) acts on the adrenal medulla.
    b. Follicle-stimulating hormone (FSH) stimulates sperm production in men.
    c. Growth hormone promotes protein catabolism.
    d. Vasopressin decreases systolic blood pressure.

16. Which statement about the gonads is correct?
    a. Gonads are reproductive glands found in males only.
    b. The function of the hormones begins at birth in low, undetectable levels.
    c. The placenta secretes testosterone for the development of male external genitalia.
    d. External genitalia maturation is stimulated by gonadotropins during puberty.

17. Which statements about the adrenal glands are correct? **Select all that apply.**
    a. The cortex secretes androgens in men and women.
    b. Catecholamines are secreted from the cortex.
    c. Glucocorticoids are secreted by the medulla.
    d. The medulla secretes hormones essential for life.
    e. The cortex secretes aldosterone that maintains extracellular fluid volume.
    f. Serum potassium level affects the release of aldosterone from the adrenal cortex.

18. Which is the major function of the hormones produced by the adrenal cortex?
    a. "Fight-or-flight" response
    b. Control of potassium, sodium, and water
    c. Regulation of cell growth
    d. Calcium and stress regulation

19. Which statements about the hormone cortisol being secreted by the adrenal cortex are accurate? **Select all that apply.**
    a. Cortisol peaks occur late in the day, with lowest points 12 hours after each peak.
    b. Cortisol has an effect on the body's immune function.
    c. Stress causes an increase in the production of cortisol.
    d. Blood levels of cortisol have no effect on its secretion.
    e. Cortisol affects carbohydrate, protein, and fat metabolism.
    f. Emotional stability is affected by a person's cortisol level.

20. Which assessment findings does the nurse monitor in response to catecholamines released by the adrenal medulla? **Select all that apply.**
    a. Increased heart rate
    b. Increased blood pressure
    c. Increased perspiration
    d. Constriction of pupils
    e. Increased blood glucose
    f. Increased motility in the gastrointestinal tract

21. Which statements about the thyroid gland and its hormones are correct? **Select all that apply.**
    a. The gland is located in the posterior neck below the cricoid cartilage.
    b. The gland has two lobes joined by a thin tissue called the isthmus.
    c. T_4 and T_3 are two thyroid hormones.
    d. Thyroid hormones increase red blood cell production.
    e. Thyroid hormone production depends on dietary intake of iodine and potassium.
    f. Respiratory rate and drive are affected by thyroid hormones in adults.

22. Which hormone responds to a low serum calcium blood level by increasing bone resorption?
    a. Parathyroid hormone (PTH)
    b. T_4
    c. T_3
    d. Calcitonin

23. Which hormone responds to an elevated serum calcium blood level by decreasing bone resorption?
    a. Parathyroid hormone (PTH)
    b. T_4
    c. T_3
    d. Calcitonin

24. Which statements about T_3 and T_4 hormones are correct? **Select all that apply.**
    a. The hormones affect basal metabolic rate.
    b. Hypothalamus is stimulated by cold and stress to secrete thyrotropin-releasing hormone (TRH).
    c. These hormones need intake of protein and iodine for production.
    d. Circulating hormone in the blood directly affects the production of thyroid stimulating hormone (TSH).
    e. T_3 and T_4 increase oxygen use in tissues.
    f. Very little circulating T_3 and T_4 is bound to plasma proteins.

25. Which are the target organs of parathyroid hormone (PTH) in the regulation of calcium and phosphorus? **Select all that apply.**
    a. Stomach
    b. Kidney
    c. Bone
    d. Gastrointestinal tract
    e. Thyroid gland
    f. Pancreas

26. Which statement about the pancreas is correct?
    a. Endocrine functions of the pancreas include secretion of digestive enzymes.
    b. Exocrine functions of the pancreas include secretion of glucagon and insulin.
    c. The islets of Langerhans are the only source of somatostatin secretion.
    d. Somatostatin inhibits pancreatic secretion of glucagon and insulin.

27. Which statement about glucagon secretion is correct?
    a. It is stimulated by an increase in blood glucose levels.
    b. It is stimulated by a decrease in amino acid levels.
    c. It exerts its primary effect on the pancreas.
    d. It acts to increase blood glucose levels.

28. Which statements about insulin secretion are correct? **Select all that apply.**
    a. Insulin levels increase following the ingestion of a meal.
    b. Insulin is stimulated primarily by fat ingestion.
    c. Basal levels are secreted continuously.
    d. Insulin promotes glycogenolysis and gluconeogenesis.
    e. Carbohydrate intake is the main trigger for insulin secretion.
    f. Insulin increases glucose uptake by the cells.

29. In addition to the pancreas that secretes insulin, which gland secretes hormones that affect protein, carbohydrate, and fat metabolism?
    a. Posterior pituitary
    b. Thyroid
    c. Ovaries
    d. Parathyroid

30. The bloodstream delivers glucose to the cells for energy production. Which hormone controls the cells' use of glucose?
    a. T_4
    b. Growth hormone
    c. Adrenal steroids
    d. Insulin

31. Which disease involves a disorder of the islets of Langerhans?
    a. Diabetes insipidus
    b. Diabetes mellitus
    c. Addison's disease
    d. Cushing's disease

32. Which endocrine tissues are most commonly found to have reduced function as a result of aging? **Select all that apply.**
    a. Hypothalamus
    b. Ovaries
    c. Testes
    d. Pancreas
    e. Thyroid gland
    f. Parathyroid glands

33. Which statement about age-related changes in older adults and the endocrine system is true?
    a. All hormone levels are elevated.
    b. Thyroid hormone levels decrease.
    c. Adrenal glands enlarge.
    d. The thyroid gland enlarges.

34. In the older adult female, which physiologic changes occur as a result of decreased function of the ovaries?
    a. Decreased bone density and estrogen production
    b. Decreased sensitivity of peripheral tissues to the effects of insulin
    c. Decreased urine-concentrating ability of the kidneys
    d. Decreased metabolic rate

35. An older adult reports a lack of energy and not being able to do the usual daily activities without several naps during the day. Which problem may these symptoms indicate that is often seen in the older adult?
    a. Hypothyroidism
    b. Hyperparathyroidism
    c. Overproduction of cortisol
    d. Underproduction of glucagon

36. The nurse is performing a physical assessment of a patient's endocrine system. Which gland can be palpated?
    a. Pancreas
    b. Thyroid
    c. Adrenal glands
    d. Parathyroids

37. Which statement about performing a physical assessment of the thyroid gland is correct?
    a. The thyroid gland is easily palpated in all patients.
    b. The patient is instructed to swallow sips of water to aid palpation.
    c. The anterior approach is preferred for thyroid palpation.
    d. The thumbs are used to palpate the thyroid lobes.

38. Which are diagnostic methods to measure patient hormone levels? **Select all that apply.**
    a. MRI scans
    b. Suppression testing
    c. 24-hour urine testing
    d. Chromatographic assay
    e. Needle biopsy
    f. Stimulation testing

39. What is the correct nursing action before beginning a 24-hour urine collection for endocrine studies?
    a. Place each voided specimen in a separate collection container.
    b. Check whether any preservatives are needed in the collection container.
    c. Start the collection with the first voided urine.
    d. Weigh the patient before beginning the collection.

40. Which instructions are included when teaching a patient about urine collection for endocrine studies? **Select all that apply.**
    a. Fast before starting the urine collection.
    b. Measure the urine in mL rather than ounces.
    c. Empty the bladder completely and then start timing.
    d. Time the test for exactly the instructed number of hours.
    e. Avoid taking any unnecessary drugs during endocrine testing.
    f. Empty the bladder at the end of the time period and keep that specimen.

41. Which are the types of imaging tests that may be used for an endocrine assessment? **Select all that apply.**
    a. Ultrasonography
    b. Skull x-ray
    c. Chest x-ray
    d. Magnetic resonance imaging (MRI)
    e. Computed tomography (CT)
    f. Abdominal x-ray

42. A patient is suspected of having a pituitary tumor. Which radiographic test aids in determining this diagnosis?
    a. Skull x-rays
    b. Magnetic resonance imaging (MRI) with contrast
    c. Angiography
    d. Ultrasound

43. After an ultrasound of the thyroid gland, which diagnostic test determines the need for surgical intervention for thyroid nodules?
    a. CT scan
    b. Magnetic resonance imaging (MRI)
    c. Angiography
    d. Needle biopsy

44. A patient is at risk for falling related to the effect of pathologic fractures as a result of bone demineralization. Which endocrine problem is this pertinent to?
    a. Underproduction of PTH
    b. Overproduction of PTH
    c. Underproduction of thyroid hormone
    d. Overproduction of thyroid hormone

45. When blood glucose levels start to rise above normal insulin is secreted. Insulin increases glucose uptake by the cells, causing a decrease in blood glucose levels. Which phenomenon does this exemplify?
    a. Simple negative feedback hormone response
    b. Complex interaction for negative feedback
    c. Simple positive feedback hormone response
    d. Complex interaction for positive feedback

46. A patient develops an endocrine disorder related to insufficient intake of iodide-containing foods. The nurse recognizes that this is an example of which priority concept related to the endocrine system?
    a. Fluid and electrolyte imbalance
    b. Nutrition
    c. Elimination
    d. Acid-base balance

62 CHAPTER

Care of Patients with Pituitary and Adrenal Gland Problems

1. Decreased production of all of the anterior pituitary hormones results in which condition?
   a. Adenohypophysis
   b. Panhypopituitarism
   c. Primary pituitary dysfunction
   d. Secondary pituitary dysfunction

2. A malfunctioning posterior pituitary gland can result in which disorders? **Select all that apply.**
   a. Hypothyroidism
   b. Altered sexual function
   c. Diabetes insipidus (DI)
   d. Growth retardation
   e. Syndrome of inappropriate antidiuretic hormone (SIADH)
   f. Virilization

3. A malfunctioning anterior pituitary gland can result in which disorders? **Select all that apply.**
   a. Pituitary hypofunction
   b. Pituitary hyperfunction
   c. Diabetes insipidus
   d. Hypothyroidism
   e. Osteoporosis
   f. Syndrome of inappropriate antidiuretic hormone secretion

4. The assessment findings of a male patient with an anterior pituitary tumor include reports of changes in secondary sex characteristics, such as episodes of impotence and decreased libido. The nurse explains to the patient that these findings are a result of overproduction of which hormone?
   a. Gonadotropins inhibiting prolactin (PRL)
   b. Thyroid hormone inhibiting prolactin (PRL)
   c. Prolactin (PRL) inhibiting secretion of gonadotropins
   d. Steroids inhibiting production of sex hormones

5. When reviewing the medication record for a patient being treated for a PRL-secreting tumor, the nurse is **most** likely to note the use of which medication?
   a. Dopamine agonists
   b. Antidiuretic hormone
   c. Corticosteroids
   d. Growth hormone (GH)

6. A 30-year-old female patient is prescribed bromocriptine. Which information does the nurse teach the patient? **Select all that apply.**
   a. Get up slowly from a lying position.
   b. Take medication on an empty stomach.
   c. Take daily for purposes of raising GH levels to reduce symptoms of acromegaly.
   d. Begin therapy with a maintenance level dose.
   e. Report watery nasal discharge to the health care provider immediately.
   f. If pregnancy occurs the drug is stopped immediately.

7. Patients diagnosed with an anterior pituitary tumor can have symptoms of acromegaly. These symptoms are a result of overproduction of which hormone?
   a. ACTH
   b. PRL
   c. Gonadotropins
   d. GH

8. The nurse is performing an assessment of an adult patient with new-onset acromegaly. What does the nurse expect to find?
   a. Extremely long arms and legs
   b. Thickened lips
   c. Changes in menses with infertility
   d. Rough, extremely dry skin

9. When analyzing laboratory values, the nurse expects to find which value as a direct result of overproduction of GH?
   a. Hyperglycemia
   b. Hyperphosphatemia
   c. Hypocalcemia
   d. Hypercalcemia

10. In caring for a patient with hyperpituitarism, which symptoms does the nurse expect the patient to report? **Select all that apply.**
    a. Joint pain
    b. Visual disturbances
    c. Changes in menstruation
    d. Increased libido
    e. Headache
    f. Fatigue

11. A deficiency of which anterior pituitary hormones is considered life-threatening? **Select all that apply.**
    a. Growth hormone (GH)
    b. Melanocyte-stimulating hormone (MSH)
    c. Prolactin (PRL)
    d. Thyroid-stimulating hormone (TSH)
    e. Adrenocorticotropic hormone (ACTH)
    f. Luteinizing hormone (LH)

12. Which statements about the etiology of hypopituitarism are correct? **Select all that apply.**
    a. Dysfunction can result from radiation treatment to the head or brain.
    b. Dysfunction can result from infection or a brain tumor.
    c. Infarction following systemic shock can result in hypopituitarism.
    d. Severe malnutrition and body fat depletion can depress pituitary gland function.
    e. There is always an underlying cause of hypopituitarism.
    f. Pituitary tumors are the most common cause of hypopituitarism.

13. Which statement about hormone replacement therapy for hypopituitarism is correct?
    a. Once manifestations of hypofunction are corrected, treatment is no longer needed.
    b. The most effective route of androgen replacement is the oral route.
    c. Testosterone replacement therapy is contraindicated in men with prostate cancer.
    d. Clomiphene citrate is used to suppress ovulation in women.

14. A female patient has been prescribed hormone replacement therapy. What does the nurse instruct the patient to do regarding this therapy? **Select all that apply.**
    a. Report any recurrence of symptoms, such as decreased libido, between injections.
    b. Avoid smoking because of the increased risk for cardiovascular complications.
    c. Treat leg pain, especially in the calves, with gentle muscle stretching.
    d. Take measures to reduce risk for hypertension and thrombosis.
    e. Monitor blood pressure at least weekly for potential hypotension.
    f. Regular follow-up visits with the health care provider are essential.

15. A patient requires 100 grams of oral glucose for suppression testing and growth hormone (GH) levels are measured serially for 120 minutes. The results of the suppression testing are abnormal. The nurse assesses for the signs and symptoms of which endocrine disorder?
    a. Adrenal insufficiency
    b. Diabetes insipidus
    c. Hyperpituitarism
    d. Hypothyroidism

16. A patient is recovering from a transsphenoidal hypophysectomy. What postoperative nursing interventions apply to this patient? **Select all that apply.**
    a. Encouraging the patient to perform deep-breathing exercises
    b. Vigorous coughing and deep-breathing exercises
    c. Instructing on the use of a soft-bristled toothbrush for brushing the teeth
    d. Strict monitoring of fluid balance
    e. Hourly neurologic checks for first 24 hours
    f. Instructing the patient to alert the nurse regarding postnasal drip

17. Following a complete hypophysectomy, the patient requires instruction on hormone replacement for which hormones? **Select all that apply.**
    a. Cortisol
    b. Thyroid
    c. Gonadal
    d. Aldosterone
    e. Prolactin (PRL)
    f. Vasopressin

18. After a hypophysectomy, focused assessment and monitoring by the nurse include which factors? **Select all that apply.**
    a. Cognition and mental status
    b. Maintaining bedrest with bedside commode
    c. Possible leakage of cerebrospinal fluid (CSF)
    d. 24-hour intake of fluids and urine output
    e. 24-hour diet recall
    f. Headaches or visual disturbances

19. The nurse is providing care for a patient who had an hypophysectomy by the minimally invasive endoscopic transnasal approach. How is care different for this patient as opposed to a patient with a transsphenoidal hypophysectomy?
    a. The patient is encouraged to cough and deep-breathe to decrease pulmonary complications.
    b. The patient does not have nasal packing of a mustache dressing.
    c. The patient should be taught to floss and rinse his or her mouth frequently.
    d. The patient must be taught that hormone replacement is lifelong.

20. While caring for a postoperative patient following a transsphenoidal hypophysectomy, the nurse observes nasal drainage that is clear with yellow color at the edge. This "halo sign" is indicative of which condition?
    a. Worsening neurologic status of the patient
    b. Drainage of CSF from the patient's nose
    c. Onset of postoperative infection
    d. An expected finding following this surgery

21. A patient with a hypophysectomy can postoperatively experience transient diabetes insipidus (DI). Which manifestation alerts the nurse to this problem?
    a. Urine output much greater than intake
    b. Change in mental status indicating confusion
    c. Laboratory results indicating hyponatremia
    d. Nonpitting edema of the lower extremities

22. The action of antidiuretic hormone (ADH) influences normal kidney function by stimulating which mechanism?
    a. Glomerulus to control the filtration rate
    b. Proximal nephron tubules to reabsorb water
    c. Distal nephron tubules and collecting ducts to reabsorb water
    d. Constriction of glomerular capillaries to prevent loss of protein in urine

23. What is the disorder that results from a deficiency of vasopressin (ADH) from the posterior pituitary gland called?
    a. SIADH
    b. Diabetes insipidus (DI)
    c. Cushing's syndrome
    d. Addison's disease

24. Which statements about diabetes insipidus (DI) are accurate? **Select all that apply.**
    a. It is caused by ADH deficiency.
    b. It is characterized by a decrease in urination.
    c. Urine output of greater than 4 L/24 hours is the first diagnostic indication.
    d. The water loss increases plasma osmolarity.
    e. Nephrogenic DI can be caused by lithium (Eskalith).
    f. Increased thirst is a mechanism of the body to attempt maintaining fluid balance.

25. What does the nurse instruct patients with permanent diabetes insipidus (DI) to do? **Select all that apply.**
    a. Continue vasopressin therapy until symptoms disappear.
    b. Monitor for recurrence of polydipsia and polyuria.
    c. Monitor and record weight daily.
    d. Check urine specific gravity three times a week.
    e. Wear a medical alert bracelet.
    f. Urge the patient to drink fluids in an amount equal to urine output.

26. A hospitalized patient is prescribed desmopressin acetate metered dose spray as a replacement hormone for vasopressin (ADH). Which is an indication for another dose? **Select all that apply.**
    a. Excessive urination
    b. Specific gravity of 1.003
    c. Dark, concentrated urine
    d. Edema in the legs
    e. Decreased urination
    f. Shortness of breath

27. The nurse is caring for a patient with diabetes insipidus (DI). What is the **priority** goal of collaborative care?
    a. Correct the water metabolism problem.
    b. Control blood sugar and blood pH.
    c. Measure urine output, specific gravity, and osmolality hourly.
    d. Monitor closely for respiratory distress.

28. Which medication is used to treat diabetes insipidus (DI)?
    a. Desmopressin acetate
    b. Lithium
    c. Vasopressin
    d. Demeclocycline

29. Which patient's history puts him or her at risk for developing SIADH?
    a. 27-year-old patient on high-dose steroids
    b. 47-year-old hospitalized adult patient with acute renal failure
    c. 58-year-old with small cell lung cancer
    d. Older adult with history of a stroke within the last year

30. Which statement about the pathophysiology of SIADH is correct?
    a. ADH secretion is inhibited in the presence of low plasma osmolality.
    b. Water retention results in dilutional hyponatremia and expanded extracellular fluid (ECF) volume.
    c. The glomerulus is unable to increase its filtration rate to reduce the excess plasma volume.
    d. Renin and aldosterone are released and help decrease the loss of urinary sodium.

31. The effect of increased ADH in the blood results in which effect on the kidney?
    a. Urine concentration tends to decrease.
    b. Glomerular filtration tends to decrease.
    c. Tubular reabsorption of water increases.
    d. Tubular reabsorption of sodium increases.

32. In SIADH, as a result of water retention from excess ADH, which laboratory values does the nurse expect to find? **Select all that apply.**
    a. Increased sodium in urine
    b. Elevated serum sodium level
    c. Increased urine specific gravity
    d. Decreased serum osmolarity
    e. Decreased urine specific gravity
    f. Decreased serum sodium level

33. Which nursing intervention is the **priority** for a patient with SIADH?
    a. Restrict fluid intake.
    b. Monitor neurologic status at least every 2 hours.
    c. Offer ice chips frequently to ease discomfort of dry mouth.
    d. Monitor urine tests for decreased sodium levels and low specific gravity.

34. Which type of IV fluid does the nurse use to treat a patient with SIADH when the serum sodium level is very low?
    a. $D_5$1/2 normal saline
    b. D_5W
    c. 3% normal saline
    d. Normal saline

35. In addition to IV fluids, a patient with SIADH is on a fluid restriction as low as 500 to 600 mL/24 hours. Which serum and urine results demonstrate effectiveness of this treatment? **Select all that apply.**
    a. Decreased urine specific gravity
    b. Decreased serum sodium
    c. Increased urine output
    d. Increased urine specific gravity
    e. Increased serum sodium
    f. Decreased urine output

36. Which medications are used in SIADH to promote water excretion without causing sodium loss? **Select all that apply.**
    a. Tolvaptan
    b. Demeclocycline
    c. Furosemide
    d. Conivaptan
    e. Spironolactone
    f. Hydrochlorothiazide

37. Which statement about pheochromocytoma is correct?
    a. It is most often malignant.
    b. It is a catecholamine-producing tumor.
    c. It is found only in the adrenal medulla.
    d. It is manifested by hypotension.

38. A patient in the emergency department is diagnosed with possible pheochromocytoma. What is the **priority** nursing intervention for this patient?
    a. Monitor the patient's intake and output and urine specific gravity.
    b. Monitor blood pressure for severe hypertension.
    c. Monitor blood pressure for severe hypotension.
    d. Administer medication to increase cardiac output.

39. The nurse expects to perform which diagnostic test for pheochromocytoma?
    a. 24-hour urine collection for sodium, potassium, and glucose
    b. Catecholamine-stimulation test
    c. Administration of beta-adrenergic blocking agent and monitor results
    d. 24-hour urine collection for fractionated metanephrine and catecholamine levels

40. Which intervention applies to a patient with pheochromocytoma?
    a. Assist to sit in a chair for blood pressure monitoring.
    b. Instruct not to smoke, drink coffee, or change positions suddenly.
    c. Encourage to maintain an active exercise schedule including activity such as running.
    d. Encourage one glass of red wine nightly to promote rest.

41. Which intervention is contraindicated for a patient with pheochromocytoma?
    a. Monitoring blood pressure
    b. Palpating the abdomen
    c. Collecting 24-hour urine specimens
    d. Instructing the patient to limit activity

42. Which diuretic is ordered by the health care provider to treat hyperaldosteronism?
    a. Furosemide
    b. Ethacrynic acid
    c. Bumetanide
    d. Spironolactone

43. Which statement about hyperaldosteronism is correct?
    a. Painful "charley horses" are common from hyperkalemia.
    b. It occurs more often in men than in women.
    c. It is a common cause of hypertension in the population.
    d. Hypokalemia and hypertension are the main issues.

44. When diagnosed with Cushing's syndrome, the patient's manifestations are **most likely** related to an excess production of which hormone?
    a. Insulin from the pancreas
    b. ADH from posterior pituitary gland
    c. PRL from anterior pituitary gland
    d. Cortisol from the adrenal cortex

45. What is the **most common** cause of endogenous hypercortisolism, or Cushing's disease?
    a. Pituitary hypoplasia
    b. Insufficient ACTH production
    c. Adrenocortical hormone deficiency
    d. Hyperplasia of the adrenal cortex

46. Which are physical findings of Cushing's disease? **Select all that apply.**
    a. "Moon-faced" appearance
    b. Decreased amount of body hair
    c. Truncal obesity
    d. Coarse facial features
    e. Thin, easily damaged skin
    f. Extremity muscle wasting

47. Which laboratory findings does the nurse expect to find with Cushing's syndrome? **Select all that apply.**
    a. Decreased serum sodium
    b. Increased serum glucose
    c. Increased serum sodium
    d. Increased serum potassium
    e. Decreased serum calcium
    f. Increased lymphocyte count

48. The female patient with Cushing's syndrome expresses concern about the changes in her general appearance. What is the expected outcome for this patient?
    a. To verbalize an understanding that treatment will reverse many of the problems
    b. To ventilate about the frustration of these lifelong physical changes
    c. To verbalize ways to cope with the changes such as joining a support group or changing style of dress
    d. To achieve a personal desired level of sexual functioning

49. Which drug is an adrenal cytotoxic agent used for inoperable adrenal tumors?
    a. Mitotane
    b. Aminoglutethimide
    c. Cyproheptadine
    d. Fludrocortisone

50. Which drug decreases cortisol production?
    a. Mitotane
    b. Aminoglutethimide
    c. Cyproheptadine
    d. Hydrocortisone

51. A patient is scheduled for bilateral adrenalectomy. Steroids will be given before surgery. What is the reasoning behind the administration of this drug?
    a. To promote glycogen storage by the liver for body energy reserves
    b. To compensate for sudden lack of adrenal hormones following surgery
    c. To increase the body's inflammatory response to promote scar formation
    d. To enhance urinary excretion of salt and water following surgery

52. The nurse is teaching a patient being discharged after bilateral adrenalectomy. What medication information does the nurse emphasize in the teaching plan?
    a. The dosage of steroid replacement drugs will be consistent throughout the patient's lifetime.
    b. The steroid drugs should be taken in the evening so as not to interfere with sleep.
    c. The patient should take the drugs on an empty stomach.
    d. The patient should learn how to give himself an intramuscular injection of hydrocortisone.

53. Which statement about a patient with hyperaldosteronism after a successful unilateral adrenalectomy is correct?
    a. The low-sodium diet must be continued postoperatively.
    b. Glucocorticoid replacement therapy is temporary.
    c. Spironolactone must be taken for life.
    d. Additional measures are needed to control hypertension.

54. Which patient is at risk for developing secondary adrenal insufficiency?
    a. Patient who suddenly stops taking high-dose steroid therapy
    b. Patient who tapers the dosages of steroid therapy
    c. Patient deficient in ADH
    d. Patient with an adrenal tumor causing excessive secretion of ACTH

55. An ACTH stimulation test is the **most definitive** test for which disorder?
    a. Adrenal insufficiency
    b. Cushing's syndrome
    c. Pheochromocytoma
    d. Acromegaly

56. Which interventions are necessary for a patient with acute adrenal insufficiency (addisonian crisis)? **Select all that apply.**
    a. IV infusion of normal saline
    b. IV infusion of 3% saline
    c. Hourly glucose monitoring
    d. Insulin administration
    e. IV potassium therapy
    f. Administer IV hydrocortisone sodium

57. A patient in the emergency department who reports lethargy, muscle weakness, nausea, vomiting, and weight loss over the past weeks is diagnosed with addisonian crisis (acute adrenal insufficiency). Which drug(s) does the nurse expect to administer to this patient?
    a. Beta-blocker to control hypertension and dysrhythmias
    b. Hydrocortisone sodium IV along with IM injections of hydrocortisone
    c. IV fluids of $D_5 NS$ with KCl added for dehydration
    d. Spironolactone to promote diuresis

58. The nurse determines that the administration of hydrocortisone for addisonian crisis is effective when which outcome is assessed?
    a. Increased urine output
    b. No signs of pitting edema
    c. Weight gain
    d. Lethargy improving; patient alert and oriented

59. Which interdisciplinary intervention is a preventive measure for adrenocortical insufficiency?
    a. Maintaining diuretic therapy
    b. Instructing the patient on salt restriction
    c. Reducing high-dose glucocorticoid therapy quickly
    d. Reducing high-dose glucocorticoid doses gradually

60. The nurse should instruct a patient who is taking hydrocortisone to report which symptoms to the health care provider for possible dosage adjustment? **Select all that apply.**
    a. Rapid weight gain
    b. Changes in blood pressure
    c. Fluid retention
    d. Gastrointestinal irritation
    e. Urinary incontinence
    f. Round face

61. The patient who is to be discharged with a prescription for prednisone asks the nurse why it is necessary to report any illness to the health care provider. What is the nurse's **best** response?
    a. Because the usual daily dosage may not be adequate during periods of illness or severe stress.
    b. Because you need to be protected from the risk for infection.
    c. Because the health care provider needs to know whenever you are ill.
    d. Because you will need to have your dosage tapered to safely come off of this drug.

62. Which are causes of secondary adrenal insufficiency? **Select all that apply.**
    a. Tuberculosis
    b. Pituitary tumors
    c. Adrenalectomy
    d. Hypophysectomy
    e. Metastatic cancer
    f. High-dose pituitary radiation

63. The patient with pheochromocytoma has intermittent episodes of hypertension. What manifestations does the nurse expect?
    a. Confusion, abdominal pain, and unsteady gait
    b. Severe headaches, palpitations, and diaphoresis
    c. Visual disturbances, decreased pulses, and nausea
    d. Tachycardia, cold intolerance, and decreased urine output

64. Which patient care tasks could the nurse delegate to the unlicensed assistive personnel (UAP) in the care of a patient with acute adrenal insufficiency that is immobile? **Select all that apply.**
    a. Turn the patient every 1-2 hours.
    b. Apply skin lubricants.
    c. Assess lung sounds every 2-4 hours.
    d. Provide mouth care every 2 hours while awake.
    e. Record accurate intake and output.
    f. Teach the patient to cough and deep breathe.

65. The unlicensed assistive personnel (UAP) asks the nurse why it is necessary to check temperature every 4 hours for a patient with acute adrenal insufficiency. What is the nurse's **best** response?
    a. The temperature on all patients with endocrine disorders should be checked every 4 hours.
    b. The patient is at risk for infection; a temperature elevation of 1°F (or 0.5°C) above baseline is significant.
    c. It is essential to monitor all patients with endocrine disorders carefully to prevent infection.
    d. Because the patient is in the hospital, he is exposed to many infectious organisms.

66. The patient with hypercortisolism asks the nurse why she is prescribed the drug ranitidine. What is the nurse's **best** response?
    a. This drug inhibits the gastric proton pump and prevents the formation of hydrochloric acid in your stomach.
    b. Gastrointestinal bleeding is common complication in patients with hypercortisolism.
    c. Ranitidine blocks the H2-receptor site to decrease formation of hydrochloric acid and prevent GI bleeding.
    d. This drug buffers stomach acids and protects the gastrointestinal mucosa.

67. The nurse is supervising a student nurse providing care for a patient with adrenal insufficiency. Which action by the student nurse requires that the nurse intervene?
    a. The student nurse records patient intake and output for lunch.
    b. The student nurse weighs the patient in the morning before breakfast.
    c. The student nurse checks the patient's serum electrolyte results.
    d. The student nurse prepares to administer prednisolone instead of prednisone.

63 CHAPTER

Care of Patients with Problems of the Thyroid and Parathyroid Glands

1. The nurse is performing a physical examination of a patient's thyroid gland. Precautions are taken in performing the correct technique because palpation can result in which occurrence?
   a. Damage to the esophagus causing gastric reflux
   b. Obstruction of the carotid arteries causing a stroke
   c. Pressure on the trachea and laryngeal nerve causing hoarseness
   d. Exacerbation of symptoms by releasing additional thyroid hormone

2. Which assessment findings indicate hyperthyroidism? **Select all that apply.**
   a. Weight loss with increased appetite
   b. Constipation
   c. Increased heart rate
   d. Insomnia
   e. Decreased libido
   f. Heat intolerance

3. The nurse assesses a patient in the emergency department (ED) and finds the following: constipation, fatigue with increased sleeping time, impaired memory, facial puffiness, and weight gain. Which deficiency does the nurse recognize?
   a. Hyperthyroidism
   b. Hypothyroidism
   c. Hyperparathyroidism
   d. Hypoparathyroidism

4. Which factor is a **hallmark** assessment finding that signifies hyperthyroidism?
   a. Weight loss
   b. Increased libido
   c. Heat intolerance
   d. Diarrhea

5. Which factor is a **key** assessment finding that signifies hypothyroidism?
   a. Irritability
   b. Cold intolerance
   c. Diarrhea
   d. Fatigue

6. Which sign/symptom is one of the **first** indicators of hyperthyroidism that is often noticed by the patient?
   a. Eyelid or globe lag
   b. Vision changes or tiring of the eyes
   c. Protruding eyes
   d. Photophobia

7. Which laboratory result is consistent with a diagnosis of hyperthyroidism?
   a. Decreased serum triiodothyronine (T_3) and thyroxine (T_4) levels
   b. Elevated serum thyrotropin-releasing hormone (TRH) level
   c. Decreased radioactive iodine uptake
   d. Increased serum T_3 and T_4

8. The laboratory results for a 53-year-old patient indicate a low T_3 level and elevated thyroid-stimulating hormone (TSH). What do these results indicate?
   a. Hyperthyroidism
   b. Hypothyroidism
   c. Malfunctioning pituitary gland
   d. Normal laboratory values for this age

9. The clinical manifestations of hyperthyroidism are known as which condition?
   a. Thyrotoxicosis
   b. Euthyroid function
   c. Graves' disease
   d. Hypermetabolism

10. What is the **most** common cause of hyperthyroidism?
    a. Radiation to thyroid
    b. Graves' disease
    c. Thyroid cancer
    d. Thyroiditis

11. The nurse assessing a patient palpates enlargement of the thyroid gland, along with noticeable swelling of the neck. How does the nurse interpret this finding?
    a. Globe lag
    b. Myxedema
    c. Exophthalmos
    d. Goiter

12. The nurse is assessing a patient diagnosed with hyperthyroidism and observes dry, waxy swelling of the front surfaces of the lower legs. How does the nurse interpret this finding?
    a. Globe lag
    b. Pretibial myxedema
    c. Exophthalmos
    d. Goiter

13. Which statement **best** describes globe lag in a patient with hyperthyroidism?
    a. Abnormal protrusion of the eyes
    b. Upper eyelid fails to descend when the patient gazes downward
    c. Upper eyelid pulls back faster than the eyeball when the patient gazes upward
    d. Inability of both eyes to focus on an object simultaneously

14. The nurse is assessing a patient with Graves' disease and observes an abnormal protrusion of both eyeballs. How does the nurse document this assessment finding?
    a. Globe lag
    b. Pretibial myxedema
    c. Exophthalmos
    d. Goiter

15. Which statements about hyperthyroidism are accurate? **Select all that apply.**
    a. It is most commonly caused by Graves' disease.
    b. It can be caused by overuse of thyroid replacement medication.
    c. It occurs more often in men between the ages of 20-40.
    d. Weight gain is a common manifestation.
    e. Serum T_3 and T_4 results will be elevated.
    f. There may be an increase in number of bowel movements per day.

16. The nurse is providing instructions to a patient taking levothyroxine. What **key** information about dosing does the nurse tell the patient about this medication?
    a. It is started at a high dose and gradually decreased based on symptom relief.
    b. With myxedema coma, the drug is crushed and given through a feeding tube.
    c. Starting at too high a dose or increasing the dose too rapidly can cause severe hypertension, heart failure, and myocardial infarction.
    d. The patient requires this therapy until all symptoms are completely relieved.

17. The nurse is providing instructions to a patient who is taking the antithyroid medication propylthiouracil (PTU). The nurse instructs the patient to notify the health care provider **immediately** if which sign/symptom occurs?
    a. Weight gain
    b. Dark-colored urine
    c. Cold intolerance
    d. Headache

18. The patient who is prescribed methimazole 4 mg orally every 8 hours tells the nurse that his heart rate is slow (60/minute), he has gained 7 pounds, and wears a sweater even on warm days. What does the nurse suspect?
    a. Indications of hypothyroidism will require a lower dosage.
    b. Indications of hypothyroidism will require a higher dosage.
    c. Indications of hyperthyroidism will require a lower dosage.
    d. Indications of hyperthyroidism will require a higher dosage.

19. A patient who has been diagnosed with Graves' disease is to receive radioactive iodine (RAI) in the oral form of ^{131}I. What does the nurse teach the patient about how this drug works?
    a. It destroys the hormones T_3 and T_4.
    b. It destroys the tissue that produces thyroid hormones.
    c. It blocks thyroid hormone production.
    d. It prevents T_4 from being converted to T_3.

20. A patient who has been diagnosed with Graves' disease is to receive radioactive iodine (RAI) in the oral form of ^{131}I as a treatment. What instructions does the nurse include in the teaching plan about preventing radiation exposure to others? **Select all that apply.**
    a. Do not share a toilet with others for 2 weeks after treatment.
    b. Flush the toilet three times after each use.
    c. Wash clothing separately from others in the household.
    d. Limit contact with pregnant women, infants, and children.
    e. Do not use a laxative within 2 weeks of having the treatment.
    f. It may take 6 to 8 weeks after RAI therapy for complete symptom relief.

21. Which statements about hypothyroidism are accurate? **Select all that apply.**
    a. It occurs more often in women.
    b. It can be caused by iodine deficiency.
    c. Weight loss is a common manifestation.
    d. It can be caused by autoimmune thyroid destruction.
    e. Myxedema coma is a rare but serious complication.
    f. Symptoms are the result of high levels of metabolism.

22. The nurse is assessing a patient with a diagnosis of Hashimoto's disease. What are the **primary** manifestations of this disease? **Select all that apply.**
    a. Dysphagia
    b. Painless enlargement of the thyroid gland
    c. Painful enlargement of the thyroid gland
    d. Weight loss
    e. Intolerance to heat
    f. Diagnosis based on circulating antithyroid antibodies

23. Laboratory findings of elevated T_3 and T_4, decreased TSH, and high thyrotropin receptor antibody titer indicate which condition?
    a. Multinodular goiter
    b. Hyperthyroidism related to overmedication
    c. Pituitary tumor suppressing TSH
    d. Graves' disease

24. The patient has multiple thyroid nodules resulting in thyroid hyperfunction. What is the **most** likely cause of this hyperthyroidism?
    a. Thyroid carcinoma
    b. Graves' disease
    c. Toxic multinodular goiter
    d. Pituitary hyperthyroidism

25. After a visit to the health care provider's office, a patient is diagnosed with general thyroid enlargement and elevated thyroid hormone level. Which condition do these findings indicate?
    a. Hyperthyroidism and goiter
    b. Hypothyroidism and goiter
    c. Nodules on the parathyroid gland
    d. Thyroid or parathyroid cancer

26. Which condition is a life-threatening emergency and serious complication of untreated or poorly treated hypothyroidism?
    a. Endemic goiter
    b. Myxedema coma
    c. Toxic multinodular goiter
    d. Thyroiditis

27. A patient with exophthalmos from hyperthyroidism reports dry eyes, especially in the morning. The nurse teaches the patient to perform which intervention to help correct this problem?
    a. Wear sunglasses at all times when outside in the bright sun.
    b. Use cool compresses to the eye four times a day.
    c. Tape the eyes closed with nonallergenic tape.
    d. There is nothing that can be done to relieve this problem.

28. Which factors are considered to be triggers for thyroid storm? **Select all that apply.**
    a. Infection
    b. Cold temperatures
    c. Vigorous palpation of a goiter
    d. Diabetic ketoacidosis
    e. Extremely warm temperatures
    f. Pregnancy

29. A patient has the following assessment findings: elevated TSH level, low T_3 and T_4 levels, difficulty with memory, lethargy, and muscle stiffness. These are clinical manifestations of which disorder?
    a. Hypothyroidism
    b. Hyperthyroidism
    c. Hypoparathyroidism
    d. Hyperparathyroidism

30. A patient has been prescribed thyroid hormone for treatment of hypothyroidism. Within what time frame does the patient expect improvement in mental awareness with this treatment?
    a. A few days
    b. 2 weeks
    c. 1 month
    d. 3 months

31. Which signs and symptoms are assessment findings indicative of thyroid storm? **Select all that apply.**
    a. Abdominal pain and nausea
    b. Hypothermia
    c. Elevated temperature
    d. Tachycardia
    e. Elevated systolic blood pressure
    f. Bradycardia

32. Management of the patient with hyperthyroidism focuses on which goals? **Select all that apply.**
    a. Blocking the effects of excessive thyroid secretion
    b. Treating the signs and symptoms the patient experiences
    c. Establishing euthyroid function
    d. Preventing spread of the disease
    e. Maintaining an environment of reduced stimulation
    f. Promoting comfort

33. Which are preoperative instructions for a patient having thyroid surgery? **Select all that apply.**
    a. Teach postoperative restrictions such as no coughing and deep-breathing exercises to prevent strain on the suture line.
    b. Teach the moving and turning technique of manually supporting the head and avoiding neck extension to minimize strain on the suture line.
    c. Inform the patient that hoarseness for a few days after surgery is usually the result of a breathing tube (endotracheal tube) used during surgery.
    d. Humidification of air may be helpful to promote expectoration of secretions. Suctioning may also be used.
    e. Clarify any questions regarding placement of incision, complications, and postoperative care.
    f. A supine position and lying flat will be maintained postoperatively to avoid strain on suture line.

34. The nurse is preparing for a patient to return from thyroid surgery. What **priority** equipment does the nurse ensure is immediately available? **Select all that apply.**
    a. Tracheostomy equipment
    b. Calcium gluconate or calcium chloride for IV administration
    c. Mechanical ventilator
    d. Humidified oxygen
    e. Suction equipment
    f. Pillows

35. **After** a thyroidectomy, a patient reports tingling around the mouth and muscle twitching. Which complication do these assessment findings indicate to the nurse?
    a. Hemorrhage
    b. Respiratory distress
    c. Thyroid storm
    d. Hypocalcemia

36. The nurse assesses a patient for laryngeal nerve damage after thyroidectomy. Which findings indicate this complication? **Select all that apply.**
    a. Dyspnea
    b. Sore throat
    c. Hoarseness
    d. Weak voice
    e. Dry cough
    f. Increased respiratory rate

37. The nurse is assessing a patient after thyroid surgery and discovers harsh, high-pitched respiratory sounds. What is the nurse's **best** first action?
    a. Administer oxygen at 5 L via nasal cannula.
    b. Administer IV calcium chloride.
    c. Notify the Rapid Response Team.
    d. Suction the patient for oral secretions.

38. After hospitalization for myxedema, a patient is prescribed thyroid replacement medication. Which statement by the patient demonstrates a correct understanding of this therapy?
    a. "I'll be taking this medication until my symptoms are completely resolved."
    b. "I'll be taking thyroid medication for the rest of my life."
    c. "Now that I'm feeling better, no changes in my medication will be necessary."
    d. "I'm taking this medication to prevent symptoms of an overactive thyroid gland."

39. Which statements about thyroiditis are accurate? **Select all that apply.**
    a. It is an inflammation of the thyroid gland.
    b. Hashimoto's disease is the most common type.
    c. It always resolves with antibiotic therapy.
    d. There are three types: acute, subacute, and chronic.
    e. The patient must take thyroid hormones.
    f. Subacute thyroiditis is caused by a viral infection.

40. Which statements about acute thyroiditis are accurate? **Select all that apply.**
    a. It is caused by a bacterial infection of the thyroid gland.
    b. It is treated with antibiotic therapy.
    c. It results from a viral infection of the thyroid gland.
    d. Subtotal thyroidectomy is a form of treatment.
    e. Manifestations include neck tenderness, fever, and dysphagia.
    f. It is an autoimmune disorder caused by viral infection.

41. What is a **hallmark** of thyroid cancer?
    a. Aggressive tumors
    b. Elevated serum thyroglobulin level
    c. Metastasis to other organs
    d. Invasion of blood vessels

42. Serum calcium levels are maintained by which hormone?
    a. Cortisol
    b. Luteinizing hormone
    c. Antidiuretic hormone (ADH)
    d. Parathyroid hormone (PTH)

43. Production of which hormone causes lower levels of calcium?
    a. Calcitonin
    b. Parathyroid hormone (PTH)
    c. Thyroxine (T_4)
    d. Thyroid stimulating hormone (TSH)

44. Bone changes in the older adult are often seen with endocrine dysfunction and increased secretion of which substance?
    a. Parathyroid hormone (PTH)
    b. Calcitonin
    c. Insulin
    d. Testosterone

45. In addition to regulation of calcium levels, parathyroid hormone (PTH) and calcitonin regulate the circulating blood levels of which substance?
    a. Potassium
    b. Sodium
    c. Phosphate
    d. Chloride

46. A patient has positive Trousseau's and Chvostek's signs resulting from hypoparathyroidism. What condition does this assessment finding indicate?
    a. Hypercalcemia
    b. Hypocalcemia
    c. Hyperphosphatemia
    d. Hypophosphatemia

47. Which foods will the nurse instruct a patient with hypoparathyroidism to avoid? **Select all that apply.**
    a. Canned vegetables
    b. Yogurt
    c. Fresh fruit
    d. Red meat
    e. Milk
    f. Processed cheese

48. A patient with continuous spasms of the muscles is diagnosed with hypoparathyroidism. The muscle spasms are a clinical manifestation of which condition?
    a. Nerve damage
    b. Seizures
    c. Tetany
    d. Decreased potassium

49. Which disorders/conditions can cause hyperparathyroidism? **Select all that apply.**
    a. Chronic kidney disease
    b. Neck trauma
    c. Thyroidectomy
    d. Vitamin D deficiency
    e. Parathyroidectomy
    f. Congenital hyperplasia

50. A patient has hyperparathyroidism and high levels of serum calcium. Which initial medication does the nurse prepare to administer to the patient?
    a. Furosemide with IV saline
    b. Calcitonin
    c. Oral phosphates
    d. Mithramycin

51. Which are assessment findings of hypocalcemia? **Select all that apply.**
    a. Numbness and tingling around the mouth
    b. Muscle cramping
    c. Bone fractures
    d. Fever
    e. Tachycardia
    f. Trousseau's and Chvostek's signs

52. Which medication therapies does the nurse expect patients with hypoparathyroidism to receive? **Select all that apply.**
    a. Calcium chloride
    b. Calcium gluconate
    c. Calcitriol
    d. Propranolol
    e. Ergocalciferol
    f. Furosemide

53. Discharge planning for a patient with chronic hypoparathyroidism includes which instructions? **Select all that apply.**
    a. Take prescribed medications for the rest of the patient's life.
    b. Eat foods low in vitamin D and high in phosphorus.
    c. Eat foods high in calcium, but low in phosphorus.
    d. Discontinue medication after several weeks.
    e. Kidney stones are no longer a risk to the patient.
    f. Interventions to reduce anxiety.

54. In older adults, assessment findings of fatigue, altered thought processes, dry skin, and constipation are often mistaken for signs of aging rather than assessment findings for which endocrine disorder?
    a. Hyperthyroidism
    b. Hypothyroidism
    c. Hyperparathyroidism
    d. Hypoparathyroidism

55. What is the **most** common cause of death from myxedema coma?
    a. Myocardial infarction
    b. Acute kidney failure
    c. High serum level of iodide
    d. Respiratory failure

56. Which conditions may precipitate myxedema coma? **Select all that apply.**
    a. Rapid withdrawal of thyroid medication
    b. Vitamin D deficiency
    c. Untreated hypothyroidism
    d. Surgery
    e. Excessive exposure to iodine
    f. Radioactive iodine (RAI) treatment

57. The nurse is caring for a young female patient with papillary carcinoma of the thyroid gland. Which treatment is **most** likely to be prescribed for this patient?
    a. Radiation therapy
    b. Ablation
    c. Chemotherapy
    d. Thyroidectomy

58. Which patient care task would the nurse supervise but delegate to unlicensed assistive personnel (UAP) when providing care for a patient with hyperthyroidism? **Select all that apply.**
    a. Check vital signs and report any temperature elevation immediately.
    b. Administer methimazole (Tapazole) as ordered.
    c. Ensure that the patient has a pitcher of fresh ice water at the bedside.
    d. Teach the patient about thyroid replacement therapy.
    e. Change the bed linen whenever it becomes damp.
    f. Remind the patient to take a cool shower if sweating occurs.

59. The unlicensed assistive personnel (UAP) is providing a bath for a patient with hyperparathyroidism. What essential teaching must the nurse provide to the UAP?
    a. Handle the patient carefully and use a lift sheet for repositioning.
    b. Be sure to use a bath blanket to keep the patient from shivering.
    c. Remind the patient about the importance of consuming foods rich in potassium.
    d. Allow the patient to get out of bed and walk to the bathroom without assistance.

CHAPTER 64

Care of Patients with Diabetes Mellitus

1. Which statements about type 2 diabetes mellitus (DM) are **most** characteristic? **Select all that apply.**
   a. Autoimmune process causes beta cell destruction.
   b. Cells have decreased ability to respond to insulin.
   c. Diagnosis is based on results of 100-g glucose tolerance test.
   d. Most patients diagnosed are obese adults.
   e. Usually has abrupt onset of thirst and weight loss.
   f. Most patients are not dependent on insulin.

2. Which statement is true about insulin?
   a. It is secreted by alpha cells in the islets of Langerhans.
   b. It is a catabolic hormone that builds up glucagon reserves.
   c. It is necessary for glucose transport across cell membranes.
   d. It is stored in muscles and converted to fat for storage.

3. Why is glucose vital to the body's cells?
   a. It is used to build cell membranes.
   b. It is used by cells to produce energy.
   c. It affects the process of protein metabolism.
   d. It provides nutrients for genetic material.

4. A patient with type I diabetes mellitus presents to the emergency department (ED) with a blood sugar of 640 mg/dL and reports being constantly thirsty and having to urinate "all of the time." How does the nurse document this subjective finding?
   a. Polydipsia and polyphagia
   b. Polydipsia and polyuria
   c. Polycoria and polyuria
   d. Polyphagia and polyesthesia

5. People from which cultures tend to have a higher incidence of DM? **Select all that apply.**
   a. Mexican American
   b. African American
   c. Caucasian
   d. American Indian
   e. Eastern European
   f. Alaskan Indian

6. Which individual is at greatest risk for developing type 2 DM?
   a. 25-year-old African American woman
   b. 36-year-old African American man
   c. 56-year-old Hispanic woman
   d. 40-year-old Hispanic man

7. According to the American Diabetes Association (ADA), which laboratory finding is most indicative of DM?
   a. Fasting blood glucose = 80 mg/dL
   b. 2-hour postprandial blood glucose = 110 mg/dL
   c. 1-hour glucose tolerance blood glucose = 110 mg/dL
   d. 2-hour glucose tolerance blood glucose = 210 mg/dL

8. The nurse would observe the patient with untreated hyperglycemia for which condition?
   a. Respiratory acidosis
   b. Metabolic alkalosis
   c. Respiratory alkalosis
   d. Metabolic acidosis

9. A patient with hyperglycemia displays a rapid and deep respiratory pattern. The nurse would describe this as which respiratory pattern?
   a. Tachypnea
   b. Cheyne-Stokes respiration
   c. Kussmaul respiration
   d. Biot respiration

10. When assessing a patient with hyperglycemia the nurse would evaluate the patient for changes in which electrolyte?
    a. Sodium
    b. Chloride
    c. Potassium
    d. Magnesium

11. Which complications of DM are considered emergencies? **Select all that apply.**
    a. Diabetic ketoacidosis (DKA)
    b. Hypoglycemia
    c. Diabetic retinopathy
    d. Hyperglycemic-hyperosmolar state (HHS)
    e. Diabetic neuropathy
    f. Diabetic nephropathy

12. In determining if a patient is hypoglycemic, in addition to checking the patient's blood glucose, the nurse assesses the patient for which characteristics? **Select all that apply.**
    a. Nausea
    b. Hunger
    c. Irritability
    d. Tremors
    e. Profuse perspiration
    f. Rapid, deep respirations

13. Which factors differentiate diabetic ketoacidosis (DKA) from hyperglycemic-hyperosmolar state (HHS)? **Select all that apply.**
    a. Sudden versus gradual onset
    b. Amount of ketones produced
    c. Serum bicarbonate levels
    d. Amount of volume depletion
    e. Dosage of insulin needed
    f. Level of hyperglycemia

14. A patient is admitted with a blood glucose level of 900 mg/dL. IV fluids and insulin are administered. Two hours after treatment is initiated, the blood glucose level is 400 mg/dL. Which complication is the patient **most** at risk for developing?
    a. Hypoglycemia
    b. Pulmonary embolus
    c. Renal shutdown
    d. Pulmonary edema

15. What type of insulin is used in the emergency treatment of diabetic ketoacidosis (DKA) and hyperglycemic-hyperosmolar state (HHS)?
    a. NPH
    b. Lente
    c. Regular
    d. Protamine zinc

16. Early treatment of diabetic ketoacidosis (DKA) and hyperglycemic-hyperosmolar state (HHS) includes IV administration of which fluid?
    a. Glucagon
    b. Potassium
    c. Bicarbonate
    d. Saline

17. Glucagon is used primarily to treat the patient with which disorder?
    a. Diabetic ketoacidosis (DKA)
    b. Idiosyncratic reaction to insulin
    c. Severe hypoglycemia
    d. Hyperglycemic-hyperosmolar state (HHS)

18. In which situations does the nurse teach a patient to perform urine ketone testing? **Select all that apply.**
    a. Acute illness or stress
    b. When blood glucose levels are above 200 mg/dL
    c. When symptoms of diabetic ketoacidosis (DKA) are present
    d. To evaluate the effectiveness of diabetic ketoacidosis (DKA) treatment
    e. When a diabetic patient is in a weight-loss program
    f. When a diabetic patient has a diagnosis of hyperglycemic-hyperosmolar state (HHS)

19. The patient asks the nurse "Why am I getting glucagon?" Which response by the nurse is **most** accurate?
    a. Glucagon competes for insulin at the receptor sites.
    b. Glucagon frees glucose from hepatic stores of glycogen.
    c. Glucagon supplies glycogen directly to the vital tissues.
    d. Glucagon is a glucose substitute for rapid replacement.

20. Which statements about type 1 DM are accurate? **Select all that apply.**
    a. It is an autoimmune disorder.
    b. Most people with type 1 DM are obese.
    c. Age of onset is typically younger than 30.
    d. Etiology may be attributed to viral infections.
    e. It can be treated with oral antidiabetic medications and insulin.
    f. It involves insulin resistance that progresses leading to decreased beta cell secretion of insulin.

21. Which statements about type 2 DM are accurate? **Select all that apply.**
    a. It peaks at about the age of 50.
    b. Most people with type 2 DM are obese.
    c. It typically has an abrupt onset.
    d. People with type 2 DM have insulin resistance.
    e. It can be treated with oral antidiabetic medications and insulin.
    f. Presence of metabolic syndrome increases the risk for type 2 DM.

22. The nurse is teaching people in a community education class about modifiable risk factors for type 2 DM. Which factors would the nurse discuss? **Select all that apply.**
    a. Age
    b. Family history
    c. Working in a low-stress environment
    d. Maintaining ideal body weight
    e. Maintaining adequate physical activity
    f. Lack of exercise

23. A patient with diabetes is scheduled to have a blood glucose test the next morning. Which instruction does the nurse give the patient?
    a. Eat the usual diet but have nothing after midnight.
    b. Take the usual oral hypoglycemic tablet in the morning.
    c. Eat a clear liquid breakfast in the morning.
    d. Follow the usual diet and medication regimen.

24. The nurse is providing discharge teaching to a patient about self-monitoring of blood glucose (SMBG). What information does the nurse include? **Select all that apply.**
    a. Only perform SMBG before breakfast.
    b. Wash hands before using the meter.
    c. Do a retest if the results seem unusual.
    d. It is okay to reuse lancets in the home setting.
    e. Do not share the meter.
    f. How to calibrate the machine

25. Which are considered the early signs of diabetic nephropathy? **Select all that apply.**
    a. Positive urine red blood cells
    b. Microalbuminuria
    c. Positive urine glucose
    d. Positive urine white blood cells
    e. Elevated serum uric acid
    f. Hypertension

26. Which class of antidiabetic medication should be taken with the **first** bite of a meal to be fully effective?
    a. Alpha-glucosidase inhibitors, which include miglitol
    b. Biguanides, which include metformin
    c. Meglitinides, which include nateglinide
    d. Second-generation sulfonylureas, which include glipizide

27. Which class of antidiabetic medication must be held after using contrast media until adequate kidney function is established?
    a. Alpha-glucosidase inhibitors, which include miglitol
    b. Biguanides, which include metformin
    c. Meglitinides, which include nateglinide
    d. Second-generation sulfonylureas, which include glipizide

28. Which class of antidiabetic medication is **most likely** to cause hypoglycemia even when hyperglycemia is not present?
    a. Alpha-glucosidase inhibitors, which include miglitol
    b. Biguanides, which include metformin
    c. Meglitinides, which include nateglinide
    d. Second-generation sulfonylureas, which include glipizide

29. Which class of antidiabetic medication should be taken **just before** or with meals?
    a. Alpha-glucosidase inhibitors, which include miglitol
    b. Biguanides, which include metformin
    c. Meglitinides, which include nateglinide
    d. Sulfonylureas, which include chlorpromazine

30. Which oral agent may cause lactic acidosis in patients with kidney impairment?
    a. Nateglinide
    b. Repaglinide
    c. Metformin
    d. Miglitol

31. For which patient should the health care provider avoid prescribing rosiglitazone?
    a. Patient with symptomatic heart failure
    b. Patient with new-onset asthma
    c. Patient with kidney disease
    d. Patient with hyperthyroidism

32. The patient with type 2 diabetes is prescribed sitagliptin for glucose regulation. Which key changes does the nurse teach a patient to report to the health care provider immediately? **Select all that apply.**
    a. Report any signs of jaundice.
    b. Report any signs of bleeding.
    c. Report any blue-gray discoloration of the abdomen.
    d. Report any cough or flu symptoms.
    e. Report any sudden onset of abdominal pain.
    f. Report any rash or other signs of allergic reaction.

33. Which statement about insulin is true?
    a. Exogenous insulin is necessary for management of all cases of type 2 DM.
    b. Insulin's effectiveness depends on the patient's absorption of the drug.
    c. Insulin doses should be regulated according to self-monitoring urine glucose levels.
    d. Insulin administered in multiple doses per day decreases the flexibility of a patient's lifestyle.

34. Which statement about insulin administration is correct?
    a. Insulin may be given orally, intravenously, or subcutaneously.
    b. Insulin injections should be spaced no closer than one-half inch apart.
    c. Insulin absorption is fastest in the abdomen except for a 2-inch radius around the navel.
    d. Shake the bottle of intermediate-acting insulin and then draw it into the syringe.

35. A diabetic patient is on a mixed-dose insulin protocol of 8 units regular insulin and 12 units NPH insulin at 7 AM. At 10:30 AM, the patient reports feeling uneasy, shaky, and has a headache. Which is the probable explanation for this?
    a. The NPH insulin's action is peaking, and there is an insufficient blood glucose level.
    b. The regular insulin's action is peaking, and there is an insufficient blood glucose level.
    c. The patient consumed too many calories at breakfast and now has an elevated blood glucose level.
    d. The symptoms are unrelated to the insulin administered in the early morning or food taken in at lunchtime.

36. A patient asks the nurse how insulin injection site rotation should be accomplished. What is the nurse's **best** response?
    a. "Rotation within one site is preferred to avoid changes in insulin absorption."
    b. "Change rotation sites after a week or two to avoid lipohypertrophy."
    c. "Rotation from site to site each day is best for the most insulin absorption."
    d. "Always rotate insulin injection sites within 4-5 inches from the umbilicus."

37. A patient will be using an external insulin pump. What instruction does the nurse give the patient about the pump?
    a. SMBG levels should be done three or more times a day.
    b. The insulin supply must be replaced every 2-4 weeks.
    c. The pump's battery should be checked on a regular weekly schedule.
    d. The needle site must be changed every day.

38. A 47-year-old patient with a history of type 2 DM and emphysema who reports smoking three packs of cigarettes per day is admitted to the hospital with a diagnosis of acute pneumonia. The patient is placed on his regular oral antidiabetic agents, sliding-scale insulin, and antibiotic medications. On day 2 of hospitalization, the health care provider orders prednisone therapy. What does the nurse expect the blood glucose to do?
    a. Decrease
    b. Stay the same
    c. Increase
    d. Return to normal

39. Which laboratory test is the best indicator of a patient's average blood glucose level and/or compliance with the DM regimen over the last 3 months?
    a. Postprandial blood glucose test
    b. Oral glucose tolerance test (OGTT)
    c. Casual blood glucose test
    d. Glycosylated hemoglobin (HbA$_{1c}$)

40. A patient with diabetic ketoacidosis is on an insulin drip of 50 units of regular insulin in 250 mL of normal saline. The current blood glucose level is 549 mg/dL. According to insulin protocol, the insulin drip needs to be changed to 8 units per hour. At what rate does the nurse set the pump?
    a. 40 mL/hr
    b. 50 mL/hr
    c. 60 mL/hr
    d. 75 mL/hr

41. Which insulins are considered to have a rapid onset of action? **Select all that apply.**
    a. Novolin 70/30
    b. Glulisine
    c. Humulin N
    d. Aspart
    e. Lispro
    f. Glargine

42. A patient with type 2 DM, usually controlled with a second-generation sulfonylurea, develops a urinary tract infection. Due to the stress of the infection, the patient must be treated with insulin. What additional information about this treatment does the nurse explain to the patient?
    a. The sulfonylurea must be discontinued and insulin taken until the infection clears.
    b. Insulin will now be necessary to control the patient's diabetes for life.
    c. The sulfonylurea dose must be reduced until the infection clears.
    d. The insulin is necessary to supplement the second-generation sulfonylurea until the infection clears.

43. The diabetic patient experiences early morning hyperglycemia (Somogyi effect) as a result of the counterregulatory response to hypoglycemia. What action will the nurse expect for this condition? **Select all that apply.**
    a. Administer a 10 PM dose of intermediate-acting insulin.
    b. Provide an evening snack to ensure adequate dietary intake.
    c. Evaluate insulin dosage and exercise program.
    d. Add an oral antidiabetic drug to patient's regimen.
    e. Increase blood glucose checks to every 2 hours around the clock.
    f. Diagnosis is accomplished by blood glucose monitoring during the night.

44. Which diabetic complication is associated with diabetic peripheral neuropathy?
    a. End-stage kidney disease
    b. Muscle weakness
    c. Permanent blindness
    d. Retinal hemorrhage

45. A patient will be using rapid acting insulin injected by an external insulin pump. What does the nurse tell the patient about the pump?
    a. SMBG levels can be done only twice a day.
    b. The insulin supply must be replaced every 2-4 weeks.
    c. The pump's battery should be checked on a regular weekly schedule.
    d. Be sure to match your insulin dose to the carbohydrate (CHO) content of your diet.

46. The patient's urinalysis shows proteinuria. Which pathophysiology does the nurse suspect?
    a. Nephropathy
    b. Neuropathy
    c. Retinopathy
    d. Gastroparesis

47. Which infection control measures must the nurse teach a patient who will be performing SMBG? **Select all that apply.**
    a. Always wash hands before monitoring glucose.
    b. Regular cleaning of the meter is critical.
    c. Do not reuse lancets.
    d. Do not share blood glucose monitoring equipment.
    e. Sterilize blood glucose monitor before each use.
    f. Family members who help with testing should wear gloves.

48. Which statements about sensory alteration in patients with diabetes are accurate? **Select all that apply.**
    a. Very few patients with diabetic foot ulcers have peripheral sensory neuropathy.
    b. Loss of pain, pressure, and temperature sensation in the foot increases the risk for injury.
    c. Sensory neuropathy causes loss of normal sweating and skin temperature regulation.
    d. Sensory alterations can be delayed by keeping the blood glucose level as close to normal as possible.
    e. Reduced blood flow to the foot results in increased risk for ulcer formation.
    f. Healing of foot wounds is reduced because of impaired sensation.

49. Intensive therapy with good glucose control results in delayed occurrence in which diabetic complications? **Select all that apply.**
    a. Macrovascular disease
    b. Cardiovascular disease
    c. Stroke
    d. Retinopathy
    e. Nephropathy
    f. Neuropathy

50. The patient with diabetes has a foot that is warm, swollen, and painful. Walking causes the arch of the foot to collapse and gives the foot a "rocker bottom" shape. Which foot deformity does the nurse recognize?
    a. Hallux valgus
    b. Claw-toe deformity
    c. Charcot foot
    d. Diabetic foot ulcer

51. In developing an individualized meal plan for a patient with diabetes, which goals will be focal points of the plan? **Select all that apply.**
    a. Maintain blood glucose levels at or as close to the normal range as possible.
    b. Allow patient food preferences.
    c. Permit patients to eat as much as they desire.
    d. Honor patient cultural preferences.
    e. Limit food choices only when guided by scientific evidence.
    f. Include the family member who buys groceries and prepares meals in the teaching.

52. What is the basic principle of meal planning for a patient with type 1 DM?
    a. Five small meals per day plus a bedtime snack
    b. Taking extra insulin when planning to eat sweet foods
    c. High-protein, low-carbohydrate, and low-fiber foods
    d. Considering the effects and peak action times of the patient's insulin

53. Which statement about dietary concepts for a patient with diabetes is true?
    a. Alcoholic beverage consumption is unrestricted.
    b. Carbohydrate counting is emphasized when adjusting dietary intake of nutrients.
    c. Sweeteners should be avoided because of the side effects.
    d. Both soluble and insoluble fiber foods should be limited.

54. What is the recommended protocol for patients with type 2 DM who must lose weight?
    a. Participate in an aerobic program twice a week for 20 minutes each session.
    b. Slowly increase insulin dosage until mild hypoglycemia occurs.
    c. Reduce calorie intake moderately and increase exercise.
    d. Reduce daily calorie intake to 1000 calories and monitor urine for ketones.

55. Along with exercise, what is the recommended calorie reduction for a patient with diabetes who needs to lose weight?
    a. 100-200 calories/day
    b. 250-500 calories/day
    c. 501-600 calories/day
    d. 601-750 calories/day

56. What type of exercise does the nurse recommend for the patient with diabetic retinopathy?
    a. Non–weight-bearing activities such as swimming
    b. Weight-bearing activities such as jogging
    c. Vigorous aerobic and resistance exercises
    d. Weight training and heavy lifting

57. The nurse is teaching a patient with diabetes about proper foot care. Which instructions does the nurse include? **Select all that apply.**
    a. Inspect feet daily.
    b. Wear open-toed shoes or sandals in warm weather to prevent perspiration.
    c. Apply moisturizing cream to the feet after bathing but not between the toes.
    d. Use cold water for bathing the feet to prevent inadvertent thermal injury.
    e. Do not go barefoot.
    f. Use rubbing alcohol to toughen the skin on the soles of the feet.

58. A 25-year-old female patient with type 1 DM tells the nurse, "I have two kidneys and I'm still young. I expect to be around for a long time, so why should I worry about my blood sugar?" What is the nurse's **best** response?
    a. "You have little to worry about as long as your kidneys keep making urine."
    b. "You should discuss this with your provider because you are being unrealistic."
    c. "You would be right if your diabetes was managed with insulin."
    d. "Keeping your blood sugar under control now can help to prevent damage to both kidneys."

59. SMBG levels is most important in which patients? **Select all that apply.**
    a. Patients taking multiple daily insulin injections
    b. Patients with mild well-controlled type 2 diabetes
    c. Patients with hypoglycemic unawareness
    d. Patients using a portable infusion device for insulin administration
    e. Patients with acute illnesses
    f. Pregnant patients

60. Which statement about sexual intercourse for patients with diabetes is true?
    a. The incidence of sexual dysfunction is lower in men than women.
    b. Retrograde ejaculation does not interfere with male fertility.
    c. Impotence is associated with DM in male patients.
    d. Sexual dysfunction in female patients includes inability to achieve pregnancy.

61. A patient with type 1 DM is planning to travel by air and asks the nurse about preparations for the trip. What does the nurse tell the patient to do?
    a. Pack insulin and syringes in a labeled, crushproof kit in the checked luggage.
    b. Carry all necessary diabetes supplies in a clearly identified pack aboard the plane.
    c. Ask the flight attendant to put the insulin in the galley refrigerator once on the plane.
    d. Take only minimal supplies and get the prescription filled at his or her destination.

62. Which statement by a patient with DM indicates an understanding of the principles of self-care?
    a. "I don't like the idea of sticking myself so often to measure my sugar."
    b. "I plan to measure the sugar in my urine at least four times a day."
    c. "I plan to get my spouse to exercise with me to keep me company."
    d. "If I get a cold, I can take my regular cough medication until I feel better."

63. After a 2-hour glucose challenge, which result demonstrates impaired glucose tolerance?
    a. Less than 100 mg/dL
    b. Less than 140 mg/dL
    c. Greater than 140 mg/dL
    d. Greater than 250 mg/dL

64. The nurse is caring for a patient with DM. The patient's urine is positive for ketones. What does the nurse instruct the patient with regard to exercise?
    a. "When urine ketones are present, you should not exercise."
    b. "You may exercise as long as serum ketones are low positive."
    c. "If you exercise now, be sure to perform aerobic exercises."
    d. "Exercise is always a good option because it helps with glucose utilization."

65. A patient with type 2 DM often has which laboratory value?
    a. Elevated thyroid studies
    b. Elevated triglycerides
    c. Ketones in the urine
    d. Low hemoglobin

66. A patient has been diagnosed with DM. Which aspects does the nurse consider in formulating the teaching plan for this patient? **Select all that apply.**
    a. Covering all needed information in one teaching session
    b. Assessing visual impairment regarding insulin labels and markings on syringes
    c. Assessing manual dexterity to determine if the patient is able to draw insulin into a syringe
    d. Assessing patient motivation to learn and comprehend instructions
    e. Assessing the patient's ability to read printed material
    f. Assisting patients to choose an SMBG device that is best for their level of visual impairment.

67. Which are signs and symptoms of mild hypoglycemia? **Select all that apply.**
    a. Headache
    b. Weakness
    c. Cold, clammy skin
    d. Irritability
    e. Pallor
    f. Tachycardia

68. The older adult with DM asks the nurse for advice about beginning an exercise program. What is the nurse's best response? **Select all that apply.**
    a. Begin with high-intensity activities.
    b. Start low-intensity activities in short sessions.
    c. Be sure to include warm-up and cool-down periods.
    d. Start with exercise periods of 20 minutes or less.
    e. Gradually change activities.
    f. Exercise programs should avoid causing hypoglycemia.

69. A patient with type 1 DM is taking a mixture of NPH and regular insulin at home. The patient has been NPO for surgery since midnight. What action does the nurse take regarding the patient's morning dose of insulin?
    a. Administer the dose that is routinely prescribed at home because the patient has type 1 DM and needs the insulin.
    b. Administer half the dose because the patient is NPO.
    c. Hold the insulin with all the other medications because the patient is NPO and there is no need for insulin.
    d. Contact the health care provider for an order regarding the insulin.

70. What glucose level range does the American Association of Clinical Endocrinologists recommend for a critically ill patient?
    a. Between 100 and 130 mg/dL
    b. Between 140 and 180 mg/dL
    c. Between 180 and 200 mg/dL
    d. Between 200 and 240 mg/dL

71. The patient with DM had a pancreas transplant and takes daily doses of cyclosporine. For which key lab assessment does the nurse monitor?
    a. Serum electrolytes
    b. CBC with differential count
    c. Serum creatinine
    d. Clotting studies

72. Which diabetic patient is at greatest risk for diabetic foot ulcer formation?
    a. 75-year-old African American male with history of cardiovascular disease
    b. 53-year-old Caucasian female with history of renal insufficiency
    c. 38-year-old American Indian with history of gastric ulcers
    d. 28-year-old Caucasian male with history of chronic kidney disease

73. A patient with DM has signs and symptoms of hypoglycemia. The patient is alert and oriented with a blood glucose of 56 mg/dL. What does the nurse do **next**?
    a. Give a glass of orange juice with two packets of sugar and continue to monitor the patient.
    b. Give 8 oz of skim milk, then a carbohydrate and protein snack if next meal is more than an hour away.
    c. Give a complex carbohydrate and continue to monitor the patient.
    d. Administer D50 IV push and give the patient something to eat.

74. A patient with diabetes has signs and symptoms of hypoglycemia. The patient has a blood glucose of 18 mg/dL, is not alert but responds to voice, and is confused and is unable to swallow fluids. What does the nurse do **next**?
    a. Give a glass of orange juice with two packets of sugar and continue to monitor the patient.
    b. Give a glass of orange or other type of juice and continue to monitor the patient.
    c. Give a complex carbohydrate and continue to monitor the patient.
    d. Administer subcutaneous or IM glucagon and 50% IV dextrose.

75. A patient has been receiving insulin in the abdomen for 3 days. On day 4, where does the nurse give the insulin injection?
    a. Deltoid
    b. Thigh
    c. Abdomen, but in an area different from the previous day's injection
    d. Abdomen, in the same area as the previous day's injection

76. From which injection site is insulin absorbed most rapidly?
    a. Buttocks
    b. Abdomen
    c. Deltoid
    d. Thigh

77. Which are characteristics of regular insulin?
Select all that apply.
a. This insulin does not have a peak time.
b. When mixing types of insulin, this insulin is always drawn up first.
c. This insulin is given once daily for basal insulin coverage.
d. This insulin should be given 30 minutes before meals.
e. This insulin should not be diluted or mixed with any other insulin.
f. This insulin should be gently rolled between the hands before it is drawn up.

78. The nurse is preparing to teach a diabetic patient how to select appropriate shoes. Which points must be included in the teaching plan?
Select all that apply.
a. "It is best to have the shoes fitted by an experienced shoe fitter such as a podiatrist."
b. "The shoes should be 1 to 1.5 inches longer than your longest toe."
c. "The heels of the shoes should be less than 2 inches high."
d. "Avoid tight-fitting shoes, which can cause tissue damage to your feet."
e. "You should get at least two pairs of shoes so you can change them at mid-day and in the evening."
f. "Buy your shoes later in the day, when feet are normally larger."

79. The male diabetic patient asks the nurse for advice about alcohol consumption. What is the nurse's **best** response?
a. "It is best to have alcohol near bedtime."
b. "As long as your diabetes is under control you can drink as much as you like."
c. "You should drink only one alcoholic beverage with each meal."
d. "Avoid more than two drinks a day and have them with or shortly after meals."

80. The nurse is caring for a diabetic patient in the ED. The patient's lab values include serum glucose 353 mg/dL, positive serum ketones, and positive urine ketones. What complication does the nurse suspect?
a. DKA
b. HHS
c. Hyperglycemia
d. Hypoglycemia

81. The critical care nurse is caring for an older patient admitted with HHS. What is the **first priority** in caring for this patient?
a. Slowly decreasing blood glucose
b. Fluid replacement to increase blood volume
c. Potassium replacement to prevent hypokalemia
d. Diuretic therapy to maintain kidney function

82. The patient has an HbA_{1c} level of 8.0. The nurse understands that this means the patient's mean glucose level is which of the following?
a. 126 mg/dL (7.0 mmol/L)
b. 154 mg/dL (8.6 mmol/L)
c. 183 mg/dL (10.2 mmol/L)
d. 212 mg/dL (13.4 mmol/L)

83. The female patient has type 2 DM. Which types of sexual dysfunction should the nurse teach may occur for this patient? **Select all that apply.**
a. Decreased libido
b. Excessive vaginal lubrication
c. Painful intercourse
d. Failure to achieve orgasm
e. Decreased sexual response
f. Increased fear of sexual encounters

84. On assessment, the patient has abdominal obesity (waist 40 inches/100 cm), a fasting blood glucose level of 100 mg/dL, blood pressure 140/92, and a triglyceride level of 150 mg/dL. Which condition is indicated by these findings?
a. Metabolic syndrome
b. Kidney failure
c. Gestational diabetes
d. Atherosclerosis

85. Which characteristic describes a needleless insulin injection system?
    a. The patient must be able to operate the pump, adjust the settings, and respond to alarms.
    b. Insulin is given by jet injection, is absorbed at a faster rate, and has a shorter duration of action.
    c. A continuous subcutaneous infusion of a basal dose of insulin is provided.
    d. If a meal is skipped, an additional mealtime dose of insulin is not given.

86. What must the nurse teach a patient with type 1 DM about preventing the loss of insulin potency? **Select all that apply.**
    a. "Avoid exposing insulin to temperatures below 36°F (2.2°C) or above 86°F (30°C)."
    b. "Freeze bottles of insulin for long-term storage."
    c. "Always shake NPH insulin to assure it is evenly cloudy."
    d. "Do not expose insulin to heat or light."
    e. "Insulin glargine (Lantus) should be stored in a refrigerator."
    f. "A slight loss in potency may occur for bottles in use for more than 30 days."

87. The patient has a history of hypoglycemic unawareness. What specific information must the nurse stress when teaching this patient about SMBG?
    a. "Alternative site monitoring will allow you to use other sites than your fingers."
    b. "SMBG monitoring will help you to avoid episodes of hypoglycemia."
    c. "You should avoid the use of alternative site monitoring when doing SMBG."
    d. "Today's meter systems require a very small blood sample."

88. The postoperative patient with DM has experienced relatively good glucose control during hospitalization. Suddenly the patient has an unexpected increase in blood glucose level. What should the nurse suspect?
    a. Family bringing in food for patient consumption
    b. Wound infection occurring before fever
    c. Postoperative rise in glucose due to new drugs
    d. Respiratory infection acquired from a visitor

89. Which are symptoms of diabetic neuropathy? **Select all that apply.**
    a. Metatarsalgia
    b. Hyperalgesia
    c. Loss of vision
    d. Decreased urine output
    e. Allodynia
    f. Numbness and tingling in legs

90. Which drug does the nurse expect will be prescribed for a patient with burning neuropathy?
    a. Gabapentin
    b. Amitriptyline hydrochloride
    c. Duloxetine
    d. Capsaicin cream 0.075%

91. The patient with DM is prescribed an angiotensin-converting enzyme inhibitor (ACEI). What lab value does the nurse expect will be checked while the patient is on this drug?
    a. Serum sodium
    b. Urine albumin
    c. Serum calcium
    d. Urine potassium

92. Which are common causes of hypoglycemia? **Select all that apply.**
    a. Too much insulin compared with food intake and physical activity
    b. Increased food intake especially after missed or delayed meals
    c. Insulin injected at the wrong time relative to food intake and physical activity
    d. Decreased insulin sensitivity as a result of regular exercise and weight loss
    e. Decreased insulin clearance from progressive kidney failure
    f. Decrease liver glucose production after alcohol ingestion

93. The nurse is caring for a patient recovering from DKA. Which patient care task could be delegated to the unlicensed assistive personnel (UAP)?
    a. Record urine output every hour.
    b. Assess mental status every hour.
    c. Assess central venous pressure every 30 minutes.
    d. Teach patient about causes of DKA.

94. The nurse is teaching a newly diagnosed patient with type 1 DM. Which topics are considered survival information to be taught during the initial phase of DM education? **Select all that apply.**
    a. In-depth discussion of DM pathophysiology
    b. Learning how to prepare and administer insulin
    c. Sick day management rules
    d. Recognition of hypoglycemia and hyperglycemia
    e. Discussion of the actions of insulin
    f. Monitoring blood glucose and urine ketones

95. A patient with type 2 DM is prescribed albiglutide. What **key** information must the nurse provide about this drug?
    a. "Take this drug with the first bite of your meal."
    b. "Albiglutide comes in pill form and is taken every morning before breakfast."
    c. "This drug is administered subcutaneously once a week."
    d. "Be sure to carry a glucose source with you at all times."

96. The health care provider prescribes empagliflozin for the patient with diabetes. For which complication will the nurse be sure to monitor while the patient is taking this drug?
    a. Heart failure
    b. Impaired renal function
    c. Pulmonary edema
    d. Gastrointestinal distress

65

CHAPTER

Assessment of the Renal/Urinary System

1. A patient has sustained a minor kidney injury. Which structure must remain functional in order to form urine?
   a. Medulla
   b. Nephron
   c. Calyx
   d. Capsule

2. Which event is **most likely** to trigger renin production?
   a. Patient drinks an excessive amount of fluid.
   b. Patient becomes anxious and nervous.
   c. Patient has urge to urinate during the night.
   d. Patient sustains significant blood loss.

3. In which circumstance is the regulatory role of aldosterone **most important** in order for the person to maintain homeostasis?
   a. Person has a kidney stone and decreased urine output.
   b. Person has been hiking in the desert for several hours.
   c. Person experiences stress incontinence when coughing.
   d. Person eats excessive citrus and urine becomes alkaline.

4. In which circumstance would vasopressin be released to maintain blood osmolality?
   a. Person exercises for a long period without drinking any fluid.
   b. Person receives an intravenous fluid bolus too rapidly.
   c. Person is on a severely restricted protein diet for several days.
   d. Person becomes anxious and hyperventilates for several minutes.

5. Based on the nurse's knowledge of the normal function of the kidney, which large particles should not appear in a routine urine sample because they are too large to filter through the glomerular capillary walls? **Select all that apply.**
   a. Blood cells
   b. Albumin
   c. Other proteins
   d. Electrolytes
   e. Water
   f. Acids

6. What is the average urine output of a healthy adult for a 24-hour period?
   a. 500 mL to 1000 mL per day
   b. 1500 mL to 2000 mL per day
   c. 3000 mL to 5000 mL per day
   d. 5000 mL to 7000 mL per day

7. The nurse is caring for a patient who sustained major injuries in an automobile accident. Which blood pressure will result in compromised kidney function, in particular the glomerular filtration rate?
   a. 160/80 mm Hg
   b. 70/40 mm Hg
   c. 80/60 mm Hg
   d. 140/100 mm Hg

8. What instructions would the nurse give to unlicensed assistive personnel about the proper handling of a urine specimen?
   a. "Urine must be in a covered container and delivered to the laboratory within 1 hour."
   b. "Leave the urine specimen in the bathroom; just make sure the lid is tightly secured."
   c. "Urine should always be in a sterile container and be immediately taken to the laboratory."
   d. "Have the patient pee in a cup and tell him to tighten the lid and leave the cup by the toilet."

9. Which hematologic disorder is **most likely** to occur if the hormonal function of the kidneys is not working properly?
   a. Leukemia
   b. Thrombocytopenia
   c. Neutropenia
   d. Anemia

10. Which patient is **most likely** to exceed the renal threshold if there is noncompliance with the prescribed therapeutic regimen?
    a. Has recurrent kidney stone formation
    b. Has type 2 diabetes mellitus
    c. Has functional urinary incontinence
    d. Has biliary obstruction

11. Which personal action is **most likely** to cause the kidneys to produce and release erythropoietin?
    a. Person moves to a low desert area where the humidity is very low.
    b. Person moves to a high-altitude area where atmospheric oxygen is low.
    c. Person drinks an excessive amount of fluid that results in fluid overload.
    d. Person eats a large high-protein meal after a rigorous exercise workout.

12. Vitamin D is converted to its active form in the kidney; if this function fails, which electrolyte imbalance will occur?
    a. Hyperkalemia
    b. Hypocalcemia
    c. Hypernatremia
    d. Hypoglycemia

13. Which patient is the **least likely** to have control over voluntary micturition?
    a. A 25-year-old with a spinal cord injury
    b. A 56-year-old woman who has microalbuminuria
    c. A 40-year-old who has recurrent pyelonephritis
    d. An 18-year-old who has a urine specific gravity of 1.030

14. An elderly patient has been in bed for several days after a fall. The nurse encourages ambulation to stimulate the movement of urine through the ureter by which physiologic phenomenon?
    a. Peristalsis
    b. Gravity
    c. Exercise
    d. Backflow

15. Which renal change associated with aging does the nurse expect an older adult patient to report?
    a. Nocturnal polyuria
    b. Anuria
    c. Hematuria
    d. Dysuria

16. An older adult male patient has a history of an enlarged prostate. The patient is **most likely** to report which symptom associated with this condition?
    a. Inability to sense the urge to void
    b. Difficulty starting the urine stream
    c. Passing large amounts of very dilute urine
    d. Burning sensation when urinating

17. Impairment in the thirst mechanism associated with aging makes an older adult patient more vulnerable to which disorder?
    a. Hypernatremia
    b. Hypocalcemia
    c. Hyperkalemia
    d. Hypoglycemia

18. The nurse is talking to a group of older women about changes in the urinary system related to aging. What sign/symptom is likely to be the **common** concern for this group?
    a. Incontinence
    b. Hematuria
    c. Retention
    d. Dysuria

19. African Americans have the highest risk for kidney failure. Which topics are related to kidney health and require special attention during patient teaching with this group?
    a. Hypertension and sodium intake
    b. Diabetes mellitus and calcium intake
    c. Weight loss and vitamin D intake
    d. Osteoporosis and potassium intake

20. The nurse is taking a history on a patient with a change in urinary patterns. In addition to the medical and surgical history, what does the nurse ask about in order to complete the assessment? **Select all that apply.**
    a. Occupational exposure to toxins
    b. Use of illicit substances, such as cocaine
    c. Financial resources for payment of treatments
    d. Likelihood of complying with treatment recommendations
    e. Recent travel to geographic regions that pose infectious disease risks
    f. History of chronic health problems, especially diabetes mellitus or hypertension

21. Which patient narrative describes the symptom of dysuria?
    a. "I have to pee all the time."
    b. "I have to wait before the pee starts."
    c. "It hurts when I pee."
    d. "It feels like I am going to pee in my pants."

22. The nurse is interviewing a 35-year-old woman who needs evaluation for a potential kidney problem. The woman reports she has been pregnant twice and has two healthy children. Which question would the nurse ask about potential health issues that occurred during pregnancy?
    a. "How much weight did you gain during the pregnancy?"
    b. "Were you treated for gestational diabetes?"
    c. "Did both of your pregnancies go to full-term?"
    d. "Did you have a urinary catheter inserted during labor?"

23. The health care provider recommends a fluid intake of at least 2 liters per day. The patient reports fluid intake over the past 24 hours: 15 ounces of coffee and 10 ounces of juice for breakfast, 10 ounces of skim milk for a snack, 12 ounces of protein shake for lunch, ½ liter of sports drink in the afternoon, and 3 ounces of wine for dinner. After calculating the 24-hour fluid intake, what does the nurse tell the patient?
    a. Fluid consumption should be increased by at least 2 more servings.
    b. Fluid consumption is meeting the 2 liter/day recommendation.
    c. Fluid consumption exceeds recommendation; therefore, eliminate the wine.
    d. Fluid consumption includes only liquids such as water, juice, or milk.

24. The nurse is taking a history on a 55-year-old patient who denies any serious chronic health problems. Which **sudden** onset sign/symptom most strongly suggests possible kidney disease in this patient?
    a. Weakness
    b. High blood pressure
    c. Fever
    d. Rapid pulse

25. Which over-the-counter product used by a patient does the nurse further explore for potential impact on kidney function?
    a. Mouthwash with alcohol
    b. Fiber supplement
    c. Vitamin C
    d. Acetaminophen

26. A patient appears very uncomfortable with the nurse's questions about urinary functions and patterns. What is the **best** technique for the nurse to use to elicit relevant information and decrease the patient's discomfort?
    a. Defer the questions until a later time.
    b. Direct the questions toward a family member.
    c. Use professional medical terminology.
    d. Use the patient's own terminology.

27. The nurse is taking a nutritional history on a patient. The patient states, "I really don't drink as much water as I should." What is the nurse's **best** response?
    a. "That's okay. Most of us should drink more water than we do."
    b. "It's an easy thing to forget; just try to remember to drink more."
    c. "What would encourage you to drink the recommended 2 liters per day?"
    d. "Would you like to read this brochure about kidney health and fluids?"

28. When patients have problems with the kidneys or urinary tract, what is the **most common** symptom that prompts them to seek medical attention?
    a. Change in the frequency or amount of urination
    b. Pain in flank or abdomen or pain when urinating
    c. Change in color, clarity, or odor of the urine
    d. Exposure to a nephrotoxic substance

29. The nurse is determining whether a patient has a history of hypertension because of the potential for kidney problems. Which question is **best** to elicit this information?
    a. "Do you have high blood pressure?"
    b. "Do you take any blood pressure medications?"
    c. "Have you ever been told that your blood pressure was high?"
    d. "When was the last time you had your blood pressure checked?"

30. The nurse is performing an assessment of the renal system. What is the **first** step in the assessment process?
    a. Percuss the lower abdomen; continue toward the umbilicus.
    b. Observe the flank region for asymmetry or discoloration.
    c. Listen for a bruit over each renal artery.
    d. Lightly palpate the abdomen in all quadrants.

31. A patient with chronic kidney disease develops anorexia, nausea and vomiting, muscle cramping, and pruritus. How does the nurse interpret these findings?
    a. Oliguria
    b. Azotemia
    c. Anuria
    d. Uremia

32. The nurse hears in report that the patient is having renal colic pain. When performing the physical assessment of this patient during a severe pain episode, what additional sign/symptom may the nurse expect to observe?
    a. Diaphoresis
    b. Ecchymosis
    c. Jaundice
    d. Bruit

33. The nurse is assessing a patient with a chronic kidney problem. The nurse notes that the patient has pedal and periorbital edema. What additional assessments will the nurse make to assess for fluid overload? **Select all that apply.**
    a. Obtain a urine specimen.
    b. Compare current blood pressure to baseline.
    c. Measure the residual urine with a bladder scanner.
    d. Weigh the patient and compare to baseline.
    e. Auscultate lung fields to determine if fluid is present.
    f. Check the sacral area, particular if patient is sedentary

34. A patient is diagnosed with renal artery stenosis. Which sound does the nurse expect to hear by auscultation when a bruit is present in a renal artery?
    a. Quiet, pulsating sound
    b. Swishing sound
    c. Occasional gurgling
    d. Faint wheezing

35. The nurse is assisting an inexperienced health care provider to assess a patient who has an aneurysm. The nurse would intervene if the provider performed which action?
    a. Inspected the flank for bruising or redness
    b. Listened for a bruit over the renal artery
    c. Auscultated the abdomen for bowel sounds
    d. Palpated deeply to locate masses or tenderness

36. The nurse reads in the assessment note made by the advanced-practice nurse that the "left kidney cannot be palpated." How does the nurse interpret this notation?
    a. The left kidney is smaller than normal, which indicates kidney disease.
    b. The left kidney is normally deeper and may not be palpable.
    c. The palpation of kidneys should be repeated by another provider.
    d. The patient is too obese for this type of examination.

37. The nurse is assessing a patient for bladder distention. What technique does the nurse use?
    a. Gently palpate for outline of bladder and percuss lower abdomen toward umbilicus until dull sounds are no longer produced.
    b. Locate the symphysis pubis, gently palpate for outline of bladder, auscultate for bowel sounds in the lower abdomen.
    c. Place one hand under back and palpate with other hand over bladder and percuss lower abdomen until tympanic sounds are no longer produced.
    d. Use hand to gently depress the bladder as the patient inhales a deep breath, then percuss as the patient slowly exhales.

38. A patient reports flank pain and tenderness. What technique does the nurse use to assess for costovertebral angle (CVA) tenderness?
    a. Percuss the nontender CVA area and assess for rebound.
    b. Massage the CVA area with the flat surface of the hand.
    c. Quickly thump the CVA area with a clenched fist.
    d. Place one palm over the CVA area, thump with other fist.

39. The nurse is preparing to assess a female patient's urethra prior to the insertion of an indwelling urinary catheter. In addition to gloves, which equipment does the nurse obtain to perform the initial assessment?
    a. Clean glass slide
    b. Good light source
    c. Disposable speculum
    d. Water-based lubricant

40. A healthy female patient has no physical symptoms, but urinalysis results reveal a protein level of 0.8 mg/dL and a white blood cell count of 4 per high-powered field. What question would the nurse ask the patient in order to assist the health care provider to correctly interpret the urinalysis results?
    a. "Have you ever been treated for a urinary tract infection?"
    b. "Do you have a family history of cardiac or biliary disease?"
    c. "Are you sexually active and if so, do you use condoms?"
    d. "Have you recently performed any strenuous exercise?"

41. How does the nurse interpret presence of ketones in the urine?
    a. Glomerular filtration rate has decreased.
    b. Patient has a chronic kidney infection.
    c. Fat is being used for cellular energy.
    d. Urinary tract infection is likely.

42. The nurse and nutritionist are evaluating the diet and nutritional therapies for a patient with kidney problems. Blood urea nitrogen levels for this patient are tracked because of the direct relationship to the intake and metabolism of which substance?
    a. Lipids
    b. Carbohydrates
    c. Protein
    d. Fluids

43. The nurse is caring for a patient with dehydration. Which laboratory test results does the nurse anticipate to observe in this patient?
    a. Blood urea nitrogen and creatinine ratio stay the same.
    b. Blood urea nitrogen rises faster than creatinine level.
    c. Creatinine will be higher than blood urea nitrogen.
    d. Blood urea nitrogen and creatinine are always inverse.

44. The nurse sees that the patient with known kidney dysfunction has a decreased blood urea nitrogen (BUN). Which major organ could be dysfunctional and therefore contributing to the decreased BUN?
    a. Heart
    b. Pancreas
    c. Liver
    d. Gallbladder

45. A healthy 34-year-old male with no physical complaints has a blood urea nitrogen of 26 mg/dL. Which questions would the nurse ask to identify nonrenal factors that could be contributing to this laboratory result? **Select all that apply.**
    a. "Did you drink a lot of extra fluid before the blood sample was drawn?"
    b. "Have you been on a high protein diet or been drinking high protein drinks?"
    c. "Are you taking or have you recently taken any steroid medications?"
    d. "Have you recently experienced any physical or emotional stress?"
    e. "Have you noticed any blood in the stool or have you vomited any blood?"
    f. "Have you been trying to lose weight with severe calorie restrictions?

46. The nurse sees that an older patient has a blood osmolarity of 303 mOsm/L. Which additional assessment is the nurse **most likely** to perform before notifying the health care provider about the laboratory results?
    a. Respiratory status
    b. Signs of dehydration
    c. Any discomfort or pain
    d. Odor of the urine

47. Which patient is **most likely** to have a decreased serum calcium level?
    a. Has kidney disease
    b. Has a bladder infection
    c. Has urinary incontinence
    d. Has urinary retention

48. The nurse performs a dipstick urine test for a patient being evaluated for kidney problems. Glucose is present in the urine. How does the nurse interpret this result?
    a. Blood glucose level is greater than 220 mg/dL.
    b. Kidneys are failing to filter any glucose.
    c. Patient is at risk for hypoglycemia.
    d. Renal threshold has not been exceeded.

49. In addition to kidney disease, which patient condition causes the blood urea nitrogen to rise above the normal range?
    a. Anemia
    b. Asthma
    c. Infection
    d. Malnutrition

50. The community health nurse is talking to a group of African American adults about renal health. The nurse encourages the participants to have which type of yearly examination to screen for kidney problems?
    a. Kidney ultrasound, blood urea nitrogen, and serum glucose
    b. Serum creatinine, blood urea nitrogen, and renal scan
    c. Urinalysis, microalbuminuria, and serum creatinine
    d. 24-hour urine collection, blood urea nitrogen, and urinalysis

51. During the shift, the nursing student is measuring urine output and observing for urine characteristics in a patient. Which abnormal finding is the **most urgent** and should be immediately reported to the supervising nurse?
    a. Specific gravity is decreased.
    b. Output is decreased.
    c. pH is decreased.
    d. Color has changed.

52. Which patient is **most likely** to produce urine with a specific gravity of less than 1.005?
    a. Takes diuretic medication every day.
    b. Has dehydration secondary to vomiting.
    c. Is hypovolemic due to blood loss.
    d. Has syndrome of inappropriate antidiuretic hormone.

53. What does an increase in the ratio of blood urea nitrogen (BUN) to serum creatinine indicate?
    a. Highly suggestive of kidney dysfunction
    b. Definitive for kidney dysfunction secondary to infection
    c. Suggests nonkidney factors causing an elevation in BUN
    d. Suggests kidney factors causing an elevation in serum creatinine

54. Which urine characteristic listed on a urinalysis report arouses the nurse's suspicion of a problem in the urinary tract?
    a. Cloudiness
    b. Straw color
    c. Ammonia odor
    d. One cast per high-powered field

55. A patient has a urinalysis ordered. When is the **best** time for the nurse to collect the specimen?
    a. In the evening
    b. After a meal
    c. In the morning
    d. After a fluid bolus

56. Which test is the **best** indicator of kidney function?
    a. Urine osmolarity
    b. Serum creatinine
    c. Urine pH
    d. Blood urea nitrogen

57. A 24-hour urine specimen is required from a patient. Which strategy is **best** to ensure that all the urine is collected for the full 24-hour period?
    a. Instruct unlicensed assistive personnel to collect and save all urine.
    b. Put a bedpan or commode next to the bed as a reminder.
    c. Place a sign in the bathroom reminding everyone to save all urine.
    d. Make the patient responsible for collecting the urine specimen.

58. A patient requires measurement of residual urine after voiding. Place the steps of using the bedside bladder scanner in the correct order. **1 being the first step and 6 being the last step.**

    _____ a. Select the male or female icon on the bladder scanner.

    _____ b. Aim the scan head toward the expected location of the bladder.

    _____ c. Place the probe midline about 1.5 inches (4 cm) above the pubic bone.

    _____ d. Explain the purpose and what sensations to expect.

    _____ e. Place the ultrasound probe with gel right above the symphysis pubis.

    _____ f. Press and release the scan button.

59. A patient is scheduled for a computed tomography with iodinated contrast medium. Which medication is discontinued 24 hours before the procedure and for at least 48 hours until kidney function has been reevaluated?
    a. Glucophage
    b. Morphine
    c. Furosemide
    d. Oral acetylcysteine

60. Several patients are scheduled for testing to diagnose potential kidney problems. Which test **requires** a patient to have a urinary catheter inserted before the test?
    a. Urine stream testing
    b. Computed tomography
    c. Cystography
    d. Renal scan

61. What is included in the postprocedural care for a patient who had a renal scan?
    a. Administer laxatives to cleanse the bowel.
    b. Encourage oral fluids to assist excretion of isotope.
    c. Administer captopril to increase renal blood flow.
    d. Insert a urinary catheter to measure urine output.

62. The patient is scheduled to have computed tomography with contrast at 10:00 AM. At 3:00 AM the night shift nurse receives laboratory results that show the patient's serum creatinine is 1.1 mg/dL. What should the nurse do?
    a. Ask the day shift nurse to inform the radiologist about the results as within normal limits.
    b. Call the health care provider because the creatinine level is too high to use contrast dye.
    c. Inform the night shift radiology technician that the diagnostic test will need to be cancelled.
    d. Document the results; no further action is needed because results do not impact the procedure.

63. The nurse sees a radiology report that the ultrasound of the patient's kidney showed an enlarged kidney. Which serial assessment is the nurse **most likely** to initiate?
    a. Monitoring hourly urinary output
    b. Monitoring for dehydration every 4 hours
    c. Assessing hourly for hemorrhage
    d. Checking for incontinence every 2 hours

64. A patient returns to the unit after a renal scan. Which instruction about the patient's urine does the nurse give to unlicensed assistive personnel?
    a. There is radioactive urine, so use special biohazard precautions for disposal.
    b. There is no danger because the amount of radioactive material is very small.
    c. There is danger of radioactive exposure but only for those who are pregnant.
    d. There is potential danger of radioactivity if the urine is not immediately flushed.

65. What is an advantage of a renal scan compared to computed tomography (CT) for diagnosing the perfusion, function, and structure of the kidneys?
    a. Renal scan is more readily tolerated by elderly patients and small children.
    b. Renal scan is preferred if the patient is allergic to iodine or has impaired kidney function.
    c. Renal scans are more likely to detect pathologic changes that CT scans do not detect.
    d. Renal scan requires less pre- and postprocedural care than CT scan.

66. The nurse is teaching a patient scheduled for an ultrasonography. What preprocedural instruction does the nurse give the patient?
    a. Void just before the test begins.
    b. Drink water to fill the bladder.
    c. Stop routine medications.
    d. Have nothing to eat or drink after midnight.

67. A patient had a cystoscopy. After the procedure, what does the nurse expect to see in this patient?
    a. Pink-tinged urine
    b. Bloody urine
    c. Very dilute urine
    d. Decreased urine output

68. A patient is scheduled for retrograde urethrography. Postprocedural care is similar to postprocedural care given for which test?
    a. Ultrasonography
    b. Computed tomography
    c. Renal angiogram
    d. Cystoscopy

69. A patient has undergone a kidney biopsy. What is the **priority** post procedural assessment?
    a. Observe for nephrotoxicity
    b. Check for hemorrhage
    c. Monitor for urinary retention
    d. Assess for hypertension

70. The health care provider informs the nurse that there is a change in orders because the patient has a decrease in creatinine clearance rate. What change does the nurse anticipate?
    a. Fluid restriction
    b. Reduction of drug dosages
    c. Limitations on activity level
    d. Delay in discharge

71. The nurse is planning the care for several patients who are undergoing diagnostic testing. Which patient is likely to need the **most time** for postprocedural care?
    a. Will have a kidney, ureter, and bladder x-ray
    b. Needs a kidney ultrasound
    c. Will have a cystoscopy
    d. Needs urine for culture and sensitivity

72. A patient has undergone a kidney biopsy. In the **immediate** postprocedural period, the nurse notifies the health care provider about which findings? **Select all that apply.**
    a. Hematuria with blood clots
    b. Localized pain at the site
    c. "Tamponade effect"
    d. Decreasing urine output
    e. Flank pain
    f. Decreasing blood pressure

73. Limiting fluid intake would have what effect on urine?
    a. Increases the specific gravity of urine.
    b. Increases the pH of urine.
    c. Decreases the risk for urine infection.
    d. Decreases the osmolality of urine.

74. Which **abnormal** finding would be associated with chronic kidney disease?
    a. Hematuria
    b. Pus in the urine
    c. Blood at the urethral meatus
    d. Decreased urine specific gravity

75. For which circumstance, would it be appropriate to select the male icon when performing a bladder scan on a female patient?
    a. Female who identifies self as a male
    b. Woman with a history of hysterectomy
    c. Woman who is 5 years postmenopausal
    d. Female with a history of bladder cancer

76. A patient is newly diagnosed with type 2 diabetes mellitus. Which screening can be done for the **early** detection of diabetic kidney disease?
    a. Urine should be tested for protein and microalbuminuria.
    b. Blood urea nitrogen and serum creatinine should be tested within 5 years.
    c. Urine should be tested for ketones and protein.
    d. Urine should be tested annually for glucose, and blood.

66 CHAPTER

Care of Patients with Urinary Problems

1. The home health nurse reads in the patient's chart that the patient has asymptomatic bacterial urinary tract infection (ABUTI). Which intervention will the nurse perform?
   a. Obtain an order for urinalysis and urine culture and sensitivity.
   b. Check the patient's medication list for appropriate antibiotic order.
   c. Closely monitor for conditions that cause progression to acute infection.
   d. Ask the patient when the ABUTI first started and when it was diagnosed.

2. Which group has the **highest** prevalence of urinary tract infections?
   a. Postpartum women
   b. Older women
   c. Older men
   d. Adolescent girls

3. Which patient has the **highest** risk for developing a complicated urinary tract infection?
   a. 26-year-old man who is sexually active but inconsistently uses condoms
   b. 22-year-old man who has a neurogenic bladder due to spinal cord injury
   c. 35-year-old woman who had three full-term pregnancies and a miscarriage
   d. 53-year-old woman who is having some menstrual irregularities

4. The nurse is working in a long-term care facility. Which circumstance is cause for **greatest** concern, because the facility has a large number of residents who are developing urinary tract infections?
   a. Residents are not drinking enough fluids with meals.
   b. Unlicensed personnel are not assisting with toileting in a timely fashion.
   c. A large percentage of residents have indwelling urinary catheters.
   d. Many residents have severe dementia and functional incontinence.

5. The nurse is caring for a patient with an indwelling catheter. What intervention does the nurse use to minimize catheter-related infections?
   a. Assess the patient daily to determine need for catheter.
   b. Irrigate the catheter daily with sterile solution to remove debris.
   c. Use sterile technique to open the system to obtain urine samples.
   d. Apply antiseptic solutions or antibiotic ointments to the perineal area.

6. Which task related to care of patients who have indwelling catheters can be delegated to unlicensed assistive personnel?
   a. Wash the perineum daily and frequently empty the drainage bag using a separate, clean container for each patient.
   b. Use sterile technique when cleaning urinary catheters or when helping the patients with genital or rectal hygiene.
   c. Determine whether use of condom catheters is appropriate for male patients and apply the devices accordingly.
   d. Keep urine collection bag in a place that is readily visible to the patient so that the patient is reassured of kidney function.

7. In which patient circumstance would the nurse **question** the order for the insertion of an indwelling catheter?
   a. Patient is critically ill and at risk for hypovolemic shock.
   b. Patient has urinary retention with beginnings of hydronephrosis.
   c. Patient was in a car accident and has a possible spinal cord injury.
   d. Patient has functional incontinence related to Alzheimer's disease.

8. For a patient who needs an indwelling catheter for at least 2 weeks, which intervention would help reduce the bacterial colonization along the catheter?
   a. Secure the catheter to the female patient's thigh.
   b. Obtain an order to insert an antiseptic catheter.
   c. Wash the urine bag and outflow tube every day.
   d. Apply antiseptic ointment to the catheter tubing.

9. The nurse hears in report that the patient is being treated for a fungal urinary tract infection (UTI). In addition to performing routine care and assessments, the nurse is extra-vigilant for signs/symptoms of which systemic disorder that may underlie the fungal UTI?
   a. Chronic cardiac disease
   b. Immune system compromise
   c. Chronic skin condition
   d. Connective tissue disorder

10. The nurse is caring for a patient who has an indwelling catheter and subsequently developed a urinary tract infection. The patient has been receiving antibiotics for several days but develops hypotension, a rapid pulse, and confusion. The nurse suspects urosepsis and alerts the health care provider. Which diagnostic test is the provider **most likely** to order to confirm sepsis?
    a. Culture of the urinary meatus
    b. Culture of the catheter tip
    c. Blood cultures
    d. Repeat urinalysis

11. The nurse is teaching a woman how to prevent urinary tract infections. What information does the nurse include?
    a. Clean the perineal area from front to back.
    b. Douche before and after sexual intercourse.
    c. Take oral estrogen to decrease vaginal dryness.
    d. Avoid urinary stasis by urinating every 6 to 8 hours.

12. The nurse is teaching a man about how to prevent urinary tract infections. What information does the nurse include?
    a. "Drink adequate fluid before and after intercourse."
    b. "Empty your bladder before and after intercourse."
    c. "Make sure that spermicides are used with condoms."
    d. "Gently wash the genital area before intercourse."

13. Patients who have central nervous system lesions from stroke, multiple sclerosis, or parasacral spinal cord lesions may develop which type of urinary incontinence?
    a. Detrusor hyperreflexia
    b. Mixed
    c. Stress
    d. Functional

14. A patient reports intense urgency, frequency, and bladder pain. Urinalysis results show no white blood cells and no red blood cells and urine culture results are negative for infection. How does the nurse interpret these findings?
    a. These findings are associated with a diagnosis of interstitial cystitis.
    b. Patient could have urethritis due to sexually transmitted disease.
    c. Signs and symptoms suggest kidney stones; pain is likely to intensify.
    d. Findings suggest bacterial cystitis that is partially treated by antibiotics.

15. The nurse sees that the patient was recently started on oxybutynin. Which question is the nurse **most likely** to ask to evaluate whether or not the medication is having the desired effect?
    a. "Are you still losing small amounts of urine during your daily jogging activity?
    b. "Have you had any episodes of flank pain or difficult passing your urine?
    c. "Have you had any problems with fever or noticed any burning when you urinate?"
    d. "Are you still having a sudden strong urge to void and leaking large amounts of urine?"

16. A young female patient reports burning with urination. What question does the nurse ask to differentiate between a vaginal infection and a urinary infection?
    a. "Have you noticed any blood in the urine?"
    b. "Have you recently had sexual intercourse?"
    c. "Have you noticed any vaginal discharge?"
    d. "Have you had fever or chills?"

17. A patient reports symptoms indicating a urinary tract infection (UTI). Which urine test results **most strongly** indicates a UTI?
    a. Presence of leukocyte esterase and nitrate
    b. Presence of glucose and ketones
    c. Presence of epithelial cells and red blood cells
    d. Low urine specific gravity and low urine pH

18. A patient is diagnosed with a fungal urinary tract infection. Which drug does the nurse anticipate the patient will be treated with?
    a. Trimethoprim/sulfamethoxazole
    b. Ciprofloxacin
    c. Fluconazole
    d. Amoxicillin

19. The nurse is teaching a patient about self-care measures to prevent urinary tract infections. Which daily fluid intake does the nurse recommend to the patient to prevent a bladder infection?
    a. 2-3 L of water
    b. 3-6 glasses of iced tea
    c. 4-6 cups of electrolyte fluid
    d. 3-4 glasses of juice

20. The nursing student sees an order for a urinalysis for a patient with frequency, urgency, and dysuria. In order to collect the specimen, what does the student do?
    a. Use sterile technique to insert a small-diameter (6 Fr) catheter.
    b. Instruct the patient on how to collect a clean-catch specimen.
    c. Tell the patient to urinate approximately 10 mL into a specimen cup.
    d. Take the urine from a bedpan and transfer it into a specimen cup.

21. The nurse is reviewing the laboratory results for an older adult patient with an indwelling catheter. The urine culture is pending, but the urinalysis shows greater than 10^5 colony-forming units, and the differential white blood cell count shows a "left shift." The nurse will monitor for additional signs/symptoms associated with which condition?
    a. Interstitial cystitis
    b. Urosepsis
    c. Complicated cystitis
    d. Bladder cancer

22. A patient has urinary tract infection symptoms but there are no bacteria in the urine. The health care provider suspects interstitial cystitis. The nurse prepares patient teaching material for which diagnostic test?
    a. Voiding cystourethrography
    b. Ultrasonography
    c. Computed tomography
    d. Cystoscopy

23. Several patients at the clinic have just been diagnosed with urinary tract infections. Which patients may need longer antibiotic treatment (7-21 days) or different agents than the typical first-line medications? **Select all that apply.**
    a. Postmenopausal female patient
    b. Female patient with urethritis
    c. Diabetic female patient
    d. Immunosuppressed male patient
    e. Pregnant female patient
    f. Older male patient who engages in anal intercourse

24. The nurse is counseling a patient with recurrent symptomatic urinary tract infections (UTIs) about diet therapy. What information does the nurse give to the patient?
    a. Drink cranberry juice but avoid products with high fructose.
    b. Low consumption of protein may prevent recurrent UTIs.
    c. Caffeine, carbonated beverages, and tomato products cause UTI.
    d. Cranberry tablets are more effective than juice or fluids.

25. A patient received an antibiotic prescription several hours ago and has started the medication but requests "some relief from the burning." What comfort measures does the nurse suggest to the patient?
    a. Take over-the-counter acetaminophen.
    b. Sit in a sitz bath and urinate into the warm water.
    c. Place a cold pack over the perineal area.
    d. Rest in a recumbent position with legs elevated.

26. A patient's recurrent cystitis appears to be related to sexual intercourse. The patient seems uncomfortable talking about the situation. What communication technique does the nurse use to assist the patient?
    a. Have an open and sensitive discussion with the patient.
    b. Give the patient reading material with instructions to call with any questions.
    c. Call the patient's partner and invite the partner to discuss the problem.
    d. Talk about other topics until the patient feels more comfortable disclosing.

27. Which factor is the **strongest** predictor for a patient to develop a catheter-associated urinary tract infection ?
    a. Previous history of urinary tract infection
    b. Length of time that catheter dwells in patient
    c. Qualifications of health care worker inserting the catheter
    d. Lack of daily perineal hygiene and daily bathing

28. A male college student comes to the clinic reporting burning or difficulty with urination and a discharge from the urethral meatus. Based on the patient's report, what is the **most** logical question for the nurse to ask?
    a. "Do you have a history of a narrow urethra or a stricture?"
    b. "Could you have been exposed to a sexually transmitted disease?"
    c. "Do you have a history of kidney stones?"
    d. "Have you been drinking an adequate amount of fluids?"

29. The health care provider verbally informs the nurse that the patient needs a fluoroquinolone antibiotic to treat a urinary tract infection. The pharmacy delivers gabapentin. What should the nurse do **first**?
    a. Administer the medication as ordered.
    b. Call the pharmacist and ask for a read back of the order.
    c. Call the health care provider for clarification of the order.
    d. Look at the written order and take steps to correct the error.

30. Which patient should not be advised to take cranberry juice?
    a. 26-year-old pregnant woman with an uncomplicated urinary tract infection
    b. 23-year-old man with history of recurrent kidney stones
    c. 65-year-old man with urinary retention secondary to enlarged prostate
    d. 33-year-old woman with dysuria associated with interstitial cystitis

31. Which urine characteristic suggests that the patient is drinking a sufficient amount of fluid?
    a. Urine pH is between 6 to 6.5.
    b. Urine has a high specific gravity.
    c. Urine has a faint ammonia odor.
    d. Urine is a pale yellow color.

32. A young woman tells the nurse that she gets frequent urinary tract infections that seem to follow sexual intercourse. Which questions would the nurse ask? **Select all that apply.**
    a. "Do you use a diaphragm or spermicides for contraception?"
    b. "Do you feel guilty or embarrassed about your sexual activities?"
    c. "Have you considered abstaining from intercourse?"
    d. "Do you and your partner(s) wash the perineal area before intercourse?"
    e. "Some positions cause more irritation during sex. Have you noticed this?"
    f. "Do you and your partner(s) ever engage in anal intercourse?"

33. A patient is diagnosed with urethral stricture. What is the **priority** assessment?
    a. Monitor for pain during urination.
    b. Monitor urinary output.
    c. Assess for swelling at meatus.
    d. Observe for hematuria.

34. The nurse is caring for a patient who had a mid-urethral sling procedure. What instructions would the nurse give to unlicensed assistive personnel to prevent postoperative complications?
    a. Bedrest with bathroom privileges must be maintained for 2-3 days.
    b. Urethral catheter must be secured in place with a tube holder.
    c. Food and fluid restriction must be maintained for 24 hours.
    d. Watch for and report any drainage on the urethral catheter dressing.

35. A patient reports the loss of small amounts of urine during coughing, sneezing, jogging, or lifting. Which type of incontinence is the patient describing?
    a. Urge
    b. Overflow
    c. Functional
    d. Stress

36. The nurse is caring for an obese older adult patient with dementia. The patient is alert and ambulatory but has functional incontinence. Which nursing intervention is **best** for this patient?
    a. Help the patient to lose weight.
    b. Help the patient apply an estrogen cream.
    c. Offer assistance with toileting every 2 hours.
    d. Intermittently catheterize the patient.

37. Which patient is **mostly likely** to have mixed incontinence?
    a. 62-year-old woman who had four full-term pregnancies
    b. 40-year-old man who had a stroke with neurologic deficits
    c. 76-year-old man with benign prostatic hyperplasia
    d. 25-year-old woman who has a pelvic fracture

38. The nurse is caring for an older adult patient with urinary incontinence. The patient is alert and oriented but refuses to use the call bell and has fallen several times while trying to get to the bathroom. What is the nurse's **priority** concern for this patient?
    a. Managing noncompliance
    b. Accurately measuring urinary output
    c. Initiating fall prevention measures
    d. Managing urinary incontinence

39. The nurse is performing an assessment on a patient with probable stress incontinence. Which assessment technique does the nurse use to validate stress incontinence?
    a. Assess the abdomen to estimate bladder fullness.
    b. Check for residual urine using a portable ultrasound.
    c. Catheterize the patient immediately after voiding.
    d. Ask the patient to cough while wearing a perineal pad.

40. The nurse reads in the documentation that the advanced practice nurse performed a digital rectal examination and found that the rectal sphincter did not contract on digital insertion. Based on this information, which assessment is the nurse **most likely** to perform?
    a. Monitor the urinary output every 4 hours.
    b. Assess for bowel and bladder incontinence.
    c. Palpate the bladder and monitor for distention.
    d. Check the stool and urine for occult blood.

41. A middle-aged woman has urinary stress incontinence related to weak pelvic muscles. Which interventions does the nurse include in the treatment plan? **Select all that apply.**
    a. Suggest keeping a detailed diary of urine leakage, activities, and foods eaten.
    b. Suggest wearing absorbent undergarments during the assessment process.
    c. Teach pelvic floor (Kegel) exercise therapy.
    d. Teach about vaginal cone therapy.
    e. Encourage drinking orange juice every day for 4-6 weeks.
    f. Refer to a nutritionist for diet therapy for weight reduction.

42. A patient has been performing Kegel exercises for 2 months. Which outcome statement indicates that the goal of therapy has been met?
    a. Incontinence is still present, but there is decrease in frequency.
    b. Patient is able to voluntarily stop the urinary stream.
    c. Patient states that there are no problems with dysuria.
    d. The patient is using fewer absorbent undergarments for protection.

43. The home health nurse is assessing an older adult patient who refuses to leave the house to see friends or participate in usual activities. She reports taking a bath several times a day and becomes very upset when she has an incontinent episode. What is the **priority** problem for this patient?
    a. Negative self-image
    b. Stress urinary incontinence
    c. Decreased opportunities to socialize
    d. Potential for skin breakdown

44. The nurse is evaluating outcome criteria for a patient being treated for urge incontinence. Which statement indicates the treatment has been successful?
    a. "I'm doing the exercises, but I think surgery is my best choice."
    b. "I lose a little urine when I sneeze, but I wear a thin pad."
    c. "I had trouble at first, but now I go to the toilet every 3 hours."
    d. "I have been using the bladder compression technique and it works."

45. The nurse is teaching a patient with urge incontinence about dietary modifications. What is the **best** information for the nurse to give about fluid intake?
    a. Drink at least 2000 mL of water every day unless you have a heart problem.
    b. Drink 120 mL every hour or 240 mL every 2 hours and limit fluids after dinner.
    c. Drink fluid freely in the morning hours but limit intake before going to bed.
    d. Drinking water is especially good for bladder health; drink as much as you can.

46. A patient has agreed to try a bladder training program. What is the **priority** nursing intervention in starting this therapy?
    a. Advise the patient to plan and start a schedule for voiding every 2-3 hours.
    b. Teach the patient how to be alert, aware, and able to resist the urge to urinate.
    c. Convince the patient that the bladder issues are controlling his/her lifestyle.
    d. Give a thorough explanation of the problem of stress incontinence.

47. An older adult patient with a cognitive impairment is living in an extended-care facility. The patient is incontinent, but as the family points out, "he will urinate in the toilet if somebody helps him." Which type of incontinence does the nurse suspect in this patient?
    a. Urge
    b. Overflow
    c. Functional
    d. Stress

48. The nurse is designing a habit training bladder program for an older adult patient who is alert but mildly confused. What task associated with the training program is delegated to unlicensed assistive personnel?
    a. Tell the patient it is time to go to the toilet and assist him to go on a regular schedule.
    b. Help the patient record the incidents of incontinence in a bladder diary.
    c. Change the patient's incontinence pants (or pad) every 4 hours.
    d. Gradually encourage independence and increase the intervals between voidings.

49. Which patient with incontinence is **most likely** to benefit from a surgical sling or bladder suspension procedure?
    a. Has stress incontinence and altered urethral competency.
    b. Has reflex (overflow) incontinence caused by obstruction.
    c. Has functional incontinence related to musculoskeletal weakness.
    d. Has overactive bladder and declines bladder training program.

50. The nurse is teaching a patient a behavioral intervention for bladder compression. In order to correctly perform the Credé method, what does the nurse teach the patient to do?
    a. Insert the fingers into the vagina and gently push against the vaginal wall.
    b. Breathe in deeply and direct the pressure towards the bladder during exhalation.
    c. Empty the bladder, wait a few minutes, and attempt a second bladder emptying.
    d. Apply firm and steady pressure over the bladder area with the palm of the hand.

51. The health care provider has recommended intermittent self-catheterization for a patient with long-term problems of incomplete bladder emptying. Which information does the nurse give the patient about the procedure?
    a. Perform proper handwashing and cleaning of the catheter to reduce the risk for infection.
    b. Use a large-lumen catheter and good lubrication for rapid emptying of the bladder.
    c. Catheterize yourself when you are incontinent or when the bladder gets distended.
    d. Use sterile technique, especially if catheterization is done by a family member.

52. The nurse is reviewing a care plan for a patient who has functional incontinence. There is a note that containment is recommended, especially at night. What is the **major** concern with this approach?
    a. Skin integrity
    b. Cost of materials
    c. Self-esteem of patient
    d. Risk for falls

53. The nurse is caring for a patient with functional incontinence. The unlicensed assistive personnel (UAP) reports that "the linens have been changed four times within the past 6 hours, but the patient refuses to wear a diaper." What does the nurse do next?
    a. Thank the UAP for the hard work and advise to continue to change the linens.
    b. Call the health care provider to obtain an order for an indwelling catheter.
    c. Instruct the UAP to stop using the term "diaper" and instead use "incontinence pants."
    d. Assess the patient for any new urinary problems and ask about toileting preferences.

54. Which dietary changes does the nurse suggest to a patient with urge incontinence?
    a. Limit fluid intake to no more than 2 L/day.
    b. Peel all fruit before consuming.
    c. Avoid alcohol and caffeine.
    d. Avoid smoked or salted foods.

55. A patient with stress incontinence has been attempting vaginal cone therapy for several weeks but is discouraged. She says, "It isn't working. I want to try something else." What is the nurse's **best** response?
    a. "Don't give up yet. Let's review the process and you can try for a few more weeks."
    b. "The cones are hard to use. I'll ask the health care provider to write you a prescription."
    c. "Tell me about your experiences with the cones and how you are tracking your progress."
    d. "Let me give you some more information about exercises to strengthen the pelvic floor muscles."

56. A patient with urinary incontinence is prescribed oxybutynin. What precautions or instructions does the nurse provide related to this therapy?
    a. Avoid aspirin or aspirin-containing products.
    b. Increase fluids and dietary fiber intake.
    c. Report any unusual vaginal bleeding.
    d. Change positions slowly, especially in the morning.

57. Teaching intermittent self-catheterization for incontinence is appropriate for which patient?
    a. 25-year-old male patient with paraplegia
    b. 35-year-old female patient with stress incontinence
    c. 70-year-old patient who wears absorbent briefs
    d. 18-year-old patient with a severe head injury

58. A patient with reflex (overflow) urinary incontinence had surgery to relieve an obstruction. Postoperatively the nurse observes and reports that the patient is having urinary retention. Which drug has a role in addressing this problem?
    a. Captopril is given to lower urine cystine levels.
    b. Levofloxacin is given to prevent infection due to retention.
    c. Mirabegron is given to increase bladder capacity.
    d. Bethanechol chloride may be used short-term after surgery.

59. A patient is admitted for an elective orthopedic surgical procedure. The patient also has a personal and family history for urolithiasis. Which circumstance creates the **greatest** risk for recurrent urolithiasis?
    a. Giving the patient milk with every meal tray
    b. Restricting food and fluids for extended periods
    c. Giving the patient an opioid narcotic for pain
    d. Inserting an indwelling catheter for the procedure

60. A patient reports severe flank pain. The report indicates that urine is turbid, malodorous, and rust-colored; red blood cells, white blood cells, and bacteria are present; and microscopic analysis shows crystals. What does this data suggest?
    a. Pyuria and cystitis
    b. Staghorn calculus with infection
    c. Urolithiasis and infection
    d. Dysuria and urinary retention

61. A patient comes to the clinic and reports severe flank pain, bladder distention, and nausea and vomiting with increasingly smaller amounts of urine with frank blood. The patient states, "I have kidney stones and I just need a prescription for pain medication." What is the **priority** concern in the interdisciplinary care of this patient?
    a. Controlling the patient's pain
    b. Checking the quantity of blood in the urine
    c. Flushing the kidneys with oral fluids
    d. Determining if there is an obstruction

62. The nurse is caring for a patient with urolithiasis. Which type of medication is likely to be given in the acute phase to relieve the patient's severe pain?
    a. Nonsteroidal anti-inflammatory drugs
    b. Spasmolytic drugs
    c. Antibiotics
    d. Opioid analgesics

63. A patient returns to the medical-surgical unit after having shock wave lithotripsy. What is an appropriate nursing intervention for the postprocedural care of this patient?
    a. Strain the urine to monitor the passage of stone fragments.
    b. Report bruising that occurs on the flank of the affected side.
    c. Continuously monitor electrocardiogram for dysrhythmias.
    d. Apply a local anesthetic cream to the skin of the affected side.

64. The nurse is teaching self-care measures to a patient who had shock wave lithotripsy for kidney stones. What information does the nurse include? **Select all that apply.**
    a. Finish the entire prescription of antibiotics to prevent infection.
    b. Balance regular exercise with sleep and rest.
    c. Drink at least 3 L of fluid a day.
    d. Watch for and immediately report bruising after lithotripsy.
    e. Urine may be bloody for several days.
    f. Pain in the region of the kidneys or bladder is expected.

65. A patient with a history of kidney stones presents with severe flank pain, nausea, vomiting, pallor, and diaphoresis. He reports freely passing urine, but it is bloody. What is the **priority** concern?
    a. Possible hemorrhage
    b. Impaired tissue perfusion
    c. Impaired urinary elimination
    d. Severe pain

66. Which clinical manifestation indicates to the nurse that interventions for the patient's renal colic are effective?
    a. Urine is pink-tinged.
    b. Patient reports that pain is relieved.
    c. Urine output is 50 mL/min.
    d. Bladder scan shows no residual urine.

67. The urine output of a patient with a kidney stone has decreased from 40 mL/hr to 5 mL/hr. What is the nurse's **priority** action?
    a. Check patency of IV access and notify the health care provider.
    b. Perform the Credé maneuver on the patient's bladder.
    c. Test the urine for ketone bodies.
    d. Document the finding and continue monitoring.

68. Several attempts to obtain a clean-catch urine specimen from an older patient are unsuccessful because the patient has poor manual dexterity and poor control over stopping and starting the stream. What is the nurse's **best** action?
    a. Assist patient to void directly into a container and label as "voided but not midstream."
    b. Obtain an order for straight catheterization and use a small-diameter (6 Fr) catheter.
    c. Obtain an order to insert an indwelling catheter and use an 18 Fr catheter with a bag.
    d. Call the health care provider and report that the patient is unable to produce the specimen.

69. Which patient has the **highest** risk for bladder cancer?
    a. 60-year-old female patient with malnutrition secondary to chronic alcoholism and self-neglect
    b. 25-year-old male patient with type 1 diabetes mellitus who is noncompliant with therapeutic regimen
    c. 60-year-old male patient who smokes two packs of cigarettes per day and works in a chemical factory
    d. 25-year-old female patient who had three episodes of bacterial cystitis in the past year

70. The nurse is talking to a 68-year-old male patient who has lifestyle choices and occupational exposure that put him at high risk for bladder cancer. The nurse is **most** concerned about which urinary characteristic?
    a. Frequency
    b. Nocturia
    c. Painless hematuria
    d. Incontinence

71. To prevent recurrence of superficial bladder cancer, the patient receives intravesical instillation of bacille Calmette-Guérin at the outpatient cancer clinic. What home care instructions should be given to the patient?
    a. Flush the toilet after every voiding and remind all family members about hand hygiene.
    b. Drink a lot of extra fluid to flush your bladder, but otherwise there are no special instructions.
    c. Your urine will be radioactive for 24 hours, so avoid exposing children and pregnant women.
    d. For 24 hours, others should not share your toilet; afterward clean the toilet with 10% bleach.

72. Which statement by a patient indicates effective coping with a Kock's pouch?
    a. "I don't have any discomfort, but the pouch frequently overflows."
    b. "My wife has been irrigating the pouch daily. She likes to do it."
    c. "I check the pouch every 2 to 3 hours and use a catheter as needed."
    d. "I never undress in front of anyone anymore, but I guess that is okay."

73. A patient has had a bladder suspension and a suprapubic catheter is in place. The patient wants to know how long the catheter will remain in place. What is the nurse's **best** response?
    a. "For most patients, it remains for 24 hours postoperatively."
    b. "It will be removed at your first clinic visit, unless there are complications."
    c. "When you have the urge and can void on your own, it will be removed."
    d. "It is removed when you void and residual urine is less than 50 mL."

74. The employee health nurse is conducting a presentation for employees who work in a paint manufacturing plant. In order to protect against bladder cancer, what advice does the nurse give to personnel who directly work with chemicals?
    a. Shower with mild soap and rinse well before coming to work.
    b. Use personal protective equipment such as gloves and masks.
    c. Limit exposure to chemicals and fumes at all times.
    d. Avoid hobbies such as oil painting that increase exposure to chemicals.

75. A patient is returning from the postanesthesia care unit after surgery for bladder cancer and has a cutaneous ureterostomy. Where does the nurse expect the stoma to be located?
    a. On the perineum
    b. At the beltline
    c. On the posterior flank
    d. In the midabdominal area

67
CHAPTER

Care of Patients with Kidney Disorders

1. Which manifestation is **primarily** associated with acute pyelonephritis?
   a. Obstruction caused by hydroureter
   b. Active bacterial infection
   c. Increased urinary retention
   d. Peripheral and facial edema

2. The health care provider informs the nurse that the patient has acute pyelonephritis that appears to have been caused by a bacterial infection in the blood. For this patient, what is the **priority** concept?
   a. Immunity
   b. Elimination
   c. Fluid and electrolyte imbalance
   d. Cellular regulation

3. What might the nurse notice if the patient is experiencing problems with urinary elimination as a result of acute pyelonephritis? **Select all that apply.**
   a. Patient urinates large amounts of dilute urine.
   b. Patient reports pain and burning on urination.
   c. Patient reports back or flank pain.
   d. Urine is cloudy and foul smelling.
   e. Urine may be darker or smoky or have obvious blood in it.
   f. Patient reports nocturia.

4. What laboratory values would the nurse observe in a patient experiencing problems with urinary elimination as a result of acute pyelonephritis? **Select all that apply.**
   a. Complete blood count for elevation of differentials.
   b. Blood urea nitrogen and serum creatinine levels for elevation.
   c. Electrolyte deficiencies, such as hypokalemia and hyponatremia.
   d. Urine culture to identify specific organisms causing infection.
   e. Urinalysis for bacteria, leukocyte esterase, nitrate, or red blood cells.
   f. C-reactive protein and erythrocyte sedimentation rate for immune response.

5. Which patient has the **greatest** risk for developing acute pyelonephritis?
   a. 80-year-old woman who takes diuretics for mild heart failure
   b. 80-year-old man who drinks four cans of beer per day
   c. 36-year-old woman with diabetes mellitus who is pregnant
   d. 36-year-old man with diabetes insipidus

6. A patient is admitted to the medical-surgical unit for acute pyelonephritis. What is the **priority** concept to consider in the immediate nursing care of this patient?
   a. Oxygenation
   b. Acid-base balance
   c. Pain
   d. Cellular regulation

7. What are the key features associated with chronic pyelonephritis? **Select all that apply.**
   a. Abscess formation
   b. Hypertension
   c. Inability to conserve sodium
   d. Decreased urine-concentrating ability, resulting in nocturia
   e. Tendency to develop hyperkalemia and acidosis
   f. Sudden onset of massive proteinuria

8. A patient with chronic pyelonephritis returns to the clinic for follow up. Which behavior indicates the patient is performing the self-care measures to conserve existing kidney function?
   a. Drinks a liter of fluid every day
   b. Considers buying a home blood pressure cuff
   c. Reports taking antibiotics as prescribed
   d. Takes pain medication on a regular basis

9. A patient has come to the clinic for follow up of acute pyelonephritis. Which action does the nurse reinforce to the patient?
   a. Complete all antibiotic regimens.
   b. Report episodes of nocturia.
   c. Wash hands to prevent spreading infection.
   d. Avoid taking any over-the-counter drugs.

10. The nurse is assessing a patient who reports chills, high fever, and flank pain with urinary urgency and frequency. On physical examination, the patient has costovertebral angle tenderness, pulse is 110 beats/min, and respirations are 28/min. How does the nurse interpret these findings?
    a. Complicated cystitis
    b. Acute pyelonephritis
    c. Chronic pyelonephritis
    d. Acute glomerulonephritis

11. Which patient has the **greatest** risk for developing chronic pyelonephritis?
    a. Patient is bedridden and has prostate enlargement with reflux.
    b. Patient has hematuria and dysuria related to a urinary tract infection.
    c. Patient had a nephrectomy secondary to severe kidney trauma.
    d. Patient reports limiting fluids in the evening to control nocturia.

12. The nurse is reviewing the medical history of a patient who was admitted for acute glomerulonephritis. Which systemic conditions may have caused acute glomerulonephritis and should be included in the overall plan of care?
    a. Systemic lupus erythematosus and diabetic glomerulopathy
    b. Myocardial infarction and atrial fibrillation
    c. Ischemic stroke and hemiparesis
    d. Blunt trauma to the kidney with hematuria

13. The nurse is assessing a patient with possible acute glomerulonephritis. During the inspection of the hands, face, and eyelids, what is the nurse **primarily** observing for?
    a. Redness
    b. Edema
    c. Rashes
    d. Dryness

14. The nurse is assessing a patient with glomerulonephritis and notes crackles in the lung fields and neck vein distention. The patient reports mild shortness of breath. Based on these findings, what does the nurse do **next**?
    a. Check for costovertebral angle tenderness or flank pain.
    b. Obtain a urine sample to check for proteinuria.
    c. Assess for additional signs of fluid overload.
    d. Alert the health care provider about the respiratory symptoms.

15. The nurse is interviewing and assessing a patient who has the signs/symptoms of acute glomerulonephritis. Which disorder is **most likely** to mimic similar signs/symptoms?
    a. Acute flare up of rheumatoid arthritis
    b. Metastasis of renal carcinoma to distal sites
    c. Urinary obstruction due to hydroureter
    d. Acute exacerbation of heart failure

16. For a patient with acute glomerulonephritis, a 24-hour urine test was initiated and the glomerular filtration rate (GFR) results are pending. What is the correct clinical implication of GFR results?
    a. GFR is normal; the therapy can be discontinued.
    b. GFR is low; the patient is at risk for retention.
    c. GFR is high; the patient is at risk for infection.
    d. GFR is low; the patient is at risk for fluid overload.

17. A patient is very ill and is admitted to the intensive care unit with rapidly progressing glomerulonephritis. The nurse monitors for manifestations of which prognosis?
    a. End-stage kidney disease
    b. Gradual improvement after IV fluids
    c. Stroke due to malignant hypertension
    d. Full recovery if aggressively treated

18. The health care provider writes an order, to give the patient a fluid allowance equal to the 24-hour urine output plus 500 to 600 mL. Urine output was 60mL at 8:00 AM; 260 mL 12:00 PM; 200 mL at 4:00 PM; 280 mL at 8:00 PM; 100 mL at 12:00 AM; 100 mL at 4:00 AM; and 50 mL at 7:00 AM. How much fluid can the patient have over the next 24 hours?
    a. 500 to 600 mL
    b. 1050 to 1060 mL
    c. 1550 to 1650 mL
    d. 2500 to 2600 mL

19. A patient is diagnosed with chronic glomerulonephritis. The patient's spouse reports that the patient is irritable, forgetful, and has trouble concentrating. Which assessment finding does the nurse expect on further examination?
    a. Increased respiratory rate
    b. Elevated blood urea nitrogen
    c. Hypokalemia
    d. Low blood pressure

20. The nurse is reviewing the laboratory results for a patient with chronic glomerulonephritis. The serum albumin level is low. What else does the nurse expect to see?
    a. Proteinuria
    b. Elevated hematocrit
    c. High specific gravity
    d. Low white blood cell count

21. A patient has chronic glomerulonephritis. In order to assess for uremic symptoms, what does the nurse do?
    a. Evaluate the blood urea nitrogen.
    b. Ask the patient to extend the arms and hyperextend the wrists.
    c. Gently palpate the flank for asymmetry and tenderness.
    d. Auscultate for the presence of an S₃ heart sound.

22. The nurse is reviewing the laboratory results of a patient with chronic glomerulonephritis. The phosphorus level is 5.3 mg/dL. What else does the nurse expect to see?
    a. Serum calcium level below the normal range
    b. Serum potassium level below the normal range
    c. Falsely elevated serum sodium level
    d. Elevated serum levels for all other electrolytes

23. The nurse is reviewing arterial blood gas results of a patient with acute glomerulonephritis. The pH of the sample is 7.35. As acidosis is likely to be present because of hydrogen ion retention and loss of bicarbonate, how does the nurse interpret this data?
    a. Normal pH with respiratory compensation
    b. Acidosis with failure of respiratory compensation
    c. Alkalosis with failure of metabolic compensation
    d. Normal pH with metabolic compensation

24. The nurse is taking a history on a patient with chronic glomerulonephritis. What is the patient **most likely** to report?
    a. History of antibiotic allergy
    b. Intense flank pain
    c. Poor appetite and weight loss
    d. Occasional edema and fatigue

25. Which patient history factor is considered causative for acute glomerulonephritis?
    a. Urinary incontinence for 6 months
    b. Strep throat 3 weeks ago
    c. Kidney stones 2 years ago
    d. Mild hypertension diagnosed 1 year ago

26. A patient with acute glomerulonephritis has edema of the face. The blood pressure is moderately elevated and the patient has gained 2 pounds within the past 24 hours. The patient reports fatigue and refuses to eat. What is the **priority** for nursing care?
    a. Cluster care to allow rest periods for the patient.
    b. Obtain a dietary consult to plan an adequate nutritional diet.
    c. Monitor urine output with accurate intake and output amounts.
    d. Assess for signs and symptoms of fluid volume overload.

27. A patient with acute glomerulonephritis is required to provide a 24-hour urine specimen. What does the nurse expect to see when looking at the specimen?
    a. Smoky or cola-colored urine
    b. Clear and very dilute urine
    c. Urine that is full of pus and very thick
    d. Bright orange-colored urine

28. Which nursing intervention is applicable for a patient with acute glomerulonephritis?
    a. Restricting visitors who have infections
    b. Assessing the incision site
    c. Inspecting the vascular access
    d. Measuring weight daily

29. Which diagnostic test results does the nurse expect to see with acute glomerulonephritis? **Select all that apply.**
    a. Hematuria
    b. Proteinuria
    c. Microscopic red blood cell casts in urine
    d. Serum albumin level decreased
    e. Serum potassium decreased
    f. Serum phosphorus decreased

30. A patient has late-stage chronic glomerulonephritis. Which educational brochure would be the **most** appropriate to prepare for the patient?
    a. "How to Take Your Anti-infective Medications"
    b. "Important Points to Know about Dialysis"
    c. "What Are the Side Effects of Radiation Therapy?"
    d. "Precautions to Take During Immunosuppressive Therapy"

31. The nurse is caring for a patient with nephrotic syndrome. What interventions are included in the plan of care for this patient? **Select all that apply.**
    a. Fluids should be restricted.
    b. Administer mild diuretics.
    c. Assess for edema.
    d. Administer antihypertensive medications.
    e. Assess for dysuria
    f. Assess hydration status.

32. The nurse is reviewing the patient's history, assessment findings, and laboratory results for a patient with suspected kidney problems. Which manifestation is the **main** feature of nephrotic syndrome?
    a. Abrupt onset flank asymmetry
    b. Proteinuria greater than 3.5 g in 24 hours
    c. Serum sodium greater than 148 mmol/L
    d. Serum cholesterol (total) 190 mg/dL

33. A patient is newly admitted with nephrotic syndrome and has proteinuria, edema, hyperlipidemia, and hypertension. What is the **priority** for nursing care?
    a. Consult the dietitian to provide adequate nutritional intake.
    b. Prevent kidney and urinary tract infection.
    c. Monitor fluid volume and the patient's hydration status.
    d. Prepare the patient for a renal biopsy.

34. Which ethnic or cultural groups are **mostly likely** to develop end-stage kidney disease related to hypertension? **Select all that apply.**
    a. Caucasian Americans
    b. Jewish Americans
    c. American Indians
    d. African Americans
    e. Hispanic Americans
    f. Bisexual Americans

35. Which patient has the **greatest** risk of developing a kidney abscess?
    a. Patient is diagnosed with acute pyelonephritis.
    b. Patient has flank asymmetry related to hydronephrosis.
    c. Patient developed a urinary tract infection secondary to a urinary catheter.
    d. Patient is diagnosed with hypertension and nephrosclerosis.

36. The health care provider advises the patient that diagnostic testing is needed to identify the possible presence of a renal abscess. Which test does the nurse prepare the patient for?
    a. Renal arteriography
    b. Cystourethrogram
    c. Renal scan
    d. Urodynamic flow studies

37. A patient is diagnosed with nephrosclerosis. Which factors would promote long-term adherence to the prescribed antihypertensive medication therapy? **Select all that apply.**
    a. Once-a-day dosing
    b. Annual reminders
    c. Minimal side effects
    d. Eliminating dietary restrictions
    e. Low cost
    f. Drug brochures

38. Insertion of an indwelling urinary catheter increases the patient's risk for developing what type of kidney disorder?
    a. Polycystic kidney disease
    b. Acute pyelonephritis
    c. Renal stenosis
    d. Nephrosclerosis

39. Under what circumstances would it be appropriate for the nurse to seek an order for catheter replacement if the health care provider fails to order it?
    a. Family requests a long-term catheter to prevent urinary incontinence for a confused relative.
    b. Patient has had current catheter for two weeks and new antibiotics were just ordered.
    c. Patient has an existing catheter but exterior of closed system becomes soiled.
    d. Nurse notices a large amount of dark amber urine in the drainage bag.

40. A 22-year-old patient comes to the clinic for a wellness check-up. History reveals that the patient's parent has the autosomal-dominant form of polycystic kidney disease (PKD). Which vital sign suggests that the patient should be evaluated for PKD?
    a. Pulse of 95 beats/min
    b. Temperature of 100.6°F
    c. Blood pressure of 136/88 mm Hg
    d. Respiratory rate of 26/min

41. The nurse is interviewing a patient with suspected polycystic kidney disease (PKD). What questions does the nurse ask the patient? **Select all that apply.**
    a. "Is there any family history of PKD or kidney disease?"
    b. "Do you have a history of sexually transmitted disease?"
    c. "Have you had any constipation or abdominal discomfort?"
    d. "Have you noticed a change in urine color or frequency?"
    e. "Have you had any problems with headaches?"
    f. "Have you had any problems with muscles aches or joint pain?"

42. A patient has a family history of the autosomal-dominant form of polycystic kidney disease (PKD) and has been advised to monitor for and report symptoms. What is an **early** symptom of PKD?
    a. Headache
    b. Pruritus
    c. Edema
    d. Nocturia

43. A patient with a history of polycystic kidney disease reports dull, aching flank pain and the urinalysis is negative for infection. The health care provider tells the nurse that the pain is chronic and related to enlarging kidneys compressing abdominal contents. What nursing intervention is **best** for this patient?
    a. Administer an angiotensin-converting enzyme inhibitor such as lisinopril.
    b. Apply cool compresses to the abdomen or flank.
    c. Teach methods of relaxation such as deep-breathing.
    d. Administer around-the-clock nonsteroidal anti-inflammatory drugs.

44. Why may a patient with polycystic kidney disease (PKD) experience constipation?
    a. Polycystic kidneys enlarge and put pressure on the large intestine.
    b. Patient becomes dehydrated because the kidneys are dysfunctional.
    c. Constipation is a side effect from the medications given to treat PKD.
    d. Patients with PKD have special dietary restrictions that cause constipation.

45. The nurse is developing a teaching plan for a patient with polycystic kidney disease. Which topics does the nurse include? **Select all that apply.**
    a. Instruct how to measure and record blood pressure.
    b. Assist to develop a schedule for self-administering drugs.
    c. Teach about daily weights, same time of day, and same amount of clothing.
    d. Review the potential side effects of the drugs.
    e. Explain high-protein, low-fat diet plan.
    f. Teach to take pulse before and after taking medications.

46. A patient with polycystic kidney disease reports sharp flank pain followed by blood in the urine. How does the nurse interpret these signs/symptoms?
    a. Infection of cyst
    b. Ruptured cyst
    c. Ruptured berry aneurysm
    d. Increased kidney size

47. A patient with polycystic kidney disease is at risk for a berry aneurysm and reports a severe headache. What is the nurse's **priority** action?
    a. Assess the pain and give a prn pain medication.
    b. Reassure that this is an expected symptom of the disease.
    c. Assess for neurologic changes and check vital signs.
    d. Monitor for hematuria and decreased urinary output.

48. A patient with polycystic kidney disease reports nocturia. What is the nocturia caused by?
    a. Increased fluid intake in the evening
    b. Increased hypertension
    c. Decreased urine-concentrating ability
    d. Detrusor irritability

49. A patient is suspected of having polycystic kidney disease (PKD). Which diagnostic study has minimal risks and is used to provide initial screening for PKD?
    a. Kidneys-ureters-bladder x-ray
    b. Computed tomography with angiography
    c. Renal ultrasonography
    d. Renal biopsy

50. Which pain management strategy does the nurse teach a patient with polycystic kidney disease who has chronic pain related to the kidney cysts?
    a. Rest and sleep in a prone position
    b. Increase dosage of nonsteroidal anti-inflammatory.
    c. Gently rub or massage the flank area.
    d. Apply dry heat to the abdomen or flank.

51. A patient with polycystic kidney disease usually experiences constipation. What does the nurse recommend?
    a. Increased dietary fiber and increased fluids
    b. Drinking water until constipation resolves
    c. Daily laxatives and increased exercise
    d. Tap-water enemas and fiber supplements

52. A patient with polycystic kidney disease reports nocturia and cloudy urine. What does the nurse encourage the patient to do?
    a. Drink at least 2 liters of fluid daily.
    b. Restrict fluids to decrease urination.
    c. Drink 1000 mL early in the morning
    d. Add a pinch of salt to water in the evenings.

53. For the patient with polycystic kidney disease (PKD), which type of antihypertensive medication may be used because it helps control the cell growth aspects of PKD and reduce microalbuminuria?
    a. Angiotensin-converting enzyme inhibitors
    b. Beta blockers
    c. Calcium channel blockers
    d. Vasodilators

54. After the nurse instructs a patient with polycystic kidney disease on home care, the patient knows to contact the health care provider **immediately** when what sign/symptom occurs?
    a. Urine is a clear, pale yellow color.
    b. Weight has increased by 5 pounds in 2 days.
    c. Two days have passed since the last bowel movement.
    d. Morning systolic blood pressure has decreased by 5 mm Hg.

55. The health care provider tells the nurse that the patient with polycystic kidney disease has salt wasting. Which intervention is the nurse likely to use related to nutrition therapy?
    a. Talk to the patient about seasonings that are alternatives for salt.
    b. Help the patient select a lunch tray with low-sodium items.
    c. Obtain an order for fluid restriction to prevent loss of sodium during urination.
    d. Advise that a low-sodium diet is not currently necessary.

56. The health care team is using a collaborative and interdisciplinary approach to design a treatment plan for a patient with polycystic kidney disease. What is the **top** priority?
    a. Controlling hypertension
    b. Preventing rupture of cysts
    c. Providing genetic counseling
    d. Identifying community resources

57. A patient with polycystic kidney disease would exhibit which signs/symptoms? **Select all that apply.**
    a. Frequent urination
    b. Increased abdominal girth
    c. Hypertension
    d. Kidney stones
    e. Diarrhea
    f. Bloody or cloudy urine

58. In polycystic kidney disease, the effect on the renin-angiotensin system in the kidney has which result?
    a. Adrenal insufficiency
    b. Increased blood pressure
    c. Increased urine output
    d. Oliguria

59. What is the main concern for patients who have hydronephrosis, hydroureter, or urethral stricture?
    a. Dilute urine
    b. Pain on urination
    c. Dehydration
    d. Obstruction

60. An older adult male patient calls the clinic because he has "not passed any urine all day long." What is the nurse's **best** response?
    a. "Try drinking several large glasses of water and waiting a few more hours."
    b. "If you develop flank pain or fever, then you should probably come in."
    c. "You could have an obstruction, so you should come in to be checked."
    d. "I am sorry, but I really can't comment about your problem over the phone."

61. A patient reports straining to pass very small amounts of urine today, despite a normal fluid intake, and reports having the urge to urinate. The nurse palpates the bladder and finds that it is distended. Which condition is **most likely** to be associated with these findings?
    a. Urethral stricture
    b. Hydroureter
    c. Hydronephrosis
    d. Polycystic kidney disease

62. A patient is diagnosed with hydronephrosis. What is the **primary** complication that could result from this condition?
    a. Damage to blood vessels and kidney tubules
    b. Kidney stone disease with retained stones
    c. Hypertension and diabetic nephropathy
    d. Pyelonephritis with vesicoureteral reflux

63. Which clinical manifestation in a patient with an obstruction in the urinary system is associated **specifically** with a hydronephrosis?
    a. Flank asymmetry
    b. Chills and fever
    c. Urge incontinence
    d. Bladder distention

64. An older adult male patient reports an acute problem with urine retention. The nurse advises the patient to seek medical attention because permanent kidney damage can occur in what time frame?
    a. In less than 6 hours
    b. In less than 48 hours
    c. Within several weeks
    d. Within several years

65. The nurse is reviewing the laboratory results for a patient being evaluated for difficulties with passing urine. The urinalysis shows tubular epithelial cells on microscopic examination. How does the nurse interpret this finding?
    a. Blood chemistries should be evaluated.
    b. The obstruction is prolonged.
    c. The patient has a urinary tract infection.
    d. Glomerular filtration rate is reduced.

66. A patient had a nephrostomy and a nephrostomy tube is in place. What is included in the postoperative care of this patient?
    a. Assess the amount of drainage in the collection bag.
    b. Irrigate the tube until the return drainage is clear.
    c. Keep the patient NPO for 6 to 8 hours.
    d. Instruct to sleep with operative side downward.

67. The nurse is caring for a patient with a nephrostomy. The nurse notifies the health care provider about which assessment finding?
    a. Urine drainage is red-tinged 4 hours after surgery.
    b. Amount of drainage decreases and the patient has back pain.
    c. There is a small steady drainage for the first 4 hours postsurgery.
    d. The nephrostomy site looks dry and intact.

68. The off-going nurse is giving shift report to the oncoming nurse about the care of a patient who had a nephrostomy tube placed 12 hours ago. What is the **most important** point to clearly communicate about the urine drainage?
    a. "Urine is draining only into the collection bag, not the bladder; therefore the amount of drainage must be assessed hourly for the first 24 hours."
    b. "The intake and urinary output have been monitored hourly and the patient has not shown any signs/symptoms of dehydration."
    c. "The surgeon placed ureteral tubes so all of the urine will pass through the bladder; therefore perform hourly bladder scans to measure residual."
    d. "The nephrostomy site has not been leaking any blood or urine and you should continue to monitor the site for leakage."

69. A patient with diabetic nephropathy reports having frequent hypoglycemic episodes "so my doctor reduced my insulin, which means my diabetes is improving." What is the nurse's **best** response?
    a. "Congratulations! That's great news. You must be carefully following the diet and lifestyle recommendations."
    b. "When kidney function is reduced, the insulin is available for a longer time and thus less of it is needed."
    c. "You should talk to your doctor again. You have been diagnosed with nephropathy and that changes the situation."
    d. "Let me get you a brochure about the relationship of diabetes and kidney disease. It can be hard to understand."

70. The student nurse is assisting in the postoperative care of a patient who had a recent nephrectomy. The student demonstrates a reluctance to move the patient to change the linens because "the patient seems so tired." The nurse reminds the student that a **priority** assessment for this patient is to assess for which factor?
    a. Skin breakdown on the patient's back
    b. Blood on the linens beneath the patient
    c. Urinary incontinence and moisture
    d. The patient's ability to move self in bed

71. After a nephrectomy, a patient has a large urine output because of adrenal insufficiency. What does the nurse anticipate the **priority** intervention for this patient will be?
    a. Angiotensin-converting enzyme inhibitor to control hypertension and decrease protein loss in urine
    b. Straight catheterization or bedside bladder scan to measure residual urine
    c. IV fluid replacement because of subsequent hypotension and oliguria
    d. IV infusion of temsirolimus, to inhibit cell division and cell cycle progression

72. A 53-year-old patient is newly diagnosed with renal artery stenosis. Which clinical manifestation is the nurse **most likely** to observe when the patient **first** seeks health care?
    a. Sudden onset of hypertension
    b. Urinary frequency and dysuria
    c. Nausea and vomiting
    d. Flank pain and hematuria

73. What are key features of renovascular disease? **Select all that apply.**
    a. Sodium wasting
    b. Flank pain
    c. Decreased glomerular filtration rate
    d. Elevated serum creatinine
    e. Poorly controlled diabetes or sustained hyperglycemia
    f. Significant, difficult-to-control high blood pressure

74. What change in diabetic therapy may be needed for a patient who has diabetic nephropathy?
    a. Fluid restriction
    b. Decreased activity level
    c. Decreased insulin dosages
    d. Increased caloric intake

75. A patient has renal cell carcinoma that has metastasized to the lungs. What stage is the cancer?
    a. I
    b. II
    c. III
    d. IV

76. A patient has had one kidney removed as a treatment for kidney cancer. The patient's spouse asks, "Does the good kidney take over immediately? I know a person can live with just one kidney." What is the nurse's **best** response?
    a. "The other kidney will provide adequate function, but this may take days or weeks."
    b. "The other kidney isn't able to provide adequate function, so other therapies are needed."
    c. "That's a good question. Remember to ask your doctor next time he or she comes in."
    d. "It varies a lot, but within a few days we expect everything to normalize."

77. After a nephrectomy, one adrenal gland remains. Based on this knowledge, which type of medication replacement therapy does the nurse expect if the remaining adrenal gland function is insufficient?
    a. Potassium
    b. Steroid
    c. Calcium
    d. Estrogen

78. The nurse is caring for a patient with kidney cell carcinoma who manifests paraneoplastic syndromes. What findings does the nurse expect to see in this patient? **Select all that apply.**
    a. Urinary tract infection
    b. Erythrocytosis
    c. Hypercalcemia
    d. Liver dysfunction
    e. Decreased sedimentation rate
    f. Hypertension

79. The nurse is caring for a patient with kidney cell carcinoma. What does the nurse expect to find documented about the patient's initial assessment?
    a. Flank pain, gross hematuria, palpable kidney mass, and renal bruit
    b. Gross hematuria, hypertension, diabetes, and oliguria
    c. Dysuria, polyuria, dehydration, and palpable kidney mass
    d. Nocturia and urinary retention with difficulty starting stream

80. A patient is diagnosed with kidney cancer and the health care provider recommends the best therapy. Which treatment does the nurse anticipate teaching the patient about?
    a. Chemotherapy
    b. Surgical removal
    c. Hormonal therapy
    d. Radiation therapy

81. A patient returning to the unit after a left radical nephrectomy for kidney cell carcinoma reports having some soreness on the right side. What does the nurse tell the patient?
    a. "The right kidney was repositioned to take over the function of both kidneys."
    b. "I'll call your doctor for an order to increase your pain medication."
    c. "The soreness is likely to be from being positioned on your right side during surgery."
    d. "You are having referred pain. It's expected, but you can take mild pain medication."

82. The nurse is caring for a postoperative nephrectomy patient. The nurse notes during the first several hours of the shift, a marked and steady **downward** trend in blood pressure. How does the nurse interpret this finding?
    a. Hypertension has been corrected.
    b. Internal hemorrhage is possible.
    c. The other kidney is failing.
    d. Fluids are shifting into the interstitial space.

83. The nurse is caring for a patient after a nephrectomy. The nurse notes that the urine flow was 50 mL/hr at the beginning of the shift but several hours later has dropped to 30 mL. What would the nurse do **first**?
    a. Notify the health care provider for an order for an IV fluid bolus.
    b. Document the finding and continue to monitor for downward trend.
    c. Check the drainage system for kinks or obstructions to flow.
    d. Obtain the patient's weight and compare it to baseline.

84. The nurse is caring for a patient who had a nephrectomy yesterday. To manage the patient's pain, what is the **best** plan for analgesia therapy?
    a. Limit narcotics because of respiratory depression.
    b. Give an oral analgesic when the patient can eat.
    c. Alternate parenteral and oral medications.
    d. Give parenteral medications on a schedule.

85. A patient is brought to the emergency department because he was in a fight and was repeatedly kicked and punched in the back. What does the nurse include in the initial physical assessment? **Select all that apply.**
    a. Take complete vital signs.
    b. Check apical and peripheral pulses.
    c. Inspect flanks for bruising, asymmetry, or penetrating injuries.
    d. Inspect abdomen, chest, and lower back for bruising or penetrating wounds.
    e. Deeply palpate the abdomen for signs of rigidity.
    f. Inspect the urethra for gross bleeding.

86. The emergency department nurse is preparing a patient with kidney trauma for emergency surgery. What is the **best** task to delegate to unlicensed assistive personnel?
    a. Set the automated blood pressure machine to cycle every 2 hours.
    b. Inform the family about surgery and assist them to the surgery waiting area.
    c. Pick up the units of packed red cells from the blood bank.
    d. Insert a urinary catheter if there is no gross bleeding at the urethra.

87. The patient sustained traumatic injury and needs the best diagnostic test to determine the extent of injury to the kidney. What does the nurse do?
    a. Obtain a clean-catch urine specimen for urinalysis.
    b. Give an IV fluid bolus before renal arteriography.
    c. Explain computed tomography.
    d. Obtain a blood sample for hemoglobin and hematocrit.

68 CHAPTER

Care of Patients with Acute Kidney Injury and Chronic Kidney Disease

1. What criteria are included in the current definition of acute kidney injury? **Select all that apply.**
   a. Increase in serum creatinine by 0.3 mg/dL (26.2 μmol/L) or more within 48 hours
   b. Presence of polyuria, and nocturia with very dilute pale yellow urine
   c. Signs and symptoms of fluid overload, such as edema, and crackles on auscultation
   d. Increase in serum creatinine to 1.5 times or more from baseline in the previous 7 days
   e. Hypotension and tachycardia with progressively decreased amounts of urine
   f. Urine volume of less than 0.5 mL/kilogram/hour for 6 hours

2. The community health nurse is designing programs to reduce kidney problems and kidney injury among the general public. In order to do so, the nurse targets health promotion and compliance with therapy for people with which conditions?
   a. Diabetes mellitus and hypertension
   b. Frequent episodes of sexually transmitted disease
   c. Osteoporosis and other bone diseases
   d. Gastroenteritis and poor eating habits

3. The nurse is caring for a patient who developed acute prerenal kidney injury secondary to severe and extensive burn injuries. What is the **primary** concept that underlies the etiology of the acute kidney injury?
   a. Elimination
   b. Tissue integrity
   c. Immunity
   d. Perfusion

4. A patient can develop intrarenal kidney injury from which causes? **Select all that apply.**
   a. Vasculitis
   b. Pyelonephritis
   c. Strenuous exercise
   d. Exposure to nephrotoxins
   e. Bladder cancer
   f. Systemic infection (sepsis)

5. The nurse is caring for patients who have cancers of the bladder, cervix, colon and prostate. These patients have a risk for developing which type of acute kidney injury?
   a. Prerenal injury
   b. Intrarenal injury
   c. Postrenal injury
   d. Intrinsic renal failure

6. When shock or other problems cause an acute reduction in blood flow to the kidneys, how do the kidneys compensate? **Select all that apply.**
   a. Constrict blood vessels in the kidneys.
   b. Activate the renin-angiotensin-aldosterone pathway.
   c. Release beta blockers.
   d. Dilate arteries throughout the body.
   e. Release antidiuretic hormones.
   f. Restrict secretion of glucocorticoids.

7. What might the nurse notice if the patient is experiencing reduced perfusion and altered urinary elimination related to acute kidney injury? **Select all that apply.**
   a. Hemodynamic instability, especially persistent hypotension and tachycardia
   b. Urine output of less than 0.5 mL/kg/hour for 6 or more hours
   c. Serum creatinine below baseline or admission values
   d. Urine may be clear or have a pale yellow color
   e. Abnormal urine sodium values
   f. Bladder distention and flank pain

8. The nurse is talking to a group of healthy young athletes about maintaining good kidney health and preventing acute kidney injury. Which health promotion point is the nurse **most likely** to emphasize with this group?
   a. "Have your blood pressure checked regularly."
   b. "Find out if you have a family history of diabetes."
   c. "Avoid dehydration by drinking at least 2 to 3 L of water daily."
   d. "Have annual testing for protein and glucose in urine."

9. The nurse is caring for a patient who has hypovolemic shock secondary to trauma. Based on the pathophysiology of hypovolemia and prerenal azotemia, what does the nurse assess at least every hour?
   a. Urinary output
   b. Presence of edema
   c. Urine color
   d. Presence of pain

10. The nurse is talking to an older adult male patient who is reasonably healthy for his age, but has benign prostatic hyperplasia (BPH). Which condition does the BPH potentially place him at risk for?
    a. Prerenal acute kidney injury
    b. Postrenal acute kidney injury
    c. Polycystic kidney disease
    d. Acute glomerulonephritis

11. The nurse is taking a history of a patient at risk for kidney failure. What does the nurse ask the patient about during the interview? **Select all that apply.**
    a. Exposure to nephrotoxic chemicals
    b. Unexpected weight loss
    c. History of diabetes mellitus, hypertension, systemic lupus erythematosus
    d. Recent surgery, trauma, or transfusions
    e. Leakage of urine when coughing or laughing
    f. Recent or prolonged use of nonsteroidal anti-inflammatory drugs

12. The nurse is caring for several patients at a walk-in clinic. None of the patients currently has any acute or chronic kidney problems. Which patient has the **greatest** risk to develop acute kidney injury?
    a. 73-year-old male who has hypertension and peripheral vascular disease
    b. 32-year-old female who is pregnant and has gestational diabetes
    c. 49-year-old male who is obese and has a history of skin cancer
    d. 23-year-old female who has been treated for a urinary tract infection

13. For a patient with acute kidney injury, the nurse would consider **questioning** the order for which diagnostic test?
    a. Kidney biopsy
    b. Ultrasonography
    c. Computed tomography with contrast dye
    d. Kidney, ureter, bladder x-ray

14. The nurse is caring for a postoperative patient and is evaluating the patient's intake and output as a measure to prevent acute kidney injury. The patient weighs 60 kg and has an intake of 120 mL and 180 mL of urine in the past 4 hours. What should the nurse do?
    a. Perform other assessments related to fluid status and record the output.
    b. Call the health care provider and obtain an order for a fluid bolus.
    c. Encourage the patient to drink more fluid, so that the output is increased.
    d. Compare the patient's weight to baseline to determine fluid retention.

15. The nurse is caring for a patient receiving gentamicin. Which laboratory results does the nurse monitor? **Select all that apply.**
    a. Blood urea nitrogen
    b. Creatinine
    c. Drug peak and trough levels
    d. Prothrombin time
    e. Platelet count
    f. Hemoglobin and hematocrit

16. According to the KDIGO classification (Kidney Disease: Improving Global Outcomes), how would the nurse interpret the following data? Serum creatinine increased × 1.5 over baseline with urine output of <0.5 mL/kg/hr for ≥6 hours.
    a. Stage 1
    b. Stage 2
    c. Stage 3
    d. End-stage kidney disease

17. A patient has been diagnosed with acute kidney injury, but the cause is uncertain. The nurse prepares patient educational material about which diagnostic test?
    a. Flat plate of the abdomen
    b. Renal ultrasonography
    c. Computed tomography
    d. Kidney biopsy

18. When a patient is in the diuretic phase of acute kidney injury, the nurse is mainly concerned about implementing which intervention?
    a. Assessing for hypertension and fluid overload
    b. Monitoring for hypovolemia and electrolyte loss
    c. Adjusting the dosage of diuretic medications
    d. Balancing diuretic therapy with intake

19. A patient with prerenal azotemia receives a fluid challenge. In evaluating response to the therapy, which outcome indicates that the goal was met?
    a. Patient reports feeling better and appetite is improved.
    b. Patient produces urine soon after the initial bolus.
    c. The therapy is completed without adverse effects.
    d. The health care provider discharges the patient.

20. The nurse is caring for a patient with acute kidney injury and notes a trend of increasingly elevated blood urea nitrogen levels. How does the nurse interpret this information?
    a. Breakdown of muscle for protein which leads to an increase in azotemia
    b. Sign of urinary retention and decreased urinary output
    c. Expected trend that can be reversed by discontinuing diuretics
    d. Ominous sign of irreversible kidney failure

21. The nurse is caring for a patient with acute kidney injury that developed after a severe anaphylactic reaction. What is a primary treatment goal of the initial phase that will help to prevent permanent kidney damage for this patient?
    a. Correct fluid volume by administering IV normal saline.
    b. Maintain a minimal mean arterial pressure of 65 mm Hg.
    c. Prevent kidney infections by administering antibiotics.
    d. Give antihistamines to prevent allergic response.

22. A patient sustained extensive burns and depletion of vascular volume. The nurse expects which changes in vital signs and urinary function?
    a. Decreased urine output, hypotension, tachycardia
    b. Increased urine output, hypertension, tachycardia
    c. Bradycardia, hypotension, polyuria
    d. Dysrhythmias, hypertension, oliguria

23. Which combination of drugs is the **most** nephrotoxic?
    a. Angiotensin-converting enzyme inhibitors and aspirin
    b. Angiotensin II receptor blockers and antacids
    c. Aminoglycoside antibiotics and nonsteroidal anti-inflammatory drugs
    d. Calcium channel blockers and antihistamines

24. Which disorder could be a complication from acute kidney injury?
    a. Heart failure
    b. Diabetes mellitus
    c. Kidney cancer
    d. Compartment syndrome

25. A patient with acute kidney injury has a poor appetite. What would the health care team try **first**?
    a. Parenteral nutrition (PN or hyperalimentation)
    b. Familiar comfort foods brought by the family
    c. Nasogastric tube enteral liquids for kidney patients
    d. Oral supplements designed for kidney patients

26. The nurse is caring for a patient with acute kidney injury who does not have signs or symptoms of fluid overload. Which intervention would be most effective as a fluid challenge to promote kidney perfusion?
    a. Administering normal saline 500 to 1000 mL infused over 1 hour
    b. Administering drugs to suppress aldosterone release
    c. Instilling 500 to 1000 mL normal saline through a nasogastric tube
    d. Having the patient drink several large glasses of water

27. The emergency department (ED) nurse is assessing a healthy young marathon runner who was brought to the hospital for transient syncope and dizziness that occurred after the race. The nurse notes that the patient has low urine output, decreased systolic blood pressure, decreased pulse pressure, orthostatic hypotension, and thirst. Before obtaining orders from the ED provider, which additional assessment is the **most** important?
    a. Auscultate lungs for crackles.
    b. Assess gag reflex and ability to swallow.
    c. Palpate peripheral pulses.
    d. Ask about family history of kidney disease.

28. A patient has acute kidney injury related to nephrotoxins. To improve glomerular filtration rate and improve blood flow to the kidneys, which type of medication does the nurse anticipate the health care provider will prescribe?
    a. Loop diuretics
    b. Phosphate binders
    c. Erythropoietin stimulating agents
    d. Calcium channel blockers

29. A patient with acute kidney injury has a high rate of catabolism with an increase in blood levels of catecholamines, cortisol, and glucagon. How will this pathophysiology manifest?
    a. Blood urea nitrogen will reflect buildup of nitrogenous wastes in the blood
    b. Elevated blood sugar will cause hyperglycemia-induced diuresis
    c. Falsely low sodium level is associated with fluid overload.
    d. Weight gain occurs in response to increased calorie consumption.

30. The nurse requests a dietary consult to address the patient's high rate of catabolism. Which nutritional element is directly related to this metabolic process?
    a. Carbohydrates
    b. Proteins
    c. Liquids
    d. Fats

31. The nurse is caring for a patient in the intensive care unit who sustained blood loss during a traumatic accident. To detect signs and symptoms that suggest the development of kidney dysfunction, the nurse observes for which data? **Select all that apply.**
    a. Hypotension
    b. Bradycardia
    c. Decreased urine output
    d. Decreased cardiac output
    e. Increased central venous pressure
    f. Jugular vein distention

32. A patient with acute kidney injury is receiving total parenteral nutrition (TPN). What is the therapeutic goal of using TPN?
    a. Preserve lean body mass
    b. Promote tubular reabsorption
    c. Create a negative nitrogen balance
    d. Prevent infection

33. The nurse and the dietitian are planning dietary intake for a patient with acute kidney injury who is currently not on dialysis therapy. The dietitian informs the nurse that 0.6 g/kg of body weight of protein are needed. The patient weighs 130 pounds. How many grams of protein should the patient receive? **Round grams to the nearest whole number.**
    _____ grams

34. The patient with chronic kidney disease has consistently weighed 63 kilograms at each clinic visit. Patient reports eating "a lot of good, salty food" and drinking "too many beers" during the weekend. Today, the patient weighs 65 kilograms. How much fluid has the patient retained?
    a. 1 liter
    b. 2 liters
    c. 2 kilograms
    d. 3 kilograms

35. The patient had a diagnostic imaging test with contrast media. IV fluids were ordered before and after the procedure to prevent contrast-induced nephropathy. Which outcome statement indicates that the goal of giving IV therapy has been met?
    a. Lung sounds are clear and there are no signs/symptoms of fluid overload.
    b. Patient does not show signs/symptoms of contrast-induced immune response.
    c. Urine output is 150 mL/hour for the first 6 hours after use of contrast agent
    d. Urine is 0.5 mL/kilogram/hour for 6 hours and patient remains euvolemic.

36. The nurse is taking a history on a patient with diabetes and hypertension. Because of the patient's high risk for developing kidney problems, which early **sign** of chronic kidney disease does the nurse assess for?
    a. Decreased output with subjective thirst
    b. Urinary frequency of very small amounts
    c. Pink or blood-tinged urine
    d. Increased output of very dilute urine

37. The health care provider orders IV fluids at a rate of 1 mL/kg/hr for 12 hours prior to an imaging test. The patient weighs 152 pounds. What should the nurse do?
    a. Set the IV pump to deliver 69 mL/hr.
    b. Set the IV pump to deliver 152 mL/hr.
    c. Set the IV pump to deliver 1 mL for 12 hours.
    d. Call provider to clarify the order in mL/hour.

38. A patient's laboratory results show an elevated creatinine level. The patient's history reveals no risk factors for kidney disease. Which question does the nurse ask the patient to shed further light on the laboratory result?
    a. "How many hours of sleep did you get the night before the test?"
    b. "How much fluid did you drink before the test?"
    c. "Did you take any type of antibiotics before taking the test?"
    d. "When and how much did you last urinate before having the test?"

39. Which abnormal electrolyte imbalance is **most likely** to develop in the **early** phase of chronic kidney disease?
    a. Hyperkalemia
    b. Hyponatremia
    c. Hypercalcemia
    d. Hypokalemia

40. A patient with chronic kidney disease has a potassium level of 8 mEq/L. The nurse notifies the health care provider after assessing for which sign/symptom?
    a. Cardiac dysrhythmias
    b. Respiratory depression
    c. Tremors or seizures
    d. Decreased urine output

41. The nurse is assessing a patient with kidney injury and notes that the patient is having Kussmaul respirations. What condition is the body attempting to compensate for?
    a. Hypoxia
    b. Alkalosis
    c. Acidosis
    d. Hypoxemia

42. A patient is diagnosed with renal osteodystrophy. What does the nurse instruct unlicensed assistive personnel to do in relation to this patient's diagnosis?
    a. Assist the patient with toileting every 2 hours.
    b. Gently wash the patient's skin with a mild soap and rinse well.
    c. Handle the patient gently because of risk for fractures.
    d. Assist the patient with eating because of loss of coordination.

43. A patient with chronic kidney disease develops severe chest pain, an increased pulse, low-grade fever, and a pericardial friction rub with a cardiac dysrhythmia and muffled heart tones. The nurse **immediately** alerts the health care provider and prepares for which emergency procedure?
    a. Pericardiocentesis
    b. Continuous venovenous hemofiltration
    c. Kidney dialysis
    d. Endotracheal intubation

44. A patient is instructed by the dietitian to restrict protein to 0.6 g/kg of body weight. The patient weighs 121 pounds and reports consuming milk and eggs or meat for every meal. What should the nurse do?
    a. Instruct the patient to carefully review and follow the dietary plan as instructed by the dietician.
    b. Advise the patient that protein intake is excessive and consult the dietitian for reeducation.
    c. Ask the patient to describe what he used to eat prior to being told about the dietary plan.
    d. Give the patient a brochure that explains how to calculate grams of protein in typical foods.

45. The nurse is reviewing urinalysis results for a patient who is in the **early** stages of chronic kidney disease. What results might the nurse expect to see?
    a. Excessive protein, glucose, red blood cells, and white blood cells
    b. Increased specific gravity with a dark amber discoloration
    c. Dramatically increased urine osmolarity
    d. Pink-tinged urine with obvious small blood clots

46. The night shift nurse sees a patient with kidney failure sitting up in bed. The patient states, "I feel a little short of breath at night or when I get up to walk to the bathroom." What assessment does the nurse do?
    a. Check for orthostatic hypotension because of potential volume depletion.
    b. Auscultate the lungs for crackles, which indicate fluid overload.
    c. Check the pulse and blood pressure for possible decreased cardiac output.
    d. Assess for normal sleep pattern and need for a prn sedative.

47. What type of breath odor is **most likely** to be noted in a patient with chronic kidney disease?
    a. Fruity smell
    b. Fecal smell
    c. Smells like urine
    d. Smells like blood

48. The patient with chronic kidney disease reports chronic fatigue, lethargy with weakness, and mild shortness of breath with dizziness when rising to a standing position. In addition, the nurse notes pale mucous membranes. Based on the patient's illness and the presenting symptoms, which laboratory result does the nurse expect to see?
    a. Low hemoglobin and hematocrit
    b. Low white cell count
    c. Low blood glucose
    d. Low oxygen saturation

49. The nurse is assessing the skin of a patient with end-stage kidney disease. Which clinical manifestation is considered a sign of **very late**, premorbid, advanced uremic syndrome?
    a. Ecchymoses
    b. Sallowness
    c. Pallor
    d. Uremic frost

50. The nurse notes an abnormal laboratory test finding for a patient with chronic kidney disease and alerts the health care provider. The nurse also consults with the registered dietitian because an excessive dietary protein intake is directly related to which factor?
    a. Elevated serum creatinine level
    b. Protein presence in the urine
    c. Elevated blood urea nitrogen level
    d. Elevated serum potassium level

51. In collaboration with the registered dietitian, the nurse teaches the patient about which dietary recommendations for management of chronic kidney disease? **Select all that apply.**
    a. Controlling protein intake
    b. Limiting fluid intake
    c. Restricting potassium
    d. Increasing sodium
    e. Restricting phosphorus
    f. Reducing calories

52. The health care provider has ordered sodium restriction to 3 g daily for a patient receiving dialysis therapy. What does the nurse teach the patient?
    a. Add smaller amounts of salt at the table or during cooking.
    b. Identify foods that are high in sodium (e.g., bacon, potato chips, fast foods).
    c. Avoid foods that have a metallic, salty, or bitter taste.
    d. Eat larger amounts of bland foods with very minimal amounts of spicing.

53. In order to assist a patient in the prevention of osteodystrophy, which intervention does the nurse perform?
    a. Administer phosphate binders with meals.
    b. Encourage high-quality protein foods.
    c. Administer iron supplements.
    d. Encourage extra milk at mealtimes.

54. The home health nurse is reviewing the medication list of a patient with chronic kidney disease. The nurse calls the health care provider as a reminder that the patient might need which nutritional supplements? **Select all that apply.**
    a. Iron
    b. Magnesium
    c. Phosphorus
    d. Calcium
    e. Vitamin D
    f. Water-soluble vitamins

55. A patient has been receiving erythropoietin. Which statement by the patient indicates that the therapy is producing the desired effect?
    a. "I can do my housework with less fatigue."
    b. "I have been passing more urine than I was before."
    c. "I have less pain and discomfort now."
    d. "I can swallow and eat much better than before."

56. The nurse monitors the daily weights for a patient with chronic kidney disease because of the risk for fluid retention. What instructions does the nurse give to unlicensed assistive personnel?
    a. Weigh the patient daily at the same time each day, same scale, with the same amount of clothing.
    b. Weigh the patient daily and add 1 kilogram of weight for the intake of each liter of fluid.
    c. Weigh the patient in the morning before breakfast and weigh the patient at night just before bedtime.
    d. Ask the patient about normal weight and weigh the patient before and after each voiding.

57. A patient with chronic kidney disease has hypertension and the health care provider has tried different medications, combinations, and adjustment of dosages. Which outcome statement indicates that the goal of drug therapy is being met?
    a. Patient reports compliance with regimen as prescribed.
    b. Patient reports feeling well and having good urine output.
    c. Blood pressure readings are consistently below 135/85.
    d. Blood pressure readings are never higher than 150/90.

58. The nurse is reviewing the medication list and appropriate dose adjustments made for a patient with chronic kidney disease. The nurse would **question** the use and/or dosage adjustment of which type of medication?
    a. Antibiotics
    b. Magnesium antacids
    c. Oral antidiabetics
    d. Opioids

59. The nurse is evaluating a patient's treatment response to erythropoietin. Which hemoglobin reading indicates that the goal is being met?
    a. Around 10 g/dL
    b. Greater than 20 g/dL
    c. Upward trend
    d. At baseline for gender

60. The nurse is caring for a patient with end-stage kidney disease and dialysis has been initiated. Which drug order does the nurse **question**?
    a. Erythropoietin
    b. Diuretic
    c. Angiotensin-converting enzyme inhibitor
    d. Calcium channel blocker

61. Which behavior is the **strongest** indicator that a patient with end stage kidney disease is not coping well with the illness and may need a referral for psychological counseling?
    a. Displays irritability when the meal tray arrives.
    b. Refuses to take a drug because it causes nausea.
    c. Repeatedly misses dialysis appointments.
    d. Is quiet when the health care provider talks about prognosis.

62. A patient with chronic kidney disease is restless, anxious, and short of breath. The nurse hears crackles that begin at the base of the lungs. The pulse rate is increased and the patient has frothy, blood-tinged sputum. What does the nurse do **first**?
    a. Facilitate transfer to intensive care for aggressive treatment.
    b. Place the patient in a high-Fowler's position.
    c. Continue to monitor vital signs and assess breath sounds.
    d. Administer a loop diuretic such as furosemide.

63. Which patient is the **most likely** candidate for continuous venovenous hemofiltration?
    a. Patient with fluid volume overload
    b. Patient who needs long-term management
    c. Patient who is critically ill
    d. Patient who is ready for discharge

64. If a patient with end-stage kidney disease experiences isosthenuria, what must the nurse be alert for?
    a. Massive diuresis
    b. Fluid volume overload
    c. Oliguria
    d. Alkalosis

65. The nurse is caring for a patient with chronic kidney disease. The family asks about when renal replacement therapy will begin. What is the nurse's **best** response?
    a. "As early as possible to prevent further damage in stage 1."
    b. "When there is reduced kidney function and metabolic wastes accumulate."
    c. "When the kidneys are unable to maintain a balance in body functions."
    d. "It will be started with diuretic therapy to enhance the remaining function."

66. What should the nurse do in order to monitor kidney function in the patient with chronic kidney disease? **Select all that apply.**
    a. Monitor intake and output.
    b. Check urine specific gravity.
    c. Review blood urea nitrogen and serum creatinine levels.
    d. Review x-ray reports.
    e. Monitor serum potassium and sodium levels.
    f. Observe albumin-creatinine ratio.

67. As a result of kidney failure, excessive hydrogen ions cannot be excreted. With acid retention, the nurse is **most likely** to observe what type of respiratory compensation?
    a. Cheyne-Stokes respiratory pattern
    b. Increased depth of breathing
    c. Decreased respiratory rate and depth
    d. Increased arterial carbon dioxide levels

68. The nurse is assessing a patient with uremia. Which gastrointestinal changes does the nurse expect to find? **Select all that apply.**
   a. Halitosis
   b. Hiccups
   c. Anorexia
   d. Nausea
   e. Vomiting
   f. Salivation

69. Which patients with chronic kidney disease are candidates for intermittent hemodialysis? **Select all that apply.**
   a. Patient with fluid overload who does not respond to diuretics
   b. Patient with stage 1 injury according to the KDIGO classification
   c. Patient with symptomatic toxin ingestion
   d. Patient with uremic manifestations, such as decreased cognition
   e. Patient with symptomatic hyperkalemia and calciphylaxis
   f. Patient with increased creatinine and blood urea nitrogen

70. The home health nurse is evaluating the home setting for a patient who wishes to have in-home hemodialysis. What is important to have in the home setting to support this therapy?
   a. Specialized water treatment system to provide a safe, purified water supply
   b. Large dust-free space to accommodate and store the dialysis equipment
   c. Modified electrical system to provide high voltage to power the equipment
   d. Specialized cooling system to maintain strict temperature control

71. The nursing student is explaining principles of hemodialysis to the nursing instructor. Which statement by the student indicates a need for additional study and research on the topic?
   a. "Dialysis works as molecules from an area of higher concentration move to an area of lower concentration."
   b. "Blood and dialyzing solution flow in opposite directions across an enclosed semipermeable membrane."
   c. "Excess water, waste products, and excess electrolytes are removed from the blood."
   d. "Bacteria and other organisms can also pass through the membrane, so the dialysate must be kept sterile."

72. A patient and family are trying to plan a schedule that coordinates with the patient's hemodialysis regimen. The patient asks, "How often will I have to go and how long does it take?" What is the nurse's **best** response?
   a. "If you follow diet and fluid therapies, you spend less time in dialysis, about 12 hours a week."
   b. "Most patients require about 12 hours per week; this is usually divided into three 4-hour treatments."
   c. "It varies. You will have to call your health care provider for specific instructions."
   d. "Many patients prefer to have treatments that occur every night while sleeping."

73. A patient is undergoing a dialysis treatment and exhibits a progression of symptoms which include headache, nausea and vomiting, and fatigue. How does the nurse interpret these symptoms?
   a. Mild dialysis disequilibrium syndrome
   b. Expected manifestations in end stage kidney disease
   c. Transient symptoms in a new dialysis patient
   d. Adverse reaction to the dialysate

74. The nurse is caring for a patient with an arteriovenous fistula. What instructions are given to unlicensed assistive personnel regarding the care of this patient?
    a. Palpate for thrills and auscultate for bruits every 4 hours.
    b. Check for bleeding at needle insertion sites.
    c. Assess the patient's distal pulses and circulation.
    d. Avoid taking blood pressure readings in the arm with the fistula.

75. The nurse is assessing a patient's extremity with an arteriovenous graft. The nurse notes a thrill and a bruit, and the patient reports numbness and a cool feeling in the fingers. How does the nurse interpret this information with regards to the graft?
    a. The graft is functional and these symptoms are expected.
    b. The patient has "steal syndrome" and may need surgical intervention.
    c. The graft is patent, but the blood is flowing in the wrong direction.
    d. The patient needs to increase active use of hands and fingers.

76. The nurse is providing postdialysis care for a patient. In comparing vital signs and weight measurements to the predialysis data, what does the nurse expect to find?
    a. Blood pressure and weight are reduced.
    b. Blood pressure is increased and weight is reduced.
    c. Blood pressure and weight are slightly increased.
    d. Blood pressure is low and weight is the same.

77. The nurse is assessing a patient who has just returned from hemodialysis. Which assessment finding is cause for **greatest** concern?
    a. Feeling of malaise
    b. Headache
    c. Muscle cramps in the legs
    d. Bleeding at the access site

78. The nurse is caring for a patient with an arteriovenous fistula. What is included in the nursing care for this patient? **Select all that apply.**
    a. Assess the patient's distal pulses and circulation in the arm with the access.
    b. Encourage routine range-of-motion exercises.
    c. Avoid venipuncture or IV administration on the arm with the access device.
    d. Instruct the patient to carry heavy objects to build muscular strength.
    e. Assess for manifestations of infection of the fistula.
    f. Instruct the patient to sleep on affected side with arm in the dependent position.

79. A patient has returned to the medical-surgical unit after having a dialysis treatment. The nurse notes that the patient is also scheduled for an invasive procedure on the same day. What is the **primary** rationale for delaying the procedure for 4 to 6 hours?
    a. The patient was heparinized during dialysis.
    b. The patient will have cardiac dysrhythmias after dialysis.
    c. The patient will be incoherent and unable to give consent.
    d. The patient needs routine medications that were delayed.

80. The nurse is talking to a patient with end-stage kidney disease. The patient frequently displays weight gain and increased blood pressure beyond the baseline measurements. Which question is the nurse **most likely** to ask to determine if the patient is doing something that is contributing to these assessment findings?
    a. "Are you controlling your salt intake?"
    b. "Are you following the protein restrictions?"
    c. "Have you been eating a lot of sweets?"
    d. "Have you been exercising regularly?"

81. Which patient with kidney problems is the **best** candidate for peritoneal dialysis?
    a. Patient with peritoneal adhesions
    b. Patient with a history of extensive abdominal surgery
    c. Patient with peritoneal membrane fibrosis
    d. Patient with a history of difficulty with anticoagulants

82. The nurse is teaching the patient to perform continuous ambulatory peritoneal dialysis. Place the steps in the correct order. **1 being the first step and 4 being the last step.**

    _____ a. Fluid stays in the cavity for a specified time prescribed by the health care provider.

    _____ b. 1 to 2 L of dialysate is infused by gravity over a 10-20-minute period.

    _____ c. Fluid flows out of the body by gravity into a drainage bag.

    _____ d. Warm the dialysate bags before instillation by using a heating pad to wrap the bag.

83. The health care provider has ordered intraperitoneal heparin for a patient with a new peritoneal dialysis catheter to prevent clotting of the catheter by blood and fibrin formation. What advice does the nurse give the patient?
    a. Watch for bruising or bleeding from the gums.
    b. Make a follow-up appointment for coagulation studies.
    c. Intraperitoneal heparin does not affect clotting times.
    d. Certain foods can interact with heparin to alter clotting.

84. Patients with diabetes or hypertension should be encouraged to have which tests annually?
    a. Glomerular filtration rate, urinalysis, and urine osmolality
    b. Urine albumin-to creatinine ratio, serum creatinine, and blood urea nitrogen.
    c. Urine specific gravity, albumin-creatinine ratio, and electrolytes
    d. Blood urea nitrogen, serum creatinine, urine sodium, and kidney ultrasound

85. The home health nurse is visiting a patient who independently performs peritoneal dialysis (PD). Which question does the nurse ask the patient to assess for the **major** complication associated with PD?
    a. "Have you noticed any signs or symptoms of infection?"
    b. "Are you having any pain during the dialysis treatments?"
    c. "Is the dialysate fluid slow or sluggish?"
    d. "Have you noticed any leakage around the catheter?"

86. The nurse is teaching a patient about performing peritoneal dialysis (PD) at home. In order to identify the **earliest** manifestation of peritonitis, what does the nurse instruct the patient to do?
    a. Monitor temperature before starting PD.
    b. Check the effluent for cloudiness.
    c. Be aware of feelings of malaise.
    d. Monitor for abdominal pain.

87. During peritoneal dialysis, the nurse notes slowed dialysate outflow. What does the nurse do to troubleshoot the system? **Select all that apply.**
    a. Ensure that the drainage bag is elevated.
    b. Inspect the tubing for kinking or twisting.
    c. Ensure that clamps are open.
    d. Turn the patient to the other side.
    e. Make sure the patient has good body alignment.
    f. Instruct the patient to stand or cough.

88. A patient has recently started peritoneal dialysis therapy and reports some mild pain when the dialysate is flowing in. What does the nurse do **next**?
    a. Immediately report the pain to the health care provider.
    b. Warm the dialysate in the microwave oven.
    c. Reassure that pain should subside after the first week or two.
    d. Assess the connection tubing for kinking or twisting.

89. The nurse is caring for a patient requiring peritoneal dialysis. In order to monitor the patient's weight, what does the nurse do?
    a. Check the weight after a drain and before the next fill to monitor the patient's "dry weight."
    b. Calculate the "dry weight" by comparing daily weights to baseline weights.
    c. Determine "dry weight" by comparing the patient's weight to a standard weight chart.
    d. Weigh the patient daily and subtract fluid intake and dialysate volume to determine "dry weight."

90. The nurse is monitoring a patient's peritoneal dialysis treatment. The total outflow is slightly less than the inflow. What does the nurse do next?
    a. Instruct the patient to ambulate.
    b. Notify the health care provider.
    c. Record the difference as intake.
    d. Put the patient on fluid restriction.

91. Which patients are likely to be excluded from receiving a transplant? **Select all that apply.**
    a. Patient with breast cancer that has metastasized to lungs
    b. Patient with advanced and uncorrectable heart disease
    c. Patient with a chemical dependency
    d. Patient who is 70 years old and has a living related donor
    e. Patient with type 2 diabetes mellitus
    f. Patient who is receiving treatment for peptic ulcer disease

92. The intensive care nurse is caring for a patient who just received a kidney transplant from a related donor. The nurse notices hypotension and excessive diuresis, 1000 mL greater than intake over the past 12 hours. At this point, what is the **primary** concept that affects graft survival?
    a. Infection
    b. Perfusion
    c. Elimination
    d. Cellular regulation

93. The nurse is caring for the kidney transplant patient in the **immediate** postoperative period. During this initial period, the nurse will assess the urine output at least every hour for how many hours?
    a. First 8 hours
    b. First 12 hours
    c. First 24 hours
    d. First 48 hours

94. The intensive care nurse is caring for the kidney transplant patient who was just transferred from the recovery unit. Which finding is the **most serious** within the first 12 hours after surgery and warrants **immediate** notification of the transplant surgeon?
    a. Diuresis with increased output
    b. Pink or dark reddish urine
    c. Abrupt decrease in urine
    d. Small clots in bladder irrigation fluid

95. The nurse is caring for a patient who had kidney transplant surgery 3 days ago. The nurse notes a sudden and abrupt decrease in urine. The nurse alerts the health care provider for suspected thrombosis. What is the **priority** concept that underlies this complication?
    a. Infection
    b. Perfusion
    c. Elimination
    d. Cellular regulation

69 CHAPTER

Assessment of the Reproductive System

1. If the function of normal vaginal flora is disrupted, the female patient is **most likely** to experience which condition?
   a. Vaginal dryness
   b. Vaginal infection
   c. "Hot flashes"
   d. Irregular menses

2. The nurse is interviewing a 56-year-old woman who reports irregular and decreased flow of menses for several months. Which question does the nurse ask the patient?
   a. "Have you been exposed to sexually transmitted disease?"
   b. "Are you having any discomfort during intercourse?"
   c. "Have you noticed any lumps or tenderness in your breasts?"
   d. "Do you have a history of frequent urinary tract infections?"

3. The nurse reads in the patient's chart that there is a history of blockage in the fallopian tubes. Based on this history, what is the patient **most likely** to report?
   a. Vaginal discharge
   b. Amenorrhea
   c. Difficulty conceiving
   d. Difficulty controlling weight

4. Females with an insufficient estrogen level should be assessed for which condition?
   a. Osteoporosis
   b. Diabetes mellitus
   c. Endometriosis
   d. Decreased immune function

5. A male patient had mumps as a child which caused orchitis. Which potential complication could result?
   a. Decreased libido
   b. Chronic urinary infection
   c. Enlarged prostate gland
   d. Testicular atrophy

6. A male patient reports that he has a decreased libido. The nurse assesses for which factors related to this condition? **Select all that apply.**
   a. Tobacco use
   b. Type of exercise
   c. Alcohol consumption
   d. Occupation
   e. Illicit drug use
   f. Weight gain

7. Disorders that alter a woman's metabolism or nutrition can result in which condition?
   a. Excessive bleeding
   b. Endometriosis
   c. Amenorrhea
   d. Pelvic inflammatory disease

8. A 60-year-old female patient informs the nurse that she has experienced some vaginal changes since menopause. What gynecologic change is the patient **most likely** to report?
   a. Thin, white vaginal drainage
   b. Vaginal odor
   c. Excessive vaginal bleeding
   d. Vaginal dryness

9. The mother of a 17-year-old adolescent girl tells the nurse that her daughter has been purging, showing anorexic behavior, and continuously exercising. Based on the mother's report, which question related to the reproductive system would the nurse ask the girl?
   a. "When was your last normal menstrual period?"
   b. "Are you sexually active?"
   c. "Are you having any unusual vaginal discharge?"
   d. "Do you have any questions about contraception?"

10. A 29-year-old patient has strictures and adhesions in her fallopian tubes. This can be the result of which condition?
    a. Pelvic inflammatory disease
    b. Frequent episodes of colitis
    c. Gallbladder disease
    d. Frequent urinary tract infections

11. In a patient with a reproductive health problem, what health and lifestyle habits would the nurse assess? **Select all that apply.**
    a. Diet
    b. Socioeconomic status
    c. Exercise pattern
    d. Occupation
    e. Sleep pattern
    f. Sexual practices

12. A 23-year-old woman is diagnosed with a chlamydial infection but is reluctant to spend the money for treatment because she is asymptomatic and does not have a job or health insurance. The nurse advises her that chlamydial infections can result in which condition?
    a. Female infertility
    b. Male partner infertility
    c. Amenorrhea
    d. Teratogenic effects

13. A 40-year-old woman has heavy vaginal bleeding. Which question is the **priority** in evaluating the patient's condition?
    a. "Is the bleeding related to the menstrual cycle or intercourse?"
    b. "Are you having any sensations of pain or cramping?"
    c. "Are you sexually active and do you use oral contraceptives?"
    d. "Are you feeling weak, dizzy, or lightheaded?"

14. A 37-year-old patient reports abnormal vaginal bleeding not related to her menstrual cycle. The nurse would ask the patient about which associated symptoms? **Select all that apply.**
    a. Pain
    b. Change in bowel habits
    c. Breast mass
    d. Abdominal fullness
    e. Urinary difficulties
    f. Fluid intake

15. According to the American Cancer Society recommendations, which healthy woman with no previous history of an abnormal Pap test should be advised to have a Pap test every 3 years?
    a. 18-year-old
    b. 21-year-old
    c. 35-year-old
    d. 70-year-old

16. The health care provider has just informed the patient about the diagnosis and complications of salpingitis. Which intervention is the nurse **most likely** to use with this patient?
    a. Review nonpharmacologic methods to control chronic pain.
    b. Use empathetic listening for feelings related to possible infertility.
    c. Inform that annual Pap smears are recommended for salpingitis.
    d. Review expected changes that will occur with menstrual flow.

17. For a patient with a low testosterone level, what is the patient **most likely** to report?
    a. Increased weight and muscle mass
    b. Changes in urinary pattern
    c. Problems with sexual performance
    d. Testicular pain with nausea

18. What features would be considered normal findings for the scrotum of a young white male? **Select all that apply.**
    a. Suspended below the pubic bone
    b. Tenderness with gentle palpation
    c. Contracts with exposure to cold
    d. Sparse hair follicles
    e. Skin of pouch is thin walled
    f. Warm compared to surrounding tissues

19. If the prostate gland is not functioning correctly, which statement typifies what the patient is **most likely** to report?
    a. "Well, I am not as strong or as muscular as I was when I was younger."
    b. "My wife and I have been trying to conceive a child for several years."
    c. "Occasionally, if I am tired I have problems getting an erection."
    d. "My libido is fine, but sometimes I have premature ejaculation."

20. A 72-year-old patient admitted to the medical-surgical unit tells the nurse that he has benign prostatic hyperplasia. Which question will the nurse ask?
    a. "Have you had chemotherapy or radiation treatments?"
    b. "Were you recently diagnosed with benign prostatic hyperplasia?"
    c. "Would you like to review information about nutrition therapy?"
    d. "Are you having urinary incontinence or frequency at night?"

21. A young woman reports that she has a genital discharge causing irritation and odor. She feels embarrassed, but insists that she has not had recent sexual relations. Which question is the nurse **most likely** to ask?
    a. "Have you recently taken any antibiotic medications?"
    b. "Do you have a family history for cervical cancer?"
    c. "How old were you when you first had sexual intercourse?"
    d. "Have you had a change of diet or noticed weight loss?"

22. The nurse is interviewing a patient who reports a discharge from his penis that started 3 days ago. What does the nurse ask the patient regarding this problem? **Select all that apply.**
    a. "Has your sexual partner(s) noticed a discharge?"
    b. "Does the discharge have an odor?"
    c. "Have you noticed a mass or lump in the scrotum?"
    d. "Are you having any pain or burning during urination?"
    e. "What is the consistency of the discharge?"
    f. "Can you describe the color of the discharge?"

23. A nurse is working at an ambulatory clinic. Which patient is **most likely** to need a pelvic examination?
    a. 12-year-old whose mother desires a "virgin check"
    b. 25-year-old with a possible urinary tract infection
    c. 62-year-old who reports resumption of menses
    d. 53-year-old who reports decreased libido

24. On the figure below, indicate the surfaces of the cervix and the canal, which are the sites for Papanicolaou (Pap) testing.

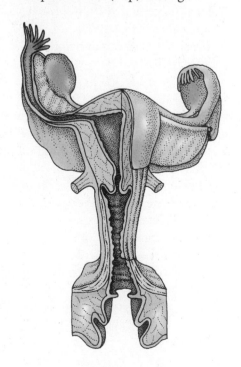

25. The nurse is taking a history on a patient who has risk for problems related to reproductive health. Despite the nurse's best attempts to establish rapport and trust, the patient absolutely refuses to answer questions about sexual practices. What should the nurse do?
    a. Tell the patient that all information is confidential.
    b. Advise the patient that withholding information can be dangerous.
    c. Rephrase questions to make them less offensive.
    d. Respect the patient's choice to refuse to answer questions.

26. Which test detects cancerous and precancerous cells of the cervix?
    a. Serologic studies
    b. Vaginal culture
    c. Pap smear
    d. Human papillomavirus test

27. A patient calls to make an appointment for a routine pelvic exam which includes a Pap smear. What type of instructions does the nurse give the patient about preparing for the exam?
    a. "Do not have intercourse for at least 24 hours before the exam."
    b. "Do not eat or drink anything after midnight."
    c. "Clean the genitals with mild soap and water before the exam."
    d. "Do not wear a tampon if you are menstruating."

28. According to the American Cancer Society guidelines, annual screening mammograms are not recommended for women less than 40 years old. What is the underlying rationale for this recommendation?
    a. Breast tumors are not very common among women under the age of 40 years.
    b. Amount of radiation exposure outweighs the benefit for women of childbearing age
    c. In younger women, there is little difference in the density of normal tissue and malignant tumors.
    d. In younger women, the tumors are likely to be too small to be detected by mammography.

29. An African American male patient has a prostate-specific antigen (PSA) level less than 2.5 ng/mL. Which information should the nurse give to the patient?
    a. African American men typically have lower-than-normal PSA levels.
    b. Level indicates a need for follow-up for possible prostate cancer.
    c. PSA level of less than 2.5 ng/mL is generally considered normal.
    d. Test should be repeated on an annual basis to monitor the abnormality.

30. Which woman has the **highest** risk for developing cervical cancer?
    a. Has normal Pap test result and decreased luteinizing hormone
    b. Has an abnormal Pap test result and a positive human papillomavirus test
    c. Has decreased levels of estradiol, total estrogens, and estriol
    d. Has abnormal findings on hysterosalpingography

31. The patient reports fatigue and low libido. Based on the patient's report of symptoms, which laboratory result would the nurse seek out **first**?
    a. Pap smear results
    b. Rubella titer
    c. Red blood cell count
    d. Luteinizing hormone level

32. Which patient is **most likely** to require an iron supplement?
    a. 53-year-old woman who is entering menopause and has a breast mass
    b. 32-year-old female with heavy menstrual bleeding and an intrauterine device
    c. 70-year-old male who is diagnosed with benign prostatic hyperplasia
    d. 23-year-old woman who has pelvic inflammatory disease

33. The health care provider tells the nurse that the patient is being evaluated for galactorrhea and to please call with the relevant laboratory results. Which laboratory result will the nurse look for?
    a. Prolactin level
    b. Endometrial biopsy results
    c. Follicle-stimulating hormone level
    d. Progesterone level

34. A 23-year-old female has a decreased level of follicle-stimulating hormone. What may this finding indicate?
    a. Midcycle of menses
    b. Pregnancy
    c. Premature menopause
    d. Infertility

35. Which patient is **most likely** to report problems with impotence?
    a. Patient has prostate specific antigen of 2 ng/mL.
    b. Patient has diabetes mellitus.
    c. Patient has a history of orchitis.
    d. Patient has testosterone of 500 ng/dL.

36. The nurse is teaching a patient about the contraindications for hysteroscopy. What does the nurse tell the patient?
    a. "During the procedure, normal or abnormal cells can be pushed through the fallopian tubes and into the pelvic cavity; therefore pregnancy is a contraindication."
    b. "The procedure causes irritation and can be very painful if your vaginal tissue is dry or fragile; therefore, the procedure is not recommended for postmenopausal women."
    c. "The procedure can cause a lot of bleeding so a recent prescription of an anticoagulant is a contraindication."
    d. "During the procedure, an iodine-based dye is used, so allergies to shellfish or iodine are contraindications."

37. A patient received treatment for prostate cancer. Which test is **most likely** to be ordered to monitor the disease after treatment?
    a. Transrectal biopsy
    b. Prostate-specific antigen test
    c. Human papillomavirus test
    d. Routine prostate examination

38. The nurse is caring for a patient who had a laparoscopy. What is included in the postoperative care for this patient? **Select all that apply.**
    a. Administer oral analgesics for incisional pain.
    b. Notify the health care provider of postoperative shoulder pain.
    c. Reassure the patient that most painful sensations disappear within 4-6 weeks.
    d. Instruct the patient to change the small adhesive bandage as needed.
    e. Teach the patient to observe the incision for signs of infection or hematoma.
    f. Remind the patient to avoid strenuous activity for 4-6 weeks after the procedure.

39. The nurse is helping a patient schedule an appointment for a hysteroscopy. When should the procedure be done?
    a. 5 days after menses have ceased
    b. 5 days before the beginning of menses
    c. During the menstrual period
    d. Whenever she can take 3-4 days off of work

40. A patient has just been informed by the health care provider that she has specific BRCA1 and BRCA2 gene mutations. Which brochure would the nurse prepare for the patient?
    a. "Role of Nutrition Therapy in Reproductive Health"
    b. "Risk Factors and Treatments for Infertility"
    c. "Risk Factors and Treatments for Breast Cancer"
    d. "Colposcopy and Other Tests for Cervical Cancer"

41. Which man has the **greatest** risk for developing prostate cancer?
    a. Patient's grandfather, age 82 years, has benign prostatic hyperplasia.
    b. Patient's father was diagnosed and treated for prostate cancer at age 50.
    c. Patient's mother took diethylstilbestrol to control bleeding during pregnancy.
    d. Patient's brother had delayed development of sexual characteristics.

42. The nurse is assisting a patient who needs a pelvic examination. Which action will the nurse perform?
    a. Clean perineum with antiseptic solution.
    b. Administer a mild analgesic.
    c. Assess for allergies to iodine.
    d. Instruct to empty the urinary bladder.

43. A patient has just been informed that she has an abnormal Pap smear and a positive human papillomavirus test. The nurse should be prepared to provide information about which topic?
    a. Increased risk for cervical cancer
    b. Increased risk for endometrial cancer
    c. Increased risk for herpes simplex virus type 2
    d. Increased risk for human immunodeficiency virus

44. The nurse is talking to a patient who is about to undergo a hysterosalpingogram. The patient discloses information that may not have been available to the health care provider when the test was initially scheduled. Which disclosure could cause the provider to **cancel or reschedule** the test?
    a. Took over-the-counter acetaminophen 1 hour ago.
    b. Has fever with malodorous vaginal discharge.
    c. Has a family history of uterine fibroids.
    d. Is on day 10 of the menstrual cycle.

45. What preprocedural instructions would the nurse give the patient about a mammogram?
    a. Do not eat or drink anything 6-7 hours before the test.
    b. Abstain from sexual relations prior to test to avoid pregnancy.
    c. Do not use lotions, creams, or powder on breasts before the study.
    d. Wear a supportive bra and bring a breast pad for use after testing.

46. What postprocedure instructions would the nurse give to a patient who just had a colposcopy?
    a. Do not drive or operate heavy machinery while taking prescribed pain medication.
    b. Do not use tampons and abstain from sexual intercourse for at least 1 week.
    c. Wear a perineal pad and expect bleeding with small clots for the first 24 hours.
    d. Perform breast self-examination every month and report changes to provider.

47. The patient needs to be scheduled for an endometrial biopsy to assess unusually heavy menstrual bleeding. Which question is the **most important** to ask, in relation to scheduling the examination?
    a. "Have you ever had a spontaneous miscarriage or an elective abortion?"
    b. "How many pads per day are you using during the heaviest flow?"
    c. "What was the date of your last menstrual period and are you regular?"
    d. "Do any unexpected symptoms accompany the heavy menstrual flow?"

48. What postprocedure instructions would the nurse give to a patient who had a prostate biopsy?
    a. Light rectal bleeding and blood in the urine or stools is expected for a few days.
    b. Swelling of the biopsy area and difficulty urinating are expected for 1 week.
    c. Low-grade fever and bright-red penile discharge are normal for several days.
    d. Return to see the health care provider in 1 week for recheck of biopsy site.

70
CHAPTER

Care of Patients with Breast Disorders

1. For a patient with mild discomfort from a fibrocystic breast condition, what will the nurse teach the patient about self-care measures?
   a. Avoid or limit reaching upward or lifting objects above the head.
   b. Avoid wearing a bra to decrease the pressure on the breast tissue.
   c. Take analgesics and limit salt before menses to help decrease swelling.
   d. Take selective estrogen receptor modulator as prescribed.

2. A 22-year-old woman is being seen for a self-detected mass in her right breast. Clinical examination reveals an oval-shaped, freely mobile, and rubbery lesion. What type of tumor is this **most likely** to be?
   a. Ductal ectasia
   b. Papilloma
   c. Fibroadenoma
   d. Macrocyst

3. Regarding the diagnosis and treatment of breast cancer, what are important considerations for young women? **Select all that apply.**
   a. Genetic predisposition is a stronger risk factor for young women compared to older women
   b. Young women frequently have more aggressive forms of the disease.
   c. Prognosis is usually better for young women because they have fewer chronic conditions.
   d. Screening tools can be less effective because young women have denser breast tissue.
   e. Young women are less likely to be concerned about cancer, so they delay seeking treatment.
   f. Early menopause, infertility, and sexual dysfunction are concerns for young women.

4. Which patient is describing an ominous sign associated with inflammatory breast cancer, which is a highly aggressive invasive breast cancer?
   a. Patient reports breast pain and a rapidly growing breast lump.
   b. Patient notices numerous small tender lumps before menses.
   c. Patient says her breasts feel similar to when she breastfed.
   d. Patient reports noticing a change in the color of her nipple.

5. Which patient should be advised to have an annual clinical breast examination?
   a. 42-year-old woman who is not having any symptoms
   b. 25-year-old woman who is nursing a newborn
   c. 35-year-old woman with no known health problems
   d. 28-year-old woman who recently had breast reduction.

6. A patient with a fibrocystic breast condition has just undergone fine needle aspiration to drain the cyst fluid and reduce pressure and pain. When would the nurse prepare patient education material about breast biopsy? **Select all that apply.**
   a. If hormonal replacement therapy is prescribed
   b. If fluid is not aspirated
   c. If the mammogram shows suspicious findings
   d. If fluid buildup recurs
   e. If the mass remains palpable after aspiration
   f. If aspirated fluid reveals cancer cells

7. A patient with a fibrocystic breast condition is prescribed hormonal therapy to manage symptoms. Which teaching materials will the nurse prepare for the patient related to the therapy?
    a. Signs/symptoms of stroke, liver disease, and increased intracranial pressure
    b. Signs/symptoms of acute renal failure, fluid retention, or electrolyte imbalances
    c. Signs/symptoms of problems with coagulation or other hematologic disorders
    d. Signs/symptoms of cardiotoxicity, cardiac failure, or fluid overload

8. A 54-year-old woman has identified a hard breast mass with irregular borders, redness, and edema. She reports a nipple discharge and enlarged axillary nodes. Based on the patient's age and description of the symptoms, what does the nurse suspect?
    a. Fibroadenoma
    b. Fibrocystic breast condition
    c. Ductal ectasia
    d. Intraductal papilloma

9. The nurse is examining the breasts of an older woman. What would be considered a normal finding?
    a. Gentle palpation elicits reports of pain or discomfort.
    b. Tissue is difficult to palpate because of fat deposits.
    c. Nipples are retracted and there is a brownish discharge.
    d. Breasts are atrophied, flattened, and elongated.

10. The nurse is reviewing discharge instructions for a patient who had breast augmentation surgery. What does the nurse include in these instructions? **Select all that apply.**
    a. Expect soreness in chest and arms for several months.
    b. Breasts will feel tight and sensitive; the breast skin may feel warm or itchy.
    c. Anticipate having difficulty raising the arms over the head.
    d. Perform lifting, pushing, and pulling exercises several times a day.
    e. Walk every few hours to prevent deep vein thrombosis.
    f. Expect some swelling for 3-4 weeks after surgery.

11. In males who have breast cancer, what is the **most typical** presenting sign/symptom?
    a. Nipple discharge with gross blood
    b. Localized red and painful lump
    c. Dimpling or orange peel appearance
    d. Hard, painless, subareolar mass

12. What does the nurse instruct the patient to do before a scheduled breast augmentation surgery? **Select all that apply.**
    a. Stop oral contraceptives.
    b. Stop smoking.
    c. Avoid taking NSAIDs.
    d. Avoid taking ginseng.
    e. Wear a supportive bra.
    f. Bathe with a mild soap.

13. After surgery, a female patient has been told her breast tumor contains estrogen receptors. What is the clinical significance of this information and how will this type of cancer be treated?
    a. This is a triple-negative breast cancer and additional surgery is the best option.
    b. This type of cancer has a better prognosis and usually responds to hormonal therapy.
    c. This tumor is localized; therefore radiation therapy should effectively eradicate the cancer.
    d. There are metastases, so long-term survival rate is low; systemic therapy is the only option.

14. Based on risk factors and personal history, which woman has the **greatest** risk of developing breast cancer?
    a. Physician, age 56, who had her first child at age 38
    b. Ballet dancer, age 25, who has a 5-year-old son
    c. Radiation technician, age 24, who had her menarche at age 13
    d. Housewife, age 42, who had breast reduction surgery at age 26

15. The nurse is counseling a woman who was recently diagnosed with breast cancer. Which factor has the **most** influence on the choice for treatment?
    a. Age at the time of diagnosis
    b. Overall health status
    c. Personal choice and self-care capacity
    d. Extent and location of metastases

16. A young woman is suspected of having invasive breast cancer. Based on the types and frequencies of breast cancer, what is the **most likely** diagnosis?
    a. Fibrocystic breast condition
    b. Infiltrating ductal carcinoma
    c. Lobular carcinoma in situ
    d. Ductal carcinoma in situ

17. Which factor is the incidence of breast cancer **most closely** related to?
    a. Lifestyle choices
    b. Aging
    c. Ethnic background
    d. Socioeconomic status

18. During clinical breast exam, the examiner observes a small mass in the breast. What is the **most** important item to include in the documentation of this finding?
    a. "Face of the clock" location of the mass
    b. Amount of pressure required to detect the mass
    c. Patient's self-awareness of the location
    d. Method used to examine the breast

19. Cancer surveillance for high-risk women is used to detect cancer in its early stages and is referred to as what kind of prevention?
    a. Primary
    b. Secondary
    c. Tertiary
    d. Prophylactic

20. According to the American Cancer Society, what are the recommendations for early detection by screening for breast masses?
    a. Women aged 45-54 should have an annual mammogram, then every 2 years at age 55 and older.
    b. High-risk women should have biannual mammograms and magnetic resonance imaging.
    c. High-risk women should be screened for breast cancer annually starting at age 21.
    d. Women aged 60 years or older should have a mammogram every 10 years.

21. The nurse is teaching a 24-year-old patient about breast self-examination (BSE). What does the nurse tell the patient about the best time to perform BSE?
    a. Day before her menstrual flow is due
    b. Third day after menstrual flow starts
    c. Whenever ovulation occurs
    d. One week after her menstrual period

22. Which factor makes the mammogram a more sensitive screening tool than other tests?
    a. Higher compliance rate because it is done annually
    b. Less expensive than other tests that identify tumor markers
    c. Able to reveal masses too small to be palpated manually
    d. Able to differentiate between fluid and solid masses

23. A patient stopped having menses about a year ago. When does the nurse advise the patient to perform breast self-examination (BSE)?
    a. The first day of every other month
    b. After menopause, BSE does not detect masses
    c. The last day of each month
    d. Any day of the month, but follow a consistent schedule

24. The nurse is teaching the patient about breast self-examination. Which correct actions are included in the procedure? **Select all that apply.**
    a. "Lie down on your back and place your right arm behind your head."
    b. "Use the palm of your left hand to feel for lumps in the right breast."
    c. "Use three different levels of pressure to feel all the breast tissue."
    d. "Move around the breast in an up and down pattern."
    e. "Repeat the exam on your left breast."
    f. "Stand in front of a mirror, press your hands firmly down on your hips, and observe breasts."

25. Which combination of screening techniques is best for **early** detection of breast cancer?
    a. Mammogram, clinical breast exam, and breast self-awareness
    b. Magnetic resonance imaging, breast self-examination, and mammogram
    c. Breast biopsy, clinical breast exam, and mammogram
    d. Mammogram, breast self-examination, and breast tomosynthesis

26. Which sign/symptom detected during clinical breast examination suggests **advanced** breast disease?
    a. Gynecomastia
    b. Oval-shaped, mobile, rubbery mass
    c. Thin, milky discharge from the nipple
    d. Skin change of peau d'orange

27. Women who have a personal history of breast cancer are at high risk for developing a recurrence. Which factors contribute to recurrence? **Select all that apply.**
    a. BRCA3 genetic mutation
    b. Strong family history of breast cancer
    c. BRCA2 genetic mutation
    d. BRCA1 genetic mutation
    e. History of breast reduction
    f. History of fibrocystic breast condition

28. A patient is recently diagnosed with a fibrocystic breast condition (FBC) and she is very fearful that she will develop breast cancer. What does the nurse tell the patient?
    a. "FBC is considered precancerous, so monitoring is essential."
    b. "There is no increased risk of developing breast cancer."
    c. "Features of FBC automatically rule out cancer."
    d. "We can review lifestyle changes that will reduce the risk."

29. A patient had breast reconstruction surgery two days ago. A Jackson-Pratt drain was placed to collect serosanguineous fluid. The nurse notices at 7:00 AM that the drainage container contains 150 mL. It was last emptied at 6:00 AM. What is the **priority** nursing intervention?
    a. Notify the health care provider about amount and appearance of drainage for the past hour.
    b. Empty the drain every 2 hours and flush the tubing so the suction will be more effective.
    c. Assess for pain, or other symptoms; chart the type and amount of drainage and continue to monitor.
    d. Reinforce the drainage site with a sterile bulky dressing and recheck the site in one hour.

30. A patient had a partial mastectomy yesterday and the nurse notes that the patient is very anxious because of removal of breast tissue. What is the nurse's **priority** intervention?
    a. Use distraction until the patient improves and can think more clearly.
    b. Encourage the patient to have a positive attitude so she will heal faster.
    c. Ensure that the patient takes prn anxiolytic medication every 4-6 hours.
    d. Encourage the patient to discuss her fears and ask questions about her concerns.

31. A patient had a partial mastectomy. When teaching about care of the arm on the affected side, what does the nurse tell the patient?
    a. Do not start any arm or hand exercises until the drains are removed from the incision.
    b. Begin using your arm for normal activities, such as eating or combing your hair.
    c. No one should take a blood pressure on the affected arm for 6 months after surgery.
    d. Do push-ups and arm circles on a routine basis for a full recovery.

32. A patient has just been diagnosed with breast cancer and informed that surgery is likely to be needed. The patient seems anxious and upset. What is the **priority** nursing care for this patient?
    a. Provide patient education about treatment options.
    b. Assist the patient to make independent decisions.
    c. Provide reassurance about long-term outcomes.
    d. Allow patient to talk openly about feelings.

33. Which intervention would be used for a patient after a modified radical mastectomy?
    a. Position the patient on the affected side to aid flow of drainage from the incision site.
    b. Place arm on the affected side in a dependent position postoperatively.
    c. Give pain medication so that arm exercises can begin as soon as possible.
    d. Teach signs and symptoms of infection and how to monitor for altered wound healing.

34. A patient who had surgery for breast cancer appears in need of continued community support. The nurse refers the patient to which organization?
    a. Reach to Recovery
    b. Empty Arms
    c. Resolve to Reach
    d. Evolve

35. A woman has had several discussions with the health care provider about her risk for breast cancer. What would the nurse say in order to reinforce the role of prophylactic mastectomy on the risk for developing breast cancer?
    a. "Prophylactic mastectomy has no impact for some women."
    b. "The procedure eliminates the risk completely."
    c. "The surgery reduces the risk for breast cancer."
    d. "An added benefit is the decreased risk for uterine cancer."

36. Which woman has the **highest** risk for developing breast cancer?
    a. 68-year-old who takes hormone replacement therapy
    b. 35-year-old who has three children and had one miscarriage
    c. 23-year-old who started menstruating at age 12
    d. 40-year-old who has two cousins who had breast cancer

37. A patient reports finding a mass in her breast 6 months ago. What question does the nurse ask related to possible metastases of a potential cancer?
    a. "Why did you wait 6 months before seeking medical attention?"
    b. "Have you noticed any joint or bone pain or other changes in your body?"
    c. "Have you ever had any exposure to radiation or toxic chemicals?"
    d. "Has your sister or mother ever been diagnosed with breast cancer?"

38. A patient has just been diagnosed with advanced breast cancer. Which behavior by the patient is the **strongest** indicator of readiness for additional patient teaching and information?
    a. Cheerfully talking about her family and the vacation they will take to Europe
    b. Being hostile and angrily throwing her belongings into her suitcase
    c. Crying and being upset, asking the nurse to call a spiritual counselor
    d. Being quiet and thoughtfully fingering the lace on her new bra

39. A patient in the medical-surgical unit says to the nurse, "My doctor told me I have advanced breast cancer and I want to give you this bracelet because you have been so sweet to me today." What does the nurse do **first**?
    a. Contact the health care provider because the comment signals suicide intent.
    b. Sit with the patient and allow her to take the lead in the conversation.
    c. Suggest that the bracelet should be given to a daughter or other family member.
    d. Explain to the patient that it is unethical for nurses to accept expensive gifts.

40. The nurse is reviewing the laboratory results from a postmenopausal woman being evaluated for a breast mass. What type of metastasis does the increased serum calcium and alkaline phosphatase levels suggest?
    a. Brain
    b. Bone
    c. Lung
    d. Liver

41. A woman recently diagnosed with breast cancer confides, "I am going to use nutritional and herbal therapy instead of taking drugs and radiation that would make my hair fall out." What is the nurse's **best** response?
    a. "Research does not support the use of complementary therapy."
    b. "Have you reviewed all treatment options with your health care provider?"
    c. "Alternative nutritional therapies would delay or interfere with treatment."
    d. "Where did you hear about this nutritional and herbal treatment?"

42. The nurse is caring for a patient who had a right-sided modified radical mastectomy. Which task does the nurse delegate to unlicensed assist personnel?
    a. Observe the drainage in the Jackson-Pratt drain.
    b. Take blood pressure on the right arm only.
    c. Assist the patient to ambulate the day after surgery.
    d. Instruct the patient about arm positioning.

43. A patient is lying in bed after a mastectomy. How does the nurse position the patient?
    a. Head of the bed up at least 30 degrees with the affected arm elevated on a pillow
    b. Supine body position with the affected arm positioned straight by the side
    c. Any position that is the most comfortable to the patient
    d. Side-lying position with the unaffected side down toward mattress

44. A patient is one day postsurgery after a mastectomy and is anxious to begin the prescribed exercises. Which exercise is appropriate for the patient's **first** efforts?
    a. Flex the fingers so that the hands slowly "walk" up the wall.
    b. Squeeze the affected hand around a soft, round object.
    c. Swing a rope in small circles and gradually increase to larger circles.
    d. Grab the ends of a rope and extend the arms until they are straight.

45. A patient is being discharged with a prescription for tamoxifen to decrease the chance of breast cancer recurrence. Because of the common side effect, what does the nurse suggest to the patient?
    a. Have soda crackers and ginger ale on hand.
    b. Install a handrail around the bathtub.
    c. Purchase a scale to monitor body weight.
    d. Buy a soft-bristle toothbrush.

46. A patient is prescribed trastuzumab for breast cancer. What is the **priority** nursing intervention for this patient?
    a. Assess for signs of cardiotoxicity
    b. Assess for signs of bleeding.
    c. Premedicate with an antiemetic.
    d. Rotate injection sites.

47. The nurse is caring for a patient who is diagnosed with ductal ectasia. What is the primary goal of the nursing care?
    a. Reduce the anxiety associated with the threat of breast cancer.
    b. Review side effects of radiation and chemotherapy treatments.
    c. Give support for decision-making about prophylactic mastectomy.
    d. Assess for readiness and willingness to seek a support group.

48. The nurse is assessing a woman with very large breasts. In addition to the routine assessment of the breasts, what specific assessment will the nurse perform on this patient?
    a. Pay special attention to the size and shape of the nipples.
    b. Observe underneath the breasts for fungal infection.
    c. Ask if the patient has considered reduction mammoplasty.
    d. Assess for pain in the joints or bones.

49. What is important information regarding breast cancer surveillance for a patient who had breast augmentation surgery?
    a. Prosthesis interferes with lump detection by breast self-examination.
    b. Mammograms are not useful because implant material is artificial.
    c. Implant displacement views allow more complete examination.
    d. Breast augmentation increases the risk for breast cancer.

50. For women with genetic risk factors for breast cancer, which intervention would address one of the modifiable risk factors?
    a. Discuss strategies to avoid weight gain and obesity.
    b. Encourage frequent genetic testing for tumors.
    c. Have testing for BRCA1 and BRCA2 gene mutations.
    d. Consider hormone replacement therapy.

51. The nurse hears in shift report that a 32-year-old patient had a prophylactic oophorectomy. What subjective symptom(s) does the nurse anticipate that the patient would report?
    a. Swelling of upper arms
    b. Tenderness of breasts
    c. Menopausal symptoms
    d. Nausea related to medications

52. Which diagnostic test is considered the **most** definitive for diagnosing breast cancer?
    a. Magnetic resonance imaging
    b. Mammography
    c. Breast tomosynthesis
    d. Breast biopsy

53. The nurse is talking to a woman who was diagnosed with breast cancer at the age of 30. The woman has a 6-year-old daughter. What advice does the nurse give about breast cancer screenings for the daughter?
    a. Your pediatrician should begin annual screenings even at age 6.
    b. When your daughter starts menstruating, screenings should start.
    c. Screenings should begin when she turns 29 or 30 years old.
    d. Screenings should begin when she turns 20 years old.

54. What is the major advantage of neoadjuvant therapy?
    a. It is the newest chemotherapy for several different types of breast cancer.
    b. It has fewer and milder side effects than conventional chemotherapy.
    c. Shrinkage of tumor allows lumpectomy rather than mastectomy.
    d. Tumor frequently resolves spontaneously without surgical intervention.

55. The nurse must assign unlicensed assistive personnel (UAP) to assist a patient who is undergoing brachytherapy for breast cancer treatment. What is the **most** important question that the nurse will ask the UAP prior to making the assignment?
    a. "Do you know how to dispose of radioactive body fluids?"
    b. "Is there any chance that you could be pregnant?"
    c. "Have you ever cared for a patient during brachytherapy?"
    d. "Have you ever had any radiation exposure?"

56. The nurse is designing a teaching plan for a patient who had surgery for breast cancer. What information does the nurse include in the plan? **Select all that apply.**
    a. Do not use lotions or ointments on the area.
    b. Delay using deodorant under the affected arm until healing is complete.
    c. Swelling and redness of the scar itself are considered normal and permanent.
    d. Report any increased heat and tenderness of the area to the surgeon.
    e. Wear loose pajamas at home for 6-8 weeks.
    f. Begin active range-of-motion exercises 1 week after surgery.

57. A patient had a mastectomy several years ago and calls the nurse to report sensations of heaviness, aching, fatigue, numbness, tingling, and swelling in the affected arm and upper chest. Which intervention would the nurse use?
    a. Arrange an immediate appointment with a lymphedema specialist.
    b. Tell patient to elevate the arm during sleep until symptoms resolve.
    c. Advise use of a supportive sling for at least 10-12 hours a day.
    d. Advise restarting postoperative exercises that were taught at the hospital.

71

CHAPTER

Care of Patients with Gynecologic Problems

1. Which laboratory result indicates that the **primary** goal of treatment of the patient's uterine fibroids has been successful?
   a. Vaginal smears show no bacterial growth.
   b. Red blood cell count is within normal limits.
   c. Human chorionic gonadotropin is negative.
   d. White blood cell count is within normal limits.

2. A 20-year-old woman is being evaluated for possible toxic shock syndrome. What question would the nurse ask?
   a. "How many pads do you use on heavy flow days?"
   b. "Have you ever used intravaginal estrogen therapy?"
   c. "Do you have a history of multiple sexual partners?"
   d. "Do you use internal contraceptives?"

3. The nurse is interviewing a young woman who is considering the option of uterine artery embolization for the treatment of uterine fibroids. Which question would the nurse ask to assist the patient in making a decision?
   a. "How has the uterine fibroid condition been affecting your lifestyle?"
   b. "Do you have a family history of breast or uterine cancer?"
   c. "What did the health care provider tell you about the procedure?
   d. "Would you like a brochure about planning future pregnancies?"

4. Which therapies would the nurse expect to use for a patient who is being treated for a rectocele?
   a. High-fiber diet, stool softeners, and laxatives
   b. Intravaginal estrogen and a pessary
   c. Oral contraceptives and antibiotics
   d. Doxorubicin and cisplatin

5. What self-management strategy would the nurse recommend to a patient to prevent vulvovaginitis?
   a. Wear lightweight nylon underwear.
   b. Cleanse inner labial mucosa with antiseptic soap.
   c. Apply antiseptic cream daily to perineal area.
   d. Wear breathable fabrics, such as cotton.

6. Which patient has the **greatest need** for evaluation of possible endometrial cancer?
   a. 63-year-old woman who is having painless vaginal bleeding
   b. 33-year-old woman who reports a past history of multiple sex partners.
   c. 23-year-old woman who has not had a menstrual period for 3 months
   d. 52-year-old woman who is having irregular menses for 3 months

7. The nurse is teaching self-care management to a 39-year-old woman who had an abdominal hysterectomy. Which point would be emphasized to avoid complications of this surgery?
   a. Bathe and douche daily to prevent infection.
   b. Take temperature twice a day for 3 days after surgery.
   c. Resume typical exercise routines as soon as possible.
   d. Gently massage calves if tenderness or swelling occurs.

8. The nurse is teaching a class about laparoscopic or hysteroscopic myomectomy. Which patient should be invited to attend the teaching session?
   a. 23-year-old woman with uterine fibroids who would like to have children in the future
   b. 65-year-old woman who was diagnosed with uterine cancer but also has a bleeding disorder
   c. 43-year-old African American woman with early diagnosed endometrial cancer
   d. 73-year-old woman with urinary incontinence secondary to a cystocele

9. Which woman is at **greatest risk** for pelvic organ prolapse?
   a. 16-year-old adolescent caring for her first child
   b. 25-year-old who became sexually active at age 15
   c. 34-year-old who has a history of endometriosis
   d. 48-year-old obese mother of four children

10. A young woman had minimally invasive surgery for the removal of uterine fibroids. The nurse emphasizes that this information should be included when giving health history; however for which future scenario is the history **most essential**?
    a. Becomes pregnant and is looking forward to a home delivery with midwife assistance
    b. Potentially needs a hysterosalpingogram for evaluation of fallopian tube patency
    c. Develops recurrent and frequent episodes of vulvovaginitis related to *Candida albicans*
    d. Plans to take oral contraceptives for several years to delay pregnancy

11. Following a uterine embolization using a vascular closure device, what patient care would the nurse provide? **Select all that apply.**
    a. Assist the patient to ambulate 2 hours after the procedure.
    b. Keep the patient on bedrest with the leg immobilized for 4 hours before ambulating.
    c. Encourage the patient to drink a lot of fluids.
    d. Assess for constipation and administer laxatives as needed.
    e. Raise the head of the bed.
    f. Assess pain level and provide analgesics as needed.

12. An obese 59-year-old patient describes excessive menstrual bleeding that occurs approximately every 10 days. Which question should the nurse ask **first**?
    a. "Have you noticed fever or signs of infection?"
    b. "Did you ever use oral contraceptives?"
    c. "When was the last time you had intercourse?"
    d. "How many pads (or tampons) do you use each day?"

13. A 36-year-old patient is diagnosed with dysfunctional uterine bleeding. During the pelvic exam, the health care provider determines that the bleeding is acute. What is the nurse's **priority** action?
    a. Prepare the patient for transfer to the operating room.
    b. Prepare to assist with a dilation and curettage.
    c. Anticipate an order for oral contraceptive therapy.
    d. Obtain an order for injectable medroxyprogesterone acetate.

14. The nurse is caring for a patient who had hysteroscopic surgery. The nurse is vigilant to assess for signs and symptoms of which potential complications? **Select all that apply.**
    a. Postembolectomy syndrome
    b. Fluid overload
    c. Embolism
    d. Perforation of uterus
    e. Hemorrhage
    f. Ureter injury

15. The nurse reads in the patient's chart that the patient is experiencing surgical menopause after having a total hysterectomy and bilateral salpingo-oophorectomy. What expected sign/symptom does the nurse anticipate that the patient will report?
    a. Masculinization
    b. Vaginal changes
    c. Rejection by partner
    d. Weight gain

16. The nurse is caring for a patient who is one day post-op for a total abdominal hysterectomy. Which assessment finding is cause for **greatest concern**?
    a. Urinary catheter is in place with a moderate amount of dark amber urine.
    b. Patient reports saturating one pad in an hour with dark red blood.
    c. Patient reports difficulty with bowels and asks for a stool softener.
    d. Incision is intact but appears more inflamed than previously.

17. Which patient is **most likely** to be accepting of surgery and demonstrate better coping behaviors?
    a. 62-year-old woman with an active social and work life has an abdominal hysterectomy for advanced ovarian cancer.
    b. 23-year-old woman with BRCA1 and BRCA2 genes elects to have a prophylactic bilateral salpingo-oophorectomy.
    c. 58-year-old woman with one supportive adult child has ovarian cancer which was treated with cytoreduction.
    d. 44-year-old woman with two children and supportive partner had an abdominal hysterectomy for uterine fibroids.

18. A patient has undergone a total hysterectomy with vaginal repair. Which over-the-counter product will the nurse recommend to decrease sexual discomfort related to intercourse?
    a. Hydrocortisone cream
    b. Water-based lubricants
    c. Petroleum jelly
    d. Vitamin A and D ointment

19. The nurse is caring for a patient who had hysteroscopic surgery. The patient reports severe lower abdominal pain, appears pale, and has trouble focusing on the nurse's questions about the pain. Vital signs show T 98.6°F, P 120/min, R 24/min, BP 103/60. Which complication does the nurse suspect?
    a. Hemorrhage
    b. Embolism
    c. Fluid overload
    d. Incomplete suppression of menstruation

20. The patient reports itching, change in vaginal discharge, and an odor. The nurse suspects that the patient has vulvovaginitis. Based on knowledge about the common causes of vulvovaginitis, which questions would the nurse ask? **Select all that apply.**
    a. "Have you recently been taking antibiotics?"
    b. "Have you been swimming in a lake or pond?"
    c. "Do you consistently wipe from front to back?"
    d. "Do you use tampons?"
    e. "Do you douche or use vaginal sprays?"
    f. "Have you had problems with vaginal yeast infections?"

21. The nurse sees that a patient has been advised by the health care provider to apply lindane to the affected area. What is a self-care measure for this patient to ensure that the symptoms **do not return** after using the medication?
    a. Wash the area daily with hydrogen peroxide.
    b. Take a sitz bath for 30 minutes several times a day.
    c. Wash clothes and linens, and disinfect the home environment.
    d. Remove any irritants or allergens (e.g., change detergents).

22. A patient with a fever, myalgia, sore throat, and sunburn-like rash is admitted with the diagnosis of toxic shock syndrome. What additional clinical manifestation should the nurse assess for?
    a. Hypotension
    b. Vaginal bleeding
    c. Bradycardia
    d. Polyuria

23. The nurse is teaching a group of women about prevention of toxic shock syndrome. What preventive measure does the nurse include?
    a. "Use superabsorbent tampons at night."
    b. "Use sanitary napkins on heavy flow days."
    c. "Change your tampon every 3-6 hours."
    d. "Void immediately after intercourse."

24. A patient is admitted with toxic shock syndrome. What organism is frequently associated with this syndrome when it occurs as a menstrual-related infection?
    a. *Escherichia coli*
    b. *Staphylococcus aureus*
    c. *Haemophilus influenzae*
    d. Beta-hemolytic streptococcus

25. A patient reports the sensation of feeling as if "something is falling out" along with painful intercourse, backache, and a feeling of heaviness or pressure in the pelvis. Which question does the nurse ask to assess for a cystocele?
    a. "Are you having urinary frequency or urgency?"
    b. "Do you feel constipated?"
    c. "Have you had problems with hemorrhoids?"
    d. "Have you had any heavy vaginal bleeding?"

26. A patient had an anterior colporrhaphy and is returning to the clinic for the follow-up appointment. Which patient statement indicates that the procedure has achieved the desired therapeutic outcome?
    a. "The abdominal pain is almost gone."
    b. "I have good control over my urination."
    c. "That constipated feeling has resolved."
    d. "My vaginal bleeding has resolved."

27. A patient has had a posterior colporrhaphy. What is included in the nursing care of this patient?
    a. Give pain medication before a bowel movement.
    b. Obtain an order for prn laxatives.
    c. Resume regular activities after discharge.
    d. Promote a high-fiber diet.

28. The nurse is giving discharge teaching to a patient who had a transvaginal repair for pelvic organ prolapse using a surgical mesh. What does the nurse include?
    a. Avoid cigarette smoking for at least 1 month.
    b. Abstain from sexual intercourse for 6 weeks.
    c. Reduce calories to lose 2 pounds a month.
    d. Avoid tub baths to prevent soaking the mesh.

29. A patient is diagnosed with uterine leiomyomas. What does the nurse expect to see in the documentation as the patient's chief presenting symptom?
    a. Foul-smelling vaginal discharge
    b. Heavy vaginal bleeding
    c. Intermittent abdominal pain
    d. Urinary incontinence

30. A patient with uterine leiomyomas reports a feeling of pelvic pressure, constipation, and urinary retention. She says, "I can't button my pants anymore." What does the nurse do to further evaluate the patient's condition?
    a. Check the lower extremities for fluid retention.
    b. Assess the abdomen for distention or enlargement.
    c. Measure the fluid intake and urine output.
    d. Palpate the urinary meatus for inflammation.

31. A patient had a pelvic examination and needs an additional diagnostic test for possible uterine leiomyomas. The nurse prepares the patient for which diagnostic test?
    a. Transvaginal ultrasound
    b. Laparoscopy
    c. Hysteroscopy
    d. Endometrial biopsy

32. What is the **priority** preoperative and postoperative nursing care for a patient with leiomyomas?
    a. Preventing infection
    b. Managing severe pain
    c. Monitoring for bleeding
    d. Assessing for and managing anxiety

33. Which disorder is strongly associated with prolonged exposure to estrogen without the protective effects of progesterone?
    a. Endometriosis
    b. Uterine cancer
    c. Leiomyomas
    d. Endometrial cancer

34. Three years after the patient was diagnosed and treated for endometrial cancer, the patient and family are told that the cancer is recurring. Which intervention is the nurse **most likely** to use?
    a. Arrange for the patient to speak to other patients with recurring cancer.
    b. Assess for readiness to explore palliative care and hospice.
    c. Assist the patient to identify complementary therapies for palliation.
    d. Teach about radical hysterectomy followed by brachytherapy.

35. A patient who had a total abdominal hysterectomy is anxious to resume her activities because she has young children at home. What postprocedure information does the nurse provide to the patient? **Select all that apply.**
    a. Climb stairs to build strength and endurance.
    b. Avoid sitting for prolonged periods.
    c. Do not lift anything heavier than 5-10 lbs.
    d. Walk or jog at least 1-2 miles every day.
    e. When sitting, do not cross the legs.
    f. Resume regular household chores and activities.

36. The nurse is caring for several patients who had total abdominal hysterectomies. All patients are coming to the clinic for their 6-week follow-up appointment. Which patient demeanor is the **strongest** indicator that there is a need for psychological referral?
    a. Quiet and withdrawn but asks appropriate questions
    b. Tense and impatient but answers questions correctly
    c. Disheveled and lackluster and displays a lack of interest in questions
    d. Cheerful and distractible and answers questions with excessive detail

37. The nurse is giving discharge teaching to a woman who had local cervical ablation. What information would be included?
    a. Sexual activity may be resumed usually in 1 week.
    b. Change tampons every 4 hours.
    c. Report heavy vaginal bleeding or foul-smelling drainage.
    d. Avoid lifting heavy objects for several days.

38. The nurse is caring for a patient who had a posterior colporrhaphy. Which task is **most appropriate** to delegate to unlicensed assistive personnel?
    a. Assist the patient with a sitz bath to relieve discomfort
    b. Assist the patient to select menu items that are low residue.
    c. Change the bed linens every 4 hours or more as needed.
    d. Supervise and teach the patient to turn every 2 hours.

39. The patient needs diagnostic testing to determine the presence of endometrial thickening and possible cancer. Which brochure will the nurse prepare for the patient?
    a. "How Transvaginal Ultrasound and Endometrial Biopsy Are Used in Cancer Diagnosis."
    b. "The Role of Abdominal Ultrasound and Magnetic Resonance Imaging in Cancer Diagnosis."
    c. "Advances in the Diagnosis of Cancer Using Computed Tomography and Cystography."
    d. "What the Presence of BRCA1 or BRCA2 Gene Mutations Means in the Diagnosis of Cancer."

40. The surgical procedure for stage I disease of endometrial cancer involves removal of which components? **Select all that apply.**
    a. Uterus
    b. Vagina
    c. Fallopian tubes
    d. Rectum
    e. Ovaries
    f. Peritoneum fluid for cytologic examination

41. The nurse is caring for a patient with a radioactive implant in the uterus. Which instruction will the nurse give to unlicensed assistive personnel?
    a. Patient is on bedrest and excessive movement is restricted.
    b. Assist the patient to ambulate in the hall at least three times per shift.
    c. Assist the patient to get up to the toilet or the commode chair.
    d. Linens and patient gown should be frequently changed for drainage.

42. A patient is receiving external radiation therapy for treatment of endometrial cancer. What task does the nurse delegate to unlicensed assistive personnel?
    a. Gently wash the markings outlining the treatment site.
    b. Monitor for signs of skin breakdown, especially in the perineal area.
    c. Assist the patient to ambulate if she feels fatigue or tiredness.
    d. Clean the urinary catheter and meatus with mild soap and water.

43. A patient receiving chemotherapy treatments reports fatigue, loss of energy, and experiencing an "emotional crisis every day and my hair is falling out." What does the nurse do **first** to help the patient adapt to body changes?
    a. Suggest participation in self-management.
    b. Encourage the patient to ventilate feelings.
    c. Help the patient to select a wig or scarf.
    d. Encourage the patient to talk to her family.

44. The nurse encourages a teenage patient to receive the human papillomavirus (HPV) vaccine because it protects against which type of cancer?
    a. Endometrial cancer
    b. Cervical cancer
    c. Ovarian cancer
    d. Uterine cancer

45. What information would the nurse give to a sexually active 35-year-old woman about conventional Papanicolaou (Pap) smear and human papillomavirus (HPV) testing?
    a. Every 5 years is sufficient.
    b. Annual screening is recommended.
    c. Testing can stop after three normal Pap smears.
    d. If there are no risk factors, testing is not necessary.

46. Which classic symptom is indicative of invasive gynecologic cancer?
    a. Swelling of the lymph nodes in groin area
    b. Dark and foul-smelling vaginal discharge
    c. Painless vaginal bleeding unrelated to menses
    d. Flank pain with dysuria and dark urine

47. The nurse is taking a history on a patient with probable gynecologic cancer. Which clinical manifestation is a sign of metastasis?
    a. Watery vaginal discharge
    b. Constipation
    c. Dyspareunia
    d. Dysuria

48. A patient had loop electrosurgical excision procedure for treatment and diagnosis of cervical cancer. In the discharge instructions, what does the nurse tell the patient to expect after the procedure?
    a. Spotting
    b. Menses-like vaginal bleeding
    c. Cramps lasting 24 hours
    d. Watery discharge

49. The nurse is teaching a patient who is being discharged after having a total abdominal hysterectomy. Which conditions does the nurse tell the patient to immediately report to the surgeon? **Select all that apply.**
    a. Vaginal drainage that becomes thicker or foul-smelling
    b. Hot flashes and night sweats
    c. Temperature over 100°F (38°C)
    d. Burning during urination
    e. Feeling more tired and sleeping longer
    f. Pain, tenderness, redness, or swelling in calves

50. A patient had a total abdominal hysterectomy. Which patient behavior is the **best** indicator that she is coping and adapting successfully?
    a. Refuses to look at the wound but encourages the nursing students to look.
    b. Sits quietly and passively while the nurse performs wound care.
    c. Asks questions about the wound care but seems reluctant to do self-care.
    d. Frequently stares at the wound site but refuses to touch the area.

51. The home health nurse is reviewing the patient's medication list and sees that the patient was given doxorubicin at the hospital. What gynecologic diagnosis would the nurse expect to see as part of the patient's history?
    a. Endometrial cancer
    b. Cervical polyps
    c. Endometriosis
    d. Dysfunctional uterine bleeding

52. The nurse is preparing patient teaching for several young women who will undergo surgical procedures for gynecologic problems. Which surgical procedure is **most likely** to induce menopausal symptoms?
    a. Bilateral salpingo-oophorectomy
    b. Radioablation
    c. Uterine artery embolization
    d. Hysteroscopic myomectomy

53. The nurse is giving instructions to a patient who is undergoing brachytherapy for cervical cancer. What information does the nurse include?
    a. "Limit interactions with others between treatments for their protection."
    b. "We will give you pain medication prior to every treatment."
    c. "Report any blood in the urine or severe diarrhea immediately."
    d. "Expect heavy vaginal bleeding during this time."

54. What is the **primary** factor for the low survival rates for patients who are diagnosed with ovarian cancer?
    a. Ovarian cancer develops in patients with underlying immunosuppression and poor health.
    b. Ovarian cancer does not respond well to conventional radiation and chemotherapy treatments.
    c. Symptoms are mild and vague; therefore, the cancer is often not detected until its late stage.
    d. There are no specific diagnostic tests that can confirm or rule out ovarian cancer.

55. Young women who have intercourse as teenagers and/or have multiple sex partners are at high risk for which disease/disorder?
    a. Endometriosis
    b. Cervical cancer
    c. Amenorrhea
    d. Ovarian cancer

56. In recalling dietary intake for a recent 24-hour period, a female patient describes eating eggs, whole milk, and bacon for breakfast; fried chicken and French fries for lunch; three-cheese pizza and ice cream for dinner. This type of diet places her at increased risk for which disorder?
    a. Dysfunctional uterine bleeding
    b. Dyspareunia
    c. Early menopause
    d. Cancer of the ovaries

72
CHAPTER

Care of Patients with Male Reproductive Problems

1. A patient tells the nurse that he was diagnosed with benign prostatic hyperplasia. Based on this diagnosis, which symptom is the patient **most likely** to report?
   a. Pain in the scrotum
   b. Trouble passing urine
   c. Erectile dysfunction
   d. Constipation

2. The nurse teaches a patient with benign prostatic hyperplasia to follow which instructions? **Select all that apply.**
   a. Take diuretics to increase output
   b. Avoid sexual intercourse.
   c. Avoid antihistamines.
   d. Avoid caffeine.
   e. Avoid drinking large amounts of fluid in a short time.
   f. Void when the urge occurs.

3. The nurse is talking with an older patient who has benign prostatic hyperplasia. Which report by the patient requires emergent care?
   a. "I leak and dribble urine."
   b. "I have to get up at night to pee."
   c. "I can't pass my urine today."
   d. "I am passing dark yellow urine."

4. The nurse is preparing to assess an obese patient who reports subjective symptoms and urinary patterns associated with benign prostatic hyperplasia. Which technique does the nurse use to perform the physical assessment?
   a. Instruct the patient to undress from the waist down, then inspect and palpate the bladder.
   b. Have the patient drink several large glasses of water and percuss the bladder.
   c. Apply gentle pressure to the bladder to elicit urgency, then instruct the patient to void.
   d. Instruct the patient to void and then use the bedside ultrasound bladder scanner.

5. The nurse is interviewing a patient to determine the presence of lower urinary tract symptoms associated with benign prostatic hyperplasia. Which questions would the nurse ask? **Select all that apply.**
   a. "Do you have difficulty starting and continuing urination?"
   b. "Have you ever had a testicular infection?"
   c. "Do you have reduced force and size of the urinary stream?"
   d. "Have you noticed dribbling or leaking after urinating?"
   e. "How many times do you have to get up during the night to urinate?"
   f. "Have you noticed blood at the start or at the end of urinating?"

6. The advanced-practice nurse is preparing to examine a patient's prostate gland. Before the exam, what does the nurse tell the patient?
   a. He may feel the urge to defecate or faint as the prostate is palpated.
   b. He should lie supine with knees bent in a fully flexed position.
   c. The examination is very painful, but it only lasts a few seconds.
   d. The gland will be massaged to obtain a fluid sample for possible prostatitis.

7. The nurse is reviewing the laboratory results from a patient being evaluated for lower urinary tract symptoms. What does an elevated prostate-specific antigen (PSA) level and serum acid phosphatase level in this patient indicate?
   a. Infection
   b. Prostate cancer
   c. Benign prostatic hyperplasia
   d. Infertility

8. The nurse sees that the patient is taking tamsulosin. Which question would the nurse ask to determine if the medication is achieving the desired therapeutic effect?
   a. "Are you still having trouble passing urine?"
   b. "Does your urine have a strong odor or appear cloudy?"
   c. "Are you having any problems with achieving an erection?"
   d. "Have you had a green or yellow discharge from your penis?"

9. The nurse is using the International Prostate Symptom Score to assess a patient. Which data does the nurse intend to obtain through the use of this assessment tool?
   a. Patient's attitudes and beliefs about prostate surgery
   b. Pattern of growth of prostate and correlation with symptoms
   c. Data in aggregate that can be used for prostate research
   d. Effect of urinary symptoms on the quality of life

10. A patient has an enlarged prostate. Which procedure does the nurse anticipate that the health care provider will order to test for bladder outlet obstruction?
    a. Urodynamic pressure-flow study
    b. Bladder scan
    c. Transrectal ultrasound
    d. Computer tomography scan

11. The nurse is designing a teaching plan for a patient with an enlarged prostate with obstructive symptoms. What action could the patient perform that might help to relieve the obstruction?
    a. Increase frequency of sexual intercourse.
    b. Void before going to bed and upon waking.
    c. Urinate forcefully after drinking fluids.
    d. Spread fluid intake throughout the day.

12. Which conditions meet the criteria for a having a surgical intervention for benign prostatic hyperplasia? **Select all that apply.**
    a. Acute urinary retention
    b. Hydronephrosis
    c. Acute urinary tract infection that does not respond to first-line antibiotics
    d. Recurrent kidney stones
    e. Hematuria
    f. Chronic urinary tract infections secondary to residual urine in the bladder

13. An older adult patient had a transurethral resection of the prostate at 8:00 AM. At 3:00 PM, the nurse assesses the patient. Which finding does the nurse report to the health care provider?
    a. Patient reports a continuous urge to void.
    b. Patient keeps attempting to void around catheter.
    c. Patient wants to get out of bed
    d. Patient keeps moving and ketchup-like urine output is noted.

14. An older patient is scheduled for an annual physical including a prostate-specific antigen (PSA) and a digital rectal examination (DRE). How are these two tests scheduled for the patient?
    a. PSA is drawn before the DRE is performed.
    b. DRE is done several weeks before the PSA.
    c. PSA is reviewed first because DRE may be unnecessary.
    d. Both tests can be done at the convenience of the patient.

15. A patient had a transurethral resection of the prostate and has a three-way urinary catheter taped to the left thigh. What does the nurse instruct about the position of the left leg?
    a. Maintain slight abduction.
    b. Maintain slight flexion of the hip.
    c. Keep the leg elevated.
    d. Keep the leg straight.

16. The nurse notes bright-red blood with numerous clots in the urinary drainage bag for a patient who had a transurethral resection of the prostate. Besides notifying the surgeon, what is the nurse's **best** action?
    a. Irrigate the catheter with normal saline per protocol.
    b. Remove the urinary catheter and save the tip to culture.
    c. Start an IV infusion and draw blood for type and cross.
    d. Empty the drainage bag and record the appearance of output.

17. The nurse is giving discharge instructions to a patient who had a transurethral resection of the prostate. What does the nurse include in the instructions?
    a. Reassurance that loss of control of urination or dribbling of urine is temporary
    b. Instructions about how to apply a condom catheter and monitor for skin breakdown
    c. Advice about how to control bleeding and passage of blood clots
    d. Information about the side effects related to aminocaproic acid

18. The nurse is giving instructions to unlicensed assistive personnel (UAP) about hygienic care for an older adult patient who is uncircumcised. What does the nurse instruct the UAP to do?
    a. Defer cleaning the penis because of patient embarrassment.
    b. Replace the foreskin over the penis after bathing.
    c. Observe the penis and the foreskin for redness or odor.
    d. Avoid touching the foreskin because of hypersensitivity.

19. An older patient reports that he has an enlarged prostate with chronic urinary retention but declines to seek treatment because "it's been that way for a long time." The nurse would encourage a follow-up appointment to prevent which complication of this chronic condition?
    a. Prostate cancer
    b. Erectile dysfunction
    c. Hydronephrosis
    d. Testicular cancer

20. The patient had several diagnostic tests to evaluate lower urinary tract symptoms. Which finding suggests that the patient may have kidney disease?
    a. Elevated white blood cell count
    b. Elevated serum creatinine
    c. Elevated red blood cell count
    d. Elevated prostate-specific antigen

21. The nurse is caring for a patient who is taking finasteride, a 5-alpha reductase inhibitor. What question would the nurse ask to determine if the medication is having the desired therapeutic effect?
    a. "Have you had any discharge from your penis?"
    b. "Has your libido returned to the way it was before?'
    c. "Are you having any problems with urination?"
    d. "Have you gotten any relief from the testicular pain?"

22. The nurse notes that the patient has just started taking an alpha-blocker medication to treat benign prostatic hyperplasia. What instruction, related to the medication side effects, will the nurse give to unlicensed assistive personnel who will assist the patient with activities of daily living?
    a. Frequently offer the patient the urinal.
    b. Have him sit up slowly and pause before standing.
    c. Remind the patient to drink plenty of extra fluids.
    d. Frequently check the linens for soiling and moisture.

23. The nurse reads in the patient's chart that the patient had a transurethral needle ablation. Which question would the nurse ask the patient to determine if the procedure achieved the intended therapeutic goal?
    a. "Did the pain resolve completely after the procedure?"
    b. "Are you able to achieve and sustain an erection?"
    c. "Have your problems with urination been resolved?"
    d. "Have you had a follow-up prostate-specific antigen level?"

24. A patient is undergoing large-volume bladder irrigation. During and after the procedure, the nurse observes the patient for confusion, muscle weakness, and increased gastrointestinal motility related to which potentially adverse effect of large-volume irrigation?
    a. Hyponatremia
    b. Hypovolemia
    c. Hypokalemia
    d. Hypotension

25. The patient has an indwelling catheter in place following a transurethral resection of the prostate. What instructions will the nurse give to unlicensed assistive personnel regarding the catheter?
    a. Secure the catheter so there is no tension.
    b. Irrigate the catheter to prevent clotting.
    c. Maintain traction on the catheter.
    d. Defer catheter care until the patient is discharged.

26. A patient needs surgical intervention for an enlarged prostate but also needs to maintain his anticoagulant therapy. Which brochure would be the **most** appropriate to prepare for the patient?
    a. "Talking to Your Doctor About Holmium Laser Enucleation of the Prostate"
    b. "Transurethral Resection of the Prostate: The Traditional Treatment."
    c. "Is Laparoscopic Radical Prostatectomy with Robotic Assistance Right for You?"
    d. "Common Questions About the Open Surgical Technique for Radical Prostatectomy."

27. The patient has a continuous bladder irrigation via a three-way urinary catheter. At 7:00 AM, the urine drainage bag was emptied and 1000 mL of irrigation fluid was hung. At 11:00 AM, 350 mL of irrigation fluid had been administered through the catheter. The urinary drainage bag now contains 600 mL. How many mL of urine has the patient produced in the past 4 hours?
    _____ mL

28. The nurse is caring for an older patient who had an indwelling urinary catheter inserted after a transurethral resection of the prostate. The patient is intermittently confused, and picks at the IV tubing and the catheter. What should the nurse try **first**?
    a. Obtain an order to restrain the patient's hands and forearms.
    b. Sedate the patient until the IV tube and catheter can be removed.
    c. Inform the family that a family member will have to sit by the patient.
    d. Give the patient a familiar object to hold, such as a family picture.

29. The patient had a transurethral resection of the prostate (TURP) several days ago, and the urinary catheter was removed 6 hours ago. Which sign/symptom must be resolved **before** the patient is discharged?
    a. Patient has not voided since the catheter was removed.
    b. Patient reports a burning sensation with urination.
    c. Patient reports dribbling and leakage since catheter was removed.
    d. Patient reports anxiety related to sexual function because of TURP.

30. Which man has the **highest** risk for prostate cancer?
    a. A 65-year-old Caucasian American man who has two cousins with prostate cancer
    b. A 45-year-old Asian American man with a history of benign prostatic hyperplasia
    c. A 55-year-old Hispanic American man who has poor dietary practices
    d. A 75-year-old African American man whose brother had prostate cancer

31. The nurse is reviewing prostate-specific antigen (PSA) results for a patient who had a prostatectomy for prostate cancer several months ago. The PSA level is 40 ng/mL. How does the nurse interpret this data?
    a. At this stage, PSA level of 40 ng/mL is expected.
    b. The cancer was completely removed.
    c. The cancer is most likely recurring.
    d. Prostate irritation and infection are present.

32. What are common serum tumor markers that confirm a diagnosis of testicular cancer? **Select all that apply.**
    a. Lactate dehydrogenase
    b. Early prostate cancer antigen
    c. Glutathione S-transferase
    d. Alpha-fetoprotein
    e. Beta human chorionic gonadotropin
    f. BRCA1 or BRCA2 mutations

33. The nurse is reviewing the laboratory results for a patient with prostate cancer. Which laboratory result suggests metastasis to the bone?
    a. Decreased alpha fetoprotein
    b. Increased blood urea nitrogen
    c. Elevated serum alkaline phosphatase
    d. Decreased serum creatinine

34. A patient had a transrectal ultrasound with biopsy earlier in the day. What urine characteristics does the nurse expect to see?
    a. Light pink urine
    b. Bright red urine
    c. Dark urine with small clots
    d. Very pale yellow urine

35. What is the major advantage of tadalafil compared to other medications or treatments for erectile dysfunction?
    a. User is able to control erections.
    b. Erection occurs more naturally.
    c. There is no need to abstain from alcohol.
    d. Sexual stimulation is not required.

36. During the first 24 hours after prostatectomy, what is the **priority** concern?
    a. Hemorrhage
    b. Infection
    c. Hydronephrosis
    d. Confusion

37. The nurse is talking to a 35-year-old African American man about prostate-specific antigen (PSA) testing. The patient tells the nurse that his father was diagnosed with prostate cancer in his 50s. What should the nurse tell the patient?
    a. "Although authorities do not always agree, PSA testing usually starts at age 50."
    b. "Your genetic and racial risk factors suggest testing should begin at age 45."
    c. "Because of your African American heritage, you should start testing now."
    d. "PSA testing can be started at any time for all males at any age."

38. The nurse is teaching a patient at risk for prostate cancer about food sources of omega-3 fatty acids. Which food does the nurse suggest?
    a. Red meat
    b. Fish
    c. Watermelon
    d. Oatmeal

39. Which sign/symptom is associated with **advanced** prostate cancer?
    a. Difficulty starting urination
    b. Swollen lymph nodes
    c. Frequent bladder infections
    d. Erectile dysfunction

40. What are common sites of metastasis for prostate cancer? **Select all that apply.**
    a. Pancreas
    b. Bones of the pelvis
    c. Liver
    d. Lumbar spine
    e. Lungs
    f. Kidneys

41. A patient had a transrectal ultrasound with biopsy. After this procedure, what does the nurse instruct the patient to do?
    a. Report fever, chills, bloody urine, and any difficulty voiding.
    b. Limit fluid intake for several hours after the procedure.
    c. Expect decreased urine output for 24 hours after the procedure.
    d. Expect some mild perineal and abdominal pain.

42. An older patient's wife is very upset because "my husband was just told that he had prostate cancer. He feels fine now, but the doctor told him to watch and wait. Why are we just watching? What are we supposed to do?" What is the nurse's **best** response?
    a. "Prostate cancer is slow growing. Your husband needs regular prostate specific antigen testing; I'll give you a list of symptoms to watch for."
    b. "This is very upsetting news. Let's sit down and talk about how you feel and then I will have the doctor talk to you again."
    c. "It's okay, don't be upset. This is a very common way to handle prostate cancer for men who are your husband's age."
    d. "I can get you some information about prostate cancer. This will help you understand why the doctor said this to your husband."

43. The nurse is caring for a patient who had an open radical prostatectomy. During the assessment, the nurse notes that the penis and scrotum are swollen. What does the nurse do **next**?
    a. Notify the health care provider and monitor for an inability to void or increasing pain.
    b. Elevate the scrotum and penis; apply ice intermittently to the area for 24-48 hours.
    c. Assist the patient to increase mobility, especially early ambulation.
    d. Observe the urethral meatus for redness and discharge and monitor urine output.

44. The nurse is teaching a patient who had an open radical prostatectomy about how to manage the common potential long-term complications. What does the nurse teach the patient?
    a. How to perform testicular self-examination
    b. How to manage a permanent suprapubic catheter
    c. How to perform Kegel perineal exercises
    d. How to use dietary modifications to acidify the urine

45. A patient has undergone external beam radiation therapy (EBRT) for palliative treatment of prostate cancer. What suggestions does the nurse make to help the patient manage acute radiation cystitis secondary to EBRT?
    a. Limit intake of water and other fluids.
    b. Avoid consumption of caffeinated drinks.
    c. Increase consumption of dairy products.
    d. Wash genitals with mild soap and water.

46. A patient is receiving internal radiation therapy (brachytherapy) and has had a low-dose radiation seed implanted directly into the prostate gland. What nursing implication is related to this therapy?
    a. Ensure that any staff member or visitor who is pregnant is not exposed to the patient.
    b. Organize the nursing care so that exposure to the patient is limited to a few minutes.
    c. Instruct all staff that all urine specimens should be immediately discarded.
    d. Teach the patient that fatigue is common but should pass after several months.

47. A patient is prescribed leuprolide, a luteinizing hormone–releasing hormone agonist, for treatment of a prostate tumor. What possible side effect of this medication does the nurse advise the patient about?
    a. Nipple discharge
    b. Scrotal enlargement
    c. Fragility of the skin
    d. Erectile dysfunction

48. A patient reports having uncomfortable and unsettling episodes of "hot flashes" after receiving hormonal therapy for a prostate tumor. To alleviate this symptom, the nurse would obtain an order for which medication?
    a. Bisphosphonate drug such as pamidronate
    b. Antiandrogen drug such as bicalutamide
    c. Hormonal inhibitor drug such as megestrol acetate
    d. Antimuscarinic agents such as tolterodine

49. The nurse is teaching a patient about self-care following an open radical prostatectomy. What does the nurse include in the health teaching? **Select all that apply.**
    a. Teach how to care for the indwelling catheter and manifestations of infection.
    b. Instruct to walk short distances.
    c. Instruct to have prostate-specific antigen testing 12 weeks after surgery and then once a year.
    d. Advise to maintain an upright position and not to walk bent or flexed.
    e. Advise to shower rather than soak in a bathtub for the first 2-3 weeks.
    f. Teach to use enemas or laxatives as needed to prevent straining.

50. The health care provider tells the nurse that the patient needs testing for prostatitis. Which specimen needs to be obtained and sent to the laboratory?
    a. Blood sample for serum creatinine
    b. Prostatic fluid for culture and sensitivity
    c. Semen sample to test for sperm count
    d. Blood sample for prostate specific antigen

51. The nurse is talking to a patient who had the relatively new procedure, prostate artery embolization. Which patient report indicates that the intended goal of therapy has been met?
    a. "My problem with ejaculation is much better."
    b. "I used the sperm bank and now I'm less anxious."
    c. "I am not having any more urinary symptoms."
    d. "My doctor said the prostate-specific antigen was good."

52. The patient is prescribed a broad-spectrum antibiotic for prostatitis. Which laboratory result indicates that the medication is having the desired therapeutic effect?
    a. Normalization of white cell count
    b. Decreased blood urea nitrogen level
    c. Increased red blood cell count
    d. Prostate-specific antigen within normal limits

53. The nurse is taking a health history on a patient with organic erectile dysfunction. What are possible causes of this condition? **Select all that apply.**
    a. Medications for hypertension
    b. Obesity
    c. Thyroid disorders
    d. Diabetes mellitus
    e. Diverticulitis
    f. Smoking and alcohol

54. A patient reports having erectile dysfunction and is seeking a prescription for sildenafil. Because of the potential for dangerous drug-drug interactions, the nurse asks the patient specifically if he takes which type of medication?
    a. NSAIDs
    b. Nitrates
    c. Opioids
    d. Antilipemics

55. A patient who has testicular cancer is likely to have which common problem?
    a. Priapism
    b. Erectile dysfunction
    c. Azoospermia
    d. Cryptorchidism

56. The advanced practice nurse is performing a testicular exam on a young Caucasian male patient. The practitioner finds a hard, painless lump. This finding is considered the **most common** manifestation of which disease or disorder?
    a. Testicular cancer
    b. Erectile dysfunction
    c. Prostate cancer
    d. Epididymitis

57. A young patient is diagnosed with testicular cancer. He and his wife have been trying to conceive a child for several months. What information does the nurse give the couple about sperm storage?
    a. Arrangements for sperm storage should be made as soon as possible after diagnosis.
    b. Sperm collection should be completed after radiation therapy or chemotherapy.
    c. Two or three samples should be collected 6 days apart.
    d. Saving sperm helps to alleviate fears related to erectile dysfunction.

58. The nurse is caring for a patient who had minimally invasive surgery for testicular cancer. The nurse is also caring for a patient who had an open radical retroperitoneal lymph node dissection for testicular cancer. The nurse anticipates that the second patient has **greater risk** for which condition?
    a. Paralytic ileus
    b. Urinary incontinence
    c. Lower urinary tract symptoms
    d. Fluid overload

59. The nurse is teaching a patient who had an open retroperitoneal lymph node dissection. What instructions does the nurse give to the patient? **Select all that apply.**
    a. Do not lift anything over 15 lbs.
    b. Limit intake of fluids to 1000 mL per day.
    c. Do not drive a car for several weeks.
    d. Perform monthly testicular self-examination on the remaining testis.
    e. Have follow-up diagnostic testing for at least 3 years after the surgery.
    f. Report fever, drainage, or increasing tenderness or pain around the incision.

60. The nurse is interviewing a patient with erectile dysfunction. Which question would the nurse ask to assist the health care provider in differentiating the etiology as organic versus functional?
    a. "Have you ever had an elevated prostate-specific antigen level?"
    b. "Do you ever have nocturnal emissions or morning erections?"
    c. "Have you tried any medications or therapies for erectile dysfunction?
    d. "Do you have trouble passing urine or starting the stream?"

73 CHAPTER

Care of Transgender Patients

1. Which patient statement **most accurately** describes identifying oneself as transgender?
   a. "I enjoy wearing women's clothes. Women's fashions are pretty and interesting."
   b. "I think men are more powerful and influential, so I would rather be viewed as male."
   c. "Since childhood, I have always felt like I was born into the wrong body."
   d. "I have always been sexually attracted to other males and other men often reciprocate."

2. According to the American Psychiatric Association, which circumstance **best** describes gender identity?
   a. At birth, midwife informs parents that they have a healthy baby girl.
   b. Biologically, the person has obvious male sexual organs.
   c. A person takes on the social roles of mother, wife, and sister.
   d. Family, friends, and others treat the child as a little boy.

3. The nurse reads in the patient's medical record that the patient has gender dysphoria. Which question is the nurse most likely to ask **first**?
   a. "Are you seeking interventions for sex reassignment?"
   b. "How do you prefer to be addressed?"
   c. "Do you think of yourself as female or male?"
   d. "What issues of sexuality would you like to discuss?"

4. A male patient with gender dysphoria confides in the nurse that he notices that his 4-year-old son shows a preference for playing with dolls and other traditional girls' toys. What is the nurse's **best** response?
   a. "Let him choose his own toys and he will be happier."
   b. "It's normal for children to explore different gender behaviors."
   c. "When you see him playing with dolls, how does this make you feel?"
   d. "Did you play with dolls and other girls' toys when you were a child?"

5. The nursing student is writing a report about caring for a 56-year-old patient with diabetes mellitus who identified himself as transgender. Which sentence reflects proper use of terminology?
   a. "Today I learned how to properly care for a transvestite who has diabetes."
   b. "I developed a therapeutic relationship with a 56-year-old tranny with diabetes."
   c. "A 56-year-old transgender had complications related to his diabetes."
   d. "A 56-year-old transgender patient was admitted for complications due to diabetes."

6. Which comment from a family member would be **most strongly** associated with the term "natal sex"?
   a. "My little girl likes to play with her brother's toys and she admires her brother."
   b. "My brother just called me. His wife delivered a healthy baby girl this morning."
   c. "My brother seems a bit effeminate, but I wouldn't call him transgender."
   d. "My sister is unsure if she is sexually attracted to men or to women."

7. The acronym LGBTQ (lesbian, gay, bisexual, transgender, and queer/questioning) is used to describe a group of people of minority sexual and gender identities under one population category. Which of these terms refer specifically to sexual orientation? **Select all that apply.**
   a. Lesbian
   b. Gay
   c. Bisexual
   d. Transgender
   e. Queer
   f. Questioning

8. A patient identifies self as genderqueer. How does the nurse interpret this?
   a. Patient's significant other will be the same gender.
   b. Patient prefers to have male sexual partners.
   c. Patient's gender identity does not conform to male or female.
   d. Patient identifies self as female, but natal sex is identified as male.

9. A transwoman patient of color comes to the clinic for treatment because she was physically assaulted and beaten. Before the nurse begins the interview, the patient becomes angry and defensive and accuses the nurse of discrimination. How does the nurse interpret the patient's behavior?
   a. Recognizes that own verbal and/or nonverbal behavior has offend the patient.
   b. Suspects that the patient is likely to be unstable because of gender dysphoria.
   c. Realizes that the patient is reacting to bias-related violence and emotional distress.
   d. Projects a lack of understanding about the sociology of transgender issues.

10. The nurse is interviewing a transgender patient who reports depression related to continuous verbal harassment, threats, and intimidation. Which patient statement is the **greatest** concern for failure to cope with stressors?
    a. "I smoke three packs of cigarettes every day."
    b. "I have tried to commit suicide several times."
    c. "When I get really down, I drink and use recreational drugs."
    d. "Last night I went to a bar and picked up a stranger for sex."

11. The nurse is assisting a health care provider perform a genital examination on a transgender patient. During the exam, the provider is respectful and professional toward the patient. Later, the nurse hears the provider making jokes within earshot of the patient. What should the nurse do **first**?
    a. Apologize to the patient and reassure that the provider is caring and trustworthy.
    b. Report the provider to the appropriate licensing board for discipline.
    c. Take the provider aside and explain that the patient overheard what was said.
    d. Remind the provider about ethical responsibilities to treat patients with dignity.

12. In caring for transgender patients, under which circumstance would the nurse make a clinical judgment and decide to **forego** extensive questioning about gender identity?
    a. Needs treatment for a sprained ankle sustained during a soccer game.
    b. Has recurrent urinary tract infections despite medication compliance.
    c. Appears to be a male but requests a pelvic examination by a female provider.
    d. Is dressed as a man and wants information about hormones that feminize the body.

13. The nurse sees that John Smith, natal sex male, has an order for insertion of an indwelling urinary catheter for hourly measurements of urine output. However, when the nurse enters the room, the patient appears to be female. What should the nurse do **first**?
    a. Introduce self, verify patient's identity by checking name band, and explain the procedure for catheterization.
    b. Inspect the genitalia and adapt catheter insertion as appropriate while avoiding use of gender-specific language.
    c. Respectfully address the patient as Mr. Smith, and perform catheter insertion for a male patient.
    d. Politely excuse self and obtain advice from the charge nurse about whether to treat the patient as a male or a female.

14. The nurse is working in an inner-city clinic that serves a diverse population. While all patients are apt to ask for directions to restrooms, the staff is continuously debating about how to direct LGBTQ patients to public restrooms. What should the nursing staff do?
    a. Agree to give general directions to both male and female restrooms to everyone.
    b. Ask administration to post more signs so that directions to restrooms are explicit.
    c. Advocate for creation of designated unisex or single-stall restrooms.
    d. Directly ask patients if they would like directions to the male or female restrooms.

15. A new nurse has been conscientious about asking all transgender patients about preferred use of pronouns and names, but inadvertently makes an error while caring for a patient. What should the new nurse do?
    a. Apologize and explain that working with transgender patients is a new experience.
    b. Assume that the patient is used to this type of error and continue care.
    c. Watch the patient's nonverbal behavior to gauge if the error was noticed.
    d. Self-correct and continue with care rather than making a prolonged apology.

16. The nurse is taking a health history and inquiring about any interventions that the patient has had for gender reassignment. Which questions would the nurse include? **Select all that apply.**
    a. "Have you made any changes in gender expression, such as clothes or hairstyle?"
    b. "Have you ever had psychotherapy for body image or to strengthen coping mechanisms?"
    c. "Are you currently taking any hormonal therapy to feminize or masculinize your body?"
    d. "How have your parents and other people responded to changes in your appearance?"
    e. "Have you had or considered having surgery to change sexual characteristics?"
    f. "Have you tried attending a support group that would reaffirm your natal sex role?"

17. For a patient who is taking estrogen therapy, which vital sign is **most important** to assess for the detection of a health risk that can be caused by this therapy?
    a. Temperature
    b. Pulse
    c. Respiration
    d. Blood pressure

18. The nurse is caring for an older transgender adult who transitioned years ago from male-to-female. Which question is the nurse **most likely** to ask?
    a. "Have you had any hot flashes or vaginal dryness?"
    b. "Do you experience urinary retention or dribbling?"
    c. "How old were you when you went through menopause?"
    d. "Did you have any problems after your hysterectomy?"

19. The nurse must insert a urinary catheter in a transgender patient who is in early transition from female-to-male. The patient appears to be a male and identifies self as male. Why would the nurse assess the genitalia prior to opening the sterile catheter kit?
    a. The nurse would expect to see a larger-than-average–sized male penis which may require a larger catheter.
    b. The presence of hormonally enhanced clitoral tissue makes catheterization very difficult and a smaller catheter may be needed.
    c. Genitals may not match physical appearance, so technique and equipment must be modified accordingly.
    d. There is a high risk for necrosis of the neopenis, which should be reported to the provider before catheterization.

20. According to the World Professional Association for Transgender Health, which patient(s) **would not** meet the criteria for hormone therapy? **Select all that apply.**
    a. A 16-year-old who has had gender dysphoria since early childhood.
    b. A 35-year-old lesbian with history of suicide attempts.
    c. A 62-year-old with known gender dysphoria who has symptoms of dementia.
    d. A 30-year-old with gender dysphoria and no physical or mental health problems.
    e. A 22-year-old who has bisexual relationships but calls self queer/questioning.
    f. A 40-year-old who would like to temporarily try out being the opposite gender.

21. A patient is considering estrogen therapy for male-to-female transition. What is an expected physical change that will occur with this therapy?
    a. Weight loss
    b. Thicker, longer hair
    c. Decreased testicular size
    d. Feminization of vocalization

22. A patient is taking estrogen therapy. Which patient report is cause for **greatest** concern?
    a. Breast tenderness
    b. Tenderness and swelling in the calf
    c. Nausea with vomiting
    d. Decreased erectile function

23. The nurse sees that in addition to estrogen therapy, the patient is also taking spironolactone. Which laboratory result will the nurse assess to ensure the patient does not suffer adverse effects due to the medication?
    a. Blood glucose level
    b. White blood cell count
    c. Serum potassium level
    d. Platelet count

24. The female-to-male patient reports that he has been taking testosterone therapy. What is an indication that the medication is having the desired effect?
    a. Patient reports a decreased libido.
    b. Nurse observes increased body hair.
    c. Nurse observes average male penis.
    d. Patient reports breast tenderness.

25. The nurse is doing the preoperative care for an male-to-female patient who will undergo a vaginoplasty. What is included in the care for this patient? **Select all that apply.**
    a. Administer an enema and laxatives as ordered.
    b. Give nothing by mouth for 24 hours prior to surgery.
    c. Monitor and report hemoglobin and hematocrit results.
    d. Administer preoperative antimicrobials to minimize infection.
    e. Monitor and record the drainage from Jackson-Pratt drain.
    f. Instruct to ambulate, because positioning for surgery will be prolonged

26. A male-to-female patient underwent a vaginoplasty with epidural anesthesia. What is an expected assessment finding during the **first several hours** after surgery?
    a. Patient is unable to move legs.
    b. The pedal pulses are diminished.
    c. Feet and ankles are cold to the touch.
    d. Patient has a decreased level of consciousness.

27. Which patient report indicates that the patient is experiencing the **most serious** complication of vaginoplasty?
    a. Reports burning sensation during urination
    b. Reports leakage of stool from the vagina
    c. Reports urinary incontinence when sneezing
    d. Reports tenderness and bruising on labia

28. A female-to-male patient is seeking information about sex reassignment surgery. Which reconstructive surgery is the **most difficult** and the **least likely** to yield patient satisfaction?
    a. Bilateral mastectomy
    b. Hysterectomy and bilateral salpingo-oophorectomy
    c. Pectoral muscle implants
    d. Phalloplasty

29. For a patient with a vaginoplasty what would be included in the self-care measures? **Select all that apply.**
    a. Routine douching and douching after intercourse to prevent infection.
    b. Regular sexual intercourse to keep the vagina dilated.
    c. Inserting the vaginal dilator several times a day for months after surgery.
    d. Using a water-based lubrication when inserting the vaginal stent.
    e. Watching for and immediately reporting feces leaking from vagina.
    f. Applying an ice pack to the perineum twice daily for two months after surgery.

30. The health care provider informs the nurse that a male-to-female patient had a feminization laryngoplasty. The patient is requesting information on additional therapies because the surgery has not fully met her expectations. Which brochure would the nurse prepare for the patient?
    a. "Expected Effects of Testosterone Therapy in Sexual Reassignment"
    b. "How Using Estrogen Helps You to Transition Through Gender Changes"
    c. "Vocal Therapy: Voice and Communication That Reflect Gender Identity"
    d. "Thyroid Chonodroplasty for Feminization of Pitch and Intonation"

Care of Patients with Sexually Transmitted Infections

1. What is the **first** symptom of primary syphilis?
   a. Small, painless, indurated, smooth, weeping lesion
   b. Urinary frequency, burning incontinence, and dribbling
   c. Malaise, low-grade fever, and general muscular aches and pains
   d. Rash that changes from papules to squamous papules to pustules

2. A patient phones the clinic because of a one-time exposure to syphilis that occurred about 6 weeks ago. He reports being asymptomatic and abstinent since the incident. What is the nurse's **best** response?
   a. "The first sign is a chancre which will usually develop by the third week."
   b. "Continue abstinence for up to 90 days and observe the genitalia for painless sores."
   c. "Use a latex or polyurethane condom for genital and anal intercourse."
   d. "The chancre can appear and then disappear, so you should get tested."

3. A patient is admitted for emergency surgery after an accident. In addition, the patient has a pustular rash related to secondary syphilis. What instructions does the nurse give to unlicensed assistive personnel?
   a. Gloves should always be worn when caring for or touching the patient.
   b. The lesions are highly contagious, so the patient should do own hygienic care.
   c. No instructions are given because patient confidentiality is essential.
   d. If the skin is open and draining pus or fluid, use gloves during patient care.

4. A patient is diagnosed with primary syphilis. The nurse prepares to administer and educate the patient about which treatment regimen?
   a. Benzathine penicillin G given intramuscularly as a single 2.4-million-unit dose, and follow-up evaluation at 6, 12, and 24 months
   b. Benzathine penicillin G given intramuscularly for 7 days and follow-up evaluation at 6, 12, and 24 months
   c. Ceftriaxone 125 mg intramuscularly in a single dose plus azithromycin 1 g orally in a single dose, and follow-up evaluation at 6, 12, and 24 months
   d. Metronidazole 500 mg orally twice daily for 14 days and follow-up evaluation at 6, 12, and 24 months

5. A patient with a sexually transmitted disease has no reaction to a penicillin skin test, so the health care provider orders benzathine penicillin G intramuscularly. What does the nurse do **immediately after** the injection?
   a. Ask the patient to give contact information for all sexual partners.
   b. Instruct the patient to go home to rest for 2-4 hours.
   c. Observe the patient for 4 hours to detect any allergic reaction.
   d. Observe the patient for at least 30 minutes to detect any allergic reaction.

6. The health care provider tells the nurse that a patient has Jarisch-Herxheimer reaction. Which interventions does the nurse anticipate?
   a. Oxygen, epinephrine, and antihistamines
   b. Emergency IV fluid resuscitation
   c. Analgesics and antipyretics
   d. Monitoring for symptom resolution

7. A patient is diagnosed with late tertiary syphilis. In addition to benign lesions of the skin and mucous membranes, what other findings does the nurse expect to see documented in the patient's record?
   a. Chronic renal failure
   b. Latent tuberculosis
   c. Cardiovascular syphilis
   d. Contagious chancroid lesions

8. A patient is diagnosed with early latent syphilis. Which assessment will the nurse make related to the medication that is **likely** to be prescribed for the patient?
   a. Assess for allergies to penicillin.
   b. Check results of coagulation studies.
   c. Assess for history of noncompliance.
   d. Ask if the patient takes nitrates.

9. A patient reports a possible exposure to syphilis. Which screening tests are typically done **first**?
   a. Serology testing, such as glycoprotein G antibody-based, to identify either type 1 or 2
   b. Venereal Disease Research Laboratory serum test and the more sensitive rapid plasma reagin
   c. Fluorescent treponemal antibody absorption test or microhemagglutination assay for *Treponema pallidum*
   d. Viral cell culture or polymerase chain reaction assays of the lesions

10. Which sexually transmitted diseases are reportable to the local health authorities in every state? **Select all that apply.**
    a. Chlamydia
    b. Genital herpes
    c. Gonorrhea
    d. Syphilis
    e. Chancroid
    f. Human immunodeficiency virus

11. The nurse sees a laboratory report that indicates that the patient's specimen is positive for *Treponema pallidum*. The nurse will call the health care provider to obtain an order for which medication?
    a. Valacyclovir
    b. Levofloxacin
    c. Azithromycin
    d. Benzathine penicillin G

12. What sexually transmitted organisms are **most** often responsible for pelvic inflammatory disease?
    a. *Chlamydia trachomatis* and *Neisseria gonorrhoeae*
    b. Herpes simplex virus and *Escherichia coli*
    c. *Haemophilus influenzae* and staphylococcus
    d. *Treponema pallidum* and *Gardnerella vaginalis*

13. The nurse is talking to a group of college students about safer sex practices. What recommendations are included as safer sex practices? **Select all that apply.**
    a. Use a latex or polyurethane condom for genital and anal intercourse.
    b. Wash hands immediately after hand contact with vagina or rectum.
    c. Practice abstinence.
    d. Practice serial monogamy.
    e. Decrease the number of sexual partners.
    f. Men should not have sex with men.

14. The nurse is talking to a patient who reports getting genital herpes (GH) several years ago. Based on the nurse's knowledge of viral shedding, what advice would the nurse give the patient?
    a. "If you haven't had any more episodes, the GH is inactive, so you are not contagious."
    b. "GH can recur and not show symptoms; infection is still possible, so always use a condom."
    c. "If you don't have any open sores or notice any drainage, the GH is not contagious."
    d. "The majority of adults have already been exposed to GH; so don't worry about passing it."

15. The nurse is teaching a patient who received treatment for genital herpes. Which patient statement indicates a need for further teaching?
    a. "I can be contagious even when I do not have any lesions."
    b. "If I get pregnant, I need to tell my nurse midwife that I have genital herpes."
    c. "After taking acyclovir, I won't have to worry about exposing my partner."
    d. "I need an annual Pap smear because of my increased risk for cervical cancer."

16. A female patient is prescribed azithromycin 1 g orally in a single dose for the treatment of *Chlamydia trachomatis*. What additional information does the nurse give the patient about treatment issues?
    a. Abstain from sex for 7 days from the start date of treatment.
    b. Even with treatment, there is risk for meningitis and endocarditis.
    c. There is no need for rescreening unless there is new exposure.
    d. Watch for and report headache, malaise, or loss of appetite.

17. Why do women develop complications **more often** than men when being treated for gonorrhea?
    a. Treatment for the disease can leave women infertile.
    b. Men are more likely to have symptoms and will seek curative treatment.
    c. Estrogen leaves the woman more resistant to antibiotic therapy.
    d. The disease is much more difficult to cure in women.

18. The patient tells the nurse that he had unprotected sexual intercourse 1 week ago and just found out that the person might have gonorrhea. The patient reports that he has been watching for symptoms but has not noticed anything, so he is hoping that he is okay. What is the nurse's **best** response?
    a. "Symptoms usually develop in 3-10 days, but you should be tested even if there are no symptoms."
    b. "Abstain from sex for 7 more days, then come in for testing. Meanwhile, watch for symptoms."
    c. "If you are not having any symptoms after 1 week, it is unlikely that you were infected."
    d. "We can give you a prescription for antibiotics, but you must avoid sex for 2-3 months."

19. The nurse is performing a history and physical on the male patient who suspects exposure to a sexually transmitted disease. Which symptom is the **most common** in the male with chlamydia?
    a. Painful intercourse
    b. Urethritis
    c. Dark yellow urine
    d. Thick, green discharge

20. When obtaining a complete obstetric-gynecologic history, the nurse also takes a sexual history from the patient. Which approach is the **most** therapeutic to elicit information from the patient?
    a. Use a checklist to ask "yes" and "no" questions.
    b. Ask the patient to detail her sexual history.
    c. Ask directly about episodes of sexually transmitted disease.
    d. Ask open-ended questions.

21. The nurse is talking to a 25-year-old African American woman whose health history and lifestyle do not suggest an increased risk for sexually transmitted disease (STD); however, which question will the nurse ask that addresses the concept of health care disparities?
    a. "Would you like a brochure about incidence of STDs among African Americans?"
    b. "Do you have a primary care provider who you see on a regular basis?"
    c. "Can you describe safer sex practices that you and your partner(s) use?"
    d. "Do you have a family history for any type of reproductive cancers?"

22. The nurse sees that the patient was prescribed valacyclovir. Which patient statement indicates that the goal of therapy is being met?
    a. "The rash is still present, but I hardly notice it."
    b. "Pain in my joints is much less than before treatment."
    c. "Abdominal pain is no longer interfering with movement."
    d. "The sores are not as painful as they were before."

23. Women with pelvic inflammatory disease are at an **increased** risk for which condition?
    a. Amenorrhea
    b. Appendicitis
    c. Infertility
    d. Cardiac disease

24. What is the **most** common symptom that leads a patient with pelvic inflammatory disease to seek medical health care?
    a. Vaginal itching
    b. Lower abdominal pain
    c. Malaise with fever
    d. Abnormal menstrual flow

25. A patient with pelvic inflammatory disease is on bedrest with bathroom privileges. What position is **best** for the patient while on bedrest?
    a. Prone
    b. Supine
    c. Side-lying
    d. Semi-Fowler's

26. A patient with pelvic inflammatory disease is discharged home on oral antibiotics. What important measure should the nurse include in patient teaching?
    a. "Douche 3 times a week to aid healing."
    b. "Take antacids if the antibiotics upset your stomach."
    c. "Continue taking the antibiotics until the medication is gone."
    d. "Do not have intercourse until after the follow-up appointment."

27. A female patient is diagnosed and treated for sexually transmitted disease. What does the nurse teach the patient about resuming sexual relations?
    a. Douche within 24 hours after vaginal intercourse.
    b. Sexual relations are prohibited for 3 months.
    c. Intercourse should be postponed until the treatment regimen is completed.
    d. Intercourse is permitted unless there is an increase in abdominal pain.

28. What does the nurse tell a patient with pelvic inflammatory disease (PID) about the practice of vaginal douching?
    a. Douching increases the risk for developing PID.
    b. Douche daily to reduce vaginal infections.
    c. Vinegar is a safe and natural alternative.
    d. Disposable equipment is recommended.

29. Which sexually transmitted disease is detectable by urine self-collection?
    a. Chlamydia
    b. Herpes simplex type 2
    c. Syphilis
    d. Gonorrhea

30. A patient with human papillomavirus will commonly develop which disease?
    a. Human immunodeficiency virus
    b. Genital warts
    c. Vulvovaginitis
    d. Chancroid

31. The nurse is preparing an information packet about women's health considerations for sexually transmitted diseases (STDs). What information does the nurse include? **Select all that apply.**
    a. Young women generally have excellent knowledge about the risk of STDs.
    b. Young women frequently believe that they are vulnerable to STDs.
    c. Young women mistakenly believe that contraceptives protect them from STDs.
    d. Mucosal tears in postmenopausal women may also place them at greater risk for STDs.
    e. Women have more asymptomatic infections that may delay diagnosis and treatment.
    f. Young women who alcohol binge are more prone to risky behavior.

32. A young female patient requires hospitalization for a severe case of genital herpes. What information is given to the patient regarding the long-term consequences?
    a. There is an increased risk of central nervous system complications.
    b. There is a risk of neonatal transmission and an increased risk for acquiring HIV infection.
    c. There is an increased risk for scars and adhesions of the fallopian tubes.
    d. There is an increased risk for multiple types of reproductive cancers at a young age.

33. The nurse is counseling a patient who is experiencing recurrent outbreaks of genital herpes. What suggestions for symptomatic treatment does the nurse include?
    a. Oral analgesics, sitz baths, and increased oral fluid intake
    b. Topical anesthetics, nutritional therapy, and warm compresses
    c. Abstinence, frequent bathing, and fluid restriction
    d. Bedrest and application of podofilox 0.5% solution

34. A patient is diagnosed with *Condylomata acuminata*. What are the desired outcomes of management for this patient?
    a. Reduce pain and prevent recurrence.
    b. Prevent long-term complications to the cardiac system.
    c. Remove the warts and treat the symptoms.
    d. Prevent infertility and systemic infection.

35. A patient requires treatment for genital warts. Which treatment can be done by the patient at home if given the proper instructions?
    a. Imiquimod 5% cream
    b. Cryotherapy with liquid nitrogen
    c. Podophyllin resin 10% in a compound of tincture of benzoin
    d. Trichloroacetic acid or bichloracetic acid

36. Which woman has the **greatest** risk for pelvic inflammatory disease?
    a. 24-year-old who smokes and has multiple sexual partners
    b. 62-year-old who uses topical estrogen therapy for dyspareunia
    c. 35-year-old lesbian who recently entered a new relationship
    d. 45-year-old whose husband was treated for sexually transmitted disease

37. A patient had podophyllin treatment for *Condylomata acuminata*. For which sign/symptom does the nurse tell the patient to return for further treatment?
    a. Discomfort at the site
    b. Bleeding from the site
    c. Infection at the site
    d. Sloughing of parts of warts

38. A male patient reports that a female sexual partner just told him that she was treated for gonorrhea. What symptoms does the nurse ask about, because they are the **most likely** to occur in a male with gonorrhea?
    a. Small, painless lump that occurred on the penis but spontaneously disappeared
    b. Numerous small, painless, papillary growths in the genital area
    c. Painful intercourse because of scrotal swelling and epididymitis
    d. Dysuria and a profuse yellowish green or scant clear penile discharge

39. For which patient would a test of cure be recommended **after** treatment is completed?
    a. Patient is treated for gonorrhea with cefixime.
    b. Patient is treated for chlamydia with azithromycin.
    c. Patient is treated for syphilis with benzathine penicillin.
    d. Patient is being treated for gonorrhea with ceftriaxone.

40. A female patient is tested for and diagnosed with gonorrhea. The nurse advocates that the choice of drug therapy include medications that concurrently treat which condition?
    a. Genital herpes
    b. Chlamydia
    c. Syphilis
    d. Genital warts

41. A young woman discovers she has chlamydia after going to her health care provider for a routine Pap smear and pelvic exam. She is reluctant to accept the diagnosis because she is asymptomatic and "does not have any money for unnecessary treatment right now." What is the nurse's **best** response?
    a. Explain that there is a single-dose of medication which has a one-time cost.
    b. Talk to the woman about her financial situation and help her find resources.
    c. Encourage the patient to express her reluctance and disbelief.
    d. Tell her that it is possible to have chlamydia without having any symptoms.

42. A patient with a sexually transmitted disease freely admits to being a commercial sex worker. In talking to this patient, the nurse recognizes that she has not disclosed a true name, address, or partner contact information. What is the **best** treatment strategy to use with this patient?
    a. Reassure her that all health data are confidential and will be handled with discretion.
    b. Spend extra time with the patient to elicit trust so that she will give correct information.
    c. Administer a one-dose course of treatment and dispense a box of condoms.
    d. Give her all medications for a 7-day treatment and convey a nonjudgmental attitude.

43. Which factors increase the risk for pelvic inflammatory disease? **Select all that apply.**
    a. Age younger than 26 years
    b. Multiple sexual partners
    c. Smoking
    d. Caffeine use
    e. History of chlamydia or gonococcal infection
    f. Intrauterine device placed within the previous 3 weeks

44. A young female patient with a history of previous sexually transmitted disease has a hunched-over gait and has difficulty getting on the examination table. On observing this behavior, what does the nurse **first** assess for?
    a. Lower abdominal pain
    b. Lower back pain
    c. Musculoskeletal weakness
    d. Vaginal bleeding

45. The nurse is reviewing laboratory results for a patient with pelvic inflammatory disease. Which lab results does the nurse expect to see? **Select all that apply.**
    a. Elevation in white blood cell count
    b. Elevation in erythrocyte sedimentation rate
    c. Elevation of C-reactive protein
    d. Presence of human chorionic gonadotropin in urine
    e. Cervical infection with *Neisseria gonorrhoeae* or *Chlamydia trachomatis*
    f. Presence of virus in polymerase chain reaction

46. In the emergency department, a patient is diagnosed with pelvic inflammatory disease and there is an order to discharge the patient home with a prescription for antibiotics. What circumstance would cause the nurse to **question** the order for discharge to home?
    a. The patient has history of sexually transmitted disease but did not always seek treatment.
    b. The patient is nauseated but able to tolerate small amounts of oral fluids.
    c. The patient is pregnant but willing to attempt self-care if properly instructed.
    d. The patient is afraid to go home, but the sister and husband are available to help.

47. The nurse is caring for a patient admitted for pelvic inflammatory disease. Which task does the nurse delegate to unlicensed assistive personnel?
    a. Apply a heating pad to the lower abdomen or back.
    b. Place the patient in semi-Fowler's position.
    c. Ask the patient if the pain is a 2-3 on a pain scale of 0-10.
    d. Report to the nurse if the patient is anxious about infertility.

48. A patient reports an itching or tingling sensation felt in the skin 1-2 days followed by a blister on the penis which ruptured spontaneously with painful erosion. These symptoms are consistent with which condition?
    a. Syphilis
    b. Genital warts
    c. Genital herpes
    d. Gonorrhea

49. The nurse is teaching a group of high school students about the use of condoms. What information does the nurse include? **Select all that apply.**
    a. Use spermicide (nonoxynol-9) with condoms.
    b. Do not used female condoms; they are too difficult for inexperienced partners.
    c. Keep condoms (especially latex) in a cool, dry place out of direct sunlight.
    d. Do not use condoms if package is damaged or if they are brittle or discolored.
    e. Put condoms on the penis before foreplay or arousal.
    f. Make sure that lubricants are water-based.

50. Which sexually transmitted disease is associated with an increased risk for cervical cancer?
    a. Syphilis caused by *Treponema pallidum*
    b. Condylomata acuminata caused by HPV type 16
    c. Condylomata lata caused by *Treponema pallidum*
    d. Chlamydia caused by *Chlamydia trachomatis*

51. Which group has the **greatest** risk for contracting primary and secondary syphilis?
    a. Males aged 15-25 years
    b. Postmenopausal women
    c. Women who have sex with women
    d. Men who have sex with men

52. The nurse has just finished teaching an 18-year-old male patient about sexually transmitted diseases and safe sex practices. Which patient statement **most strongly** suggests that the patient will succeed in making a behavior change?
    a. "I don't intend to have sex anymore until I get married."
    b. "You have given me a lot to think about. I know I am taking risks."
    c. "I am going directly to the pharmacy and buy a supply of condoms."
    d. "Wearing gloves during foreplay seems weird, but I guess I could try it."

53. Which patient circumstance is **most appropriate** for expedited partner treatment?
    a. Partner is afraid to come to health care facility.
    b. Partners are clients of a commercial sex worker.
    c. Patient and partner are both HIV positive.
    d. Patient and partner have multiple other partners.

54. The nurse is volunteering at a walk-in clinic where, compliance, continuity of care, and limited resources are issues for patients, but the staff tries to give good service. For which circumstance, would the nurse **question** the provider's decision?
    a. Instructs on how to use podofilox 0.5% cream for self-treatment.
    b. Declines to perform biopsy and prepares to eradicate warts on patient's cervix.
    c. Prescribes a single 2.4 million-unit dose of IM benzathine penicillin G for syphilis.
    d. Declines expedited partner treatment because partner may have pelvic inflammatory disease.

55. A young patient has been diagnosed with gonorrhea. What additional testing should be offered to this patient because of possible concurrent infections? **Select all that apply.**
    a. Syphilis
    b. *Chlamydia*
    c. Hepatitis B
    d. Hepatitis C
    e. HIV infection
    f. *Candida albicans*

56. In performing a genital exam on a teenage patient, the examiner sees multiple large cauliflower-like growths in the perineal area. The patient reports these appeared about 3 months after her first sexual experience. What does the examiner suspect?
    a. *Condylomata acuminata*
    b. Genital herpes
    c. Salpingitis
    d. Gonorrhea

Answer Key

CHAPTER 1

1. b
2. b
3. d
4. a, b, e
5. b
6. d
7. a
8. b
9. a, c, d, e, f
10. c
11. a
12. c
13. a, c, d, e
14. c
15. a

CHAPTER 2

1. a
2. d
3. b
4. b, c, e, f
5. c
6. a, c, d, f
7. b
8. c
9. a
10. a, d, f
11. a
12. a
13. b, d, e
14. c
15. b
16. a, b, c, e, f
17. d
18. b
19. a
20. c
21. d
22. a, c, d, e
23. b
24. b, c, e
25. d
26. a

27. a, c, e, f
28. b
29. a, b, e
30. c
31. b
32. a, d, e
33. c
34. a, b, d, e
35. d
36. c
37. b
38. a
39. b
40. a, b, e, f

CHAPTER 3

1. d
2. a, b, d, e
3. c
4. a
5. d
6. d
7. a, c, d, e
8. a
9. a
10. a
11. b
12. a
13. b
14. c
15. d
16. b
17. a
18. c
19. d
20. b

CHAPTER 4

1. b
2. c
3. c
4. b
5. c
6. c

7. d
8. a
9. a
10. c
11. c
12. a
13. c
14. b
15. a
16. c
17. b
18. d
19. a, e, f
20. b
21. d
22. d
23. b
24. d
25. d
26. d
27. a
28. b
29. c
30. a
31. b
32. 0.4
33. c
34. a
35. c
36. d
37. b
38. c
39. b, c, e, f
40. d
41. c
42. d
43. b
44. a
45. b
46. c
47. d
48. c
49. c
50. b
51. c
52. a

53. c
54. d
55. b
56. c
57. b
58. b
59. b
60. d
61. a

CHAPTER 5

1. b
2. d
3. c
4. b
5. a, c, d
6. a, c, e, f
7. d
8. c
9. a
10. b
11. a, c, f
12. d
13. b, c, d
14. d
15. b
16. c
17. c
18. a
19. b
20. a, c, e
21. a
22. b, e, f
23. c
24. a, c, f

CHAPTER 6

1. b
2. d
3. a
4. a, c, e
5. a, b, d, e
6. d
7. c

8. a, c, d, e, f
9. a, b, d, e, f
10. c
11. b
12. a
13. a
14. d
15. a
16. a, c, d, e
17. a, c, d, e, f
18. a, c, d, f
19. a
20. b
21. c
22. a
23. c
24. a
25. c
26. a, b, c, f
27. a, b, c, e
28. c
29. c
30. b
31. b
32. c
33. a, b, c, f
34. c
35. d
36. a
37. b
38. c
39. a
40. a, c, e, f
41. b
42. a
43. c

CHAPTER 7

1. b
2. c
3. c
4. c
5. c
6. b
7. d
8. b
9. c
10. c
11. a
12. b, d, f
13. d
14. b
15. b
16. a
17. d
18. c
19. b
20. d
21. a

CHAPTER 8

1. b
2. a, b, d, e, f
3. c
4. b
5. d
6. b
7. d
8. b, d, e, f
9. d
10. d
11. b, c, e, f
12. c
13. a, c, e
14. b, c, e, f
15. c
16. b, c, e, f
17. c
18. a
19. c
20. c
21. d
22. b
23. a
24. b
25. a
26. b
27. b
28. a
29. a
30. c
31. b, c
32. c
33. d
34. b
35. b
36. b, a, c, d
37. d
38. c
39. b
40. d
41. c, b, a, d, e
42. c
43. b
44. c
45. c
46. d
47. b
48. b
49. a
50. c
51. c
52. d
53. c
54. a
55. c
56. b
57. a
58. b

59. c
60. b, c, e

CHAPTER 9

1. a
2. c
3. b
4. b
5. b
6. c
7. c
8. d
9. d
10. a
11. a
12. d
13. a, b, e, f
14. c
15. c
16. c
17. a
18. c
19. c
20. c
21. c
22. c
23. a
24. a, c, d, e, f
25. b
26. b
27. d
28. c
29. b
30. c
31. a
32. b, c, d, e, f
33. c
34. b
35. b
36. b, d, e, f
37. c
38. c
39. a, c, d
40. a
41. c
42. b
43. c
44. d
45. c
46. d
47. a, c, d, e, f
48. c
49. c
50. b, c, d
51. b
52. a, b, d, e
53. a
54. a
55. c

56. a, b, d, e, f
57. b
58. b, d, e, f
59. a
60. b
61. d
62. b
63. b
64. a
65. a, b, e
66. d
67. b
68. c
69. d
70. c, d, e
71. b, e, c, a, d
72. b
73. c
74. c
75. a
76. b
77. a, b, d
78. a, b, c, e, f
79. a, b, d, e
80. a, b, d, e

CHAPTER 10

1. d
2. a
3. c
4. b
5. a, c, d, f
6. b
7. d
8. c
9. c
10. a
11. a
12. a, c, d, e
13. c
14. d
15. c
16. a
17. a
18. a
19. d
20. d
21. a
22. a, d, e
23. c
24. a
25. b
26. a
27. b
28. c
29. c
30. d
31. c
32. d

33. c, e
34. d
35. b
36. b
37. c
38. d

CHAPTER 11

1. d
2. a, b, c, e
3. b
4. b
5. d
6. a, d, f
7. b
8. a
9. a, b, c, e, f
10. a
11. c
12. b, c, e, f
13. b
14. d
15. a
16. a
17. c
18. b
19. d
20. c
21. c
22. b
23. a
24. c
25. b
26. b, d, e, f
27. a, d, e, f
28. b, c, e, f
29. c
30. a
31. a, d, e, f
32. b, d, e
33. a, c, d, f
34. d
35. c
36. c, d, e, f
37. a
38. a
39. d
40. a
41. b
42. d, f
43. d
44. b, e, f
45. c
46. a
47. a, b, d
48. a
49. b
50. b
51. b, c, d

52. d
53. b, c, e
54. a
55. d
56. a, c, e, f
57. b
58. b
59. b
60. b
61. d
62. b, c, d, f
63. a, c, d, f
64. b
65. b, c, d
66. a
67. c
68. a, b, d
69. b, d, e
70. c
71. b
72. b
73. b
74. a
75. b, c, e, f
76. c
77. a, c, d, e
78. a, c, d, e
79. a, b, d
80. b
81. a
82. a, b, c, d, f
83. c
84. d
85. b
86. c
87. a
88. a
89. b
90. a, c, d, f
91. d
92. b, e, f
93. a
94. a, c, f
95. b, c, d
96. c
97. a, e
98. d
99. b
100. a
101. c
102. d
103. a
104. c
105. a, c, e
106. b

CHAPTER 12

1. a, c, e, f
2. a, b, d, f

3. d
4. b
5. b
6. a
7. a, c
8. b
9. b, c, d
10. a, b, e
11. a
12. b
13. b
14. a, b, e
15. b
16. c
17. a
18. b
19. b
20. c
21. a
22. c
23. b
24. b, c, f
25. c
26. a
27. a, b, d
28. b
29. a
30. c
31. a, c, f
32. a, b, c, e
33. c
34. b
35. b
36. c
37. d
38. d
39. d
40. b
41. c
42. b
43. c
44. a
45. a, c
46. b, d, f
47. a
48. d
49. c
50. b
51. b
52. b
53. c
54. c
55. c
56. b, c, e

CHAPTER 13

1. a, b, d, e, f
2. a
3. b

4. b, d, e
5. b
6. a, b, c, e, f
7. a, b, c, f
8. c
9. c, d, e, g
10. d
11. a, c, e, f
12. d
13. b
14. a
15. d
16. a
17. d
18. b
19. c
20. b
21. c
22. c
23. a, c, d, f
24. a
25. b
26. b
27. b, c, f
28. c
29. c
30. a
31. a, b, e, f
32. c
33. a
34. c, d, e
35. d
36. d
37. b
38. d
39. b, c, d
40. a
41. a, c, d, f
42. a, b, d, e
43. a, b, d, e
44. c
45. d
46. a, b, c, e, f
47. d
48. a, b, e, f
49. d
50. a
51. a, c, e, f
52. c
53. b
54. d
55. b, c, e, f
56. c
57. b, c, f
58. c
59. a
60. b
61. a, b, c, e
62. d
63. d

64. d
65. a, b, d, f
66. a
67. d
68. a
69. c
70. d
71. b
72. c

CHAPTER 14

1. c
2. b
3. b, d, e
4. a, c, d, f
5. d
6. b
7. a
8. c
9. a
10. b
11. c
12. d
13. b
14. b, c, e, f
15. d
16. b
17. a, b, c, f
18. a, b, d, e
19. a
20. b
21. b, c, e, f
22. a
23. c
24. a, b, d, e, f
25. a
26. a, b, d, e, f
27. a, d, e, f
28. c
29. a
30. a
31. c
32. a, c, d, f

CHAPTER 15

1. a
2. a, c, d
3. b, c
4. a, c, d, e, f
5. a
6. d
7. a, c, d, f
8. b
9. b
10. a, b, c, e, f
11. d
12. b, c, e, f
13. d

14. a, d, e
15. a
16. b, c, d, e
17. a, c, d
18. c
19. c
20. c
21. a, c, d, f
22. b
23. c
24. d
25. c
26. a
27. b
28. d
29. c
30. c

CHAPTER 16

1. d
2. b
3. d
4. a
5. c
6. c, d, e, f
7. c
8. b, c, e, f
9. b
10. a
11. c
12. a, b, e
13. a, b, e
14. b, c, d, e
15. b, d, f
16. a, b, d, e
17. a
18. d
19. b
20. d
21. a
22. d
23. b
24. c
25. a, b, d, e
26. b, c, e
27. b, d
28. a
29. c
30. a, b, d, e
31. a
32. c
33. a, c, d, f
34. a, b, e, f
35. c
36. b, d, e, f
37. a
38. b

CHAPTER 17

1. b
2. a, b, c, e, f
3. c
4. d
5. d
6. d
7. c
8. a, b, d
9. b
10. a, b, d, e, f
11. b
12. c
13. b
14. b
15. b, e, a, f, d, c
16. d
17. c
18. a
19. a
20. a
21. c
22. d
23. a, b, d, e, f
24. b
25. a, b, d
26. d
27. b
28. a
29. d
30. a, b, c, f
31. c
32. c
33. d
34. a
35. b
36. c, d
37. c
38. b
39. a
40. d
41. c
42. a
43. a
44. a
45. a
46. b
47. a
48. a
49. b

CHAPTER 18

1. d
2. a
3. b
4. a
5. c
6. a, c, e, f

7. b
8. a, b, d, e
9. b
10. b
11. c
12. b
13. b
14. c
15. a, b, c, d
16. c
17. a, b, c, f
18. a
19. c
20. d
21. a, b, c, e
22. a
23. b
24. a, b, d, e
25. c
26. a
27. c
28. a, b, c, e
29. d
30. c
31. b
32. c
33. a
34. a
35. c
36. b
37. a, b, d, e
38. c
39. d
40. a
41. b
42. a
43. c
44. c
45. a
46. c
47. c
48. c
49. d
50. d
51. d
52. b
53. c
54. a
55. c
56. d
57. c
58. b
59. b
60. c
61. d
62. c
63. b
64. b
65. c

66. d
67. a
68. c
69. a
70. b
71. b
72. a, c, d, f
73. c

CHAPTER 19

1. d
2. c
3. b
4. c
5. c
6. d
7. b
8. b, c, f
9. a, d, f
10. c
11. b
12. b, c, e
13. c
14. c
15. a
16. a, c, e, f
17. b
18. d
19. a
20. a
21. a
22. b
23. d
24. a, c, d
25. d
26. c, e, a, d, b, f
27. b
28. a
29. d
30. b
31. d
32. d
33. b
34. b
35. d
36. c
37. b
38. c
39. a
40. c
41. a
42. b
43. a, c, d
44. b

CHAPTER 20

1. b
2. d

3. a
4. b, d, f
5. a
6. b
7. c
8. a
9. d
10. a
11. b
12. b
13. a, b, e
14. d
15. a
16. d
17. b
18. a
19. a
20. d
21. a, d, e, f
22. b
23. a
24. d
25. d
26. a, b, d, e
27. c
28. a
29. b
30. b
31. c
32. b, d, e, f
33. c
34. a
35. b
36. d
37. a, b, f
38. d

CHAPTER 21

1. b
2. a
3. c
4. c
5. a
6. c
7. b, d, e, f
8. c
9. d
10. b
11. b
12. b, c, d, f
13. d
14. a
15. b, c, d
16. a
17. b
18. b
19. c
20. a

21. a
22. c
23. a, b, c, e
24. a
25. d
26. c
27. d
28. b
29. a
30. a
31. d
32. b
33. b
34. b
35. a
36. c

CHAPTER 22

1. b
2. b, c, e, f
3. c
4. b
5. a
6. a, b, c, f
7. a
8. c
9. a
10. b
11. b
12. d
13. d
14. a, b, f
15. d
16. a
17. b
18. c
19. a
20. b
21. a, c, d, f
22. c
23. d
24. c
25. a
26. d
27. d
28. b
29. b
30. a
31. b
32. c
33. c
34. b
35. c
36. d
37. c
38. a, c, d
39. a
40. c

41. c
42. b
43. c
44. c
45. a
46. d
47. a
48. a
49. a
50. c
51. c
52. d
53. d
54. a
55. b

CHAPTER 23

1. b
2. b
3. a
4. a
5. c
6. a, b, c, f
7. c, f
8. d
9. c
10. a, c
11. d
12. c
13. b
14. d
15. a, b, d
16. b
17. b
18. c
19. a
20. d
21. a
22. a
23. d
24. b
25. b
26. b
27. b
28. b
29. c
30. a
31. a
32. b
33. a
34. c, d
35. b, c, e, f

CHAPTER 24

1. d
2. b
3. c
4. a

5. c
6. a
7. a
8. b, c, e, f
9. d
10. b
11. a
12. a, b, d, e
13. c
14. d
15. b
16. b
17. a
18. b
19. d
20. d
21. a, b, d, f
22. a, c, f
23. a
24. c
25. a, c, e
26. b
27. c
28. a
29. c
30. a
31. b
32. c
33. a
34. a, b, c, d, f
35. d
36. b
37. c
38. d
39. a
40. c
41. a
42. a
43. c
44. a
45. b
46. d
47. b
48. c
49. c
50. b
51. b
52. c
53. b
54. a
55. b
56. d
57. a
58. d
59. b
60. c
61. a
62. c
63. d

64. b
65. b
66. a
67. b
68. a
69. a
70. b

CHAPTER 25

1. d
2. a
3. b
4. c
5. b, c, d, f
6. b
7. d
8. a
9. b
10. a, c, d, f
11. a
12. d
13. a, b, d, e
14. c
15. b, c, d, e
16. a
17. b, c, e, f
18. b
19. a
20. d
21. b
22. c
23. c
24. b
25. a, b, e, f
26. c
27. a
28. b
29. b
30. c
31. a
32. d
33. c
34. d
35. a, b, d, f
36. a
37. d
38. d
39. a
40. a, b, c, e, f
41. b
42. a, d, e
43. a, b, c, e
44. b
45. b
46. a
47. c
48. d
49. a

50. c
51. c
52. d
53. c
54. b
55. a, c, d, e
56. c
57. b
58. c
59. a
60. c
61. c
62. d
63. b
64. b
65. c
66. a
67. d
68. a
69. b
70. a
71. d
72. b
73. d
74. a
75. c
76. a
77. a
78. b

CHAPTER 26

1. a, c, e
2. a
3. c
4. b, c, d, e
5. d
6. a
7. c
8. d
9. c
10. b
11. b
12. b
13. a, c, d, e
14. b
15. a
16. b
17. c
18. b
19. b, c, d, f
20. a, b, c, f
21. b
22. d
23. c
24. d
25. c
26. d
27. b

28. d
29. b
30. b
31. a, b, c, e
32. c
33. b
34. a
35. c
36. b
37. a
38. c
39. a
40. c
41. c
42. b
43. c
44. b
45. a
46. c
47. b
48. a, c, e
49. c
50. c, d, e, f
51. d
52. a, c, e
53. a
54. b
55. a, b, c, e
56. a
57. b
58. c
59. d
60. a, b, d, e
61. b
62. a, d
63. b
64. a, b, d, f
65. c
66. a
67. a, b, d, f
68. a
69. b, c, d, f
70. a
71. a
72. a
73. a
74. a
75. c
76. c
77. b
78. b
79. b, c, d
80. c
81. c
82. d
83. b, d, f
84. a
85. a
86. d

87. b
88. a, b, e, f
89. c
90. b, c, d

CHAPTER 27

1. b
2. d
3. a
4. a
5. b, c, d
6. b
7. b
8. a
9. c
10. b, d, e, f
11. a, b, d, e, f
12. d
13. b
14. b, c, e, f
15. a
16. b
17. d
18. c
19. b
20. c
21. d
22. b
23. a, b, c, e
24. c
25. a
26. b
27. d
28. c
29. b
30. c
31. b, c, e, f
32. b
33. b
34. c
35. c
36. a
37. a, b, e, f
38. a, b, c, d, f
39. d
40. c
41. a
42. c
43. c
44. a
45. a, e
46. b
47. c
48. a, b, e, f
49. a
50. d
51. b
52. c

53. a
54. a
55. c
56. b, d, f
57. d
58. d
59. b
60. b
61. a, b, c, d
62. d
63. b
64. a
65. c
66. b

CHAPTER 28

1. c
2. a, c, e, f
3. b, d, e, f
4. b, c, e, f
5. a, d, e
6. a, b, d, e
7. c
8. d
9. b, c, e
10. b
11. b
12. b
13. c
14. a
15. c
16. a, b, c, f
17. c
18. a, c, d, f
19. c
20. a
21. b
22. a
23. a, b, d, e
24. c
25. c
26. a
27. a, b, d, e, f
28. d
29. a
30. a, c, e, f
31. a
32. c
33. d
34. c
35. a, b, d, e, f
36. b
37. a, c, d, e
38. a
39. d
40. a
41. b
42. a, b, c, f

43. a, c, d, e, f
44. a
45. b
46. d
47. a
48. d
49. d
50. d
51. a, b, e
52. c
53. d
54. a, d, e, f
55. c
56. b
57. c
58. b
59. c
60. a, c, d, e

CHAPTER 29

1. a, d
2. a, c, d, e, f
3. d
4. d
5. a, c, e, f
6. a
7. c
8. b
9. a, b, d, f
10. a
11. a
12. a, c, d
13. d
14. c
15. c
16. a
17. d
18. a
19. a
20. b
21. c
22. d
23. d
24. c
25. a
26. c
27. a
28. d
29. a, d, e, f
30. c
31. a, b, e, f
32. c
33. a
34. d
35. b
36. c
37. a
38. a, b, e, f

39. a, b, e
40. a, c, e, f
41. a
42. a
43. a, c, d
44. d
45. c
46. c
47. b
48. b
49. a
50. a
51. b
52. a, c, d, e
53. c
54. a
55. a
56. c
57. a, c, d, e, f
58. b
59. a
60. a
61. c
62. b
63. c
64. d
65. d
66. c

CHAPTER 30

1. b
2. a, d, e
3. a, b, d, f
4. a, c, d, f
5. c
6. a, b, d, e
7. a
8. d
9. b
10. a, d, f
11. d
12. a, c, d, f
13. b
14. b
15. b
16. b
17. a, c, d, e, f
18. a, d, e, f
19. c
20. d
21. a
22. c
23. c
24. c
25. b
26. c
27. d
28. c

29. a, b, c, e
30. b
31. b
32. c
33. d
34. b
35. a
36. d
37. a, c, d
38. c
39. a
40. d
41. b
42. c
43. d
44. b
45. c
46. c
47. c
48. a
49. b
50. c
51. a
52. c
53. a
54. b
55. b, c, e, f
56. a, c, d, f
57. a, b, d, f
58. d
59. a, c, e
60. b
61. a
62. c
63. d
64. a
65. b
66. a, c, e
67. c
68. a
69. b, c, e, f
70. a, c, e, f
71. c
72. d
73. c
74. b
75. c
76. d
77. a
78. d
79. c
80. c
81. d
82. b

CHAPTER 31

1. a
2. b
3. b, d, f
4. d
5. a, c, d, f
6. a, c, d, e
7. a, b, d, e
8. a, c, d, e, f
9. a
10. b, c, e
11. a, c, d, e
12. c
13. a, c, e, f
14. c, d
15. c
16. a
17. a, c, e, f
18. b
19. b, c, d, f
20. c
21. a
22. b
23. c
24. a, c, d, f
25. a
26. a, d, f
27. b
28. b
29. a, d, e, f
30. a, e, f
31. d
32. a
33. c
34. a
35. c
36. a
37. c
38. c
39. d
40. b
41. a
42. b
43. c
44. a
45. a
46. b
47. a
48. a, b, d, e
49. a, b, d, e
50. b
51. c
52. b, c, d, f
53. c
54. b
55. b, c, d, f
56. a, c, e, f
57. a, c, e, f
58. b
59. d
60. c
61. d
62. d
63. b, c, e, f
64. b
65. a, b, d
66. b
67. b
68. c
69. b, c, e, f
70. b
71. c
72. a, c, d, e

CHAPTER 32

1. b, d, e
2. b
3. c
4. a, c, e
5. c
6. c
7. a, b, c, f
8. b
9. b
10. d
11. b
12. b, d, e
13. d
14. a, d, e, f
15. a, b, e, f
16. c
17. c
18. d
19. b
20. d
21. b, c, d, f
22. c
23. c
24. b
25. a
26. c
27. b, c, d, e
28. a, b, d, e
29. b
30. a, c, d, f
31. c
32. a
33. b
34. d
35. b, c, e, f
36. a
37. c
38. b
39. d
40. b
41. b
42. a, c, d, e
43. b, c, e
44. b
45. c
46. a, b, c, e, f
47. b
48. c
49. a, c, e
50. b
51. c
52. c
53. a
54. b, c, d, e, f
55. c
56. c
57. a
58. a
59. b
60. b
61. a
62. a
63. a, b, c, e, f
64. b, c, e, f
65. a, b, d
66. a, c, e, f
67. d
68. a, b, e
69. a, d, e, f
70. c
71. d
72. d
73. b
74. a
75. d
76. d
77. d
78. a, b, d
79. b, d, e, f
80. c
81. d
82. b
83. a
84. a
85. b
86. a
87. a, d
88. a, c, e
89. a, c, e, f
90. b

CHAPTER 33

1. b
2. a, c, d, f
3. a, c, d, e
4. a
5. a
6. a, b, d, f
7. a, b, e, f
8. b
9. c
10. a
11. b, d, e
12. a, c, d, f
13. b, d, f
14. b
15. b

16. b
17. d
18. c
19. a
20. c
21. d
22. b
23. c
24. a
25. a
26. b
27. a
28. a
29. c
30. d
31. b, d, f
32. c
33. d
34. a
35. a
36. d
37. a, c, d, f
38. b
39. a, c, d, e, f
40. a, c, d, f
41. c
42. c
43. b, c, e
44. a
45. b
46. a
47. a, c, d, e
48. d
49. b
50. a
51. a, d, e, f
52. a
53. a
54. a, b, d
55. b
56. c
57. d
58. a, d
59. a, b, f
60. a
61. b
62. a
63. c
64. d
65. b, e, f
66. b, d, e
67. c, d, e
68. b
69. a, b, d, f
70. a
71. b
72. c
73. b
74. a

75. d
76. a, c, e
77. b
78. b

CHAPTER 34

1. b
2. b
3. c
4. c
5. a
6. c
7. a
8. a
9. d
10. a
11. c
12. d
13. c
14. a
15. c
16. a, c, e, f
17. d
18. b
19. a
20. b •
21. a, b, e, f
22. d
23. b, c, d, f
24. b
25. d
26. b
27. a
28. d
29. a, b, e
30. c
31. b
32. b
33. b
34. a, c, e, f
35. b
36. b
37. b
38. c
39. d
40. a, b, d, f
41. a, c, d, e
42. b, c, e, f
43. a, c, d, f
44. c
45. b
46. a, b, d, e
47. d
48. b, c, e
49. a
50. b, d, e, f
51. a
52. b

53. a
54. a, c, d, e, f
55. d
56. a
57. a
58. a, c, d, f
59. d
60. c
61. a, b, c, d
62. d
63. c
64. b
65. a
66. d
67. a
68. b
69. a
70. a
71. b, c, e, f
72. c
73. b
74. b
75. b
76. d
77. b
78. a
79. b, c, d, f
80. b
81. c
82. a
83. a, c, d, e, f
84. a, b, d, f
85. a
86. c
87. c
88. d
89. a, d, e
90. c
91. b
92. c
93. a

Rhythm strip interpretations
94. RATE: 80/min; RHYTHM: Regular; P WAVES: 1 per QRS; PR INTERVAL: 0.16 second; QRS DURATION: 0.10 second; INTERPRETATION: Normal sinus rhythm
95. RATE: about 50/min; RHYTHM: Regular except 1 complex; P WAVES: 1 per QRS; PR INTERVAL: 0.20 second; QRS DURATION: 0.08 second; INTERPRETATION: Sinus bradycardia with 1 premature atrial contraction (PAC)

96. RATE: Variable about 130/min; RHYTHM: Irregularly irregular; P WAVES: fibrillatory wave; PR INTERVAL: None; QRS DURATION: 0.08 second; INTERPRETATION: Atrial fibrillation with rapid ventricular response
97. RATE: 150/min; RHYTHM: Regular; P WAVES: 1 per QRS; PR INTERVAL: 0.12 second; QRS DURATION: 0.04 second; INTERPRETATION: Sinus tachycardia
98. RATE: About 80/min; RHYTHM: regular except 1 complex; P WAVES: 1 per QRS except for the wide complex; PR INTERVAL: 0.20 second; QRS DURATION: 0.04 second; INTERPRETATION: Sinus rhythm with 1 premature ventricular contraction (PAC)
99. RATE: About 200/min; RHYTHM: Regular with wide QRS complexes; P WAVES: None; PR INTERVAL: None; QRS DURATION: Wide 0.28 second; INTERPRETATION: Ventricular tachycardia
100. RATE: Cannot be determined; RHYTHM: Chaotic; P WAVES: None; PR INTERVAL: None; QRS DURATION: None; INTERPRETATION: Ventricular fibrillation
101. RATE: None; RHYTHM: None; P WAVES: None; PR INTERVAL: None; QRS DURATION: None; INTERPRETATION: Ventricular asystole
102. RATE: 50/min; RHYTHM: regular; P WAVES: 1 per QRS; PR INTERVAL: 0.20 second; QRS DURATION: 0.08 second; INTERPRETATION: Sinus bradycardia

CHAPTER 35

1. c
2. d
3. a

4. b
5. c
6. c
7. a, c, e
8. b, c, e, f
9. d
10. d
11. d
12. b
13. a, b, d, e, f
14. c
15. d
16. d
17. b
18. b
19. a
20. a
21. a, b, c, e
22. a, d, e
23. a
24. d
25. c
26. b
27. c
28. a
29. d
30. c
31. a
32. d
33. a
34. b
35. a
36. c
37. b
38. a, b, c, e
39. b
40. c, d, e, f
41. b
42. a
43. b, d, f
44. b, c, d, f
45. a, b, c, e
46. b
47. a
48. a
49. c
50. c
51. a
52. a
53. b
54. b
55. c
56. b
57. a
58. c
59. a
60. b, c, d, f
61. c
62. c

63. b, c, d, f
64. a, c, d, e
65. b
66. c
67. a
68. b
69. b
70. b
71. d
72. a, c, e, f
73. b
74. c
75. b
76. a
77. a, c, d, f
78. b
79. a, c, d, f
80. b
81. a, b, c, e
82. c
83. b
84. d
85. a, c, d, e
86. a, b, e, f
87. a
88. b
89. a, d, e, f
90. c
91. c

CHAPTER 36

1. a, b, c, e, f
2. a, b, d, e
3. b, c, d
4. d
5. a, d
6. a
7. b
8. d
9. b, c, e, f
10. d
11. b
12. a
13. b, c, d, f
14. b, d, f
15. a
16. b
17. b
18. b, c, d, e
19. d
20. a
21. d
22. c
23. a
24. b
25. d
26. a
27. c
28. a

29. b
30. a, b, d
31. b
32. a, c, d, e
33. b
34. b
35. d
36. a, b, c, f
37. a
38. b
39. c
40. d
41. b
42. b
43. a
44. c
45. a, b, d, f
46. c
47. a, d, e
48. a, c, d, f
49. a, c, e, f
50. b
51. a, b, c, e
52. b
53. a
54. d
55. a
56. b
57. d
58. a
59. a
60. b
61. a, b, e, f
62. b
63. a
64. c
65. a
66. b, c, f
67. b, e
68. a
69. b, d, e, f
70. a, b, d, f
71. c
72. b
73. b
74. d
75. b
76. a
77. b
78. a, b, e
79. b, c, e, f
80. c
81. c
82. d
83. c
84. c
85. a, b, e, f
86. a
87. d

88. b
89. c
90. c, d, e
91. a
92. d
93. a
94. c
95. a
96. c
97. d
98. a
99. c, d, e, f
100. c
101. c
102. a, b, c, f
103. a
104. a, b, c, d, f
105. b
106. c
107. d
108. a
109. a, b, e, f
110. a
111. c
112. b, c, e
113. a, c, e, f
114. b, c, e, f
115. b
116. a
117. a, b, d, e
118. a
119. a, c, d, f
120. a
121. c
122. a, b, d, e
123. b
124. c
125. b
126. c
127. a, d

CHAPTER 37

1. a
2. a, b, d, f
3. b, c, d, e
4. c
5. a, c, e, f
6. d
7. b, c, d, f
8. a, b, d, e
9. b, d, f
10. c
11. c
12. d
13. d
14. a, b, c, d
15. c
16. a, c, e, f
17. c

18. a, c, d, e, f
19. d
20. a
21. c
22. b, e, f
23. c
24. a, b, d, e
25. b
26. a
27. c
28. a, b, d, e, f
29. a, b, c, f
30. b
31. a, b, c, d, e
32. b
33. d
34. c
35. a
36. b
37. b
38. c
39. b, d, e
40. b
41. c
42. c
43. a
44. c
45. d
46. d
47. c
48. d
49. b
50. c
51. a
52. a
53. d
54. c
55. c
56. a, c, d, e
57. d
58. a, b, c, e, f
59. b
60. d
61. b
62. a
63. a, c, e
64. c
65. a, c, d
66. a

CHAPTER 38

1. a, e
2. c, d, e, f
3. b
4. d
5. b, c, f
6. c
7. a

8. c
9. a
10. a, d, f
11. b
12. a, c
13. b
14. b, c, d, e
15. b
16. a
17. c, d, e
18. c
19. a
20. a
21. d
22. a, c, d, e
23. d
24. c
25. b
26. a, b, c, e, f
27. a, c, d, f
28. a
29. a, b, e, f
30. d
31. b
32. c
33. b, e
34. a, b, c, d, f
35. c
36. b
37. b
38. a, b, c, e, f
39. b
40. a, d, f
41. b
42. a, c, e, f
43. b
44. b, d, f
45. b, c, d, f
46. a
47. b
48. a
49. b
50. b
51. a
52. b
53. c
54. a
55. a
56. a, b, d, e, f
57. a
58. a
59. c
60. b
61. a
62. c
63. a
64. c
65. a
66. b

67. a
68. a, c, d, f
69. b, c, e
70. b
71. b, c, d, e
72. a, b, d, e, f
73. b
74. b
75. d
76. a
77. b
78. d
79. b
80. a
81. c
82. a, b, c, e
83. b
84. b, c, d
85. c
86. a
87. b
88. a
89. a, b, d, e, f
90. b
91. c
92. a, c, f
93. d
94. b, c, e
95. a, b, d, f
96. a, c, d, f
97. b
98. a, b, d

CHAPTER 39

1. a
2. d
3. b
4. a, c, d, e
5. d
6. b
7. d
8. b
9. a
10. d
11. c
12. b
13. b
14. c
15. d
16. a, b, e
17. d
18. c
19. a, b, d, f
20. a
21. c
22. b
23. d
24. c

25. d
26. c
27. c
28. a

CHAPTER 40

1. a, d, e, f
2. a, c, d, e, f
3. d
4. a
5. c
6. a
7. a, c, e, f
8. c
9. b
10. a
11. c
12. d
13. a, b, c, d, e
14. a
15. b
16. a, b, c, e
17. a
18. a
19. c
20. b
21. a
22. a
23. a, b, c, d, e
24. a
25. c
26. b
27. c
28. a, d, e
29. c
30. b, c, d, f
31. a
32. a
33. c
34. b
35. a
36. b
37. c
38. c
39. a
40. c
41. a
42. b
43. c
44. b
45. c
46. c
47. d
48. c
49. a, b, d, f
50. a
51. c

CHAPTER 41

1. c
2. a
3. b
4. b
5. b
6. d
7. a
8. d
9. a
10. a
11. b
12. a, b, d, e
13. a, b, d, e, f
14. a
15. a
16. c
17. d
18. c
19. a
20. a
21. c
22. a
23. a
24. b
25. b
26. c
27. a
28. a
29. b
30. c
31. c
32. d
33. b
34. d
35. d
36. a, b, c, d, f
37. d
38. c
39. a
40. c
41. b
42. d
43. a
44. d
45. d

CHAPTER 42

1. d
2. a, b, c, d, e
3. a, b, d, e, f
4. d
5. d
6. a
7. b
8. a
9. c, d, e, f
10. b

11. c
12. c
13. d
14. c
15. a
16. a
17. b
18. c
19. d
20. b
21. a, b, c, d, f
22. c
23. b
24. c
25. b
26. c
27. d
28. b
29. a, b, e, f
30. c
31. b
32. c
33. a
34. b
35. a, b, c, e
36. a
37. c
38. d
39. b
40. b
41. c
42. b
43. d
44. b, c, e
45. c

CHAPTER 43

1. a
2. b
3. a
4. d
5. a, b, c, e, f
6. b
7. a, b, c, e, f
8. b
9. c
10. a
11. a
12. d
13. b
14. a, b, d, e, f
15. c
16. b
17. a
18. a
19. b
20. b, d, e
21. b

22. b
23. b
24. b, c, e, f
25. c
26. a
27. b
28. b
29. d
30. a
31. c
32. b
33. c
34. b
35. a
36. b, c, e, f
37. c
38. a
39. b
40. d
41. a, c, e
42. b
43. c
44. a, b, c, e, f
45. c

CHAPTER 44

1. b, e, f
2. c
3. c
4. d
5. c
6. a
7. c
8. a, b, d
9. d
10. c
11. a
12. b
13. b, c, d, e, f
14. a
15. b
16. a
17. a
18. c
19. a
20. a, b, e
21. a
22. c
23. d
24. a, b, d, f
25. a
26. b
27. c
28. a
29. d
30. c
31. b
32. a

33. c
34. a
35. c
36. b
37. c
38. b
39. d
40. b
41. b
42. a
43. a
44. c
45. a
46. b
47. d
48. b
49. a, c, d, e
50. a
51. c
52. c
53. b, c, e
54. a, b, c, e, f
55. a
56. a
57. a, b, c, f
58. c
59. b
60. a
61. a
62. a, b, c, d
63. a, c, e
64. c
65. b

CHAPTER 45

1. c
2. a, b, c, d, e
3. b
4. b
5. d
6. c
7. a
8. b
9. c
10. b
11. b
12. c
13. b
14. a
15. a
16. c
17. d
18. a
19. b
20. c
21. d
22. a, b, c, d, e
23. a, b, d, f

4. a, c, e
5. b, c, e
6. a, b, c, f
7. d
8. a, d
9. a, b, d, f
10. d
11. d
12. c
13. a
14. b
15. a, b, d, f
16. c
17. b, c, e, f
18. b
19. d
20. a
21. d
22. a, b, e
23. c, e, f
24. a
25. b
26. a
27. c
28. c
29. a, b, d, e
30. d
31. a, c, d, f
32. c
33. b
34. b
35. d
36. a
37. a, b, c, d
38. d
39. a, b, e, f
40. b, c, e, f
41. a, c, d, f
42. b
43. a
44. c
45. a, c, d, e

CHAPTER 53

1. a, c, d, f
2. c
3. b, c, e
4. d
5. a
6. a
7. b
8. c
9. b
10. a
11. a
12. c
13. a, b, c, f
14. b

15. a, d, e
16. b
17. a
18. c
19. a, b, d, f
20. c
21. c
22. d
23. d
24. a, c, d, f
25. c
26. b, c, e, f
27. a, b, e
28. c
29. b, d, e
30. a
31. c
32. c
33. a, b, d, f
34. a
35. a, c, d, f
36. a, b, d, f

CHAPTER 54

1. b
2. a
3. a, e, f
4. a, d
5. c
6. a, c, e
7. b
8. d
9. b
10. a
11. d
12. c
13. b, c, e, f
14. a, c, e
15. a
16. d
17. b
18. a, b, c, e, f
19. d
20. a, c, d, e
21. b
22. a
23. a, b, c, e, f
24. a
25. a, c, d, f
26. d
27. a
28. b
29. c
30. d
31. c
32. a, b, c, e, f
33. d
34. b

35. a
36. a, b, d, e
37. b
38. a
39. c
40. b
41. b
42. b
43. d
44. a, b, d, e
45. c

CHAPTER 55

1. a, b, d, f
2. a, c, d, e
3. b, d, e
4. a, c, d, f
5. a
6. b
7. d
8. a
9. b
10. d
11. a
12. d
13. b, d, e
14. a
15. d
16. d
17. c
18. a
19. b, c, d
20. a, c, d, e
21. b
22. d
23. c
24. d
25. a, c, d, f
26. b
27. c
28. a, b, c, e, f
29. a, b, d, e, f
30. a
31. c
32. a, c, e
33. a, c, f
34. d
35. b
36. c
37. a, c, d, e
38. c
39. a, c, d, e, f
40. a
41. a
42. a
43. a, c, d, e, f
44. a, c, e, f
45. d

CHAPTER 56

1. a, b, d, e
2. c
3. d
4. a
5. a
6. b, c, d, f
7. d
8. c
9. c
10. c, e, f
11. c
12. b
13. a, c, e, f
14. a, d, e
15. c
16. b
17. a
18. a, b, e
19. a, c, e
20. a
21. c
22. d
23. b
24. a
25. b, c, e, f
26. d
27. c
28. a
29. a
30. b, c, d, e
31. a
32. b
33. d
34. a
35. c
36. a
37. b, e, f
38. a, b, d
39. a, c, e
40. a, c, d
41. c
42. a, c, e
43. a, c, d, f
44. a
45. b
46. d
47. a, f
48. b
49. a, c
50. b
51. a, c, d
52. b, c, e, f
53. c
54. d
55. a
56. a, c, d, f

CHAPTER 57

1. c
2. a, b, f
3. b
4. b, c, e, f
5. d
6. a, b, d, e, f
7. c
8. a
9. b
10. c
11. a
12. c
13. b
14. a, b, d, f
15. d
16. b
17. b, c, e, f
18. d
19. c
20. b, c, f
21. b, c, d, e
22. a
23. b
24. a, b, e, f
25. b
26. d
27. a, b, c, d
28. d
29. d
30. a
31. d
32. d
33. a
34. c
35. c
36. b, c, d, e
37. a
38. b
39. b
40. a, b, c, d
41. a
42. c
43. b, c, e
44. d
45. a

CHAPTER 58

1. a, b, c, e, f
2. d
3. c
4. a
5. d
6. a, c, d, e, f
7. b
8. a, b, d
9. b
10. a

11. a, b, c, f
12. b
13. b
14. a, c, d, e, f
15. a
16. a
17. d
18. a, b, d, e
19. a
20. d
21. b, c, e
22. b, c, f
23. a, b, c, e
24. a, b, d, e, f
25. b
26. c
27. a, b, d, e
28. a
29. a, b, c, e
30. b, c, d, e
31. a, c, e, f
32. b
33. d
34. c
35. a
36. d
37. c
38. d
39. a, c, e, f
40. a, c, d, e
41. d
42. a, c, d, f
43. a
44. a, b, d, e
45. c
46. d
47. b

CHAPTER 59

1. a
2. c
3. c
4. a
5. a, c, e, f
6. c
7. d
8. b
9. d
10. a
11. b
12. a
13. a, c, d, f
14. d
15. c
16. d
17. b
18. b
19. d

20. a
21. c
22. b
23. c
24. d
25. c
26. c
27. a, b, d, f
28. b
29. a, b, d, e, f
30. c
31. b, c, d, e, f
32. b
33. b
34. a, c, d, f
35. a, b, d, f
36. a, c, d, e
37. c
38. a
39. b
40. a, c, d, e

CHAPTER 60

1. a, c, e, f
2. a, b, c, e
3. b
4. a
5. c
6. a, b, d, e, f
7. a, c, e, f
8. a
9. b
10. a, b, c, d, f
11. b
12. c
13. a
14. b
15. b, c
16. d
17. b, c, d, f
18. c, d, e, f
19. a
20. b, c, e
21. a, c, d, e
22. d
23. d
24. a
25. b
26. d
27. a
28. b
29. a, b, c, e
30. b
31. a
32. a, c, d, e
33. b
34. a
35. d

36. d
37. a, b, c, d
38. b
39. a
40. b, e, f
41. b, c, d, e, f
42. a, c, d, e, f
43. a, b, d
44. d
45. a, c, e, f
46. d
47. a
48. a, b, d, e, f
49. a, c, d, e, f
50. d
51. c
52. a
53. b
54. d
55. a
56. a, c, d, e, f
57. b

CHAPTER 61

1. a, c, d, e
2. c
3. b
4. b, d
5. a, d, f
6. b
7. d
8. a, b, e
9. a
10. c
11. a
12. b
13. a, b, e, f
14. a
15. b
16. d
17. a, e, f
18. b
19. b, c, e, f
20. a, b, d, e
21. b, c, d, f
22. a
23. d
24. a, b, c, e
25. b, c, d
26. d
27. d
28. a, c, e, f
29. b
30. d
31. b
32. b, c, d, e
33. b
34. a

35. a
36. b
37. b
38. b, c, d, f
39. b
40. c, d, e, f
41. a, b, d, e
42. b
43. d
44. b
45. a
46. b

CHAPTER 62

1. b
2. c, e
3. a, b, d, e
4. c
5. a
6. a, e, f
7. d
8. b
9. a
10. a, b, c, e, f
11. d, e
12. a, b, c, d
13. c
14. b, d, f
15. c
16. a, d, e, f
17. a, b, c, f
18. a, c, d, f
19. b
20. b
21. a
22. c
23. b
24. a, c, d, f
25. b, c, e, f
26. a, b
27. a
28. a
29. c
30. b
31. c
32. a, c, d, f
33. a
34. c
35. a, c, e
36. a, d
37. b
38. b
39. d
40. b
41. b
42. d
43. d
44. d

45. d
46. a, c, e, f
47. b, c, e
48. a
49. a
50. b
51. b
52. d
53. b
54. a
55. a
56. a, c, d, f
57. b
58. d
59. d
60. a, c, f
61. a
62. b, d, f
63. b
64. a, b, d, e
65. b
66. c
67. d

CHAPTER 63

1. d
2. a, c, d, f
3. b
4. c
5. b
6. b
7. d
8. b
9. a
10. b
11. d
12. b
13. c
14. c
15. a, b, e, f
16. c
17. b
18. a
19. b
20. a, b, c, d, f
21. a, b, d, e
22. a, b, f
23. d
24. c
25. a
26. b
27. c
28. a, c, d, f
29. a
30. b
31. a, c, d, e
32. a, b, c, e, f
33. b, c, d, e

34. a, b, d, e, f
35. d
36. c, d
37. c
38. b
39. a, b, d, e, f
40. a, b, e
41. b
42. d
43. a
44. a
45. c
46. b
47. b, e, f
48. c
49. a, b, d, f
50. a
51. a, b, f
52. a, b, c, e
53. a, c, f
54. b
55. d
56. a, c, d
57. d
58. a, c, e, f
59. a

CHAPTER 64

1. b, d, f
2. c
3. b
4. b
5. a, b, d, f
6. c
7. d
8. d
9. c
10. c
11. a, b, d
12. b, c, d, e
13. a, b, f
14. a
15. c
16. d
17. c
18. a, c, e
19. b
20. a, c, d
21. a, b, d, e, f
22. d, e, f
23. a
24. b, c, e, f
25. b, e, f
26. a
27. b
28. d
29. c
30. c

31. a
32. a, c, e, f
33. b
34. c
35. b
36. a
37. a
38. c
39. d
40. a
41. b, d, e
42. d
43. b, c, f
44. b
45. d
46. a
47. a, b, c, d, f
48. b, c, d, e
49. a, b, d, e, f
50. c
51. a, b, d, e, f
52. d
53. b
54. c
55. b
56. a
57. a, c, e
58. d
59. a, c, d, e, f
60. c
61. b
62. c
63. c
64. a
65. b
66. b, c, d, e, f
67. a, b, d
68. b, c, e, f
69. d
70. b
71. c
72. a
73. b
74. d
75. c
76. b
77. b, d
78. a, c, d, e, f
79. d
80. a
81. b
82. c
83. a, c, e
84. a
85. b
86. a, d, e
87. c
88. b
89. a, b, e, f

90. d
91. b
92. a, c, e, f
93. a
94. b, c, d, f
95. c
96. b

CHAPTER 65

1. b
2. d
3. b
4. a
5. a, b, c
6. b
7. b
8. a
9. d
10. b
11. b
12. b
13. a
14. a
15. a
16. b
17. a
18. a
19. a
20. a, b, e, f
21. c
22. b
23. b
24. b
25. d
26. d
27. c
28. b
29. c
30. b
31. d
32. a
33. b, d, e, f
34. b
35. d
36. b
37. a
38. d
39. b
40. d
41. c
42. c
43. b
44. c
45. b, c, d, e
46. b
47. a
48. a
49. c
50. c
51. b

52. a
53. c
54. a
55. c
56. b
57. c
58. a. 2, b. 5, c. 4, d. 1, e. 3, f. 6
59. a
60. c
61. b
62. a
63. a
64. b
65. b
66. b
67. a
68. d
69. b
70. b
71. c
72. a, d, e, f
73. a
74. d
75. b
76. a

CHAPTER 66

1. c
2. b
3. b
4. c
5. a
6. a
7. d
8. b
9. b
10. c
11. a
12. d
13. a
14. a
15. d
16. c
17. a
18. c
19. a
20. b
21. b
22. d
23. c, d, e, f
24. a
25. b
26. a
27. b
28. b
29. d
30. d
31. d
32. a, d, e, f

33. b
34. b
35. d
36. c
37. a
38. c
39. d
40. b
41. a, b, c, d, f
42. b
43. a
44. c
45. b
46. b
47. c
48. a
49. a
50. d
51. a
52. a
53. d
54. c
55. c
56. b
57. a
58. d
59. b
60. c
61. d
62. d
63. a
64. a, b, c, e
65. d
66. b
67. a
68. b
69. c
70. c
71. d
72. c
73. d
74. b
75. d

CHAPTER 67

1. b
2. a
3. b, c, d, e, f
4. a, b, d, e, f
5. c
6. c
7. b, c, d, e
8. c
9. a
10. b
11. a
12. a
13. b
14. c
15. d

16. d
17. a
18. c
19. b
20. a
21. b
22. a
23. a
24. d
25. b
26. d
27. a
28. d
29. a, b, c, d
30. b
31. b, c, d, f
32. b
33. c
34. c, d
35. a
36. c
37. a, c, e
38. b
39. b
40. c
41. a, c, d, e
42. d
43. c
44. a
45. a, b, c, d
46. b
47. c
48. c
49. c
50. d
51. a
52. a
53. a
54. b
55. d
56. a
57. b, c, d, f
58. b
59. d
60. c
61. a
62. a
63. a
64. b
65. b
66. a
67. b
68. a
69. b
70. b
71. c
72. a
73. c, d, e, f
74. c
75. d
76. a

77. b
78. b, c, d, f
79. a
80. b
81. c
82. b
83. c
84. d
85. a, b, c, d, f
86. c
87. c

CHAPTER 68

1. a, d, f
2. a
3. d
4. a, b, d, f
5. c
   a, b, e
   a, b, e
   c
   a

   c, d, f

   b, c

   ams

49. d
50. c
51. a, b, c, e
52. b
53. a
54. a, d, e, f
55. a
56. a
57. c
58. b
59. a
60. b
61. c
62. b
63. c
64. b
65. c
66. a, b, c, e, f
67. b
68. a, b, c, d, e
69. a, c, d, e
70. a
71. d
72. b
73. a
74. d
75. b
76. a
77. d
78. a, b, c, e
79. a
80. a
81. d
82. a. 3, b. 2, c. 4, d. 1
83. c
84. b
85. a
86. b
87. b, c, d, e
88. c
89. a
90. c
91. a, b, c
92. b
93. d
94. c
95. b

CHAPTER 69

1. b
2. b
3. c
4. a
5. d
6. a, c, e
7. c
8. d
9. a
10. a
11. a, c, e, f
12. a

13. d
14. a, b, d, e
15. b
16. b
17. c
18. a, c, d, e

24. See Figure 69-1 in textbook.

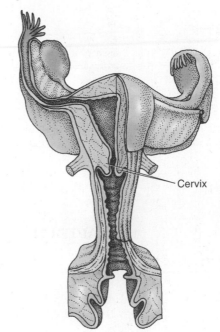
Cervix

25. d
26. c
27. a
28. c
29. c
30. b
31. c
32. b
33. a
34. d
35. b
36. a
37. b
38. a, d, e
39. a
40. c
41. b
42. d
43. a
44. b
45. c
46. b
47. c
48. a

CHAPTER 70

1. c
2. c
3. a, b, d, f

19. b
20. d
21. a
22. a, b, d, e, f
23. c

4. a
5. a
6. b, c, e, f
7. a
8. c
9. d
10. b, c, e, f
11. d
12. b, c, d
13. b
14. a
15. d
16. b
17. b
18. a
19. b
20. a
21. d
22. c
23. d
24. a, c, d, e, f
25. a
26. d
27. b, c, d
28. b
29. a
30. d
31. b
32. d
33. d

34. a
35. c
36. a
37. b
38. d
39. b
40. b
41. b
42. c
43. a
44. b
45. c
46. a
47. a
48. b
49. c
50. a
51. c
52. d
53. d
54. c
55. b
56. a, b, d, f
57. a

CHAPTER 71

1. b
2. d
3. c
4. a
5. d
6. a
7. b
8. a
9. d
10. a
11. a, e, f
12. d
13. c
14. b, c, d, e, f
15. b
16. b
17. d
18. b
19. a
20. a, c, d, e, f
21. c
22. a
23. c
24. b
25. a
26. b
27. a
28. b
29. b
30. b
31. a
32. c
33. d
34. b

35. b, c, e
36. c
37. c
38. a
39. a
40. a, c, e, f
41. a
42. c
43. b
44. b
45. a
46. c
47. d
48. a
49. a, c, d, f
50. c
51. a
52. a
53. c
54. c
55. b
56. d

CHAPTER 72

1. b
2. c, d, e, f
3. c
4. d
5. a, c, d, e, f
6. d
7. b
8. a
9. d
10. a
11. a
12. a, b, e, f
13. d
14. a
15. d
16. a
17. a
18. b
19. c
20. b
21. c
22. b
23. c
24. a
25. c
26. a
27. 250 mL
28. d
29. a
30. d
31. c
32. a, d, e
33. c
34. a
35. b
36. a

37. b
38. b
39. b
40. b, c, d, e
41. a
42. a
43. b
44. c
45. b
46. d
47. d
48. c
49. a, b, d, e
50. b
51. c
52. a
53. a, c, d, f
54. b
55. c
56. a
57. a
58. a
59. a, c, d, e, f
60. b

CHAPTER 73

1. c
2. c
3. b
4. c
5. d
6. b
7. a, b, c
8. c
9. c
10. b
11. c
12. a
13. a
14. c
15. d
16. a, b, c, e
17. d
18. b
19. c
20. a, b, c, e, f
21. c
22. b
23. c
24. b
25. a, c, d
26. a
27. b
28. d
29. a, b, c, d, e
30. c

CHAPTER 74

1. a
2. d
3. a
4. a
5. d
6. c
7. c
8. a
9. b
10. a, c, d, e, f
11. d
12. a
13. a, c, e
14. b
15. c
16. a
17. b
18. a
19. b
20. d
21. b
22. d
23. c
24. b
25. d
26. c
27. c
28. a
29. a
30. b
31. c, d, e, f
32. b
33. a
34. c
35. a
36. a
37. c
38. d
39. a
40. b
41. b
42. c
43. a, b, c, e, f
44. a
45. a, b, c, e
46. c
47. b
48. c
49. c, d, f
50. b
51. d
52. c
53. a
54. b
55. a, b, c, d, e
56. a